CONSULTANT WRITERS

ADRIENNE ARDIGO, R.N., B.S.

Instructor, Department of Health Occupations and Nursing
Los Angeles Trade Technical Community College
Los Angeles, California

INICE CHIRCO, R.N., M.A., M.S.

Chairman, Allied Health Department
Rio Hondo College
Whittier, California

BEVERLY J. RAMBO, R.N., M.A., M.N.

Assistant Professor of Nursing
Mount St. Mary's College
Los Angeles, California

BETTIE RICH, R.N., M.S.

Chairman, Health Occupations Department
Mt. San Jacinto College
Gilman Hot Springs, California

Manuscript edited by Seba Kolb

Illustrations revised by Sharon Belkin

W. B. SAUNDERS COMPANY
Philadelphia, London, Toronto

SECOND EDITION

Nursing Skills for Allied Health Services

Edited by

LUCILE A. WOOD, R.N., M.S.

Director of Nursing
Bay Area Hospital
Coos Bay, Oregon;
formerly,
Associate Director for the Nursing Occupations
Allied Health Professions Publications
University of California Extension, Los Angeles

and

BEVERLY J. RAMBO, R.N., M.A., M.N.

Assistant Professor of Nursing
Mount St. Mary's College
Los Angeles, California

W. B. Saunders Company: West Washington Square
Philadelphia, PA 19105

1 St. Anne's Road
Eastbourne, East Sussex BN21 3UN, England

1 Goldthorne Ave.
Toronto, Ontario, M8Z, 5T9, Canada

Library of Congress Cataloging in Publication Data

Wood, Lucile A
   Nursing skills for allied health services.

   1. Nursing.   2. Care of the sick.   I. Rambo, Beverly J.   II. Title.

RT41.W84 1977   610.73   76-41544

Single Vol.–ISBN 0-7216-9606-6
Vol. 1 –   ISBN 0-7216-9603-1
Vol. 2 –   ISBN 0-7216-9604-4

Nursing Skills for Allied Health Services   Volume 1 – ISBN 0–7216–9603–1
                                   Volume 2 – ISBN 0–7216–9604–X
                            Single Volume – ISBN 0–7216–9606–6

Last digit is the print number: 9   8   7   6   5   4   3

ALLIED HEALTH PROFESSIONS PROJECTS NURSING NATIONAL TECHNICAL ADVISORY COMMITTEE

J. P. Myles Black, M.D.

Clinical Instructor, College of Medicine
University of Southern California
Los Angeles, California

Mary Bruton, R.N., M.S., Assistant Professor

St. Anselm's College
Manchester, New Hampshire

Terry Crowley, Educational Coordinator

National Federation of Licensed Practical Nurses
New York, New York

Bernice Dixon, R.N., M.S., Director

School of Nursing, Grady Memorial Hospital
Atlanta, Georgia

Phyllis Drennan, R.N., M.S., Coordinator

Associate Degree Nursing Program
Kirkwood Community College
Cedar Rapids, Iowa
(Official Representative of the National League for Nursing)

Elizabeth J. Haglund

Regional Nursing Consultant for the Division of Nursing
Bureau of Health Professions Manpower Training
Department of Health, Education, and Welfare, Region IX
San Francisco, California

William F. Hartnett, R.N., M.S.

Assistant Administrator, Nursing Services
Riverside Methodist Hospital
Columbus, Ohio

Nannette Turner, L.V.N.

Past Executive Director
California Licensed Vocational Nurses Association
Los Angeles, California
(Official Representative of National Federation of Licensed Practical Nurses)

Captain Ouida Upchurch, Captain, NC, USN

Special Assistant for Education and Training R and D
Department of the Navy
Bureau of Medicine and Surgery
Washington, D.C.

George Wells, Associate Director

Health Insurance Council
Chicago, Illinois

Gerry White, R.N., M.S., Director

Allied Health Careers Institute
El Centro College of Dallas County
Dallas, Texas

Lucie Young, R.N., Ph.D., Chairman

Nursing Department of California State College, Los Angeles
Los Angeles, California
(Official Representative of the American Nurses Association)

FOREWORD

The Division of Vocational Education, University of California Extension, is an administrative unit of the University concerned with responsibilities for research, teacher education, and public service in the broad area of vocational and technical education. During 1968 the Division entered into an agreement with the U.S. Office of Education to prepare curricula and instructional materials for a variety of allied health areas. For the most part such materials are related to instruction for programs ranging from on-the-job training through the Associate degree level. They also are adapted for use in adult and continuation education.

Because of the crucial staff shortages in the nursing occupations, the Allied Health Professions Projects undertook a national occupational analysis of the activities of persons actually employed in health care facilities. This survey was designed to determine what skills and knowledge were required by personnel employed in the several nursing occupations. The results of this survey have been incorporated into the present text, which covers the activities of entry-level personnel and comprises a comprehensive introduction to nursing. It also presents material which is adaptable to the training of other allied health personnel and seeks to provide a basic introduction to patient care services wherever they may be provided.

This instructional manual is one in the series of three entitled *Nursing Skills for Allied Health Services* which completes the work undertaken in the nursing field which started with a task inventory, followed by an occupational analysis *(A Study of Nursing Occupations)*, and a curriculum guide *(A Career Model for the Nurse Practitioner)*. To implement the curriculum, these instructional materials were developed, culminating in the publication of three volumes that cover the tasks delineated in the occupational analysis and curriculum guide.

The educational philosophy exemplified in these materials is task-oriented instruction in which the emphasis is on helping the student learn to *perform* the tasks of the occupation and to *use* the basic scientific and technical knowledge related to them. This approach is designed to shorten the learning process, so that the goal of "more learning in less time with greater retention" can be achieved. If these materials make a significant contribution toward accomplishing this goal, they will help to solve the health manpower problem, and we will feel that the endless hours we have labored on the development of these manuals were not in vain.

ROBERT B. KINDRED, ED. D.
Director, Education Extension and Acting
Director, Division of Vocational Education
University of California Extension,
Los Angeles

MILES H. ANDERSON, Ed. D.
Director, Allied Health
Professions Publications
University of California Extension,
Los Angeles

PREFACE

From the time of their initial publication, *Nursing Skills For Allied Health Services, Volumes 1 and 2*, have been utilized as basic texts for teaching nursing skills in countless nursing and allied health educational programs in this country and abroad. Moreover, they are being used increasingly in hospitals, nursing homes, and other health care agencies as procedure manuals. While many of the basic nursing procedures remain the same, there have been a substantial number of changes that have been incorporated in this revised edition. The content has been updated to reflect changes in theory and in practice created by new types of equipment. As an example, the chapter on cardiopulmonary resuscitation has been rewritten in accordance with the standards recommended by the American Heart Association and the National Academy of Sciences.

The format of the book remains generally unchanged. The instructional units for Volumes 1 and 2 are built around the activities performed by all levels of workers in nursing — the nursing assistant, the licensed practical or vocational nurse, and the registered nurse. These are the skills that hospital and health agency employers expect all members of the nursing staff to perform competently. Each chapter can be used as an instructional unit that contains one or more modules covering related materials and procedures. For example, the unit on handwashing contains only one module, whereas the unit on urine elimination consists of several modules and describes procedures such as placing the patient on the bedpan, offering the urinal, collecting urine specimens, and so forth.

The key concept of each unit is performance. The student is expected to be able to perform the stated behavioral objectives satisfactorily. To prepare for meeting these objectives, information is given in the introductory portion of each unit to help the student understand the conditions or reasons for performing the task or activity. Each skill activity is divided into a logical and orderly sequence designated as "Important Steps," which are supported with practical content under the heading of "Key Points." We have attempted to include in the practical content the hints and the more subtle details that are incorporated in the art of nusing by those who have greater expertise. The Key Points also contain information related to the safety factors, communication skill, related scientific principles, suggestions for making the step easier to do, and pertinent ethical or legal concepts. The procedures in each unit are followed by the performance test, the satisfactory completion of which is crucial for a nursing skills program. For those instructors and students who wish to test for understanding of the theoretical content, additional post-test items have been included.

The sequence of units has been changed slightly. They have been rearranged on the premise that learning progresses from the general and simple to the more specific and complex. The simpler nursing skills are presented before the more complex ones, such as postoperative care and isolation techniques. The first ten units emphasize the environment where nursing takes place, handwashing, and principles of movement, serving as a foundation for most of the remaining units. Successful completion of the basic nursing skills in Volumes 1 and 2 should ensure a competent practitioner at the nursing assistant level, and provide a sound basis for all nursing students before they move on to more complex theoretical knowledge and skills in succeeding levels of nursing practice.

The units were developed in a manner to permit the students to move at their own pace through the background information on the subject and to familiarize themselves with the steps of the skills. This releases the instructor from the need to constantly repeat instructions or information for each student, and allows that time to be spent more productively and creatively in helping the students to polish their basic skills, expand their interests and understanding, and apply their knowledge and skills to the care of their patients in the clinical areas. Since the emphasis is on performance, we have found that the students experience fewer stresses in the skill learning laboratory and develop positive attitudes about their nursing activities. They become involved "up to their elbows" in their own learning.

These materials are readily adaptable to a variety of settings: they have been used in programs ranging from short courses to prepare nursing assistants to collegiate programs for professional nursing students. They are also applicable in adult education and staff development programs for nursing personnel and other allied health professionals who need these basic skills.

While preparing the revised edition of Volumes 1 and 2, we have missed Lucile Wood, former Associate Director for Nursing Occupations, U.C.L.A. Allied Health Professions Project, and her valuable contributions. Her administrative hospital duties in Coos Bay precluded her taking as active a role in the revisions as we would have liked. My co-authors and I would like to thank those who have assisted in the preparation of the new edition. We are grateful to Dr. Miles H. Anderson, who called us together as a team and coordinated the over-all effort. To Jane Kahn, former Director of Nursing at Hollywood Presbyterian Medical Center, and Frances Rogozen, Assistant Professor at Los Angeles Trade Technical Community College, we are deeply indebted for contributions they made to the first edition. Special thanks go to Seba Kolb for editing the manuscript and handling many details that helped to make the job easier for all of us. We appreciate the new illustrations prepared by Sharon Belkin and the attention she gave to the smallest details in order to reflect actual movement or appearance more accurately. To Mr. Robert Wright, Nursing Editor for W.B. Saunders Company, goes our appreciation for his guidance, interest, and help. Finally, but not least, we are indebted to the students and instructors who have used these volumes, shared their evaluations concerning the effectiveness of the program, and gained skills in providing care for their patients.

BEVERLY J. RAMBO

CONTENTS

VOLUME 1

THE HEALTH WORKER
AND THE LAW

I. DIRECTIONS TO THE STUDENT

Please read the following paragraphs carefully. They will tell you exactly what you are expected to know at the end of the unit. If you believe that your knowledge and previous experience in this area have already prepared you, please discuss with your instructor the possibility of omitting the reading of this unit and going directly to the post-test.

II. GENERAL PERFORMANCE OBJECTIVE

You will give evidence of your knowledge of the law by answering successfully a written examination based on definitions of legal terms and an understanding of legal problems that might occur during a patient–health worker relationship.

III. SPECIFIC PERFORMANCE OBJECTIVES

In the written post-test you will answer with at least 80 per cent accuracy questions related to the following capabilities. You will be able to:

1. Distinguish in a given situation who the health worker is.

2. Recognize the definition for the term "law" as used in this study.

3. List the main sources for the law, and specifically "medical" law.

4. Demonstrate your knowledge of the individual's rights under the law and how these rights might be violated if consent and medical orders are inadequate.

5. Recognize in given situations when an act can be interpreted as malpractice or negligence.

6. Distinguish civil from criminal law.

7. Demonstrate your knowledge of responsibility in relation to legal records.

8. List several basic rules to follow for the prevention of litigation.

IV. VOCABULARY

assault—either a threat or an attempt to injure another in an illegal manner.
battery—unlawful touching of another person without his consent, with or without resultant injury. Assault and battery are often charged together because of successful attempt to injure.
civil law—pertains to legal relationships between private individuals.

common law—a term given to unwritten law, customs with authority of law, or precedents established by judges and juries in past cases.

consent—permission granted by a person voluntarily and in his right mind; written consent is safer because it is easier to prove.

crime—an act that is forbidden, or the omission of a duty that is commanded by a public law and that makes the offender liable to punishment by that law.

criminal law—defines legal obligations between the individual citizen and the state; distinguished from civil law, which defines legal relationships between private individuals.

duty of care—the obligation under law for a nurse or other health worker to perform services for a patient that meet the common standards of practice expected in the community for a comparable worker.

ethics—the discipline dealing with what is good and bad, and with moral duty and obligations; a professional person is characterized by adherence to technical and ethical standards of a profession.

false imprisonment—holding or detaining a person against his will.

felony—a serious crime, for which the penalty is imprisonment in the state prison for more than one year, and possibly the death penalty.

invasion of privacy—a civil wrong that unlawfully makes public knowledge of any private or personal information without the consent of the wronged person.

libel—a civil wrong; to communicate in writing to a third party defamatory matter about an individual or group.

licensure—authorization by the state to practice one's profession or vocation; involves control of educational standards, licensing examinations, and prohibitions for individuals who are not licensed.

litigation—another word for law suit.

malpractice—literally "bad practice," improper or injurious practice; unskilled and faulty medical or surgical treatment.

misdemeanor—a crime less serious than a felony, punishable by imprisonment in the county jail for a term of less than one year.

negligence—failure to perform in a reasonably prudent manner.

privileged communication—any personal or private information related to his care that a patient gives medical personnel.

reasonable care—(refer to definition for *duty of care*); the health worker is protected by law if it can be determined that she acted reasonably as compared with fellow workers; the patient is protected by recognition of the health worker's responsibility for duty of care.

slander—spoken statement of false charges or misrepresentations that defame or damage another's reputation, as distinguished from libel, which is written.

statutory law—that law which has been enacted by a legislative branch of the government.

tort—a civil wrong; it may also be a crime.

will—a written document, legally executed, by which a person disposes of his property; to take effect after his death.

V. INTRODUCTION

As a new worker in the health field, it is important for you to become aware of problems that may occur when you care for patients. This instructional unit will provide you with information that will help you to identify and prevent medical-legal problems.

It may be disturbing to realize that although you and your classmates are here to learn specific techniques and procedures used in caring for patients, you must also be concerned about the threat of medical-legal problems that could arise in your daily work.

A health worker may be defined as anyone who comes in contact with the patient to serve him and to have access to his records. As a consequence, the patient must place great trust in the health worker. Violation of the patient's trust and confidence by the health worker may be interpreted as an illegal or immoral act.

Before presenting information relating to the health worker and the law, it is essential to take a brief look at the types of laws that are encountered in everyday living. This will serve as a foundation for the more specific instructions to follow.

The word "law" may be used in different ways. For example, there are physical laws, such as the law of gravity; moral laws, such as the law of Moses; common law (unwritten law), based on custom and precedent, which constitutes the foundation of our country's legal system; and statutory or legislative laws, which are written laws passed by the legislative branch of government, both federal and state.

You should now know and understand the following definitions: health worker, physical law, moral law, common law, and statutory law. If you cannot define these terms or think of examples of each, reread this introduction and the vocabulary. You may ask your instructor for additional resources.

ITEM 1. PROTECTIVE LAWS

When patients place themselves in our hands, they expect us to protect their comfort, life, and rights. They expect to receive the care and help they need, and to be better off as a result of that care.

In order to protect the patient, the state and federal governments have passed laws and set standards for health care. One of the responsibilities of the states is to license workers in the health occupations who can have a crucial and lasting effect on the patient's life and health. Some of the workers who must have a license to practice include dentists, dental hygienists, doctors of medicine, licensed practical or vocational nurses, medical technologists, optometrists, pharmacists, physical therapists, registered nurses, and sanitarians. In addition, hospitals, convalescent facilities, and other health care agencies must be licensed and comply with the state regulations for fire and operating safety, adequate staffing, and similar requirements.

The hospitalized patient has fundamental rights, just as any other citizen does. Even when hospitalized, the person retains his civil rights, which are guaranteed by the Bill of Rights in our Constitution. This means the patient has the right of freedom of movement, freedom of decision, and freedom to worship as he chooses, the right to vote, to make and receive phone calls, to send and receive mail, and to refuse treatment and to leave the hospital if he wishes. Exceptions are made only when (1) authorized by the courts as in the case of a criminal or a person found to be mentally incompetent, and (2) on a temporary basis when justified and ordered by the physician for medical reasons.

In taking care of patients in hospitals, health workers must guard against infringing upon their rights, especially in the following areas.

Consent. A patient's basic right of freedom is interfered with in the process of providing him with medically indicated bed rest. If bed rest is needed, there must be a patient's consent as well as a doctor's order for the health worker to follow. Patients usually sign a general admission agreement when entering a health agency for treatment. If the patient does not voluntarily agree to sign the consent, the doctor and the health agency could be guilty of false imprisonment.

Restraints. We must be doubly careful in any patient care situation that involves detaining or restraining a patient. For example, protective restraints are often used to remind a patient to hold his arm still while he is receiving intravenous fluids. Protective restraints may also be used to restrain an elderly, irritable patient. In such a case, "protective restraints" may be questionable. Are they used to protect the patient or to prevent annoyance to the health care team? However, some patients must be restrained to protect themselves and others. This is often true with confused, disoriented patients. In such cases, be sure that your judgment is correct and that you have the proper authorization to restrain.

Assault. There may be additional ways of violating a patient's rights, e.g., assault and battery. "Assault" is the handling of a patient with the threat to do harm or to restrain him forcibly. An example of a threat could be, "If you don't stay in your room, we'll put you in restraints."

Battery. As an extension of the verbal threat, there may be actual illegal bodily contact without the patient's consent; in this case the action is called "battery." An example of this situation occurs in emergency rooms when patients are brought in by the police department to have blood drawn for testing on a drunken driving charge. The procedure cannot be carried out without the patient's consent, unless he has been arrested, charged, and taken into police custody. When someone breaks the law, the status of his basic rights changes.

It is important that you understand from the foregoing paragraphs that there is protection for all. The patient is not to be coerced, and the health worker must be carrying out valid orders.

Slander and Libel. Gossiping about a patient is another important area in which you must be extremely careful of the patient's rights. Gossip may be considered "defamation of character." A carelessly spoken word can be judged "defamation by slander." A written entry in a patient's chart such as "patient was a cranky old so-and-so today" is considered written defamation and is called "libel." It can be declared an illegal act.

Privileged Communication. As you care for patients, you will often be entrusted with personal information, especially relating to their condition. This is called "privileged communication" and must be held in absolute confidence. You have heard about privileged communication in the context of clergymen, lawyers, doctors, and news reporters. Now you, too, will have this responsibility.

Invasion of Privacy. The last in our list of abuses of a patient's rights is the "invasion of privacy." An example of this could be a press photographer bursting into the patient's room following admission after a spectacular car wreck in which all other persons involved were killed. It is your responsibility as a health worker to protect your patient from this kind of trespass.

It is often difficult to analyze the patient's basic rights in light of prescribed medical services. In the next section we will consider the quality of care the patient receives and what the law says about it. However, before moving on to the next section, you should be able to define and give examples of the following terms: standards and licensing laws, Bill of Rights, false imprisonment, assault, battery, slander, libel, privileged communication, and invasion of privacy. If you cannot define these terms, reread this section. If you can, then proceed to the next item.

ITEM 2. LEGAL JUDGMENTS

Many judges have been faced with the dilemma of ascertaining that a patient is guaranteed safe care while the conscientious health worker is protected from lawsuits. The patient is legally entitled to good care; he pays for it and expects it. The law supports the patient and makes the health worker responsible for "duty of care." On the other hand, the health worker is protected by the concept of "reasonable care." This is a standard which states that the level of care must be equal to the care given by a comparable worker in similar circumstances. If the health worker does not meet this standard of reasonable care and if harm therefore comes to the patient, the worker may ultimately be judged negligent. Negligence may be failure to give reasonable care or giving unreasonable care.

Negligence and Malpractice. The differences in the meaning of the words "negligence" and "malpractice" are sometimes hard to distinguish. For most purposes, malpractice has come to mean professional care that is below the standard expected by the community—in other words, bad or faulty practice.

To clarify these terms, let's look at the following examples: When a nurse fails to give a prescribed medicine or treatment, negligence is involved because she has overlooked it or perhaps run out of time on her shift. Malpractice, on the other hand, would be giving the wrong medication or treatment to the patient.

It is customary to hold the person with the highest level of training and licensure responsible for the consequences of what has been done or what has been neglected. The registered nurse is responsible for the care of patients on her assigned list, even though other workers, such as the NA or LPN (LVN) perform some of the duties. She is the one ultimately held responsible. This is not meant to indicate, however, that persons of lesser training or licensure would not be held responsible for their own actions. It simply means that the individual with the highest level of education and licensure is the final person to be held responsible—often it may be the physician. This concept involves the chain of command, i.e., the person to whom one is directly responsible for one's actions.

Before leaving the subject of negligence and the possibility of being sued by a patient (commonly called a lawsuit or litigation), let us consider the degree of seriousness with which a lawsuit is treated by the court.

Civil and Criminal Suits. If the injury to the patient is slight and the intention of the health worker was not to harm, the entire litigation may be kept between the patient and the health worker instead of going to court. In this case, the accusation is called a "tort"; it is treated under civil law, and is known as a civil suit. On the other hand, if it is shown that the health worker intended to injure the patient, the case is removed from settlement by civil law and becomes a criminal suit. The defendant has not only injured a person (patient) but has committed an unlawful act against society.

It is understandable that the more serious the crime, the more severe the punishment. Serious crimes are called felonies, whereas lesser crimes are called misdemeanors. Both types are handled under the criminal law procedures.

You have received information on many complex concepts. Before moving on to the next section, be sure that you can give a definition and example of each of the following terms: duty of care, reasonable care, negligence, malpractice, lawsuit, litigation, tort, civil law, criminal law, felony, and misdemeanor. If you know all of them, continue with the next section.

ITEM 3. LEGAL DOCUMENTS

As a health worker, you may handle or be responsible for certain documents, records, and legal papers. Three important documents you may handle are (1) the patient's chart, (2) the written consents, and (3) his will. When the term "legal document" is used, it indicates that it is acceptable in courts of law as evidence of truth; it is above reproach, and is subject to the scrutiny and standards of any legal person.

The Chart. Let us examine a patient's chart in these respects. Is it complete? Is it signed? Is it in ink and in no way altered? These are questions asked when determining whether it is an acceptable legal document. In other words, if the health worker were to appear in court, the lawyer showing an entry in the patient's chart would be expected to ask, "Is this your signature? What did you mean by what you said here?" Later in this course you will learn to chart your nursing care on the patient's chart. With the knowledge you have gained from this unit, you will be more aware of how important it is to chart legibly, accurately, and according to prescribed charting rules.

Consents. Another highly important legal record is the "signed consent." In court action, the lawyer can be expected to ask any or all of the following questions:

"Is there a consent form available for use in this instance?"

"Was the patient competent to sign?" (He was not disoriented, confused, etc.)

"If the patient was not competent to sign, is the signature on the consent that of the legally authorized person?" (Specific information on this subject is discussed in a later unit on consents, releases, and incidents.)

"Did the patient consent to what was done, or can this consent be otherwise interpreted?"

"Was this an informed consent? Was the person told the risks, the extent of the procedure, and the expected results?"

"Was the consent signed before the treatment was given?"

Without proper consents signed by the patient, we can be accused of illegal acts. There are certain agency rules about who may witness consents; these will also be discussed in the unit on consents.

Wills. Another important document is the will. You may be asked to witness a patient's signature when he signs a will. According to law, a will must be signed in ink, signed voluntarily by the patient while in sound mind and witnessed by at least two persons over the age of 18. The health worker may be requested to witness a signature on a will. If so, follow the agency procedure. Many agencies designate one individual who may be permitted to sign as a witness to a signature on a will.

Perhaps you can think of ways in which you might prevent becoming involved in a lawsuit. If you responded with comments along the following lines, you are to be commended for your understanding of your legal responsibilities for your patient's care:

"I will be a conscientious worker because the patient is my responsibility, no matter how I feel or how distracted I am."

"I will be observant of the patient's rights and avoid any violation of them."

"I will be careful with the paperwork for which I will be responsible. I will do all in my power to see that all documents are legally correct."

"I understand what is meant by chain-of-command. In the future I will do only those things for which I have been trained and supervised to do."

ITEM 4. CONCLUSION

You have completed the lesson on the Health Worker and the Law. You should have a good idea of the law as it relates to you while performing your job of caring for patients. You are now aware of how important it is to do your best. Always be mindful that in your work you are entrusted with the care of other persons, and this is the most precious trust in life. In the next unit we will discuss ethics and how it differs from law and what your ethical responsibilities will be in caring for your patient.

When you feel sure you understand this lesson, ask your instructor to allow you to take the post-test. You will be expected to pass the test with at least 80 per cent correct answers.

VI. ADDITIONAL INFORMATION FOR ENRICHMENT

Because the material presented in this unit is complicated, you may be interested in learning more about your legal responsibilities as a health worker; if so, ask your instructor for additional reading assignments.

POST-TEST

I. Match statement on the right to the most appropriate term on the left.

_____ 1. duty of care

_____ 2. statutory law

_____ 3. invasion of privacy

_____ 4. slander

_____ 5. ethics

_____ 6. negligence

_____ 7. privileged communication

_____ 8. battery

_____ 9. tort

_____ 10. misdemeanor

a. threatening to injure another person

b. detaining unlawfully

c. the highest concept of right and wrong

d. meeting expected standards

e. illegal act between persons

f. less serious crime

g. making personal information public without due consent

h. failure to give reasonable care

i. laws made by legislature

j. verbal defamation of character

k. unlawful handling of a person without his consent

l. unwritten law

m. information kept in trust by medical personnel

II. Fill in the blanks with the term being defined.

1. If someone commits an illegal act against society, this is called a _____.

2. A lawsuit may also be called a _____.

3. A civil suit is one brought between an individual and a/ an _____.

4. Written defamation of character is called _____.

5. Detaining a person unlawfully against his will may be interpreted as _____

_____.

III. Choose and circle the one best answer.

1. A ward clerk never saw a certain patient in the hospital but was accused by his family of defamation of character. She was most likely guilty of:

   a. assault and battery

   b. felony

   c. slander

   d. negligence

2. A nurse's aide inserted a rectal thermometer in an unconscious patient and left the room to finish another task. The patient moved, broke the thermometer, and sustained injury. Which of the following might she be sued for?

   a. reasonable care

   b. felony

   c. assault

   d. negligence

3. A patient's chart after dismissal is:

   a. kept for seven years

   b. public property

   c. a legal document

   d. given to his doctor

4. The doctor orders a treatment for his patient that the registered nurse does not know how to do; however, she does it and harms the patient. The person or persons most likely to be held for negligence is the:

a. doctor

c. supervisor

b. registered nurse

d. hospital

5. A will is not valid if when signing it the patient can be proved to have been:

a. under the influence of sleeping pills

e. all of these

b. not mentally competent

f. none of these

c. coerced

g. a, b, and c

d. displeased with the witnesses

h. c and d

6. A patient may not be detained at the hospital until he pays his bill because this may be considered an illegal act of:

a. invasion of privacy

c. defamation of character

b. false imprisonment

d. libel

7. A malpractice suit can be brought against a hospital or health worker for the following:

a. a stroke patient falling from a wheelchair

e. all of these

f. a and b

b. a diabetic not receiving insulin as ordered

g. a, b, and c

c. a patient overexposed with X-ray

h. a and c

d. a patient losing a valuable ring

8. A nurse may be said to have acted with reasonable care if she:

a. is a specialist in emergencies

b. has been a supervisor

c. has nursed for 20 years

d. did what other nurses of similar background would have done in similar circumstances

9. A nurse's aide was instructed by a licensed practical nurse to place a hot water bottle for comfort at the feet of a patient who is paralyzed from the waist down. It resulted in severe tissue damage. Who will probably be held responsible for an act of negligence?

a. the hospital

c. the aide

b. the doctor

d. the licensed practical nurse

10. Which of the following will help the health worker avoid litigation?

a. consistent practicing of conscientious care

e. all of these

b. obtaining written consents

f. a and d

c. always considering human rights

g. a, b, and c

d. staying within the limits of her training

h. a and c

POST-TEST ANNOTATED ANSWER SHEET

I.   1. d   (p. 2)   6. h   (p. 2)

2. i   (p. 2)   7. m   (p. 2)

3. g   (p. 2)   8. k   (p. 1)

4. j   (p. 2)   9. e   (p. 2)

5. c   (p. 2)   10. f   (p. 2)

II. 1. crime (pp. 2 and 5)

2. litigation (pp. 2 and 5)

3. individual (or term of comparable meaning) (pp. 2 and 5)

4. libel (pp. 2 and 4)

5. false imprisonment (pp. 2 and 3)

III. 1. c   (p. 4)   6. b   (p. 3)

2. d   (p. 4)   7. c   (p. 4)

3. c   (p. 5)   8. d   (p. 4)

4. b   (p. 4)   9. d   (pp. 4–5)

5. g   (p. 6)   10. e   (p. 6)

I. DIRECTIONS TO THE STUDENT

Please read the general and specific objectives carefully. Study the vocabulary, and proceed through the lesson as directed.

II. GENERAL PERFORMANCE OBJECTIVE

You will demonstrate your understanding of the importance of ethics in the role of the health-related hospital worker. You will answer questions to demonstrate understanding of ethical behavior in health service situations.

III. SPECIFIC PERFORMANCE OBJECTIVES

In a testing situation, you should answer with 80 per cent accuracy written questions about:

1. The definition of ethics.

2. The difference between legal aspects and ethical considerations.

3. Persons who make up the health team.

4. The necessity for and utilization of ethics in hospital situations.

5. Application of ethical behavior guidelines in judging appropriate choices of action in eight hypothetical health-related situations.

IV. VOCABULARY

breach—breaking (infraction) of a law, or of any obligation, tie, or contract.
conduct—one's actions in general; behavior.
custom—long-established practice; accepted behavior.
ethics—a code of conduct for a particular group representing ideal behavior.
expire—to breathe one's last breath; to die.
hygiene—rules designed for the promotion of health; sanitary science.
hypothetical—a supposition for the purpose of reasoning; fictitious with a logical purpose.
overt—open; not hidden.
P.N. student—practical nursing student; when such students complete their course and become licensed, they are called LPN's, except in California and Texas where they are called LVN's (Licensed Vocational Nurse); all must be graduates of accredited practical nursing programs.
solvent—solution that dissolves a substance, converting it to a liquid.
unethical—not ethical; not representative of ideal behavior.
utilization—to make use of.
value system—behavior, pattern of conduct, or ideas that are accepted as worthwhile or meaningful.

V. DRAMATIZATION

MISS JOHNSON
Instructor

We're happy to have the nursing students from the Community College join our hospital orientation session for new employees. Technically, the students are not employees of our hospital, but they do have their clinical assignments here, and are therefore part of the hospital team. Our topic for discussion today is Ethics in the Healing Arts.

MISS SANDS
P.N. Student I

Miss Johnson, what does "ethics" mean?

MISS JOHNSON

It comes from a Greek word that means "custom." There are many definitions we could use, but let's try this one: "Ethics is a code of behavior that represents the ideal conduct for a particular group."

MISS McGUIRE
P.N. Student II

Well, I expect to become a Licensed Practical Nurse (LPN), so will my ethical conduct be different from yours as a Registered Nurse?

MISS JOHNSON

Each profession or vocation requiring a license in the health occupations has a written Code of Conduct that has been approved and adopted by its membership. These codes, whether for the Physician, Registered Nurse, Licensed Practical Nurse, or other group, have many things in common. For example: (1) the rules are based on reason, good judgment, and an understanding of the difference between right and wrong behavior; (2) they strive to respect the dignity and rights of the individual patient.

MISS SANDS

I've noticed that I have a tendency to judge all nurses by the actions of the few I know.

MISS JOHNSON

That's a common reaction and one good reason for each member of a group to strive for ideal behavior. Ethical conduct by the individual members of the group presents the whole group in a favorable light to the public.

MRS. DEEDS
Housekeeper Assistant

What do you mean by right and wrong? Maybe what is right for me is not right for you.

MISS JOHNSON

It is true that every person has his own "customs" and perhaps his own value system for what is right or wrong based upon his personal life experiences. However, by accepting employment in a hospital, the worker must accept the "ethics" or "customs" required by the employer.

MR. THOMAS
Orderly

Why are ethics necessary? Couldn't the employer just give us a handbook of rules when we apply for a job?

MISS JOHNSON

Sometimes this is done, but through the ages societies and groups have established codes of conduct as a method of preventing friction between people, improving personal and group status, and encouraging growth and development in one's life. For example, Hippocrates, the Greek "Father of Medicine," proposed a code of conduct for physicians before the birth of Christ.

MISS SANDS

I'd like to know how ethical conduct differs from my legal requirements as a hospital employee.

MISS JOHNSON
That is a point that needs careful explaining. Ethical conduct codes are written and adopted by the membership of the groups. Ideal behavior is encouraged through education, example, and discussion. It is to be hoped that enforcement is seldom needed. But sometimes a person whose conduct is highly unethical may be disciplined by the group or even lose his membership in the group. As one of you mentioned earlier, the group is judged by the behavior of its members, so an unethical member is expected to conform, or lose his membership privileges. None of you is as yet a member of a professional group, but you are members of the hospital group and as such, unethical conduct that reflects upon the hospital could result in reprimand or expulsion from the hospital—that is, loss of employment.

MRS. SAYRE
New LPN
Miss Johnson, could you explain this a little more and perhaps give us some examples of the difference between unethical and illegal conduct?

MISS JOHNSON
Ethics have to do with our moral responsibilities or behavior, as we said, and violation of an ethical concept means that we are not living up to ideal moral or ethical behavior. Legal requirements (laws) are set by the society as a whole, that is, by national, state, or local governments. Violation of these laws places the guilty person in trouble with the law enforcement agencies. For example: ethical conduct for a Registered Nurse or Licensed Practical Nurse requires that the uniform and cap should not be worn in public places. A nurse who does so is unethical, but she has not violated any laws that will cause her to be arrested. However, if the nurse takes money from the wallet of an unconscious patient, she has violated the law, and the action could result in her arrest and punishment. She has, of course, also committed a serious breach of ethics by her lack of ideal conduct.

MR. THOMAS
I don't seem to fit in any group. I don't wear a cap, and I'm not an RN nor an LPN. Where do I get my ethical guidelines?

MISS JOHNSON
As an orderly giving direct patient care, you belong to the Hospital Group. And since you will be working under the direct supervision of the Registered Nurse and also with the Licensed Practical Nurses, why don't you read the codes of ethics for these two groups?

(Turn to the appendix at the end of this unit and read the International Code of Nursing Ethics and the Code of Ethics for the Licensed Practical Nurse. When you have completed your study of these two codes, fill in the following blanks.)

Question 1. Ethics is a code of _____ that represents _____

behavior for a particular _____ .

Question 2. A violation of ethical behavior may result in discipline by _____ .

Question 3. A violation of a legal requirement might result in discipline by_____ .

MISS JOHNSON
Now that you have read two codes of conduct for some groups of health workers, let's continue our conversation by writing a list of specific situations in which a hospital worker would have to make a choice in his or her behavior, based upon an ethical judgment. Mr. Thomas, can you name a principle or describe a situation that you have experienced along this line?

MR. THOMAS
Yes, I must give the best possible care to each patient regardless of his financial status, religion, race, or creed.

MISS JOHNSON	Very good.
MR. THOMAS	And I must respect his religious beliefs and try not to convert him to mine.
MRS. SAYRE	That certainly follows our basic guideline of respecting the dignity and basic rights of the individual.
MISS JOHNSON	Mrs. Harmon, how do you think that "ethics" affect your relationship with your employer?
MRS. HARMON	I guess I should report for work on time, and not leave early, and not take sick time off unless I'm really ill.
MRS. WALTERS *Nurse Aide*	How about doing a day's work for a day's pay, and always doing your share of work so that your co-workers can rely on you?
MRS. HARMON	I think that would be fair to everyone.
MISS McGUIRE	Miss Johnson, I'd like to add to that list. You told us in class that we must stay with our patient if needed until relieved; isn't that part of ethical conduct, too?
MISS JOHNSON	Yes. If you were to leave before your relief came, and your patient suffered harm, it might also carry a legal penalty. So you see that the line between ethical (ideal) behavior and legal requirements is sometimes a little hazy. However, the worker who consistently holds to ideal behavior should not have to worry about meeting the requirements of the law. Miss Andrews, you had your hand up.
MISS ANDREWS	I read in the employee's handbook that I can't wear any jewelry on duty, or any nail polish except very pale or clear. Why is that in the handbook?
MISS JOHNSON	The hospital worker's uniform is designed so that it can be easily cleaned to help the worker maintain a well-groomed and immaculate appearance. Unnecessary adornment such as floppy handkerchiefs and jewelry increase the difficulty of keeping clean, and are usually not permitted with the uniform. Soiled uniforms, jewelry, and other adornments may carry germs which can cause disease or infection. It is your ethical duty to prevent the transfer of germs from patient to patient. This can be easily done by keeping your uniform and hands clean. Organized nursing has had its roots in both military and religious disciplines and adhered quite strictly to the dignity of the uniform as a "symbol" of the profession. However, a great deal more latitude is allowed now—the introduction of pantsuits and colored hose are examples. Although there is a gradual decrease in strict adherence to the symbolic uniform, you must still adhere to the basic principles of cleanliness to prevent disease and infections for your own protection as well as the protection of your patients.

In some agencies, particularly in caring for children or the emotionally ill, the nurses wear streetclothes or colored uniforms without the cap. Your employer has the right to establish the standards of apparel for his employees and, by accepting employment, you have agreed to accept such standards. Another point about uniforms—try to wear your uniform only to and from work, and not to the grocery store or on shopping errands. When a hospital worker wears his identifying uniform outside of the health setting, it is similar to a doctor wearing his stethoscope and carrying his "black bag" to do his errands. Items used in our work often become contaminated with germs, and we may carry them to the unsuspecting public when we wear our duty clothes and equipment in public places.

Nail polish is affected by some of the solvents we use and is difficult to keep undamaged and attractive. Therefore, it is usually neater and less bothersome for you if you do not wear nail polish while you are on duty.

MRS. BOYD
Nurse Assistant

Does personal grooming come under the topic of ethics?

MISS JOHNSON

I would think so. Good hygiene and careful attention to cleanliness and grooming make your patient's environment more pleasant. He surely is entitled to that. Incidentally, good grooming includes careful and minimal use of cosmetics; avoid heavy eye makeup, obvious perfumes, extremes of any sort, which are not in good taste for wear in any situation. Frequently, cosmetics have a heavy, sweet odor which may be nauseating to an ill patient. Therefore, if you are concerned about your patient's welfare, you will refrain from excessive use of cosmetics.

MRS. BOYD

Miss Johnson, last week Mr. Goldrocks tried to give me two dollars when I finished his bathtime care. I told him I wasn't permitted to accept it. How could I have handled this situation better?

MISS JOHNSON

Did you notice in the codes of ethics we read that you are supposed to accept only the money given by your employer? Tipping to ensure service could be disastrous in a hospital, couldn't it? It would violate the fundamental concepts of ethics—respect for the dignity and basic rights of the person. How do you think you would react in such a situation?

MISS SANDS

Maybe I could let my patient know that it is my pleasure, not only my job, to assist him. I can let him know this by my attitude, and how I respond to his needs.

MISS McGUIRE

I think I might suggest that if he feels like making a cash donation, perhaps he would like to give it to the hospital fund for furnishing the new patient lounge, or whatever current project the hospital has. I think there is a difference between a patient offering me a gift or money when he first comes into the hospital, and his giving me a handkerchief, card, or candy when he leaves. Is it unethical to accept the latter?

MISS JOHNSON

I don't think so, Miss McGuire, because if the patient has gone home, he could hardly expect preferential service as a result of his gift. It would be nice, though, if you received a gift, to share it with the other team members who also cared for the patient. I guess that would be following the Golden Rule.

MRS. ACALA
Diet Assistant

Something I saw yesterday bothers me. One of the hospital workers took the dessert from a patient's tray and put it in the utility room and later I saw her eating it.

MISS JOHNSON

Of course, we don't know all the circumstances, but taking what is not ours is stealing, and that is a violation of the law. I wonder if the worker would have openly eaten the dessert if the head nurse or hospital administrator had been present? You are not responsible for the actions of others, but by being responsible for your own actions, you set a good example for others. In some agencies, eating food from a patient's tray is considered cause for immediate termination.

MR. THOMAS — What should be done when a person observes someone violating either the law or ethical concepts; doesn't it show consent if nothing is done?

MISS JOHNSON — You are full of hard questions today, Mr. Thomas. No list of rules could be given that would fit every circumstance. Who is involved, the nature of the infraction, and the circumstances must all be taken into consideration. Sometimes it is best to speak directly to the person involved and allow him a chance to alter his behavior, and sometimes a private discussion with your superior will give you appropriate help in deciding what to do.

One of your most important legal and ethical responsibilities in a health care situation is to guard the privacy of your patient. Privacy is one of his basic rights. When a person is sick, he is dependent upon other people to do many things that he cannot do himself. He is entitled to privacy in all respects—about his condition, personal data, his illness, and everything that you might learn because he is a patient. Sometimes it is tempting when a hospital worker is "on the outside" to reveal information about patients. It is exciting to tell something nobody else knows. This is illegal in some instances, and unethical in all instances.

MRS. DEEDS — Sometimes patients ask me questions when I'm cleaning their rooms. Last week one of them asked me if the patient across the hall had died. I didn't know what to say, although I had just finished cleaning his unit after the body was taken away.

MISS JOHNSON — Patients are often curious about other patients, particularly about one who is very ill or who may have expired. Your ingenuity will be challenged to evade the question, and not appear rude or dishonest. How do you class members think Mrs. Deeds might have answered her patient?

MISS McGUIRE — Could she have evaded answering by saying something like, "I'm not involved with assigning patients their rooms or in moving them from one room to another"?

MISS SMITH — How about a simple, courteous "I don't know."

MISS JOHNSON — That could be a truthful reply, for perhaps the patient did not expire, but was moved to the intensive care unit, or to some other room. However, another way to handle the situation is to ask the patient in return, "Why do you ask?" The patient may only want to talk about the worries or concerns he has for his own health.

MR. TROYLE
Maintenance Man — I'm a new employee, and my neighbor was hurt in an accident and brought here. I was looking at his chart to see how he was and the head nurse jumped all over me.

MISS JOHNSON — Some of you will see information on a patient's chart. You may have reason to use the chart or see it by accident. Unless your work requires you to make notations on the chart or to use it in order to give care to the patient, do not read it or even take it from the chart rack. The chart is a legal document, belongs to the hospital, and the material in it is known as "privileged information"—that is, it is very private and is meant only for those people who need it to care for the patient. Privacy of everything surrounding the patient is his right.

Another point about privacy. It is highly unethical to discuss your patients in the cafeteria, hallways, or public places. Family and friends often overhear conversations and misunderstand what is said. Sometimes they think you are talking about their loved one or friend. Loose gossip can be very upsetting to others. Guard your conversation at all times! Discussion of your patient should be limited to those team members who assist or share in his care and then the discussion should occur in the appropriate place, so it is not overheard and misinterpreted by outsiders.

MISS BOYNE *Ward Clerk*	I think the topic of ethics is quite complex, but I'm glad we had this class today, because I have some guidelines to help me in my work. I'm going to try to be an ideal employee because it should help to keep me out of trouble with my employer and the law.
MISS JOHNSON	No doubt that is true, but aren't there other good reasons?
MRS. BOYD	Yes, I feel good when I know I'm doing the right thing and when I have done a good job.
MISS GROVES *Student Nurse*	There has been a lot in the news lately about violations of ethics, if not of law, by prominent people in many professions. Do you think that the standards for ethical conduct are changing with the times?
MISS JOHNSON	The basic principles upon which ethics are founded, that is, respecting the rights and dignity of the individual, are changeless. In fact, in some ways a greater emphasis is being placed upon the individual rights of *all* people in the fields of education and employment as well as their right to adequate health care. Although we hear about the spectacular breaches of conduct by prominent people, each of us needs to remember that we are primarily responsible for our own ethical conduct.

We have made quite a list of ethical guidelines today from our discussion. We can summarize by saying, whenever you are faced with a situation involving a moral or ethical decision, ask yourself these questions:

1. How will my action or choice affect the patient?
2. How will my action or choice affect my employer or co-workers?
3. How will my action or choice affect me?

You have probably made a sound choice if your answer to all three questions is positive. Your behavior would uphold the dignity and basic rights of the patient and your employer and maintain your own self-respect.

Let's try out our new concepts of ethics by reading the following hypothetical situations and filling in the blanks or circling the appropriate *italicized* word or words.

Situation A

A patient in Room 201 is in critical condition, and although you have not cared for him, you have heard one of the other nurses mention that the doctor feels the patient will not live much longer. A relative of the patient asks you in the corridor if Mr. Brown has improved. Your answer might be, "You probably should speak to the doctor about that." Ethically, who is being considered here?

Question 4. a. _____ b. _____

c. _____

Question 5. In any situation in which the answer is not clear to you, it is appropriate to refer the question to your *(supervisor) (co-worker)*.

Question 6. In doing the above, you recognize your *(legal) (ethical) (both legal and ethical)* limitations.

Situation B

A young girl has been brought by ambulance to the Emergency Room. You are the ward clerk there and note that she has swallowed a small glass of turpentine and is now having her stomach emptied of its contents. Since this was an attempted suicide, the police reporters were in the hallway. When you go to lunch, the other ward clerks want to know why the ambulance had its sirens sounding, how old the girl is, and why she was brought in. You were the person who recorded the emergency room notes and so you have some information. When asked why the girl took the turpentine, you might answer: (Circle the letter of the correct answer.)

Question 7. a. I assume because she is pregnant and unmarried.

b. She must have had a desire to die.

c. This information is confidential.

Question 8. In this situation, to discuss the patient not only violates her right to privacy, but could result in a *(legal action) (loss of employment) (both of these)*.

Situation C

Carol Brown, nursing assistant, has always been conscientious and reliable in her work habits. She is scheduled to work on the weekend and receives an invitation from an old friend to spend the weekend at Yosemite National Park. Carol has never been to Yosemite and does not often have such opportunities. She ponders long and hard before arriving at a decision. Persons considered in her decision-making would be:

Question 9. a. _____ b. _____

c. _____ d. _____

Situation D

Mr. Grimm in Room 410 always orders his meals from the hospital's special gourmet menu. At noon on Sunday he didn't touch any of the food although the dinner was excellent. The filet and strawberry pie were indeed tempting. You are the dietary aide who is responsible for taking trays back to the kitchen. In an effort not to waste such delectable food, you decide: (Circle correct letter.)

Question 10. a. To eat it yourself.

b. To give it to a fellow employee who is quite needy and doesn't eat properly.

c. To ask the dietitian to confer with the patient about ordering smaller portions.

Situation E

Your doctor has observed that you are very tense about your job as a ward clerk in the hospital unit, and has recommended a common tranquilizer for you to take three times a day. You know that often when patients go home, they leave their medications, which are then returned to the pharmacy. You ask the medication nurse if when these tranquilizers are left on a patient's discharge, she could give them to you, saving you the expense of having your prescription filled.

Question 11. This is a distinct breach of _____ on your part.

Question 12. Your ethical behavior is lowered. However, if the nurse grants your request, she is prescribing or dispensing medicine without a license and this is a

_____ offense.

Situation F

You are a nurse's aide and have cared daily for Mrs. Johann. She has come to rely on you and, when she is ready to go home, wants to give you a sum of money in appreciation for the "lovely things you have done for her." (Circle the correct letter.)

Question 13. a. You must explain to her that the service is part of her care.

b. You are paid a salary for giving service and patients pay for their care also.

c. Accept the gift of money and tell nobody so that no one else will feel hurt that she selected only you.

Situation G

Mrs. Johann insists you must take the money or you will hurt her feelings. Therefore you: (Circle the correct letter.)

Question 14. a. Tell her of some specific need the hospital has to which she could make a contribution.

b. Suggest a fund in her name with suitable recognition.

c. Accept the gift so that there are no hurt feelings in the situation.

CODE OF ETHICS FOR THE LICENSED PRACTICAL NURSE

Adopted by The National Federation of
Licensed Practical Nurses

The Licensed Practical Nurse shall:

1. Practice her profession with integrity.

2. Be loyal to the physician, to the patient, and to her employer.

3. Strive to know her limitations and to stay within the bounds of these limitations.

4. Be sincere in the performance of her duties and generous in rendering service.

5. Consider no duty too menial if it contributes to the welfare and comfort of her patient.

6. Accept only that monetary compensation which is provided for in the contract under which she is employed, and she does not solicit gifts.

7. Hold in confidence all information entrusted to her.

8. Be a good citizen.

9. Participate in and share responsibility of meeting health needs.

10. Faithfully carry out the orders of the physician or registered nurse under whom she serves.

11. Refrain from entering into conversation with the patient about personal experiences, personal problems, and personal ailments.

12. Abstain from administering self-medications, and in event of personal illness, take only those medications prescribed by a licensed physician.

13. Respect the dignity of the uniform by never wearing it in a public place.

14. Respect the religious beliefs of all patients.

15. Abide by the Golden Rule in her daily relationship with people in all walks of life.

16. Be a member of The National Federation of Licensed Practical Nurses, Inc., and the state and local membership associations.

17. Not identify herself with advertising, sales, or promotion of commercial products or service.

CODE FOR NURSES—ETHICAL CONCEPTS APPLIED TO NURSING*

Approved by the Council of National Representatives of the International Council of Nurses in Mexico City, May 1973

"The fundamental responsibility of the nurse is fourfold: to promote health, to prevent illness, to restore health and to alleviate suffering.

The need for nursing is universal. Inherent in nursing is respect for life, dignity and rights of man. It is unrestricted by considerations of nationality, race, creed, colour, age, sex, politics or social status.

Nurses render health services to the individual, the family and the community and coordinate their services with those of related groups.

Nurses and People

The nurse's primary responsibility is to those people who require nursing care.

The nurse, in providing care, promotes an environment in which the values, customs and spiritual beliefs of the individual are respected.

The nurse holds in confidence personal information and uses judgement in sharing this information.

Nurses and Practice

The nurse carries personal responsibility for nursing practice and for maintaining competence by continual learning.

The nurse maintains the highest standards of nursing care possible within the reality of a specific situation.

The nurse uses judgement in relation to individual competence when accepting and delegating responsibilities.

_____

*Copyright ICN. All rights reserved.

The nurse when acting in a professional capacity should at all times maintain standards of personal conduct which reflect credit upon the profession.

Nurses and Society

The nurse shares with other citizens the responsibility for initiating and supporting action to meet the health and social needs of the public.

Nurses and Co-Workers

The nurse sustains a cooperative relationship with co-workers in nursing and other fields.
The nurse takes appropriate action to safeguard the individual when his care is endangered by a co-worker or any other person.

Nurses and the Profession

The nurse plays the major role in determining and implementing desirable standards of nursing practice and nursing education.
The nurse is active in developing a core of professional knowledge.
The nurse, acting through the professional organization, participates in establishing and maintaining equitable social and economic working conditions in nursing.

WORKBOOK ANSWER SHEET

1. Ethics is a code of *behavior* that represents the *ideal* conduct for a particular group (p. 11)

2. by the group, or lose membership in the group (p. 12)

3. law enforcement agencies (p. 12)

Situation A (p. 12)

4. a. Patient — his privacy is respected

   b. Employer or group — you are representing high ideals of confidence

   c. Yourself — self-respect is maintained

5. Supervisor

6. Both legal and ethical

Situation B (pp. 12 and 15)

7. c

8. Both of these

Situation C (p. 13)

9. The following in any order: the patient, co-workers, employer, and herself (any of these)

Situation D (p. 14)

10. c

Situation E (p. 14)

11. Ethical standards

12. Legal standards

Situation F (p. 14)

13. a

Situation G (p. 14)

14. a

POST-TEST

I. True — False. Circle the letter indicating whether the statement is true or false.

T   F   1. All professions follow the same code of ethics.

T   F   2. Ethics applies only to the doctors and nurses who are licensed professionals.

T   F   3. You enter into an agreement to follow institutional policy when you take a job with the hospital.

T   F   4. Since patients are in a dependent position, they must expect their privacy to be invaded during illness.

T   F   5. Information about patients can be discussed freely as long as it is not detrimental to their character.

T   F   6. Personal hygiene and good grooming are related to ethics.

T   F   7. Wearing the symbols of your job while shopping helps to enhance your image in the community and is therefore ethical.

T   F   8. A patient's chart is simply a convenient place for everyone caring for the patient to put notes and findings.

T   F   9. Food which has been taken into a patient's room is meant only for the patient and should not be eaten by others.

II. In the statements below, indicate the word "ethical," "unethical," "legal," or "illegal" to describe what guideline or principle is being considered or violated. If two are appropriate, write in both.

____a. Mary Brown constantly comes to work in a soiled uniform which smells strongly of cigarette smoke.

____b. A patient's chart is left lying open at your desk and you as the maid read it since the patient is your neighbor and friend.

____c. At a party you tell about a prominent socialite who had given birth to an illegitimate child.

____d. You delight your classmates in the lounge with an account of the antics of a patient who was coming out of anesthesia.

____e. You ask the medicine nurse to save any unused antibiotics of a certain kind for you to give your child.

____f. When the returned medications are ready for Pharmacy, you carry them over yourself and take out whatever medicines you need for your own use, since they will not be charged to any specific patient.

____g. An elderly lady gives you $25 when she leaves the hospital and thanks you for the extra-special way you took care of her plants and flowers during her hospital stay. You accept and keep the money.

____h. Because you failed to convince a wealthy gentleman not to give you a sizeable amount of money upon his discharge without causing a scene, you accept the money and give it to the supervisor who puts it in a fund for some special equipment.

____i. Although your contract clearly states that your hours are from 8:00 A.M. to 4:40 P.M., you find you can get to work at 8:30 and leave shortly before 4:00 because your supervisor is away at a conference.

___ j.   A discharged patient leaves a lovely dinner ring in the bedside table. You find that it fits you and slip it into your pocket while cleaning the room.

III. Fill in the blanks indicated.

a. Ethics is a code of _____ for a _____ group representing ideal _____ .

b. Having to rely on another person for help or support of any kind makes a person _____ .

c. Breaking an obligation or contract, or an infraction of behavior is often called a _____ of ethics or contract.

d. A commonly used word for "die" in hospital usage is _____ .

e. Rules designed for the promotion of health and good grooming are collectively called _____ .

f. Behavior that is unethical may result in _____ from the group.

g. Ethics involve moral decision and a knowledge of the difference between _____ and _____ .

h. Ethical conduct always respects the basic _____ of the patient.

i. My hospital conduct involves myself, my employer, co-workers, and the _____ .

POST-TEST ANNOTATED ANSWER SHEET

I. 1. F (p. 11)
    2. F (p. 11)
    3. T (p. 12)
    4. F (p. 15)
    5. F (p. 16)
    6. T (p. 14)
    7. F (p. 13)
    8. F (p. 15)
    9. T (p. 14)

II. a. unethical (p. 13)
    b. unethical (p. 15)
    c. unethical (p. 16)
    d. unethical (p. 16)
    e. unethical, illegal (p. 14)
    f. unethical, illegal (p. 14)
    g. ethical (p. 14)
    h. ethical (p. 14)
    i. unethical (p. 13)
    j. unethical, illegal (p. 14)

III. a. conduct; specific; behavior (p. 11)
     b. dependent (p. 15)
     c. breach (pp. 10 and 12)
     d. expire (p. 10)
     e. hygiene (p. 10)
     f. discipline; expulsion (p. 12)
     g. right; wrong (p. 11)
     h. rights (p. 11)
     i. patient (p. 16)

Unit 3

ENVIRONMENT AND THE PATIENT

I. DIRECTIONS TO THE STUDENT

Please read the general and specific performance objectives, then proceed through the unit. At the completion of this lesson a written post-test will be given.

II. GENERAL PERFORMANCE OBJECTIVE

In a written test you will demonstrate your knowledge of ten environmental factors in a hospital which affect patients' comfort, recovery, and safety.

III. SPECIFIC PERFORMANCE OBJECTIVES

In a written post-test you will answer questions with at least 80 per cent accuracy about the following:

1. Definition of the terms presented in the vocabulary.

2. The responsibilities of the nurse in environmental management.

3. The desirable ranges for room temperature and humidity, and acceptable methods of modifying these conditions.

4. Correct methods of providing ventilation.

5. Ways to control offensive odors.

6. Common noises in the hospital and ways to minimize their effects on patients.

7. Methods of light adjustment.

8. Methods used to maintain patients' privacy.

9. Safety precautions used in the patient's environment.

IV. VOCABULARY

anesthesia—partial or complete loss of sensation, with or without loss of consciousness, such as may result from disease, injury, or administered drug or gas.
anesthetic—an agent or drug that produces insensibility to pain or touch.
anesthetized—placed under an anesthetic.
ecology—the relationship between living things and the environment.
environment—the surroundings; any condition that affects life or development.
emotional environment—the emotional surroundings affecting our life.
external environment—those conditions outside the body which affect it, such as temperature and noise.
internal environment—the fluid surrounding the body cells.
humidity—the amount of moisture in the air.

24

photophobia—fear of light; a condition in which light is painful to the eyes.

sedated—state of being calmed, usually effected by means of a drug.

ventilation—the movement of air.

V. ENVIRONMENTAL FACTORS

"Environment" is a word frequently heard in today's news media. Any condition that affects the life or development of a person is his environment or surroundings.

"Ecology" refers to relationships between living things and their environment. Environmental and ecological conditions worldwide as well as local can affect our health and that of our patients. Radiation fallout can contaminate the local food and water supply as a result of the explosion of an atom bomb thousands of miles away. Most of us are all too familiar with an unpleasant environmental factor called "pollution." Eye and respiratory irritants in the air affect all of us.

Environmental factors are not all external, i.e., outside ourselves. In nursing, the terms "therapeutic environment" and "emotional environment" are increasingly discussed. We can be surrounded by emotional factors that are helpful or detrimental. The hospital worker is responsible for using communication skills and good interpersonal relationships to reduce tensions, anxiety, and fear in order to provide a good emotional environment for the patient.

The Internal Environment. The physician is greatly concerned with our "internal environment" or the composition and volume of the fluids that surround the body cells. You will be responsible for helping the patient to maintain good internal environment by such measures as (a) keeping accurate records of fluid intake and output, or (b) restricting salt intake.

Circle the letter or letters of the appropriate answer.

Question   1.   The *interrelationship* between people and their surroundings is called:

      a.   external environment

      b.   therapeutic environment

      c.   ecology

      d.   internal environment

Question   2.   A hospital worker is helping to make a therapeutic environment for the patient when she:

      a.   gets along well with her co-workers

      b.   explains what she is going to do to the patient (to relieve his anxiety)

      c.   lessens a tense situation with her communication skills

      d.   tells the patient her honest opinion about the patient's physician

The External Environment. The rest of this lesson will be confined to those factors concerning the immediate external environment of patients for which the hospital team is responsible. In the modern hospital many people share this responsibility—for example, the engineers who maintain temperature through heating, cooling, and regulation of ventilation. Housekeeping personnel provide cleanliness and order throughout the building. This is a safety factor; cleanliness prevents the spread of disease-causing germs and a mopped-up spill will prevent an accident.

In some hospitals the housekeepers clean and restock the patient units after each patient has been discharged. Thorough, careful technique is most important, because the patient's unit is his immediate external environment.

The nursing team has a close and continuing role in patient environment. Providing safety, privacy, neatness, and order, as well as control of odor and noise, is a continuous process.

The maintenance crew keeps up the painting and repair of the building and equipment; these factors are also important to the patient's well-being and safety.

The entire hospital team works together to see that the patient's surroundings are safe, clean, and comfortable.

Question 3. The internal environment refers to the _____ and _____

of the fluids that _____ the body cells.

Question 4. The measurement of fluid intake and output and the restriction of salt in

the diet aid the physician in his management of the patient's _____ environment.

Question 5. In the following blanks, indicate a specific duty of each person which contributes to the hospital environment.

    a. Engineer: _____

    b. Housekeeper: _____

    c. Nurse's Aide: _____

    d. Maintenance: _____

Question 6. If the entire hospital team works together, the patient environment can be:

_____   _____

_____

Specific Environmental Factors. Let's examine in detail ten specific external environmental factors of concern to the nurse as she provides care to her patients.

Regulation of Temperature. Temperature affects our comfort and even our disposition. A range between 68° and 72° Fahrenheit is maintained in most air-conditioned hospitals. For the nursery, the elderly, or at bath time, a slightly higher temperature, perhaps 80°F, might be required.

When the environmental temperature is high, perspiration cools the body by evaporation. It is essential then to offer additional fluids to patients (unless contraindicated) to replace the fluids lost. Remember also to replace fluids that *you* lose when *you* are perspiring heavily.

Some air-conditioned hospitals have individual controls in the patient rooms, to allow for flexibility in temperature control. When this is not available, fans, coolers, and heaters may sometimes be used. Adding an extra blanket, shawl, or bed socks can provide warmth for the patient who feels cold. Remember that the sick person may feel cold or hot even though the temperature of the room is in the so-called ideal range. Hot water bottles are rarely used today because of the danger of burns, especially when caring for the aged, infants, diabetics, and those with decreased feeling or sensibility (such as patients who are sedated, anesthetized or paralyzed). There are effective and safe heating and cooling devices such as the K-pad and the hypothermia machine with the hypothermia blanket, which use warmed or cooled fluids circulating through tubes in the pad. The temperature is automatically maintained by thermostats. A refreshing bath or alcohol rub may temporarily cool and refresh the patient even though the room temperature cannot be lowered.

Question 7. A desirable temperature range for most hospital rooms is between _____

and _____ .

Question 8. Two occasions on which it may be desirable to raise the room temperature slightly are:

    a. _____

    b. _____

Question 9. When the environment is hot and the patient perspires freely, a nursing measure to replace lost fluids is _____ .

Question 10. List three methods of providing a patient with additional warmth (a doctor's order is required for some):

a. _____

b. _____

c. _____

Question 11. List the three types of patients who require *very special care* if external heat is applied because they could be burned easily:

a. _____ , b. _____ ,

c. _____

Humidity Control. "It's not the heat — it's the humidity," is a common expression. Humidity is the amount of moisture in the air, and a range of 30 to 50 per cent is normally comfortable. Very *low* humidity dries the respiratory passages. As the temperature increases, air can hold more water. At 50°F, saturated air holds 4.2 grains of water per cubic foot of air. At 90°F, it can exceed 14.3 grains. (A grain is a measurement of weight.) This shows that nearly three times as much water is retained in the air at the higher temperature. With the air already saturated by moisture, perspiration does not evaporate, and the patient loses one of his major cooling devices.

Unfortunately, there is no simple method of decreasing humidity; it has become a technical problem for air-conditioning experts and is accomplished by modern engineering methods. However, a vaporizer or humidifier is sometimes ordered for patients to *increase* humidity in some respiratory conditions.

Ventilation Control. Ventilation refers to the movement of air. Stale air can be oppressive. The use of fans increases comfort, even though the temperature and humidity remain unchanged because the air is in motion. In home care, opening windows—top and bottom—increases circulation when the warmer air rises to be replaced by cooler air. In most hospitals, unbalancing of air-conditioning is used for ventilation and temperature control. Windows are not used for these purposes and do not open.

Use *caution* to avoid a chilling draft on the patient. The use of screens between the source of cool air and the patient will prevent drafts.

Question 12. Circle the "T" if the statement is more true than false, and circle the "F" if the statement is more false than true.

T F a. The higher the air temperature, the more water it can hold.

T F b. Evaporation of perspiration is increased in high humidity.

T F c. The use of a vaporizer increases humidity.

T F d. A humidity of 30 to 50 per cent is considered most comfortable.

T F e. Humidity refers to movement of air.

T F f. Cold air rises.

If you are unable to answer these questions correctly, review the previous section before proceeding.

Regulation of Light. Lighting contributes to our well-being. However, some illnesses, such as measles, cause "photophobia," a condition in which light is painful to the eyes. Bright light must be avoided during the acute phase of measles. Also, patients who have had certain types of eye surgery must avoid glaring lights.

A sunny room is cheerful and can improve your patient's spirits. Adequate light should be provided for reading and all other close work. This means a light that is bright enough to see without *glare* and to avoid eye strain. Good light is *soft* and *diffused*. It does not make sharp shadows. Overhead fluorescent lighting is generally effective. You can check for glare by holding a pencil or similar object 4 to 6 inches above a piece of light-colored paper. If the outline is sharp, there is enough glare to be troublesome; if the outline is fuzzy and soft, glare should be no problem.

Most people prefer to sleep in dim light. Adjust the shades, blinds, and drapes to help regulate light. The use of a night-light provides safety for the person who gets up to go to the bathroom at night. This also has the advantage of permitting nursing personnel to observe the patient throughout his sleeping hours.

Use of Color in Patient Environment. Some bright colors stimulate; other colors are soothing. Many people have a preference for or an aversion to certain colors. The location of the source of light influences color. Decorators are aware of this, and colors in patient rooms are usually subdued pastels. In solaria and workrooms, however, bright colors may be used. It is rare now to find the cold, all-white hospital room; most have colorful bedspreads, pictures, and draperies. Many convalescent hospitals are using attractive wallpapers and color combinations to provide a cheerful, homelike atmosphere.

Question 13.   Complete the following statements:

    a.   A good light is bright enough to avoid straining the eyes in order to see,

       but it should be diffused or without _____ .

    b.   Why is a night-light desirable in a hospital room? _____

    _____ .

Circle the best response:

    c.   The colors in a room *(can) (cannot)* affect a person who is not colorblind.

    d.   Most patient rooms in hospitals have *(subdued pastel colors) (bright stimulating colors)*.

Noise Control. Noise is a negative environmental factor (one that patients frequently note and that they complain about) and can affect one's health. People who are careless or thoughtless about talking and laughing cause unnecessary noise. Voices carry loudly in corridors, which seldom have drapes or other sound-absorbing materials. Equipment and machinery, such as floor polishers and carts being rolled down hallways, are often noisy. Dropping equipment causes startling noises. Many hospitals use resilient floor materials, sound-absorbing ceilings, and plastic equipment in an effort to decrease noise. This still does not reduce the major source of noise—people. You can help to reduce "people noise." The hospital should be a place for rest and quiet.

Tact is required when one patient's radio or television is disturbing another. Skill in human relations which involves both tolerance and courtesy in dealing with people, is very important for nurses. This is a skill that you should continue to develop throughout your lifetime.

Provision of Neatness and Order. Some people seem to thrive in clutter; others are offended by a picture that hangs even slightly crooked. The unit should be kept in sufficient order to be safe, but you must avoid imposing rigid standards on the patient who enjoys being surrounded by his possesions.

Remove soiled dishes and unused equipment promptly. Check the unit several times during your tour of duty to maintain neatness and order.

Question 14. List three common sources of hospital noise.

a. _____

b. _____

c. _____

Question 15. How do you think *you* can best reduce undesirable noise in your hospital?

a. _____

b. _____

Question 16. By removing soiled dishes and unused equipment from the patient unit, you are maintaining a. _____ and b. _____ in his environment.

Prevention or Control of Odors. Odors can be pleasant or unpleasant. Unfortunately, unpleasant smells seem to predominate in a hospital. Illness alters our sensory perceptions; for example, the scent of cooking food might produce nausea rather than hunger. Some ways to reduce and control unpleasant odors follow:

a. Dispose of refuse properly. Dressings and refuse should be wrapped in paper or placed in a paper bag provided for the purpose. Place refuse in the proper container with a tight cover to prevent odors from escaping. *Do not* put such items in the patient's waste basket.

b. Remove old, disintegrated flowers and stagnant water, which may be a source of unpleasant odors.

c. Reduce offensive odors from body discharges of the sick person by covering the bedpan, urinal, and emesis basin.

d. Avoid being a source of odors: Breath—no smoking or strong foods. Perspiration—daily bath, fresh clothes. Scents—no perfumes or fragrances, which can be offensive to the sick. All of these are important. The nurse with a spotless uniform and impeccable grooming inspires confidence in her patients concerning their own care.

Good ventilation and cleanliness are far more effective in controlling odors than scented air sprays and other masking devices. "Hospital Clean" should be a reality as well as an expression. Prompt and proper disposal and scrupulous cleanliness can decrease odors. Your acceptance of unpleasant patient odors such as feces, flatus, and emesis will decrease your patient's anxiety and help maintain his therapeutic environment.

Question 17. List two ways in which the patient may be a source of unpleasant odors.

a. _____

b. _____

Question 18. List two ways in which the worker may be a source of unpleasant odors.

a. _____

b. _____

Question 19. List two ways in which the room or hospital might be a source of odors.

a. _____

b. _____

Provision of Privacy. Privacy is essential for the patient's well-being. Always knock gently when the door to a patient's room is closed, and identify yourself before entering. Closing the curtain around the patient's cubicle can spare embarrassment to the patient, worker, and visitors.

Hospital workers become accustomed to situations and functions that would be embarrassing to the nonmedical person. A discreet withdrawal from the room provides privacy for the shy patient to perform his necessary functions such as defecating, urinating, or even washing dentures.

Visitors come to see the patient. A polite greeting and withdrawal by the worker allows privacy for the patient and his guests. Lack of privacy, like noise, is a frequent source of patient irritation. The thoughtful nurse can do much to decrease these irritations.

Provision of a Safe Environment. We shall talk about SAFETY more than once—it is a fundamental guideline in the unit "Guidelines for Nursing Skills." Remember that safety also helps to prevent lawsuits.

Falls and burns are particular hazards in hospitals. Falls can be prevented by removing articles from the floor that might cause a patient to trip. Burns can be prevented by checking electrical equipment, and other means as discussed later in this unit. Handrails and grab bars should be installed in the bathroom and in the corridors to assist the weak or debilitated patient. Siderails are a common safety device. Usually the bed is left in *low* position when the patient is not receiving care that requires the high position. This decreases the danger of falls. You will learn more about siderails in future units.

Mop up spills immediately. Post "Slippery" caution signs when the floor is being mopped. Usually only one side of the floor is mopped at a time, allowing half to remain dry for use.

Soft ties and other restraints may be ordered to prevent falls. These, too, will be discussed in a later unit.

Patients who have poor vision should be given assistance in order to prevent accidents. It is especially important that scatter rugs and clutter be removed and that furniture remain in customary locations.

The danger of burns in hospitals is decreased by careful supervision of smoking (if it is permitted). The sedated patient may doze off and drop the cigarette in the bed. The confused or irrational patient may set himself or his surroundings aflame. The therapeutic use of oxygen requires "No Smoking" signs and proper use of any electrical equipment nearby. Additional safety precautions are discussed in the unit on oxygen therapy.

Inspection of all electrical plugs, cords, and equipment before use can prevent accidents. Most agencies require that any electrical appliance brought in by the patient (e.g., radio or heating pad) must be thoroughly checked by the electrician to ensure their safety.

Oily rags and other combustible materials usually are stored in metal containers which have tight lids. Oxygen and other gas containers under pressure should be secured with straps or by other means to prevent falling.

Testing the temperature of solutions used for soaks, baths, irrigations, and heating devices is necessary to prevent burns. Remember that persons with diabetes, those with impaired circulation, those who receive drugs to reduce pain, the paralyzed, and those not mentally alert can be burned much more easily than can a person in good health.

Fire in a hospital is always a possibility; therefore, know the rules for fire safety. Generally, the agency's fire regulations will be taught in the first few days of employment. Many local fire departments hold regular fire safety classes for employees in health agencies in their area. These are required in most states if a health agency is to receive its fire safety clearance from the fire department. Know the location of extinguishers, fire doors, etc. Many institutions have occasional fire drills; make sure you know what to do in case of a fire or other disaster.

The alert worker looks out for safety hazards and corrects them so that accidents can be prevented. We have discussed only falls and burns. Cuts, choking, electric shock, and drowning are other potential hazards. Prevention of accidents requires constant watchfulness by alert employees.

Some categories of patients are more likely to have accidents than other. These include:

The confused: They may be elderly, medicated, or emotionally disturbed—their safety is *your* concern.

The elderly: They may be forgetful or have decreased sensory perceptions, i.e., dimmed vision or decreased hearing which deprives them of some of their "danger warning" capabilities.

Children: They climb, touch, taste, and eagerly explore their environment. They need special protection to prevent their curiosity from causing injury.

Patients who are sedated with drugs or anesthesia: They need special safety measures such as siderails, straps, and close observation to provide safety.

Providing a pleasant and comfortable environment that contributes to the patient's safety and recovery is a challenge to the hospital worker. Manage it with skill.

Question 20. List three ways in which you can provide privacy for your patient.

a. _____

b. _____

c. _____

Question 21. Falls cause many accidents in and out of hospitals. List five ways in which you might prevent falls.

a. _____

b. _____

c. _____

d. _____

e. _____

In summary, the ten external environmental factors with which you as a health worker will need to be concerned in your care of the patient are: temperature, humidity, ventilation, light, color, noise, odor, neatness and order, privacy, and safety. It is your ethical responsibility to your patient, your co-workers, your employer and to yourself to maintain a pleasant and safe environment.

WORKBOOK ANSWER SHEET

1. c (p. 25)

2. a, b, and c (p. 25)

3. volume, composition (either order), surround (p. 25)

4. internal (p. 25)

5. a. air-conditioning, heating and cooling, ventilation (p. 25)

    b. cleanliness, order, safety (p. 25)

    c. safety, cleanliness, order, light, privacy, odor and noise control (p. 25)

    d. painting, repairs, safety (p. 26)

6. safe, clean, comfortable (any order) (p. 26)

7. $68°$ to $72°\,F$ (p. 26)

8. a. at bathtime in the nursery (p. 26)

    b. when bathing the elderly (p. 26)

9. offer fluid to drink

10. a. add blankets, shawls, bed socks, K-pad

    b. hot water bottle

    c. hypothermia machine with blanket

11. any three of the following: diabetics, infants, aged, or patients with decreased feeling or sensory abilities

12. a. T

    b. F

    c. T

    d. T

    e. F

    f. F

    g. T

13. a. glare

    b. so the patient can get up safely if he is permitted; so nurses can observe him at night

    c. can

    d. subdued pastel colors

14. any three of the following: people talking, equipment, dropping equipment, radio, TV

15. any two of the following: avoid loud talking, care in handling equipment, encourage others to be quiet, keep radios and TV at reasonable levels, avoid noisy activities during patient's rest periods (could be many other similar answers)

16. a. neatness

    b. order

17. any two of the following: discharges (feces, urine, pus, emeses), breath, perspiration, flatus, dressings, medications, and others

18. any two of the following: bad breath, strong perfumes, odor of tobacco on clothes, hands, or hair

19. any two of the following: cooking odors, improper waste disposal, lack of general cleanliness, incontinent patients who have not been kept dry and clean, use of heavy masking spray to cover odors

20. any three of the following: close door, pull screen, knock before entering, leave patient alone to use bedpan (could be many others)

21. any five of the following: remove clutter, avoid scatter rugs, mop up spills immediately, post "Slippery" signs when appropriate, encourage use of siderails and grab bars, use restraints when indicated, keep bed in low position, assist patients who have poor vision to walk, avoid moving furniture

POST-TEST

Directions: Circle the letter in front of the correct response or responses.

1. Management of hospital environment is the responsibility of:

    a. the nurse

    b. housekeeping

    c. maintenance

    d. all of these

2. The most comfortable range of temperature and humidity in a hospital room is usually:

    a. 70 to 76° F, 50 to 60 per cent humidity

    b. 65 to 70° F, 20 to 30 per cent humidity

    c. 68 to 72° F, 30 to 50 per cent humidity

    d. 72 to 80° F, 40 to 70 per cent humidity

3. Effective and desirable methods of decreasing offensive hospital odors are:

    a. prompt and proper disposal of refuse

    b. use of fragrant perfume by employees

    c. good personal hygiene by employees

    d. good ventilation

4. Bright (non-glaring) light in the room is undesirable in or during the following circumstances:

    a. when the patient is reading

    b. period of rest or sleep

    c. some types of illness (measles, eye surgery)

    d. when the patient is depressed

5. Noise can have the following effects on patients:

    a. cause irritation

    b. disturb sleep or rest

    c. increase fatigue

    d. none of these

6. Ways to provide patient privacy include:

    a. the closed door

    b. cubicle curtain

    c. visitors

    d. withdrawal from unit by nurse

7. Ventilation means:

    a. surroundings

    b. moisture in the air

    c. environment

    d. movement of air

8. A vaporizer in the room increases:

    a. temperature

    b. ventilation

    c. humidity

    d. external environment

9. The *one* major source of noise in hospitals is:

    a. equipment

    b. street noise

    c. people

    d. elevators

10. Fill in the blanks:

Safety is a fundamental responsibility for all hospital personnel. A safe environment is especially needed by certain categories of patients who cannot regulate their own environment. List four of these:

    a. _____

    b. _____

    c. _____

    d. _____

POST-TEST ANNOTATED ANSWER SHEET

1. d (p. 25)

2. c (pp. 26, 27)

3. a, c, d (p. 29)

4. b, c (pp. 27, 28)

5. a, b, c (p. 28)

6. a, b, d (p. 30)

7. d (p. 27)

8. c (p. 27)

9. c (p. 28)

10. any four of the following: infants and children, aged, mentally confused, sedated or anesthetized, unconscious, blind, deaf, or paralyzed (could be others) (p. 31)

Unit 4

I. DIRECTIONS TO THE STUDENT

Proceed through this unit on handwashing, which is one of the most important single procedures you will use. Practice the steps of the procedure in the skill laboratory and demonstrate the correct technique for your instructor.

You will need the following for this procedure:

1. A sink with hand, knee, or foot control of water supply

2. Container of liquid soap, or bar soap

3. Paper towel

4. Wastebasket

II. GENERAL PERFORMANCE OBJECTIVE

Employ the correct technique for washing the hands at all appropriate times in order to maintain standards of cleanliness that will minimize the risk of contracting or transmitting infections.

III. SPECIFIC PERFORMANCE OBJECTIVES

You will be able to:

1. Name the routes by which bacteria can be transmitted, recognize the conditions that are favorable and unfavorable to their growth, and take appropriate handwashing precautions against bacterial contamination.

2. State at least five circumstances that necessitate washing your hands as a result of direct or indirect contact with contaminated materials.

3. Wash your hands without any contamination of hands, body, or clothing.

4. Adjust water to the proper warm temperature for washing your hands.

5. Apply soap and water in the proper quantities for washing hands, fingers, wrists, and forearms in the proper sequence.

6. Use the proper rotary and frictional movements to apply firm, even pressure to each area as it is washed.

7. Rinse hands and forearms in the proper manner.

8. Clean fingernails and skin folds properly.

9. Dry hands carefully to prevent chapping.

10. Explain and demonstrate correct handwashing technique to others.

IV. VOCABULARY

abrasion—an injury resulting from scraping away a portion of skin or mucous membrane.
antiseptic—preventing or arresting the growth or action of microorganisms.
asepsis—a condition free from germs; sterile.
bacteria—one-celled microorganisms, some of which cause disease.
contaminate—to soil or pollute; to render unclean or unsterile.
debris—rubbish or ruin.
friction—the rubbing of one thing against another.
genitourinary—pertaining to the organs of reproduction and excretion.
microorganism—minute (small) living body not visible to the naked eye.
palm—concave area of the hand between base of fingers and wrist.
rotate—to turn.

V. INTRODUCTION

Hands carry germs. Germs are called microorganisms. Microorganisms are very small objects, much too small to be seen with the naked eye. They can be seen through an instrument called the microscope. Bacteria are one-celled microorganisms, some of which cause disease and are referred to as being pathogenic. Dirty or contaminated articles or surfaces provide an optimum environment in which the pathogens can grow and multiply. Infections are caused by disease-producing microorganisms (pathogens) which invade the tissues of the body and set up a chemical reaction that in turn causes the tissues to react. Some common pathogenic organisms you will be hearing about include streptococcus or "strep infection," and staphylococcus or "staph infection."

Microorganisms that do not produce disease are referred to as being nonpathogenic. Some of the common nonpathogenic organisms are *Escherichia coli (E. coli)* and *Proteus vulgaris*. They are both normal, harmless residents of the intestinal tract. However, if these organisms get into another part of the body (such as the bladder or an open wound), they may cause an infection.

The five most common methods of disease transmission are the five fingers! The fingers on your hands carry germs (or microorganisms) to the mouth, nose, eyes, and other people. Microorganisms can be spread in several ways:

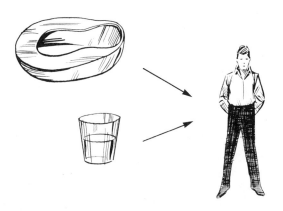

Hospital equipment to patient or worker.

How Microorganisms Are Transferred.

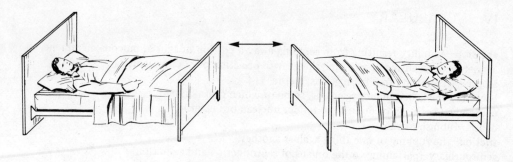

Patient to patient.

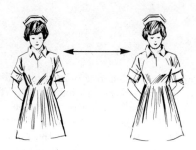

Worker to worker.

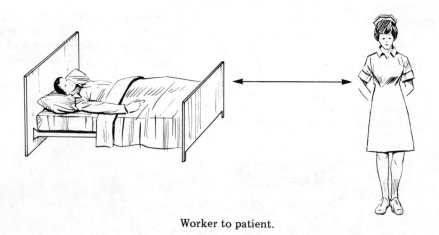

Worker to patient.

How Microorganisms Are Transferred.

Microorganisms can enter the body through the mouth and nose, the genitourinary tract, or through breaks in the skin. Breaks in the skin are frequently the means by which microorganisms enter the body. Germs are everywhere: in the air, in the soil, in the water, on plants, on food and animal life, as well as in or on human beings! Therefore, if the skin is broken, the first line of defense is broken, and germs may then enter the body.

Because germs (bacteria, microorganisms) are living organisms, they need the following environmental conditions to help them live and grow—just as you do:

Moisture: Needed in the process of nutrition to break down solid food particles to permit their utilization as nutrients for the body cells. Moisture also enables waste materials to be expelled from the body.

Food: Needed to assist in the growth process of the organism.

Oxygen: Most living organisms need an oxygen supply to live, but there are some organisms that do not; they are called anaerobic (without oxygen). Some common anaerobic pathogens you may have heard about are tetanus and gas gangrene organisms.

Temperature: The normal body temperature (98.6°F) is the best temperature for most bacteria to grow and multiply. High temperatures (over 170°F) kill most bacteria. Therefore, heat in various forms is often used to disinfect objects — to kill the germs, in other words. Below-freezing temperatures (under 32°F) inhibit the growth of bacteria, although many bacteria cannot be killed in this manner.

Darkness: Most bacteria die when exposed to light; they multiply rapidly in darkness. This is why airing and sunning of articles from a patient's home or room are highly effective ways of killing germs.

One of the most critical tasks you will encounter in the health field is providing an optimum environment for both your patient and yourself. A clean, dry, light, and airy atmosphere goes a long way toward preventing the growth of germs, or killing those that already exist.

One of the simplest methods we have to prevent the spread of disease and germs is the handwashing technique. It is a safety skill not only for you personally, but for your patient, co-workers, visitors, and your family. It assists in protecting you and others from the spread of infections and disease. You will wash your hands before and after doing any procedures that involve direct or indirect contact with a patient, after contact with any wastes or contaminated materials, before handling any food or food receptacles, and at any other time your hands could be soiled.

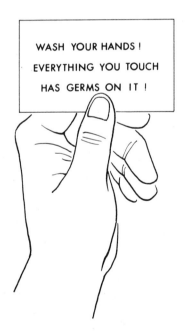

WASH YOUR HANDS !
EVERYTHING YOU TOUCH
HAS GERMS ON IT !

SPECIAL INSTRUCTIONS

There are two reasons why handwashing is absolutely essential:

1. Microorganisms that are harmful to man can be transmitted by means of direct or indirect contact.

2. Certain microorganisms are capable of causing disease.

Your hands. Jewelry should not be worn when giving patient care because bacteria become lodged in the settings or stones of rings. The only exception is a plain wedding band. Fingernails should be kept clean and short. By following these two requirements, you minimize the accumulation of bacteria on the hands or nails, which in turn can be spread to other persons. Proper hand care includes prevention of hangnails and skin abrasions, which might provide entry of bacteria into your body and cause you to become ill.

Liquid soap. Soap combines with foreign matter on the skin and lowers the surface tension (clinging effect) of grease and dirt, thus permitting them to be easily removed from the skin surfaces. Most health agencies prefer to use liquid soaps. When an investigation was made of soap bars and soap dishes in use, many bacteria were found to be growing on them. The bar of soap can be a germ-carrier itself when it is contaminated by dirty water. Care must be taken to rinse the soap well before returning it to the soap dish. This reduces the chance of germ accumulation for the next person.

Bacteria-inhibiting (bacteriostatic) liquid soaps may be used for special handwashing and disinfecting of skin surfaces. The active ingredient in these types of soaps is hexachlorophene, which has a cumulative effect in reducing bacteria on the skin; the more often it is used, and the longer it remains on the skin, the fewer the bacteria that grow. However, you should use these preparations, such as pHisoHex and others, with care and as directed, since hexachlorophene may produce other effects as well.

Running water. Running water carries away dirt and debris. If a water faucet is not available, secure a pitcher of clean water and ask someone to pour the water over your hands and forearms.

Paper towels. Paper towels are best because they are disposable. If only cloth towels are available, wipe hands on clean, unused areas and discard when soiled.

Container for soiled towels. Wastebaskets should be placed beside each lavatory for paper towel disposal. Linen hampers should be available in each wash area where linen towels are used.

Recommended handwashing routine schedule.

1. Beginning tour of duty: 2 minutes (120 strokes)

2. Between patients: 30 seconds (30 strokes) for patients not grossly contaminated; 60 seconds (60 strokes) for grossly contaminated patients.

PROCEDURE FOR 2-MINUTE HANDWASH FOR MEDICAL ASEPSIS

1. *Remove all jewelry.*

2. *Approach the sink.*

Stand in a comfortable position, leaning slightly toward the sink. Maintain good body alignment. Keep your clothes from touching the sink; usually there are many bacteria in and around the sink area. You must therefore avoid contaminating your uniform by contact with the sink. Do not splash water and get your uniform wet. Remember that bacteria thrive in moist surroundings; they grow and multiply rapidly.

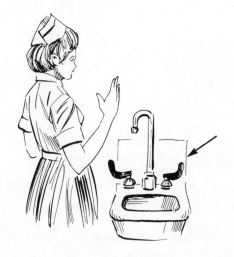

Approach sink.

3. *Turn on the water.*

Keep the water running continuously throughout the handwashing procedure. You may find one of three main types of faucets at your agency: if it is hand-operated, use a paper towel to protect your hands when turning on the faucet, then discard the towel promptly.

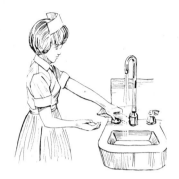

Turn on water with paper towel for hand-operated faucet.

A sink with a foot pedal is preferable because it enables you to turn on the water and regulate the flow without contaminating your hands.

A sink with elbow levers is used frequently in hospitals, particularly in the operating room area. This type of faucet also prevents contamination.

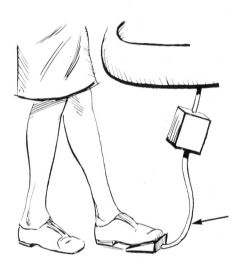

Use foot pedal.

4. *Adjust the temperature of the water.*

Warm water makes better suds than cold water and is preferred to hot water because it removes less protective oil from the skin. Extremely hot or cold water tends to dry the skin. With repeated washing, your skin may be come chapped or cracked, thus providing the prime site for germs to enter the body.

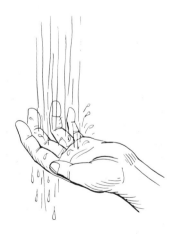

Adjust temperature of water.

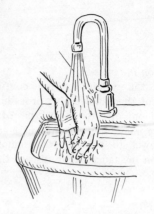

5. *Wet your hands with water.*

Hold your hands down toward the sink, lower than your elbows. Water will then drain from the wrists to the fingertips and carry the bacteria away. Be sure not to contaminate your hands by touching the faucets or the inside of the sink.

Wet hands with water.

6. *Apply soap (or detergent).*

Use approximately 2 to 4 cc (one teaspoon) of a liquid soap. This has fewer germs than bar soap and combines more easily with dirt, thus making it a more effective cleaning agent. Bar soap may retain bacteria; when used, rinse it before returning it to the soap dish. The soap dish should be the kind that permits the bar of soap to dry on all sides before reuse. (Remember that dry surfaces help to stop the growth of bacteria.)

Note: If you accidentally drop the bar of soap on the floor while washing your hands, you must pick it up, rinse it thoroughly, and then begin again at Step 1 of the handwashing procedure!

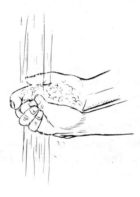

Apply soap (or detergent).

7. *Wash the palms of your hands.*

This step will take about 30 seconds. Use friction (strong rubbing movements) and rotary (circular) motions. Friction and rotary action will dislodge bacteria from your hands.

Wash the back of each hand with ten rotary motions. Be sure to apply a firm, even pressure to maintain effective friction in order to dislodge the soil.

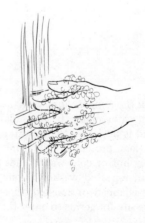

Use friction and rotary motion.

Wash your fingers with ten rotary motions. The fingers and thumbs should be interlaced. Rotation back and forth in this position cleans the interdigital spaces between the fingers quickly and efficiently.

Total of 30 seconds: 10 seconds for the palms; 10 seconds for the back of the hand; and 10 seconds for the fingers.

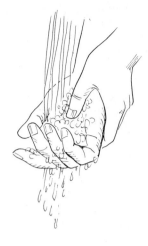

Wash fingers with ten rotary motions.

8. *Rinse well.*
   Running water should be directed so that it flows from the wrists down to the fingers, thus carrying the suds and soil down the drain.

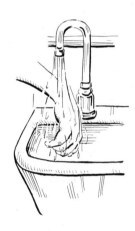

Rinse well.

9. *Again moisten your wrists and forearms with soap.*
   Use the right amount of liquid soap, about one teaspoon. Since the wrists and forearms also may come in contact with bacteria, they should also be cleaned. Wash one wrist and forearm for 10 to 15 seconds using firm rotary and friction action. Then wash the other wrist and forearm in the same manner, moving from the wrist up toward the elbow. Total strokes for both arms = 30.

10. *Rinse your arms and hands.*
    Again, remember to drain the water from the forearm to your fingertips.

11. *Repeat handwashing (60 strokes).*
Use the procedure described in Steps 5 through 9. All remaining bacteria and soil should now be gone.

12. *Inspect your knuckles.*
The knuckles frequently harbor excessive bacteria and germs in the folds of the skin and thus may need additional attention. If so, cleanse with soap, using firm friction and rotary action.

13. *Clean your fingernails.*
An orange stick or a curved end of a flat toothpick will remove the dirt and help prevent breaks in the skin; discard it after use.
Note: Fingernails should be cleaned at the beginning of your tour of duty and as needed during the shift. Normally, it will not be necessary to clean them each time you wash your hands throughout the day.

14. *Dry your hands well.*
Because you wash your hands many times throughout your tour of duty, it is necessary to dry them very gently and carefully to avoid chapping. Chapped skin frequently breaks open, thus permitting bacteria to enter your system.

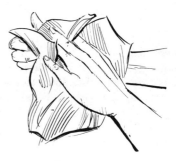

Dry hands well.

15. *Turn off the running water.*
Use a paper towel to turn off the hand faucet. Discard the towel into the wastebasket.

16. *Apply lotion.*
Use lotion as desired to keep your skin soft.

17. *Return used equipment.*
Equipment should be returned to the proper storage area, or to the appropriate area for reprocessing. Wipe the surfaces surrounding the sink with a paper towel. Remember that germs thrive on moist surfaces! Discard the towel. A clean, dry environment promotes health.

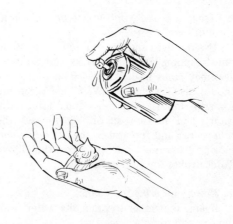

Apply lotion.

ENRICHMENT

The Nature of Bacteria and Microorganisms

There are many kinds of microorganisms; bacteria represent only one type.

You have learned that handwashing is a way of preventing the spread of bacteria and other microorganisms in order to protect the patient, others, and yourself.

You now know that bacteria enter the body through the mouth, the nose, and the genitourinary tract. Each of these tracts has secretions that serve as barriers to bacteria. Threadlike cilia (hairs) and the mucous membrane of the nose are so effective in removing dust and bacteria that the lungs are kept relatively free of these microorganisms. There is an acid reaction to urine and vaginal secretions that prevents growth of most bacteria in the genitourinary tract. Digestive juices kill some of the bacteria that enter through the mouth, and the mucous membranes of the intestines are effective in keeping bacteria from invading the tissues.

One kind of bacteria that is generally found on the skin is the staphylococcus (plural, staphylococci), commonly called "staph." This is disease-producing, and all health facilities are plagued by it. When "staph" gets into the body (through a break in the skin), it may cause local infection or soreness with pus. It may affect the entire body once it enters the blood stream, and those afflicted with it feel very ill. Staphylococcus causes such ailments as boils, styes on eyelids, infections in surgical wounds, infections around fingernails, and food poisoning.

Antibiotics are used to fight this type of infection, but staphylococcus and certain other microorganisms are highly resistant to most antibiotics, often making the patient very ill.

Staphylococci are present on your skin most of the time, even when you are in good health. This is one reason why handwashing is so important. Like all bacteria, "staph" thrives in moist, dark places. Direct sunlight is its enemy because it dries and kills "staph" when it is exposed for a given time. Remember to wash your hands well and often and to dry them thoroughly.

Escherichia coli are common inhabitants of the alimentary tract and are present in feces. This bacteria may cause an inflammatory condition of the urinary bladder, gallbladder, or peritoneal cavity. Remember to wash your hands after handling a bedpan or a bowel movement.

Pseudomonas aeruginosa is a pathogenic microorganism found in draining wounds, infant diarrhea, otitis media (ear infections), and some other conditions that cause one who is infected to become very ill. Remember to wash your hands after caring for each patient.

Harmful microorganisms are spread more by hands than any other method. Proper handwashing can prevent the spread of such germs.

PERFORMANCE TEST

Handwashing Technique for Medical Asepsis

In the skill laboratory, correctly demonstrate the handwashing procedure, carefully observing the proper sequence of steps listed in the unit.

PERFORMANCE CHECKLIST

HANDWASHING TECHNIQUE FOR MEDICAL ASEPSIS

Demonstrate the correct handwashing technique:

1. Stand away from the sink in order to keep your clothing from touching the sink.
2. Turn the water on; adjust it to warm temperature. Keep the water running during the entire procedure.
3. Wet your hands.
4. Apply soap thoroughly—under the nails and between the fingers.
5. Wash the palms and the backs of your hands with strong frictional motion (ten rotary movements for at least 20 seconds).
6. Wash the fingers and spaces between them, interlacing the fingers, rubbing them up and down for 10 seconds (ten strokes).
7. Wash the wrists and three or four inches above the wrists, using rotary action (10–15 times).
8. Repeat steps 4 through 7 (completion of two-minute scrub, 120 strokes).
9. Pay special attention to problem areas.
10. Rinse well; run the water from wrists to fingers (final rinse).
11. Dry hands thoroughly with a paper towel from wrists to fingertips.
12. Turn off the water faucet with a paper towel and discard the towel into a receptacle.
13. Use hand lotion if desired.

POST-TEST

Part I Directions: True/False. If the statement is true, circle the letter T at the left of the statement; if the statement is false, circle the letter F.

T   F   1. You can spread microorganisms to another person without touching him.

T   F   2. Initially the hands should be washed after washing the forearms.

T   F   3. Human fingers are the most common means of spreading microorganisms.

T   F   4. If the hands must be washed frequently, it is best to use cold water to avoid chapping the skin.

T   F   5. Hands should be held level with the waist during the handwashing procedure.

T   F   6. Your hands and body should not touch the sink at any time during the handwashing procedure.

T   F   7. The palms of the hands should be washed before washing the fingers.

T   F   8. An infected person can spread his bacteria to animals, food, clothing, and other objects as well as to people.

T   F   9. When washing the hands, water should not be allowed to flow down from the forearms over the palms.

T   F   10. Bacteria that enter the body through breaks in the skin are more dangerous than bacteria that enter through the nose and mouth.

T   F   11. Microorganisms must have food, moisture, and air to survive.

T   F   12. A dry bar of soap usually contains fewer bacteria than a moist one.

T   F   13. All soap film on the hands should be removed by thorough rinsing.

T   F   14. The fingertips usually contain more bacteria than other parts of the hands.

Part II Directions: Short-Answer/Completion. Please write your response in the space provided.

1. List four circumstances that necessitate handwashing.

_____   _____

_____   _____

2. Please write a brief statement explaining why ornate rings should not be worn by health care workers.

_____

_____

_____

3. List five environmental conditions that facilitate the growth of microorganisms.

_____   _____

_____   _____

_____

4. List two reasons for washing your hands in warm water.

_____

_____

POST-TEST ANNOTATED ANSWER SHEET

PART I

1. T p. 39
2. F p. 43
3. T p. 38
4. F p. 42
5. F p. 43
6. T pp. 41, 42
7. T p. 43
8. T pp. 38, 39
9. F pp. 43, 44
10. F p. 39
11. T pp. 39, 40
12. T p. 41
13. T p. 44
14. T p. 38

PART II

1. (a) Prior to handling food or food receptacles p. 40

    (b) Before and after using the bathroom p. 40

    (c) Before and after any procedure that involves direct or indirect contact with a patient p. 40

    (d) After contact with wastes or contaminated materials p. 40

2. Bacteria may become lodged in the settings or stones of jewelry p. 41

3. (a) Moisture p. 39

    (b) Food p. 40

    (c) Oxygen p. 40

    (d) Appropriate temperature range p. 40

    (e) Darkness p. 40

4. (a) Warm water makes better suds than cold water. p. 42

    (b) Warm water removes less protective oil from the skin than hot water. p. 42

GUIDELINES FOR NURSING SKILLS

I. DIRECTIONS TO THE STUDENT

Please read the General and Specific Performance Objectives carefully.

II. GENERAL PERFORMANCE OBJECTIVE

In a written test using questions representing patient situation, you will demonstrate your knowledge of the guidelines for performing a nursing skill.

III. SPECIFIC PERFORMANCE OBJECTIVES

In a written post-test of patient-situation questions, you will answer with at least 80 per cent accuracy questions about the following:

1. Given a nursing task to perform, you will recognize and apply legal and ethical concepts for the safety of the patient, worker, and employer.

2. You will communicate with the patient, co-workers, and others in such a manner as to make the task safe and effective.

3. You will apply the principles of biological and physical science that make the task safe and effective.

4. You will prepare to perform the task using the following criteria to evaluate the task:

    a. Condition of the patient.

    b. Abilities and limitations of the student.

    c. Environmental factors that could help or hinder performance.

5. You will implement the nursing task using the following guidelines:

    a. Preparing the patient physically and mentally.

    b. Preparing the required equipment.

    c. Performing the task utilizing applicable principles from biological and physical sciences.

    d. Performing follow-up care of the patient.

    e. Performing follow-up care of the equipment.

    f. Reporting and recording accurately and appropriately.

6. You will evaluate the outcome of the task by answering the following questions:

    a. Did the task accomplish the intended purpose?

    b. Was it performed safely for the patient? For the worker?

    c. Was it performed in a manner economical of time, effort, and supplies?

IV. CASE PRESENTATION

The call light is flashing at Room 212. You are about to answer it. This is your sixth week as a student in a combined Nurse Aide-LVN class at the local community college. The four hours a day you spend at Hills Memorial Hospital as a student fly by as you perform your duties.

Who is the patient in Room 212 and how can I help her? It may be Mrs. Mary Jones in bed "C" who is the reason for the flashing red light. You observe that the top bedding is pushed back, revealing a very damp drawsheet. This is your chance to be a "good nurse." Of course, you can change a drawsheet in no time at all;

but wait—

Mrs. Jones is a 76-year-old lady who is confused. She is partially paralyzed from a stroke, and she weighs 198 pounds! Are you still confident?

Try this—

Just suppose she is another Mrs. Jones, not the 198-pound lady at all. Instead, she is a 32-year-old housewife with a ruptured stomach ulcer who is getting a blood transfusion and oxygen, and has a tube in her nose leading to her stomach and connected to a suction device. Her anxious family clusters about the bed. Remember, all she needs is a dry drawsheet and, of course, you can provide that!

—Or can you?

Don't give up. Room 212 "C" might be Mrs. Jones who is a 22-year-old new mother who speaks only Spanish. She will be going home within the hour, taking that adorable baby boy from the nursery. Of course, you can handle this one—just whisk off the wet sheet and pop on a clean, dry one tight enough to satisfy old Miss Instructor.

You get the idea: It's not simply a matter of changing a drawsheet, these people have needs which require you to plan what to do and how to do it.

Circle the letter of the *best* answer.

Question 1. In order to perform even the simplest nursing skill you need to:

    a. Plan what to do.

    b. Plan how to do it.

    c. Consider the individual needs of the patient.

    d. All of these.

V. GUIDELINES

To help you plan when you are confronted with any nursing situation, consider these guidelines:

Legal and Ethical Limitations. Of course, it's legal for you to change a drawsheet, and ethical too; no problem here. Remember, nonprofessional health workers assist with care of seriously ill patients under supervision. Be sure you understand your role in performing even a simple task for a patient like our critically ill Mrs. Jones. In your role as a beginning practitioner, you can legally perform those jobs you have been trained to do according to your job description.

Safety. Always think safety. Plan safety. Anticipate safety for the patient, for you, for everyone. That wet drawsheet placed on the floor could be a safety hazard to the little old lady walking with crutches. If it were placed on the overbed table it could be a safety problem with those germs left behind.

Circle the best answer, or fill in the blanks.

Question 2. When a worker is careful to work within her legal limitations, she protects:

    a. herself

    b. the employer

    c. the patient

    d. all of these

Question 3. The nonprofessional health worker_____with the care of the seriously ill patient under _____ .

Question 4. Mrs. Jones, your patient, asks you, "What laxative would you recommend, nurse?" You *(could) (could not)* tell her because it is *(unethical) (legal) (not legal)* for a nurse to prescribe. (You should follow up on why she asked and communicate this to your team leader who can see that her needs are supplied through proper channels.)

Question 5. Remember the Mrs. Jones with the stroke? After changing her drawsheet, you make sure that the siderails were in place because nurses must provide

_____ for their patients.

Question 6. List four potential causes of accidents that the hospital worker should try to

prevent. _____ .

_____ .

_____ .

_____ .

Purpose or Goal. When you perform a task, it should accomplish its purpose. (Smoothing the top of the bed won't help if it's the drawsheet that needs changing.)

Economy of Time, Effort, and Expense. There's that budget again. But planning is especially helpful here. "Economy" means management without waste. Forgotten linen is wasteful of time and effort spent in an unnecessary trip to the linen room. Careless handling of equipment causes unnecessary expense. Using supplies for a purpose not intended can be uneconomical, e.g., wiping up a spill on the floor with a washcloth rather than a rag.

Question 7. The purpose of all your planning and implementing the plan is to accomplish

the _____ .

Question 8. Proper planning in nursing care can save: _____ ,

_____ and _____ .

Planning. Nursing is a challenge because no two situations are the same. The nurse must constantly plan, then implement (put into effect) and evaluate (judge) her actions. One very important tool used to accomplish this is communication.

Communication may be verbal (talking and listening) and nonverbal (facial and body expressions and movements). Communication is used in planning, implementing, and evaluating each nursing skill. For example, do you understand exactly what is expected of you? Tell your superior if you have doubts about your ability to perform the task. Communicate with the patient and his family; this may decrease fear.

Encourage the patient to participate. Let him know what is expected of him. (Keep in mind those legal and ethical limitations in communications.) You communicate with the other concerned members of the health team when you report and record.

Communication occurs through the knowledge gained in the classroom, ward, and conferences, and from reading and experience. It should be applied to your performance skills; this helps you develop in your vocation. Skills are improved by constantly applying theory to the nursing situation, e.g., when doing research in the library on an assigned subject, preparing for or participating in a patient care conference, or explaining to the patient what you are going to do. You applied your knowledge of physical science when you used leverage in turning Mrs. Jones. The principles learned in microbiology made your nursing care safer when you prevented contact between your uniform and the soiled drawsheet. In pulling the drawsheet tight to make Mrs. Jones comfortable, you applied the following aspects of theory from your nursing classes: moving and turning the patient, bed-making, prevention of decubiti, and good body alignment.

Question 9. Patient care involves communication. Communication may involve: (Place a checkmark before each correct answer.)

a. _____ Team leader

b. _____ The patient

c. _____ The patient's family

d. _____ The chart

Question 10. List three common ways you communicate.

a. _____ .

b. _____ .

c. _____ .

d. _____ .

Assessment. Let's get back to planning. Some factors you will need to consider when assessing the patient (determining what he can do) are these: the condition of the patient, the size of the patient, the patient's ability to assist, the patient's ability to hear, and the patient's ability to understand our language. (Remember the three different Mrs. Joneses.)

After assessing the patient, assess yourself: Is this task within the personal capacities of my training, policy, physical skills? Should I get assistance? Do I need some special equipment? (You would need help in changing the drawsheet on two of our Mrs. Joneses.)

Last, assess the environment. Will I have to move some equipment? Should I modify the temperature of the room? What are the provisions for privacy? Safety? (Changing the drawsheet would disturb the oxygen tent of the critically ill Mrs. Jones.)

These questions refer to changing the drawsheet for the Mrs. Jones who has the tubes, suction equipment, oxygen tent, and visitors.

Question 11. The presence of the oxygen tent and the location of the equipment affect the procedure of changing the drawsheet. You determined this when you

_____ the _____ .

Question 12. As a student who has been in school for six weeks, you determined the need

for assistance in changing the drawsheet when you assessed _____ .

Question 13. In turning Mrs. Jones, taking care not to disturb the tubes in her nose, you

had _____ the condition of _____ .

Implementation. After planning comes implementation, or putting your plan into action. Our guidelines for this are as follows:

Step 1. Prepare the patient. Let him know what is expected. This helps prevent fear. Provide for his safety. Pulling the curtain or closing the door provides privacy.

Step 2. Prepare the equipment. Inspect equipment for breaks, wear, and so forth (safety). Collect as much as is practical at one time (economy of time). Remember, the patient comes first—it is poor planning to bring the bath water in at the same time as the linens because it would get cold before the bedding was removed and before you are ready to bathe the patient.

Step 3. Perform the task. Some of your tasks will have been taught in great detail. Every accredited hospital has a procedure manual that can help you review if necessary. Your team leader is available for help and guidance. Strive for the minimum amount of *time*, *effort*, and *expense* that provides safe care.

Step 4. Give follow-up care to the patient. Provide cleanliness, give explanations, and take safety measures as indicated. Siderails up? Call bell handy? Necessary personal items within reach? It is best to provide for your patient *before* caring for the equipment— remember, people are more important than things.

Step 5. Give follow-up care to the equipment. Proper care of equipment can prevent the spread of infection (safety). Many items commonly used in the hospital are disposable. It is more economical to replace them than to clean and sterilize them. Nondisposable items should be stored in the proper place and carefully marked with the patient's name (economy); e.g., it is unfair that the patient be asked to pay for a second irrigation tray because the trays in the room are unlabeled and therefore unsafe to use. (You may not be sure which patient had previously used the equipment.)

Step 6. Report and record. Reporting and recording are most important. They help provide continuity of care when you are off duty. They fulfill legal requirements and provide a word picture of the patient's progress from the nursing viewpoint. The chart is a legal record. Your recording should be accurate, concise, and appropriate.

Summary. Let's list the steps required to perform a given task:

1. *Prepare the patient.* This means communicating with him before beginning.

2. *Prepare the equipment* to save time and effort.

3. *Perform the task* using the techniques acceptable to your institution.

4. *Follow-up care of the patient* for his comfort and safety.

5. *Follow-up care of equipment*: proper labeling, cleaning, or disposal.

6. *Report and record.*

Question 14. Place the numbers 1 through 6 in the blanks in the usual order of the steps for performing a nursing task.

_____ Give follow-up care to the equipment.

_____ Report and record.

_____ Prepare the patient.

_____ Explain the procedure to the patient.

_____ Give follow-up care to the patient.

_____ Perform the procedure.

Question 15.   Fill in the blanks. In explaining what you are going to do to your patient and

in _____ and _____ ,

you are using _____ skills.

Evaluation. Now that the planning and implementation are complete, let us consider evaluating the outcome. In doing this, we might ask ourselves three questions:

1. Did I accomplish the purpose of the procedure? (Changing a wet drawsheet.)

2. Was the procedure carried out with:

   a. *Safety for the patient?*
   For Mrs. Jones with the ruptured stomach ulcer, it would mean not disturbing the drainage tubes; managing the canopy of the oxygen tent to avoid losing oxygen; and moving her in such a manner as to avoid an increase in bleeding. (These are reasons why you would work under the close supervision of your team leader in this situation.)

   b. *Safety for the worker?*
   In moving the paralyzed, 198-pound Mrs. Jones, you would need to apply techniques of proper body alignment and movement. You might need assistance to reduce the risk of injuring yourself.

   c. *Safety for others?*
   You will recall from the handwashing unit that proper disposal of the soiled drawsheet and careful handwashing prevent spread of germs that might cause infection in others.

3. Did you practice economy of time, effort, and money?

   Taking all needed supplies at one trip means economy of time and effort. Also, you took only what was needed and did not waste supplies—this showed economy of expenses.

As a beginning health worker, you will constantly be faced with changing situations. This is what makes nursing interesting. Skills can be learned and improved. This lesson has provided some principles and guidelines that can help you whenever the call light flashes and you go to help many Mrs. Joneses.

In summary, we have discussed the following guidelines, which will assist you in making your work easier as well as more efficient:

1. Plan your work.

2. Consider the legal and ethical implications.

3. Practice economy of time, effort, and expense.

4. Practice good communication.

5. Assess the patient, yourself, and the environment to determine your course of action.

6. Implement your plan:

   a. Prepare the patient.

   b. Prepare the equipment.

   c. Perform the task.

   d. Give follow-up care to the patient.

   e. Give follow-up care to the equipment.

   f. Report and record.

7. Evaluate the outcome of the action:

    a. Safety for the patient, worker, and others.

    b. Was the purpose accomplished?

    c. Were you economical (time, effort, and expense)?

If you believe you understand the guidelines that have been discussed, ask your instructor to allow you to take the post-test.

U
N
I
T
5

WORKBOOK ANSWER SHEET

Question   1. d.

        2. d.

        3. assists; close supervision

        4. could not; not legal

        5. safety

        6. falls, burns, electric shock, drowning, choking, treatment for wrong patient, etc. (any order or any similar list)

        7. intended purpose (goal) of the action

        8. time, expense, effort

        9. a., b., c., d.

      10. a. verbal; b. nonverbal (gestures); c. expressions; d. charting

      11. assessed; the environment (room)

      12. your own physical skills (self)

      13. assessed; the patient

      14. 5 — Give follow-up care to the equipment

          6 — Report and record

          2 — Prepare patient

          1 — Explain procedure to the patient

          4 — Give follow-up care to the patient

          3 — Performing the procedure

      15. Reporting and recording; communication

POST-TEST

Please read the following carefully.

Mrs. Anders, a 72-year-old blind woman in Centerville Convalescent Hospital, has recently undergone surgery for a fractured hip and has a dressing on the operative area. She has been admitted from the acute hospital for convalescent and rehabilitation care. She is one of the patients assigned to your care during your clinical training.

The following questions pertain to this care situation:

1. As you assist Mrs. Anders with her oral hygiene, she tells you, "Get out my laxative pills from my overnight bag, please." Your best response would be: (Select one.)

    a. _____ Comply in a pleasant manner.

    b. _____ Explain that dependence on laxatives is harmful.

    c. _____ Offer to get her another, more effective laxative.

    d. _____ Relay Mrs. Anders' request to your team leader, assuring Mrs. Anders that you will tell the nurse that she wishes a laxative.

2. The principle in this situation is: it is (legal) (not legal) (ethical) to give any medication that is not ordered by the physician.

3. It is time for Mrs. Anders' bath. Place the number "1" in front of the activity that you would perform first. Place the number "2" in front of the activity you would do second, and so on, to the last activity.

    a. _____ Take out the soiled linen.

    b. _____ Get help to turn Mrs. Anders.

    c. _____ Remove the top bedding.

    d. _____ Put on the bath blanket.

    e. _____ Bring in the necessary clean linen.

    f. _____ Get the bath water.

    g. _____ Pull the curtain about the unit.

    h. _____ Explain what you are going to do.

    i. _____ Go to the patient's unit and check it for supplies, i.e., soap, towels, bath blanket, and so forth.

    j. _____ Turn off the cooler in the room.

    k. _____ Report that Mrs. Anders has a reddened area on her unoperated hip.

4. By reporting the reddened area to the team leader and charting accurately about it, you are: (Place an X in the appropriate blank[s].)

    a. _____ Communicating.

    b. _____ Carrying out a legal obligation.

    c. _____ Providing safety for the patient.

    d. _____ Making use of your theoretical nursing knowledge.

5. You took all of the supplies needed for the bath and linen change. In addition, you took two extra sheets to hide in the closet because the linen supply is often low and you are going to be sure your patient has what she needs. This is being economical of: (Circle letter of best answer.)

   a. Time

   b. Effort

   c. Supplies

   d. All of these

   e. None of these

   f. "a" and "b" only

6. You requested assistance from a classmate to turn Mrs. Anders carefully when you make the bottom of her bed. In getting assistance, you recognized your:

   a. Legal responsibilities

   b. Ethical responsibilities

   c. Personal limitations

   d. All of these

7. In turning off the cooler before giving the bath, you were acting upon your assessment

   of the _____ of the room for Mrs. Anders' comfort and safety.

8. Placing the soiled dressing removed from her operated hip in a paper bag and disposing of it promptly in the covered receptacle in the utility room helped to prevent spread of germs. This is an application of the theory of (biology) (social science) (physical

   science). It also was part of the follow-up care of _____ .

9. Mrs. Anders' daughter tells you, "I'm so glad when you take care of mother. The other nurses seem so uninterested and hurried." Your reply must be careful and tactful to avoid contradicting her—yet you want to support confidence in your hospital and fellow employees. A good answer would show your skill in:

   a. Legal aspects of nursing

   b. Ethics in nursing

   c. Theory of nursing

   d. "a" and "b" only

10. After completing the bath, you performed the following services. Place an "X" in front of each one that contributed to Mrs. Anders' *safety*.

   a. _____ Attached the call bell near her right hand and had her locate it.

   b. _____ Placed the bed in low position.

   c. _____ Left the siderail down so she could get up to the bathroom by herself.

   d. _____ Cleaned and filed her fingernails.

11. The guideline you would be using in putting up the siderails or placing the call bell

   within reach of the patient would be _____

   _____ .

12. After completing a nursing task, it is helpful to ask yourself three questions in order to evaluate yourself. These three questions are:

    a. _____

    b. _____

    c. _____

POST-TEST ANNOTATED ANSWER SHEET

1. d. (pp. 50, 51)

2. Not legal (pp. 50, 51)

3.
    a.   10
    b.   9
    c.   6
    d.   7
    e.   4
    f.   8
    g.   5
    h.   3
    i.   1
    j.   2
    k.   11(p. 53)

4. Mark all four blanks (pp. 50–52)

5. f. (p. 51)

6. d. (pp. 50–52)

7. environment (p. 52)

8. biology; equipment (pp. 52 and 53)

9. d. (pp. 50, 51)

10. a.; b. (p. 53)

11. the safety factor in follow-up care (p. 54)

12.
    a. Did I accomplish the purpose?

    b. Was the procedure safe for everyone?

    c. Did I economize in terms of time, effort, and expense? (p. 54)

BODY ALIGNMENT, BALANCE AND MOVEMENT

I. DIRECTIONS TO THE STUDENT

Please read the following paragraphs carefully. They will tell you exactly what you will be expected to know and do at the end of this lesson. Take the pre-test before you begin the lesson. Correct the test. If you did well on the pre-test, discuss this with your instructor, who may allow you to proceed directly to the performance and written post-tests. All students are expected to demonstrate accurately the skills required on the performance test and to demonstrate understanding of the principles of body alignment, balance, and movement.

II. GENERAL PERFORMANCE OBJECTIVE

You will demonstrate your knowledge of good body alignment, balance, and movement by a performance test and a written test.

III. SPECIFIC PERFORMANCE OBJECTIVES

After you have completed this lesson, in the skill laboratory without reference to any source material, you will be able to:

1. Position your body in alignment and balance, and state the reasons for the position of your feet, knees, buttocks, abdomen, thorax, and head, according to the standards outlined in this lesson.

2. Demonstrate accurately the body movements of flexion, extension, hyperextension, adduction, and abduction, and describe the movements using terms given in the vocabulary and in the lesson.

3. Answer with at least 85 per cent accuracy in the written post-test questions about the following:

   a. The vocabulary presented in the lesson.

   b. Principles of good body alignment as presented in this lesson.

   c. Principles of good body balance as presented in this lesson.

   d. Effects of physical forces of gravity.

IV. VOCABULARY

abdomen—part of the trunk between the chest and the pelvis.
abduct—to move a body part away from the midline of the body.

adduct—to move a body part toward the midline of the body.

antagonist—one of a pair of muscles having an action *opposite* that of the other muscle of the pair.

anterior—front side.

balance—the action of becoming stable, fixed.

body alignment—the relationship of each movable body segment to the other segments so that no undue strain is placed on the skeleton or muscles.

buttocks—the rounded prominences formed by the gluteal muscles; the seat, or rump.

circulatory system—the body system that includes the heart, blood, and blood vessels.

"corset muscles"—the layers of muscles which support the abdominal and pelvic organs.

digestive system—the body system that includes the mouth, stomach, and intestines.

endocrine system—the body system composed of the ductless glands such as the thyroid, pancreas, and adrenals.

extension—the movement that widens the angle between two adjoining parts, or brings two parts into or toward a straight line.

extremities—the limbs of the body.

flexion—the movement that narrows an angle between two adjoining parts, or the act of bending.

glucose—a simple sugar used by body cells for energy.

gluteal muscles—thick posterior muscles that form the buttocks.

gravity—a force that pulls toward the earth.

hamstring muscles—strong flexor muscles located on the posterior part of the thigh.

hormones—powerful chemicals formed by endocrine glands that regulate many body processes.

hyperextension—increasing the angle of a joint beyond its normal range (usually beyond 180°).

intervertebral disc—a cartilage found between most vertebral bones that acts as a cushion.

joint—the juncture or meeting of two or more bones.

lateral—pertaining to a side.

ligament—a tough band of tissue that attaches bone to bone at a joint.

oxygen—a colorless, odorless gas forming approximately one-fifth of the content of air.

pelvis—a basin-shaped structure of bones at the lower end of the trunk of the body that contains in its cavity the organs of the lower portion of the abdomen.

posterior—the dorsal or back portion of the human anatomy.

quadriceps femoris—the strong extensor muscles located on the anterior side of the thigh.

stability—quality of balance, firmness; not having tendency to tip or fall.

thorax—the chest portion of the body.

trunk (torso)—the body, not including the head and extremities.

urinary system—the body system that includes the kidneys, ureters, bladder, and urethra.

vertebral column—the spinal column of vertebrae; the backbone.

This may seem like a lengthy vocabulary to you, although you probably already know some of the words and understand their meaning. It may help if you pick out some of the words that go together and list them, then check to see if you know their meanings. How about listing the following?

1. Systems of the body.

2. Movements of body or joints.

3. Names of muscle groups.

ITEM 1. INTRODUCTION TO BODY MOVEMENT

Hospital workers are very active people. In performing their work, they use a variety of movements as they reach, lift, carry, push, pull, stoop, sit, stand, and walk. Your activities will require that you, too, use these movements as you reach for linen from a shelf, lift and carry objects, push wheelchairs or stretchers, stoop to pick up objects from the floor, walk, or stand at a bedside.

All of us have been performing this movements most of our lives, so why do we single them out for consideration now? What is the point? The answer is that with knowledge of proper body alignment and movement (a) your work may be easier, (b) you may prevent injury to yourself and your patient, and (c) you will present a more attractive appearance as you work. Without the knowledge of proper body alignment, balance, and movement, you may not apply the principles in your nursing activities and consequently may suffer an injury. We want you to be conscious that you are using proper body alignment for yourself and the patient at all times, that you know how to balance yourself correctly, and that you avoid strain or injury to yourself.

One of the common injuries to hospital workers is severe muscle strain, usually of the lower back, although it may occur in the shoulders or the abdomen. Low back strain is painful; it takes time to heal. It may require hospitalization, bed rest, or traction, it is costly in lost salary and medical fees, and it is preventable. Low back strain and other muscle strains are caused by improper body alignment, loss of balance, or poor body movements.

Your employer and your co-workers prefer you to be a healthy worker rather than a patient with a preventable injury. The knowledge and use of proper body alignment, balance, and movement will help you to prevent injury to yourself.

Please complete the following:

Question 1.   List five movements that you might perform in your daily hospital work.

a. _____ b. _____ c. _____

d. _____ e. _____ .

Question 2.   Give three reasons for using good body alignment, balance, and movements.

a. _____

b. _____

c. _____

Question 3.   Circle the best answer:

a. Low back strain is a *(fairly common) (uncommon)* injury among hospital workers.

b. Severe muscle strain is the result of *(lifting a heavy object) (someone else's carelessness) (poor body alignment or movements)*.

Question 4.   If you suddenly sustained this type of injury (low back strain) and were hospitalized, how do you think this might affect the workload of your co-workers? _____

_____

ITEM 2.   SYSTEMS INVOLVED IN BODY MOVEMENT

Let's take a brief look at this wonderful and complex body of ours. This will help you understand how to align and balance your body in order to perform body movements safely.

The Musculoskeletal System. The bony framework of the body is formed by the skeletal system. The bones and joints are the important parts of the skeletal system. The point where bones come together is called a joint, and it is the joint that allows the movement of the body.

Bones cannot move by themselves. Muscles attach to bones and are usually found in pairs whose members work opposite each other. If one muscle flexes or bends a joint, the other muscle can extend or straighten that joint. When the muscle contracts or shortens, it pulls one bone toward the bone on the other side of the joint.

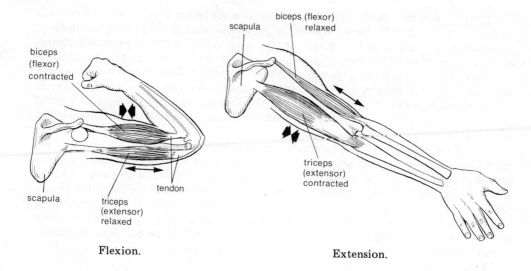

Flexion.   Extension.

These two body systems (the skeletal bones and the muscles) are often considered together and are referred to as the musculoskeletal system. In the next item, you will learn more about this system.

The Nervous System.   The brain, spinal cord, and nerves produce and conduct electrical energy impulses that allow the muscles to work in a smooth, coordinated manner. Muscles cannot function without this stimulation, or innervation, from the nervous system.

The Cardiopulmonary System.   The heart pumps the blood through a vast system of tubes called blood vessels, and the blood carries oxygen, glucose, and other vital substances to the muscles and other body tissues where they are absorbed by the cells. The respiratory system supplies the oxygen needed by the cells to convert, or change, the glucose to energy. Air that we breathe contains about 20 per cent oxygen. The air is inhaled into the lungs where the oxygen passes through very thin air sac walls and is absorbed into the blood stream. The blood is then pumped throughout the body to deliver the oxygen to the cells.

The Digestive and Urinary Systems.   The energy (or the fuel) used by the muscles is a simple sugar called glucose. The digestive system breaks down the food that we eat into simpler substances such as proteins, fats, and sugars, including glucose. In the digestive system, these substances are prepared to be absorbed into the blood stream.

When glucose is converted into energy by the body cells, not all of the substance becomes energy; some remains as waste material. When muscles have been used strenuously, waste material collects around the muscles, and this can slow down the functioning of the muscle. The waste material is absorbed into the many tiny blood vessels located throughout the muscle. These small vessels merge into larger vessels that take the blood to the kidneys where the waste products are filtered out and eliminated from the body as urine: This is the function of the urinary system.

Endocrine System.   There is one more body system that is important in providing movement—the endocrine glands. There are seven main endocrine glands. You may already know some of them. They are the thyroid, parathyroid, pituitary, adrenals, thymus, pineal, and finally, gonads (ovaries or testicles). Each gland makes one or more powerful hormones that enter the blood stream directly from the gland. These hormones regulate many of the body's activities, including that of muscle action.

Do you see why we said that your body is very complex? Even the simple movements of reaching, standing, walking, pushing, and pulling require that many systems of your body work together in harmony.

Circle the appropriate number or numbers of your answer(s) to the following questions.

Question 5. We could not align and balanace and move our body without using the:

    a. muscular system

    b. skeletal system

    c. nervous system

    d. respiratory system

    e. all of these

Question 6. Muscles need fuel to provide energy for contraction. Which statements correctly describe the nature of the "fuel" used by the body?

    a. Energy is provided by the simple sugar called glucose.

    b. The fuel is delivered to muscles by the circulatory system.

    c. The fuel comes from waste products carried in the blood.

    d. Oxygen is needed in order to release the fuel's energy.

Question 7. The glands that produce powerful chemicals that help to regulate body functions form the:

    a. digestive system

    b. endocrine system

    c. nervous system

    d. none of these

ITEM 3. THE MUSCULOSKELETAL SYSTEM

If the framework of a building should sag, the whole building would sag, be less sturdy and strong, and appear less attractive. Just so with the body. Since the skeletal system—i.e., the bones and joints—makes the body framework, it needs to be in good alignment. Good alignment reduces sagging.

The major movable body parts, called segments, are the head, the trunk, and the extremities. Each of these segments has subparts. These are shown in the picture of the skeleton on page 64.

When we describe body surface or locations, we use terms that were included in your vocabulary: anterior, posterior, lateral, midline. You will need to learn these words and what they mean because they will be used frequently in many of your assignments and in your clinical experiences. Anterior refers to the front surface of the body or its parts. Posterior refers to the back surface of the body or its parts. Lateral refers to either side of the body or its parts. Midline refers to an imaginary line that divides the body or its parts into right and left halves.

Bones are held together by tough bands of tissue that are called ligaments. Muscles are attached to bones by other strong bands of tissues called tendons. When the body parts are in proper relationship to each other, each movable segment is aligned so that the least amount of strain is placed on these tendons, ligaments, muscles, and joints. Each part should be able to perform its intended function efficiently.

The backbone, which is also called the vertebral column or spine, is not really just a "bone." The vertebral column is a series of bones, or vertebrae, that supports the head on the upper end, provides the attachment for the back of the ribs, and joins with the pelvic bones near its lower end. The vertebrae also encase the spinal cord, which is composed of nerves going to and coming from the brain.

Between each vertebra there is a cushion of cartilage called an intervertebral disc. These discs serve as shock-absorbers and decrease the jolting effect of the body movements. When the vertebrae are in good alignment, the pressure of the bones is more evenly distributed on the discs. Prolonged or severe and uneven distribution of pressure may cause the discs to become damaged.

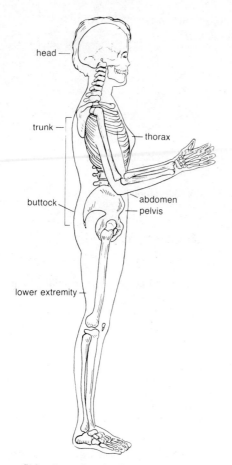

Side view of major body segments.

Some of the subparts of the head are the jaw and neck.

Some of the subparts of the upper extremities are the shoulder, upper arm, forearm, wrist, and hand.

The subparts of the trunk are the thorax or chest, abdomen, pelvis, back, and buttocks.

Subparts of the lower extremities include the hip, thigh, leg, ankle, and foot.

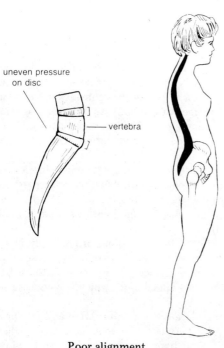

Poor alignment.

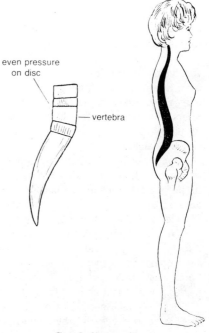

Good alignment.

This long, bony spinal column is most important in attaining proper body alignment and safe movement. The muscles that move the vertebral column are small and not very strong. They provide great flexibility of movement, but are not designed for the heaviest work. The longer, thicker, and stronger muscles used for more strenuous work are found in the shoulder, upper arm, hip, and thigh. A rule in body function is this: *Structure determines function*. As an example, to raise an object you should stoop with your back straight. Use your strong thigh muscles to rise to a standing position, instead of bending with knees straight and back bowed.

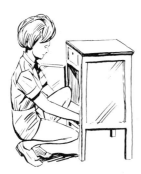

The worker will use strong thigh muscles to stand erect.

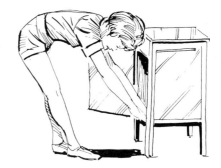

The worker is placing strain on the muscles of the back and legs.

Question 8. Place the letter from the right hand column in the appropriate blank.

1. _____ back surface

2. _____ spinal bones

3. _____ arms and legs

4. _____ bind bones together

5. _____ body without extremities

6. _____ imaginary line dividing body into equal halves

7. _____ cushions between spinal bones

8. _____ refers to side

9. _____ attaches muscles to bone

10. _____ refers to front surface

a. intervertebral disc

b. ligaments

c. anterior

d. lateral

e. midline

f. posterior

g. trunk

h. extremities

i. tendons

j. buttocks

k. skeletal

l. vertebral column

Question 9. State the rule of body function given in this part of the lesson.

_____ .

ITEM 4. BODY ALIGNMENT AND BALANCE

Alignment has been defined as the proper relationship of the body segments to one another. When the segments are properly aligned, it is easier to maintain body balance. Balanced means stable, steady, and not likely to tip or fall.

The main portions of the body (pelvis, thorax, head) are supported by structures below them that are often very small (e.g., small bones in feet, vertebrae). To maintain the proper relationship and balance of these anatomical parts, the ligaments and muscles must be used effectively. In the following figures, your common sense and past experience tell you that B is much more likely to tip or fall than A. That is, Figure A is more *stable* than Figure B.

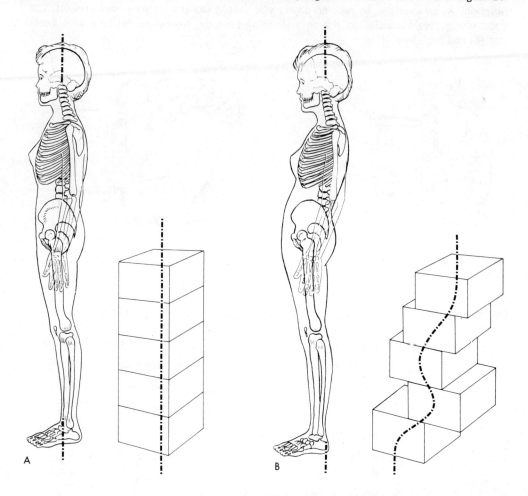

Good relationship of segments.   Poor relationship of segments.

Let us see why Figure A is more stable. The force of gravity affects balance because it is constantly pulling the body toward the earth. Three principles of gravity that affect our balance are:

1. *Center of gravity*—an area located in the pelvis about the level of the second sacral vertebrae. The exact location may vary slightly, depending on body structure.

2. *Base of support*—provides a stable stance for keeping the body from toppling over, as well as stability in movements such as lifting, pushing, or pulling.

3. *Line of gravity*—as documented by some well-known orthopedists (Lovett, Reynolds, Steindler) an imaginary line which falls in the frontal plane, i.e., it passes behind the ear downward just behind the center of the hip joint and then downward slightly in front of the knee and ankle joint. Individual variations may occur according to skeletal build and the curvatures in the spine.

When a person stands in an erect posture so that the line of gravity falls as stated above, body balance is preserved and there is minimal resistance needed to overcome the force of gravity. If the posture is out of alignment as seen in Figure B, the body weight distribution is shifted, the balance is upset, the muscles no longer work together, and the gravitational pull is increased.

To illustrate these three principles, the body may be compared to a plank of wood of the same length, or about 5 feet, 6 inches long. The body (or any object) has a point at which its "mass" or weight is centered. At this point, the weight of the upper body balances the weight of the lower body, and thus the weight of the entire body is balanced. This is called the center of gravity and it influences the stability of an object or a person.

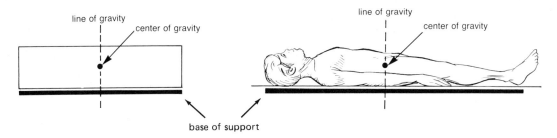

Stable objects have a broad base of support and a low center of gravity; the line of gravity passes through the base of support.

In the sketches shown above, note the center of gravity in the board and the body. It is quite low. The base of support is the part of an object in contact with the ground or other level surface. The base in the illustration is the length of the board, or the body, and is very broad. The line of gravity is an imaginary vertical line that passes through the center of gravity. Body balance is maintained when the line of gravity passes through the base.

Now let's see what happens to the center of gravity, the line of gravity, and the base when we stand up. Again, compare the body to a board of the same height.

In this illustration the mass is taller than in the previous illustration—its center of gravity is raised, the base is narrower. The board and the man therefore become more unstable and likely to fall. Think what could happen if that narrow base were perched on a ladder or a rocking chair.

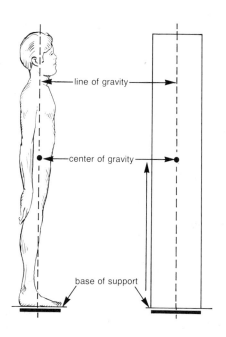

Unstable position.

In the following illustration, the figure is shown leaning over. See what happens to its stability.

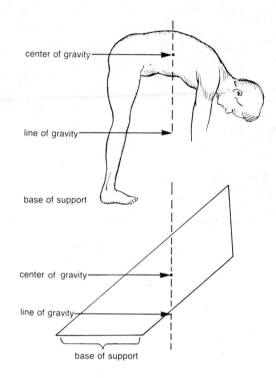

center of gravity

line of gravity

base of support

center of gravity

line of gravity

base of support

Remember! The body is most unstable when the

1. center of gravity is high,

2. base of support is narrow, and

3. line of gravity does not pass through the base of support.

This figure would fall unless an opposing force to gravity held it up. An opposing force could be the use of the arms pushing against an object to keep the body from tipping over.

Fill in the blanks with the most appropriate answer.

Question 10.   A force that pulls toward the ground is called _____.

Question 11.   The point in the body where the mass is centered is called the _____ of gravity.

Question 12.   An imaginary vertical line that passes through the center of gravity is called the _____ of gravity.

Question 13.   An object is said to be _____ if it is steady, not likely to fall.

Question 14.   We are least likely to fall if

a.   The center of gravity is _____ .

b.   We have a broad _____ , and _____ .

c.   The line of gravity passes through the _____ .

Question 15.   *A question for thought:*   Besides preventing weight bearing by an injured or weakened leg, how do crutches affect stability and balance?

ITEM 5.   BODY MOVEMENT

You have studied some of the principles of good body alignment and balance and are now ready to learn more about body movement. The joints allow the movement when the muscles contract and pull on bones. Various terms describe these joint movements. We will now take up the movements of flexion, extension, hyperextension, abduction, and adduction.

First, notice that a full circle contains 360° while a straight line has half of that, or 180°. The right angle has only 90°.

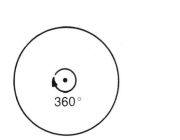

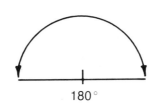

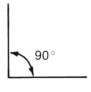

If you hold your arm out straight, the elbow joint forms a straight line—or a 180° angle. By bending the elbow joint, you decrease the angle, i.e., decrease the number of degrees from 180. This is called flexion. Extension is the joint movement opposite to flexion. When you straighten the arm that is bent at the elbow, or the leg that is bent at the knee, you are increasing the angle at the joint and extending the arm or leg.

Some joints allow for increasing the angle more than 180°, or beyond a straight line. This is called hyperextension. You hyperextend your neck each time you raise your chin and tilt your head backward. The knee joint also allows the movement of hyperextension. You can feel this movement if you stand normally with the knee joint nearly straight; then force the knee joint even straighter until the joint is locked or rigid.

Abduct is another term used to describe certain joint movements. Abduct means to move away from the midline of the body. (One way to remember this word and its meaning: if a child is kidnapped, he is abducted or taken away from his family.) The opposite movement of abduct is adduct—the movement to bring the part back toward the midline of the body. (A memory clue for this: "adds to" the body.)

The body movements are flexion, extension, adduction, and abduction. The muscles that produce the movements are called flexors, extensors, adductors, and abductors. Muscles work in pairs and are called antagonists. If one muscle flexes a joint, its antagonist will extend the joint. Abductors are antagonists of adductors. Each muscle of the pair has an action opposite to that of the other.

Question 16.   Circle the appropriate answer.

    a.   The *(skeletal system)(muscular system)* forms the framework of our body.

    b.   The *(skeletal system) (muscular system)* produces movement.

    c.   Muscles with opposite actions in pairs are called *(extensors) (antagonists).*

Question 17.   Please carry out the following movements.

    a.   Flex your lower leg (knee joint).

    b.   Extend your lower leg (knee joint).

    c.   Flex your head (neck).

    d.   Hyperextend your head (neck).

    e.   Hyperextend your lower leg (knee joint).

    f.   Flex your hip joint.

    g.   Abduct your arm.

    h.   Adduct your arm.

ITEM 6. MUSCLE GROUPS

In the movements of lifting, carrying, and stooping, we will be referring to several specific muscle groups. Since standing erect and walking are essential to these movements, we will consider two muscle groups which are the most powerful in the body. The quadriceps are extensor muscles and the hamstrings are strong flexors of the leg. The quadriceps are composed of four parts—hence the prefix "quadri." They are found on the anterior, or front, of the thigh and pass over the knee joint in order to extend the leg. Six muscles make up the hamstring group which is on the posterior of the thigh. The hamstrings oppose the action of the quadriceps, so that they work to flex the leg at the knee joint.

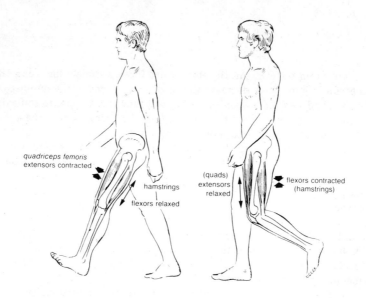

quadriceps femoris
extensors contracted

hamstrings

flexors relaxed

(quads) extensors relaxed

flexors contracted (hamstrings)

Extension of knee joint.   Flexion of knee joint.

The gluteal muscles form the seat or the rump. They are the thick muscles on which you sit. They function to extend and to hyperextend the hip joint. Several strong, broad muscles attached to the pelvis and the thigh bone produce the flexion and adduction of the hip. The gluteals, hamstrings, and quadriceps are used in walking and other movements. When you are standing, they help to keep the femur, or thighbone, erect on the shinbone (tibia), which is the large bone of the lower leg.

There are other muscles around the hip joint and knee that act to stabilize the joint rather than to move it. (Stabilize means to set or prevent unnecessary or secondary movement.) These muscles are important in walking or lifting. They allow a joint to support the shifting weight of the moving body as the center of gravity changes.

We will consider another important muscle group at this time—the "corset muscles" or the "living girdle." The corset muscles are the muscles of your abdomen which are arranged in layers to form the wall of the abdomen and support the abdominal and pelvic organs. The abdominal muscles usually work in opposition to the diaphragm so that when one is contracted, the other is relaxed. In lifting or carrying heavy objects, considerable strain is placed on the corset muscles. Before such exertion, these muscles should be contracted or "set" to provide good support and prevent possible injury.

Circle the appropriate answer to the following questions.

Question 18.   The quadriceps muscles are found on the *(anterior) (posterior) (lateral)* part of the thigh.

Question 19.   The action of the quadriceps muscles is to *(flex) (extend)* the lower leg.

Question 20. The hamstring muscles are located on the *(anterior) (posterior) (lateral)* part of the thigh.

Question 21. The hamstring muscles *(flex) (extend) (hyperextend)* the lower leg at the knee joint.

Question 22. The gluteal muscles form the *(thigh) (abdomen) (buttocks)*.

ITEM 7. CHECKPOINTS FOR GOOD BODY ALIGNMENT

Before beginning body movements, you should align and balance your body properly in order to prevent strain and injury. There are some checkpoints for you to remember and practice when aligning and balancing your body. In the skill laboratory, practice according to these checkpoints, then consciously check your alignment and balance every time you stand.

U
N
I
T
6

Important Steps	Key points
Checkpoint One	
Start from a good base of support.	Place your feet parallel and about 6 to 8 inches apart. You can widen your base if necessary, or if more comfortable. Then, for anterior-posterior stability, put one foot ahead of the other. This stable base of support will save your energy by minimizing the work the muscles must do to keep the body balanced. With your feet parallel, the joints are in good alignment. You will probably notice that the heels of your shoes will wear more evenly.
Checkpoint Two	
Distribute your weight evenly on both feet.	This permits the weight-bearing joints and their supporting structures to divide the weight and share the load.
Checkpoint Three	
Keep your knees slightly flexed.	Slight flexion produces a "shock-absorber" effect and prevents jolting movements of the entire body. It also prevents the strain caused by hyperextension of the knees, or "locked knees."
Checkpoint Four	
Tuck in your buttocks.	By tucking in the buttocks, you tilt the pelvis forward and help straighten the lumbar curve of the spine. This prevents "swayback," and allows for even distribution of pressure of the intervertebral disc cushions. If you look at yourself in a mirror with the buttocks first protruding, then tucked in, you will see that the tucked-in position presents a better appearance.

Checkpoint Five

Keep the abdomen up and in.	This will support the abdominal organs and decrease muscle strain on the back. Good abdominal muscle control permits your clothes to fit better and gives a more attractive appearance. Put your living girdle to work.

Checkpoint Six

Raise your rib cage.	By holding your chest up, you allow for more complete expansion of the lungs. Keep the shoulders relaxed; you need not stand at military attention for good body alignment and balance. By raising the rib cage, you decrease the hump-shoulder appearance.

Checkpoint Seven

Keep your head erect.	Let your head "balance" on top of your spine. Holding the chin in and up prevents exaggerated curvature of the neck and the thoracic portion of the spinal column.

In summary, these checkpoints are listed again for you:

1. Start from a stable base of support with feet separated and one slightly ahead of the other.

2. Distribute body weight evenly.

3. Flex knees slightly to act as shock-absorbers.

4. Tuck buttocks under and tilt pelvis forward to prevent swayback.

5. Keep abdominal muscles up and in to support abdominal organs.

6. Keep rib cage up to allow full expansion of the chest.

7. Hold head erect to avoid curvature of neck and thorax.

Question 23. To demonstrate body balance, you should stand and check the alignment of your body:
Are your feet parallel?
Are your feet separated for good lateral stability?
Is your weight evenly distributed on both feet?
Are your knees slightly flexed? (not locked or hyperextended)
Is your thorax up and in good alignment?
Are your shoulders relaxed?
Is your head in alignment and balanced?

Question 24. Now, maintaining the alignment of your upper body, lean forward from your hips and to the side. Now place both of your feet close together. Again lean forward from your hips and to the side.

a. Were you able to lean as far without beginning to lose your balance?

Yes _____ No _____

b. Did you feel unstable when you were leaning with your feet together?

Yes _____ No _____

c. Why do you think this was so? _____

_____.

ITEM 8. CONCLUSION OF THE LESSON

You have now completed the unit on Body Alignment, Balance, and Movement. The habit of good body alignment and balance will help you present an attractive appearance and may prevent strain or injury as you perform your duties. Obtain the written and performance post-tests. After you have completed the written test, make an appointment with your instructor to demonstrate your ability to understand and to practice good body alignment and balance.

WORKBOOK ANSWER SHEET

1. a.–e.   reach, lift, carry, push, pull, stoop, stand, sit, walk, turn (any five of these)

2. a.   attractive appearance

   b.   may prevent injury

   c.   may make work easier

   (reduce fatigue; prevent added work for fellow employees; or other similar answer)

3. a.   fairly common

   b.   poor body alignment or movements

4. It would increase their workload because they would have to perform my work as well (any similar answer).

5. e.   all of these

6. a., b., d.

7. b.

8. 1—f; 2—l; 3—h; 4—b; 5—g; 6—e; 7—a; 8—d; 9—i; 10—c

9. Structure determines function.

10. gravity

11. center

12. line

13. stable

14. a.   low

   b.   base of support

   c.   base

15. The crutches provide a broader base of support and make the body more stable.

16. a.   skeletal system

   b.   muscular system

   c.   antagonists

17. Confirm these movements by checking with the definitions in the text.

18. anterior

19. extend

20. posterior

21. flex

22. buttocks

23. The answer to each question should be *yes.*

24. a. No

    b. Yes

    c. The base of support was narrow and the line of gravity did not pass through the base.

PRE-TEST

Place a circle around the "T" if you think the statement is more true than false, and circle the "F" if the statement is more false than true.

T   F   1. As long as you do your work well, proper body alignment and balance are of no concern to your co-workers or employer.

T   F   2. Each nursing action utilizes principles of body alignment and balance.

T   F   3. Back strain and injury, although serious, are not very common among health workers.

T   F   4. Many people do not use good body alignment and balance because the proper movements appear unattractive.

T   F   5. Our weaker flexor muscles help oppose gravity and thereby maintain our upright aspect.

T   F   6. Correct alignment of body segments places added strain on ligaments, tendons and joints, there by increasing fatigue.

T   F   7. In good body alignment and balance, the shoulders should be held back firmly.

T   F   8. The knees should be firmly locked to give stability to the body.

T   F   9. The feet should be approximately two to four inches apart and rotated slightly outward for good support.

T   F   10. A "broad base stance" requires the feet to be approximately 12 to 16 inches apart with one foot slightly in front of the other.

T   F   11. We are more unstable if the vertical center of gravity passes through our base.

T   F   12. Our extensor muscles must help oppose gravity in order to help us remain upright.

T   F   13. The back is most often strained when in hyperextension.

T   F   14. The quadriceps femoris muscles flex the hip joint.

T   F   15. Joints, muscles, and ligaments can all be injured if poor body alignment and balance are used.

T   F   16. The habitual use of poor alignment and balance is fatiguing.

T   F   17. Good body mechanics are effective in reducing injury and strain, although they give the worker an awkward appearance.

PRE-TEST ANSWER SHEET

1.	F	10.	T
2.	T	11.	F
3.	F	12.	T
4.	F	13.	T
5.	F	14.	F
6.	F	15.	T
7.	F	16.	T
8.	F	17.	F
9.	F		

Note: These answers were not annotated because the student scoring less than 85 per cent will need to proceed through the unit.

PERFORMANCE TEST

In the skill laboratory, your instructor will ask you to demonstrate your ability to carry out the following instructions without reference to source material:

1. In a standing position, you are to position your body in proper alignment and describe the seven checkpoints that you are to use as a guide.

2. In a standing position using good body alignment, bend your right knee and take one step forward as you straighten your leg. Describe the body movements of the leg, and name and locate the muscles that were most involved.

3. In a standing position with good body alignment, take one step of 12 inches or more to your left, then bring the other foot parallel to your left foot. Describe the body action in the movement of the left foot and the action of the right foot.

4. You are to use your neck joints to perform these movements:

   a. flexion of the neck.

   b. hyperextension of the neck.

   c. abduction of the head.

   d. adduction of the head.

PERFORMANCE CHECKLIST

BODY ALIGNMENT, BALANCE, AND MOVEMENT

1. Student will demonstrate proper body alignment.

   - Feet in stride position, parallel or one slightly in front of the other.

   - Weight evenly distributed on both feet.

   - Knees slightly flexed.

   - Buttocks tucked in and pelvis tilted forward, spine straight, and lumbar curve reduced.

   - Abdominal muscles pulled up, held in.

   - Thorax raised, shoulders relaxed.

   - Keep head erect and balanced.

2. Student will demonstrate good posture while walking and be able to identify major muscles involved in producing the movement.

   - Body in good alignment.

   - Right knee flexed:
     Movement is flexion.
     Prime movers are the hamstring muscles.
     Location of muscles is on posterior thigh.

   - Extend right knee and step forward:
     Movement is extension.
     Prime movers are the quadriceps femoris.
     Location of muscles is on the anterior thigh.

- Shift weight to lead foot:
     Movement is extension of the hip.
     Prime movers are the gluteal muscles.
     Location of the prime muscles is the buttocks.

3. Student will perform sideward step.

   - Body in good alignment

   - With left foot, step to left side 12 or more inches:
        Movement is abduction.
        Prime movers are abductor muscles.
        Location of abductors is on outer lateral thigh.

   - Move right foot 12 or more inches to the left to parallel other foot:
        Movement is adduction.
        Prime movers are adductor muscles.
        Location of adductors is medial aspect of thigh.

4. Student will demonstrate the following movements:

   a. Flexion of the neck.

   b. Hyperextension of the neck.

   c. Abduction of the head.

   d. Adduction of the head.

POST-TEST

Vocabulary: Match the words in Column 2 with the meaning or phrase in Column 1.

Column 1   *Column 2*

___ 1.   The body without head and extemities   A.   Body alignment

___ 2.   Attaches bone to bone   B.   Gravity

___ 3.   One of a pair of muscles, having an   C.   Glucose
         action opposite from the other
                                                       D.   Hormones
___ 4.   The arms and legs
                                                       E.   Stability
___ 5.   Attaches muscle to bone
                                                       F.   Trunk
___ 6.   A simple sugar, or fuel
                                                       G.   Antagonist
___ 7.   Not likely to tip or fall
                                                       H.   Ligament
___ 8.   Formed by the gluteal muscles
                                                       I.   Buttocks
___ 9.   The relationship of movable body seg-
         ments to other segments of the body   J.   Extremities

___10.   A force that pulls toward the earth   K.   Tendon

                                                       L.   Thorax

Completion: Complete the following statements.

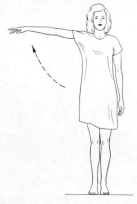

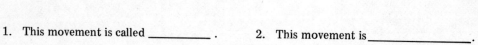

1. This movement is called _____ .   2. This movement is _____ .

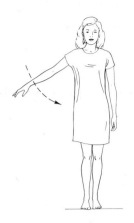

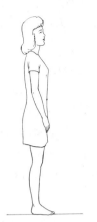

3. This body surface is the _____ view.

4. The movement is _____ .

5. This body surface is the _____ view.

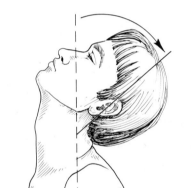

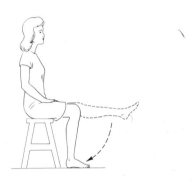

6. This movement is _____ .

7. This movement is _____ .

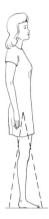

The long, narrow figure shown above is characterized by the following:

8. The base of support is _____ .

9. The center of gravity is _____ .

10. The position is one of relative _____.

Multiple Choice: Choose the best answer(s).

1. All but one of the following statements are characteristics of good body alignment and balance. The statement that is *not* characteristic is:

    ___a. The body is balanced over its base of support.

    ___b. Oxygen and glucose are used by muscles as "fuel."

    ___c. Segments of the body are in proper relationship.

    ___d. Strain on muscles and joints is minimized.

2. Balance of the body is *best* achieved by:

    ___a. a low center of gravity, a narrow base, and the line of gravity passing through the base.

    ___b. a high center of gravity, a broad base, and the line of gravity passing outside the base.

    ___c. a high center of gravity, a narrow base, and the line of gravity passing through the base.

    ___d. a low center of gravity, a broad base, and the line of gravity passing through the base.

3. Balance of the body is maintained by:

    ___a. the center of gravity passing through the base of support.

    ___b. a high center of gravity located outside a narrow base.

    ___c. a line of gravity passing through the base of support.

    ___d. a line of gravity passing outside the base of support.

4. The center of gravity in the body is a point:

    ___a. around which the body weight or mass is centered.

    ___b. located and stabilized in the chest.

    ___c. that must lie outside the base of support.

    ___d. all of the above.

5. Low back strain in the hospital worker is most often caused by:

    ___a. the carelessness of other people.

    ___b. lifting too heavy an object or person.

    ___c. using the back muscles to lift a weight.

    ___d. body segments aligned with one another.

6. The worker who suffers a muscle strain of the back or shoulder might:

    ___a. have a lot of pain.

    ___b. lose a week or more of work.

    ___c. have prevented the injury.

    ___d. all of the above.

7. Movement of the body occurs:

___a. where muscles are attached to bones.

___b. at joints that are acted upon by muscles.

___c. when bones are stimulated by nerves.

___d. at the immovable joints.

8. Ligaments are strong cartilage bands that:

___a. connect muscles and tendons.

___b. connect muscles to muscles.

___c. connect bones to bones.

___d. connect tendons and bones.

9. The trunk of the body plays an important part in body alignment and balance. The "trunk" refers to:

___a. the buttocks and the extremities.

___b. the thorax and the neck.

___c. the back and the extremities.

___d. the abdomen and the thorax.

10. The palm of the hand is a subpart of the upper extremity and its surface is referred to as:

___a. lateral

___b. midline

___c. posterior

___d. anterior

11. To ensure good stability of the base of support of the body, the feet should be positioned:

___a. parallel and very close together.

___b. about 8 inches apart, one a little ahead of the other.

___c. about 8 inches apart, toes pointed laterally.

___d. parallel and at least 2 feet apart.

12. A person with sagging abdominal muscles often has a greater curve in his back, or a "swayback." This greater curve may cause:

___a. less fatigue when doing heavy work.

___b. decreased strain on the backbone.

___c. uneven pressure on intervertebral discs.

___d. increased shock-absorber effect of the spine.

13. The large, strong muscle groups of the body include which of the following?

___a. The back muscles and the gluteals.

___b. The quadriceps femoris and the back muscles.

___c. The hamstrings and the adductors.

___d. The gluteals and the quadriceps femoris.

14. Muscles are frequently referred to by a name similar to the name of the movement produced by their action. Some of these muscles would be called:

    __a.   flexion, extensors, and adductors.

    __b.   hyperextension, abduction, and extensors.

    __c.   flexors, adductors, and abductors.

    __d.   extension, hyperextension, and flexion.

15. Groups of muscles are usually found working in pairs to produce movement at the joints of the body, and are called antagonists. One example of antagonist muscles is:

    __a.   flexor and adductor.

    __b.   quadriceps femoris and back muscles.

    __c.   abdominal muscles and diaphragm.

    __d.   extensors and hyperextension.

POST-TEST ANNOTATED ANSWER SHEET

Vocabulary

1. F.

2. H.

3. G.

4. J.

5. K.

6. C.

7. E.

8. I.

9. A.

10. B (p. 60)

Completion

1. abduction (p. 69)

2. extension (p. 69)

3. anterior (p. 63)

4. adduction (p. 69)

5. lateral (p. 63)

6. hyperextension (p. 69)

7. flexion (p. 69)

8. short or narrow (p. 67)

9. high (p. 67)

10. instability (p. 67)

Multiple Choice

1. b. (p. 72)

2. d. (p. 67)

3. c. (p. 67)

4. a. (p. 66)

5. c. (p. 65)

6. d. (p. 61)

7. b. (p. 61)

8. c. (p. 63)

9. d. (p. 64)

10. d. (p. 63)

11. b. (p. 71)

12. c. (p. 63)

13. d. (p. 70)

14. c. (p. 69)

15. c. (p. 70)

USING BODY MOVEMENT

I. DIRECTIONS TO THE STUDENT

Please read the following paragraphs carefully. They will tell you exactly what you will be expected to do and know at the end of this unit. Take the pre-test before you begin the lesson. Correct the test. If you did well on the pre-test, discuss with your instructor the possibility of progressing directly to the post-test. All students are expected to demonstrate accurately the skills required on the performance test and to indicate understanding of the knowledge and principles of body movement.

II. GENERAL PERFORMANCE OBJECTIVE

You will demonstrate your knowledge of good body movement by taking the performance test.

III. SPECIFIC PERFORMANCE OBJECTIVES

1. Given an activity to perform at floor level (e.g., mopping up a spill or placing slippers on a patient's feet), stoop, keeping the body aligned and balanced, and use the large muscles of the thighs and buttocks for the activity.

2. Given a heavy object located at least 6 inches higher than you are tall, reach and remove the object without hyperextending or straining the back, or losing your balance.

3. Given an object weighing 10 to 15 pounds, carry it for five minutes in such a manner as to minimize fatigue and prevent straining.

4. Given an object to push or pull (e.g., wheelchair, laundry cart, food cart), move the object by "setting" your muscles, using the leg muscles to supply most of the force needed and the body weight to assist the movement.

5. Given an activity that requires turning or pivoting (e.g., assisting a patient from bed to chair or turning from desk to file cabinet), position your feet and body in such a manner that you do not strain your trunk or back.

6. Be able to answer questions about the following:

    a. The five guidelines that permit good body alignment and efficient movement in the performance of your skills.

    b. The principles of body alignment, balance, and movement in reaching for an object, carrying a heavy object, making a pivoting turn, pushing or pulling an object, and performing an activity at floor level.

IV. VOCABULARY

contaminate—to soil or pollute; to render unclean or unsterile.

diaphragm—the musculomembranous wall separating the abdominal cavity and the thoracic (chest) cavity; a powerful muscle used in breathing.

friction—resistance to movement by two objects in contact.

fulcrum—the support (wedge or axis) about which a lever turns or moves.

leverage—the mechanical advantage gained by using levers.

V. INTRODUCTION

In "Body Alignment, Balance, and Movement" you learned how to position your body segments in proper alignment and balance for stability. This will serve as a "base position" or beginning point for all the movements you will make in the performance of your activities.

This lesson, "Using Body Movement," presents five guidelines to assist you in working with the natural laws of gravity, friction, and leverage, which will aid in giving patient care. It will help you to use the muscles, ligaments, and joints that are best designed for safe and effective movements.

The movements of stooping, reaching, lifting and carrying, turning, pushing, or pulling will be explained in detail so that you can (and should) practice each one carefully.

ITEM 1.   GUIDELINES FOR BODY MOVEMENTS

Guideline 1.   Maintain Alignment and Balance

You must start any body movement from a good base of support to provide stability. You can avoid twisting your back by keeping your feet pointed in the same direction as you will move and keeping your trunk aligned or in a straight position.

Before proceeding further, let's review the "key points" of our base position of good alignment and balance. These are the points to check when you assume a standing position.

1. A stable base of support with feet separated and one foot slightly ahead of the other.

2. Weight evenly distributed on both feet.

3. Both knees slightly flexed.

4. Buttocks tucked in.

5. Abdomen held up and in.

6. Rib cage raised.

7. Head held erect.

This standing posture, in good body alignment and balance, is the basis for all of the movements you will use in your work.

Guideline 2.   Work At A Comfortable Height

A comfortable working height for most people is between the waist level and a level about 6 inches below the hip joint. For most women, this level is about 30 to 32 inches from the floor. This working level minimizes muscle strain from reaching beyond the length of the arms, and allows the body to remain aligned and balanced. This working height allows us easily to flex the hip and knee joints, and to apply leverage to our work.

Working at too low a level causes strain on muscles and produces fatigue. It is more difficult to maintain your balance within your base of support, and leverage may be poor. In order to work at a low level, you may need to flex your knees and stoop so that the large thigh muscles are used rather than the weaker muscles of the back.

Working at too high a surface level adds to the demands on arms and shoulders, and this produces muscle strain and fatigue. Also, reaching a high work surface may cause hyperextension of the lower back, raises the center of gravity of your body, and results in a less stable position. Injury, such as low back strain, may occur if you reach overhead incorrectly or stretch to perform work at too high a level.

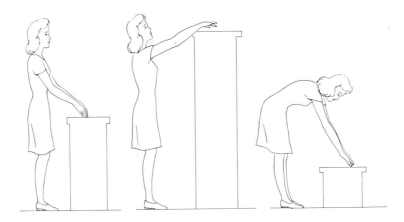

Correct work height.   Too high work level.   Too low work level.

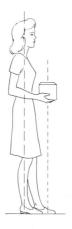

All work should be performed at the proper height when possible. You may be able to change the level of the working surface; for example, most hospital beds today can be adjusted to a higher or lower position. In the high position, the bed is about 32 inches from the floor, a good working height to provide care for the patient. If you are unable to change the height of the work surface, you may need to use a stool to raise yourself to a more suitable level or you may have to stoop down, keeping your body in good alignment.

Guideline 3.   Keep The Work Close To Your Body

You can perform tasks more easily and with less strain or fatigue if your work is close enough to your body to avoid stretching or reaching. You apply this principle when you move the patient to the side of bed nearest you before you bathe him; or when you go around to the other side of the bed rather than reach or stretch across it and hyperextend your back, or lose your balance by having your line of gravity outside your base of support.

When you carry an object during your work, you can do so more easily if the object's line of gravity falls within your base of support. The additional weight of the object may alter your center of gravity slightly, but the large, strong muscles of your thighs and buttocks will help support the weight. If the object's line of gravity is outside your base of support, the muscles of your arms or shoulders must support the weight of the object and overcome the force of gravity.

Object carried within base of support.   Object carried outside base of support.

One point of caution: Carry objects close to the body, but do not contaminate your uniform or clothing by carrying *soiled* articles next to you.

We can summarize the first three guidelines that have been presented so far:

Maintain alignment and balance.

Work at a comfortable height.

Keep work close to the body.

Question 1.   Pick up your heaviest book or a similar object and hold it out at arm's length for at least 30 seconds, Now bring it in close to your body for the same length of time.

    a.   What difference did you notice in its apparent weight?

_____

    b.   Explain why this is so. _____

_____

Question 2.   List three methods you might use in order to work at a comfortable height.

    a. _____

    b. _____

    c. _____

Question 3.   How might you avoid hyperextending your back if you were asked to support a patient's leg in a cast while the doctor adjusted the cast?

_____

_____

Question 4.   Why would you carry soiled linen slightly away from you so it would not touch your uniform?

_____

_____

Guideline 4.   *Use Smooth, Coordinated Movement*

Smooth, coordinated movements utilize the muscle contractions in an efficient way. The movements flow from one to the other in a rhythmic and graceful way, avoiding jolting and jarring, which might cause discomfort, pain, or injury. The use of smooth, coordinated movement is especially important for nurses, who will be more competent and efficient, and appear more attractive when performing any task.

Smooth movements are safer for you as a worker, and also for the patient. Uncoordinated movement produces sudden, jerky motions that may cause discomfort or injury. This is to be avoided, expecially in the case of a patient with a fracture (broken bone) where movement might cause muscle strain or separation of the bone and unnecessary pain. You can gain the patient's cooperation by explaining what you are going to do and what his part will be.

Often you will be working with another person in order to lift or move patients or objects safely. When you have a helper, one person should give the signals for moving or lifting, and thus coordinate the teamwork.

Guideline 5.   *"Set" or Prepare the Muscles for Action*

Have you ever noticed that when you prepare to move a heavy object you take a deep breath and tense your muscles, and that you let your breath out slowly as you move the object? If you have done this, you have utilized several principles of body alignment and movement: (a) you have taken in a larger supply of oxygen in the deep breath, (b) you have "set" or tensed the abdominal muscles, which are antagonists of the diaphragm muscle, and (c) as the diaphragm relaxes in releasing the breath, you have caused the abdominal and gluteal muscles to do more of the work. You have made use of the "corset muscles" or the "living girdle" to lift, pull, or push a heavy object. "Setting" the muscles, or tensing them for action, helps to distribute the workload over a larger number of muscles and to decrease the load for any one muscle. This stablizes the muscles to protect ligaments, joints, and muscles from sudden jerking and strain.

To summarize, our guidelines for body movements are:

Maintain alignment and balance.

Work at a comfortable height.

Keep the work close to your body.

Use smooth, coordinated movements.

"Set" the muscles for action.

Question 5. Give two reasons for using smooth, coordinated movements in caring for the sick.

a. _____

b. _____

Question 6. Why is it best to "set" or prepare the muscles before performing a strenuous activity?

_____

_____

ITEM 2.   LEVERAGE AND FRICTION

Knowledge of two physical forces is helpful before you study body movements in more detail. One of these forces, leverage, can make your movements easier. The other one, friction, makes your work more difficult. We will not go into detail about the physics involved in these two forces, but will describe them in simple terms.

If you tried to slide a heavy box across a damp wooden floor, friction would result from the contact between the box and the floor. This friction would make it difficult for you to slide the box. If the floor were clean, dry, and waxed, friction would be reduced and you could slide the box more easily. We can define friction as the resistance to movement by two bodies in contact with each other.

Leverage is used often in nursing to increase the amount of work that we can do and also to make it easier. A simple illustration of leverage is that of a child on a teeter-totter raising a

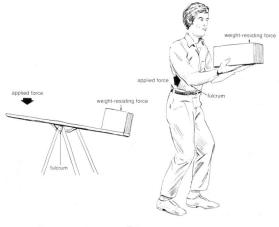

Levers

heavier child at the other end of the board. In nursing, we often brace a knee against the side of the bed in order to pull a drawsheet tight and taut under the patient. Mechanical lifts to raise or transport patients are another form of lever. Your arms act as levers when you cradle a patient or child in them in order to lift him further up in bed. In simple terms, a lever is a bar, with a fixed axis or fulcrum, acted upon at one end by an applied force, or power, and at the other by a resisting force, or weight, that moves the bar.

Question 7. _____ makes work and movements easier.

Question 8.   The resistance to movement is caused by _____ .

ITEM 3.   THE MOVEMENT OF REACHING

You are going to study in detail five body movements: reaching, stooping, turning, carrying, and pushing or pulling. These movements are basic to the performance of your hospital skills. When coupled with the five guidelines of movement you have just learned, you should be able to work with physical safety and with minimal fatigue. Each movement should be practiced step by step. Note the reason for each step. You will be asked to perform these movements and give the reason for each in your post-test.

Our first movement is reaching.

In the skill laboratory, practice reaching to place or to remove an object from a shelf that is higher than your head without hyperextending, straining your back, or losing your balance.

Important Steps	Key Points
1. Start with the basic position and stable base of support.	Check your body alignment. If the object is located or is to be placed on a high shelf, check the distance to be reached. Avoid reaching above your shoulder level when possible because this tends to hyperextend the lower back and may cause strain.
2. Stand on a footstool.	This decreases the distance to reach. Less reaching keeps the center of gravity lower in your body and increases the body's stability and balance. A ladder may be needed if the object is in a very high place.
3. Spread your feet apart.	This broadens your base and provides better lateral stability.
4. Advance one foot forward in the direction of the reach.	This provides a stable stance by broadening the anterior-posterior base of support. The toes should be parallel to the direction of body movement in order to prevent twisting of the trunk. If a footstool or ladder is used, be sure that your line of gravity is centered on it.
5. Reach in front of you rather than directly overhead to remove the object.	The stool should be placed slightly away from the area of the high shelf so that when standing on the stool you can look and reach forward. Reaching or looking overhead hyperextends the neck and spine. It also makes you less stable so that you may lose your balance. Remember to raise yourself with a stool or ladder to a comfortable working height so that you will not hyperextend your spine.
6. Stabilize your body by "setting" your muscles.	"Setting" distributes the workload over many muscles, and the tensing or contracting prepares the muscles for further action. It protects the joints and ligaments from strain or injury.

Important Steps	Key Points
7. Lower the object with smooth, coordinated movements.	Smooth movements prevent jarring or jolting of the body.
8. Look down; then step off the stool or ladder.	Step *carefully*. Watch where you are going. Deposit the article in the appropriate place.

To place an object on a high shelf, you would use the same procedure except to reverse steps 5 and 6, so that you would "set" your muscles, then reach in front of you to place the object on the shelf using smooth, coordinated movements.

Fill in the blanks.

Question 9. In reaching, the goals are to do it in such a manner that we prevent

hyperextension of the _____ and we maintain _____ .

Question 10. Why is the use of a footstool advisable when reaching?

_____

Question 11. How do you provide lateral stability while reaching?

_____

Question 12. Why is it safer to reach in front of the body rather than directly overhead?

_____

U
N
I
T
7

ITEM 4. STOOPING

It is often necessary for us to stoop in the course of our work and everyday lives. Many objects and activities may be beyond the reach of our hands when we are in a standing position. A good many people stoop incorrectly to reach these objects or perform these activities. Incorrect stooping hyperextends the knees, curves the back, and forces the weaker back muscles to pull the trunk of the body upright again.

To stoop correctly, the back must be kept as straight as possible, and the stronger gluteal and thigh muscles should be used to return the body to an upright position.

In the skill laboratory, you should practice the procedure of stooping correctly. If you have difficulty getting up from the stoop position, ask your instructor, physician, or physical education teacher to show you some exercises that will help to strengthen your quadriceps and gluteal muscle groups.

Given an activity to perform at floor level, such as wiping up spilled water or obtaining supplies from a shelf near floor level, lower and raise your body, keeping the trunk in an upright position and using the muscles of the lower extremities to do the work.

Important Steps	Key Points
1. Use good body alignment and place your feet apart with one foot advanced.	This provides a stable base of support.
2. Lower your body by flexing hip and knee joints and keeping your trunk in an upright position.	This action is *controlled* by using the thigh and leg muscles. Gravity also pulls the body downward.
3. Shift your body weight forward so that it rests on the advanced foot and on the ball of the rear foot.	The heel of your rear foot will be off the floor. This relieves the tension on the tendons of the rear foot, and helps to maintain body alignment and balance. Wipe the spill, or remove the item from the shelf.

Important Steps	Key Points
4. Keep your back straight and bend at the hips. Raise your body to standing position by extending the hip and knee joints while keeping your body aligned and balanced.	This permits use of the large, stronger extensor muscles of the hip and thigh. You can use hands to steady yourself or assist yourself to stand if extensor muscles are weak. The body works to oppose the "pulling down" force of gravity. You should be able to feel your heavy thigh muscles working as you rise to the standing position. Remember, if you are lifting an object, carry it near your body to decrease fatigue and strain.
5. Place the object in an appropriate place or discard soiled paper towels in a waste container.	

Circle the best response among the italicized word or words.

Question 13. The body is lowered by *(flexing)* *(extending)* the *(hip and knee joints)* *(trunk)*.

Question 14. *(Leverage)* *(Gravity)* pulls the body downward.

Question 15. In the stooped position, the *(rear)* *(advanced)* foot has its heel raised.

Question 16. To rise from the stooping position, the large strong muscles of *(the back)* *(buttocks and thighs)* are used.

ITEM 5.   PIVOTING TURN

A pivoting turn is used often when changing direction, when assisting a patient from the bed to a chair, or when trying to avoid hitting some object. Also, a worker who is seated in a chair frequently turns to reach a file cabinet or drawer.

Caution: An incorrect turning movement twists the trunk, and when the trunk or spine is twisted, even a relatively minor activity such as opening a drawer can cause muscle strain or injury. The body is not properly aligned if the trunk is rotated or twisted.

In a correct pivoting turn, the entire body moves and turns as a *single unit*. The trunk of the body should be like a log — not twisting, turning, or bending. The upper and lower extremities should move in the same direction and at the same time as the trunk. Later on, you may help in caring for a patient when it is vital for him to be "turned like a log" in his bed, in order to avoid injury or damage to his neck, back, or hip.

In the skill laboratory, practice making a pivoting turn until it seems natural and comfortable.

While in a standing position, make a turn laterally by placing your feet and body in such a manner as to pivot smoothly without causing your back to be twisted or strained.

Important Steps	Key Points
1. Use good body alignment. Stand with your feet apart and your knees slightly flexed.	Start with a stable base of support. This allows you to use the leg muscles and avoids "locking" or hyperextending the knees.
2. Stabilize or "set" the trunk and pelvic muscles.	The "setting" of the muscles makes it easier to turn the body as a single unit.
3. Stabilize or "set" the thigh and leg muscles.	This prepares the muscles for action.
4. Shift your weight to the ball of each foot.	The shift of weight allows the heel to lift very slightly, making the turn easier.

Important Steps	Key Points
5. Pivot, or make a rotating turn of about 90°, on the balls of your feet, in the direction you wish to turn.	Move your feet and body *as a single unit*. Use a smooth, coordinated movement to prevent twisting of the trunk.
6. When the turn is completed, distribute your weight equally on each foot.	This provides a stable base of support and balance for further movements.

To make a walking pivot turn for a right turn (Reverse directions for left turn):

1. Step forward with left foot.

2. Follow steps 4, 5, and 6 above.

3. Continue walking.

Question 17. Why would you shift your weight to the ball of each foot before making the pivoting turn?

_____

Question 18. List two activities in the hospital where a pivoting turn could be used to prevent twisting the trunk of the body.

a. _____

b. _____

ITEM 6. LIFTING AND CARRYING OBJECTS

The availability of mechanical aids and other devices now makes it less likely that you will have to lift heavy objects, but hospital workers still must lift and carry frequently. You will need to use good judgment in deciding which objects you can lift and carry alone. If in doubt, don't attempt it by yourself; leave it, or get others to help you.

In the skill laboratory, practice lifting and carrying an object. Given a box of books, a stack of linen, or other article weighing 10 to 15 pounds, lift and carry it for 5 minutes in such a manner as to minimize fatigue and prevent strain.

Important Steps	Key Points
1. Start with the stable base position.	This ensures good body alignment and balance for further movements.
2. Grasp the object firmly on either side of its approximate center of gravity.	To lift an object weighing 10 to 15 pounds, you should use both hands, grasping near its center of gravity. This helps to balance it; for example, if you are lifting a square box, place your hands near the middle of the lateral sides.
3. "Set" your abdominal muscles and arm muscles, then lift the object and bring it close to your body.	This acts to stabilize the muscles and to prepare for the action of lifting. *Note*: If you were lifting the object from a surface on or near the floor, you would use the stooping procedure to lower your body, grasp the object, and raise your body by using the buttock, thigh, and leg muscles.
4. Carry the object as close to the midline of the body as possible.	When the object's line of gravity falls within your base of support, the large, stronger muscles of the buttocks and thighs help to support the additional weight.
5. Shift the object occasionally during the 5-minute period.	This relieves strain on certain muscles by rotating their activity.

Important Steps	Key Steps
6. Put the object down periodically.	This reduces the length of time the object must be supported, and also allows the muscles a short period of rest.

Question 19. When carrying an object, why is it best to hold it close to your body?

_____

Question 20. List three ways to reduce strain if you must lift and carry heavy objects.

    a. _____

    b. _____

    c. _____

ITEM 7. PUSHING AND PULLING

Pushing and pulling are frequently involved in the activities of hospital workers. They push or pull stretchers, food carts, housekeeping carts, beds, X-ray machines, wheelchairs, tables, therapy machines — the list seems endless. When we push or pull, we avoid carrying an object (a far more tiring effort).

When we push or pull objects in the hospital, we are guided by the "rules of the road." Move your equipment down one side of the corridor so that other traffic can pass. Watch carefully when going around corners or approaching an intersection with another corridor. When you have pushed or pulled your equipment to its place of use, "park" it near the wall to avoid obstructing the hallway.

The goal of proper pushing and pulling is to move an object with minimal effort or strain. This is done by using your body weight to assist the strong muscles of the legs and trunk.

In the skill laboratory, practice the movements of pushing and pulling an object. Given a utility cart or a stretcher to push or pull, move the object with minimal force by using your body weight, trunk muscles, and extensor muscles of the leg.

Important Steps	Key Points
1. Start with a stable base of support.	Check your position for good alignment and balance.
2. Stand close to the object to be pushed or pulled.	This keeps the work close to the body, and also encourages good alignment by reducing distance of reach.
3. Position your feet: place them at least 8 inches apart, with one advanced forward in the direction you are working.	This provides for a more stable and wider base of support, as well as leverage.
4. "Set" the trunk and leg muscles.	By now this should be familiar as a guideline to stabilize the body and prepare for action.
5. To push: *Lean toward* the object to be moved.	The body weight adds greater force to the muscular action and helps to move an object.
6. To pull: *Lean away* from the object to be moved.	This is done to apply as much force as possible in the direction of the movement by using the body weight.
7. Push or pull by letting your arms, hips, and thighs do most of the work.	The large muscles of the thigh and the leg do the work. Efficient use of these muscles conserves energy and prevents strain.

Question 21. List two safety precautions to observe if you are pushing or pulling a large object in the hospital corridor.

a. _____

b. _____

Question 22. The goal in pushing or pulling an object correctly is to move it with a minimum of _____ by using the _____ to assist the strong muscles.

Question 23. What do you do in pushing an object that utilizes your body weight as an additional force?

_____

ITEM 8. CONCLUSION OF THE UNIT

You have now completed this lesson on body movements. You may need to practice some of the movements in the classroom or laboratory to be sure that you can do them correctly and know the reason for each step. When you feel confident that you have learned the body movements and related information, contact your instructor and arrange to take the performance test.

WORKBOOK ANSWER SHEET

Question 1. a. It seems lighter when held close to the body.

b. The center of gravity of the book falls within my base of support. (Any similar answer.)

2. Any three of the following:

a. raise or lower the work surface

b. raise or lower yourself

c. use stool

d. stoop

e. ladder, etc.

3. Stand on the same side of bed as the leg with the cast, then move the patient to the near side of the bed.

4. So that it does not contaminate or soil your uniform.

5. a. Avoid injury to the patient or hurting him.

b. Avoid strain or injury to the worker. (Any order.)

6. It stabilizes the muscles and joints, prepares the muscles for action, lessens danger of sudden movement or stress causing injury. (Any similar answer.)

7. Leverage

8. friction

9. back (or trunk); balance

10. It decreases the distance to be reached.

11. Spread feet apart to broaden base of support.

12. It avoids hyperextension of neck and spine; you can see what you are doing.

13. flexing; hip and knee joints

14. Gravity

15. rear

16. buttocks and thighs

17. It allows the heels to lift slightly so that a pivot turn is easier.

18. a. Assisting the patient from bed to chair.

    b. Turning to answer the phone, pick up a chart, etc. (Any answer appropriate for your job.)

19. It is more stable to carry if its center of gravity falls within your base of support.

20. a. Don't lift more than is safe; get help; use mechanical lifters.

    b. Shift your load occasionally.

    c. Put the load down occasionally.

    d. Use proper body mechanics or movements.

    e. Hold the object as near the midline of your body as practical. (Any three of these, or similar answers.)

21. a. Watch carefully when going around corners.

    b. Approach intersections carefully.

    c. Move equipment down one side of the hall or corridor.

    d. "Park" equipment close to the wall to avoid obstructing the corridor.

    e. Use care not to bump into anyone. (Any two of these, or similar answers.)

22. Effort or strain; body weight.

23. Lean toward the object being pushed.

PRE-TEST

Circle the letter "T" if you think the statement is more true than false, and circle the letter "F" if you think the statement is more false than true.

T   F   1. Many hospital workers need to do exercises before proper lifting becomes easy and natural for them.

T   F   2. Reaching places a strain on extensor muscles and can easily cause injury.

T   F   3. Carrying objects close to the body decreases muscle strain.

T   F   4. In lifting, a worker uses the strong extensor muscles of the thigh and buttocks.

T   F   5. Friction means to pull down.

T   F   6. The principles of leverage can assist the hospital worker.

T F 7. The feet should be parallel and approximately 12 to 18 inches apart for proper posture for lifting.

T F 8. Reaching overhead or away from the body places strain on the back muscles.

T F 9. In turning the body, it is best to keep the feet securely placed in one position.

T F 10. An object is easier to carry if it is held out away from the body.

T F 11. Friction can decrease movement.

T F 12. Avoid using leverage in patient care because it intensifies the force applied.

T F 13. A good working height for most workers is about 30 to 32 inches from the floor.

T F 14. Most hospital beds in the low position are about 30 inches high.

T F 15. Movement is most effective if it is smooth, rhythmic, and coordinated.

T F 16. Pushing or pulling an object is easier than lifting and carrying it because this overcomes the resistance of friction.

T F 17. The gluteal muscles are used in stooping.

T F 18. The broad, strong back muscles should be used to lift heavy objects.

T F 19. The extensor muscles of the buttocks and thighs are used to extend the lower extremity in lifting.

T F 20. Many hospital workers need special exercises before they can stoop and rise easily.

T F 21. In turning, brace the knees, use a wide stance, and turn the trunk (which is very flexible).

T F 22. The hospital worker, supporting the patient's leg, should be on the opposite side from the examining physician.

T F 23. The muscles of the back should carry most of the burden in lifting.

UNIT 7

PRE-TEST ANNOTATED ANSWER SHEET

1. F (p. 89)
2. T (p. 85)
3. T (p. 85)
4. T (p. 85)
5. F (p. 87)
6. T (p. 87)
7. T (pp. 84 and 88)
8. T (p. 88)
9. F (p. 90)
10. F (p. 85)
11. T (p. 87)
12. F (p. 87)

13. T (p. 84)
14. F (p. 85)
15. T (p. 86)
16. F (p. 87)
17. T (p. 89)
18. F (p. 89)
19. T (p. 89)
20. T (p. 90)
21. F (p. 90)
22. F (p. 86)
23. F (p. 90)

PERFORMANCE TEST

In the skill laboratory or your classroom, your instructor will ask you to demonstrate your skills in performing body movements and to state the reasons for each step in the movement. This is to be done without reference to your workbook, notes, or other source materials.

1. Given an activity to perform at floor level, such as wiping up some water or putting a slipper on a patient's foot, describe the steps and reasons for each step as you stoop, keeping the body aligned and balanced, and using the large muscles of the thighs and buttocks to return to an upright position.

2. Given an object, such as a heavy book, located on a surface at least 6 inches above your head, describe the steps and the reasons for each step as you reach and remove the object without hyperextending or straining your back, or losing your balance.

3. Given a box of books weighing 10 to 15 pounds, or similar object, located on a surface about 32 to 36 inches high, describe the steps and the reasons for each step as you lift and carry the box for 5 minutes in such a manner as to minimize fatigue and prevent muscle strain.

4. Given a utility cart or similar object to push or pull, describe the steps and the reasons for each step as you push the cart, utilizing your body weight to assist in the movement.

5. In an activity which requires turning or pivoting, describe the steps and state the reasons for each step as you position your feet and trunk in such a manner as to avoid straining your back or trunk.

PERFORMANCE CHECKLIST

USING BODY MOVEMENT

STOOPING

Demonstrate good body alignment in stooping.

1. Place feet apart, one foot slightly advanced.

2. Assume a stable base of support.

3. Lower your body to stooped position: back and trunk straight, knee and hip joints flexed.

4. Use thigh and leg muscles to control action.

5. Shift weight to advanced foot and ball of rear foot.

6. Relieve tension on rear foot and maintain balance.

7. Raise your body to standing position: keep your back straight; initiate the move by extending your hip and knee joints.

8. Work your extensor muscles to bring your body upright.

9. Identify names and locations of extensor muscles.

REACHING

Demonstrate good body alignment in reaching.

1. Start with a stable base of support.

2. Start movement with your body in good alignment and balance.

3. Check the distance to be reached in order to reach your object. Obtain footstool for use if necessary. Secure an artificial aid in order to raise yourself if necessary.

4. Describe the correct use of the footstool.

5. Utilize the footstool appropriately: line of gravity centered over center of footstool, feet in balanced position.

6. Reach up from a position directly in front of the object.

7. Lift the object from the shelf using good alignment procedures.

8. Lower the object with smooth, coordinated movement.

9. Lower yourself from the ladder or footstool, if required, using good principles of body alignment.

10. Place the object on a shelf of working height, or stoop and lower it to the floor, observing good principles of body alignment.

11. Correctly state the rationale for using the footstool or artificial aid for increasing height: to avoid hyperextension of the neck; to assist in maintaining balance.

UNIT 7

LIFTING AND CARRYING

Demonstrate correct body alignment for lifting and carrying.

1. Start with a stable base.

2. State that the body should be in good alignment before beginning your movement and demonstrate proper body alignment. (Refer to previous checklist.)

3. Grasp the object to be lifted and carried in a balanced position; state the rationale for lifting the box in its center of gravity.

4. Set your abdominal and arm muscles for action: lift a box of books; bring it close to your own line of gravity.

5. Carry the box near the midline of your body for a period of approximately 5 minutes.

6. Shift the box from side to side as required during the period of support. State the rationale for shifting the box appropriately, i.e., to relieve strain on certain sets of muscles.

7. Place box on a counter or chair for short periods of time during which you rest. Explain the rationale for utilizing rest period.

8. Complete the performance checklist as indicated by lifting and carrying the box for a period of time not to exceed 5 minutes.

PUSHING AND PULLING

Demonstrate correct body alignment in pushing and pulling.

1. Start your action with a stable base of support.

2. Indicate that good alignment and balance are necessary for pushing and pulling actions.

3. Position yourself appropriately for the desired action, observing the principles of body alignment and keeping your body erect.

4. Position your feet at least 8 inches apart with one foot slightly advanced.

5. Set your trunk and leg muscles.

6. Lean toward the utility cart in order to push. Lean away from the utility cart in order to pull. Observe the principles of good body alignment during these actions, keeping your back straight and erect.

7. Explain the rationale for leaning your body weight into the load.

8. Move the utility cart using the large muscles of your leg and thigh.

9. Identify these muscles and their specific location and action (see the previous performance checklist).

PIVOTING

Demonstrate the correct body alignment in pivoting.

1. Stand with your feet slightly apart, knees slightly flexed.

2. Explain that this allows a stable base of support for use of the leg muscles.

3. Set your trunk and pelvic muscles for action.

4. Set your thigh and leg muscles.

5. Shift your weight to the ball of each foot.

6. State that this allows you to lift your heel slightly and to pivot more easily.

7. Pivot or make a 90° turn on your feet.

8. Move your body simultaneously with your feet so that there is no twisting of your lower back.

9. State that your body and feet move together to prevent twisting your back. Explain the rationale for this log-type motion, i.e., all parts of the body move a uniform distance in a uniform period of time.

10. Distribute your weight equally on each foot following the turn.

POSITIONING THE BED PATIENT

I. DIRECTIONS FOR THE STUDENT

Study this lesson using the workbook as your guide. Practice the procedures of positioning the patient in your skill laboratory, with a fellow student or someone else as the patient. After you have completed the lesson and practiced the procedure to gain some skill, arrange with your instructor to take the performance test for this lesson.

You will need the following items for your study and practice to gain skill in positioning the patient:

1. Pillows — at least three.

2. Footboard.

3. Overbed cradle.

4. Bath blanket, sheet, or bath towel.

5. Sandbags.

6. Synthetic lamb's wool pad (decubitus pad) or foam rubber pad.

7. Protective heel (Posey).

8. Hand rolls.

9. Alternating air-pressure pad and motor if available.

Please read the following paragraphs carefully. They explain exactly what you will be expected to know and how you will be expected to position the patient in various ways. If you feel that you already have the necessary skills without studying the lesson, discuss with your instructor the possibility of advancing directly to the performance test.

II. GENERAL PERFORMANCE OBJECTIVE

Upon completing this lesson, you will be able to position the bed patient in good body alignment for his health and comfort, using various aids for support or immobilization of various body parts, as well as protective aids to reduce pressure on skin areas.

III. SPECIFIC PERFORMANCE OBJECTIVES

After you have completed this lesson, you will be able to:

1. Provide support for or immobilize various parts of the body with the use of aids such as pillows, footboards, sandbags, hand rolls, and trochanter rolls.

2. Reduce and prevent formation of pressure areas by using protective aids such as pillows, synthetic lamb's wool pads, foam rubber pads, overbed cradle, protective heel (Posey), or flotation as with the alternating air-pressure mattress pad.

3. Place the helpless bed patient in the basic supine position according to the principles of positioning, and in the variations of this position, which include Fowler's, semi-Fowler's, and Trendelenburg's.

4. Place the helpless bed patient in the basic lateral position according to the principles of positioning, and in the Sims' variation of this position.

5. Place the helpless bed patient in the basic prone position according to the principles of positioning.

6. Move the bed patient toward the head of the bed by using good body movements to prevent strain or injury to the patient or yourself.

IV. VOCABULARY

Some of the words used in this lesson may be new or unfamiliar to you. These have been listed below with their meanings. Go over this list several times, and when you see the word used in the lesson, refer to this section unless you are sure of its meaning.

alternating air-pressure pad—a plastic pad with vertical air cells that alternately fill slowly with air, then deflate.

alveoli—air sacs in the lung.

contracture—the permanent contraction of a muscle due to spasm or paralysis that leads to "freezing," or immobilization, of the affected joint(s).

decubitus (pl. decubiti)—a bedsore caused by pressure which reduces circulation to the affected part of the body.

deformity—an unnatural alteration; a misshapen or disfigured part of the body.

femur—the thigh bone, the longest and strongest bone in the body, extending from the hip to the knee.

flotation—the state of floating or the act of being buoyant.

footboard—a board placed vertically at the end of the mattress to support the sole of the foot and to help prevent foot drop.

foot drop—the hyperextension of the foot with permanent contracture of the calf muscles and tendons.

Fowler's position—a sitting position in bed with the backrest raised to a 45° angle and the knees kept flat.

fracture—a broken bone.

intravenous (IV)—within or into the vein, such as injection of fluids, or puncture to obtain blood specimens.

overbed cradle—a device made of metal or wood placed over the patient's body or lower extremities to prevent the top bed covers from pressing on him.

paralysis—the loss of sensation or voluntary muscle movement in a part of the body.

pressure—the force caused by the weight of a body or object in contact with another body or object.

prone—lying on the stomach, face downward.

sacrum—the flat triangular bone at the base of the vertebrae; it is composed of five fused vertebrae.

semi-Fowler's position—a reclining position with the backrest elevated to 45° or more and the knee rest elevated to 15°.

Sims' position—lying on one side with uppermost leg moderately flexed so it does not rest on the lower leg.

supine position—lying on the back with face upward; also referred to as dorsal recumbent position.

trochanter roll—a cylindrical cloth roll used to support the lateral hip joint or trochanter of the femur.

V. KNOWLEDGE BASIC TO POSITIONING THE PATIENT

ITEM 1. WHY IS POSITIONING IMPORTANT?

One of the basic skills that nursing workers perform most frequently is that of changing the patient's position. Any position, even the most comfortable one, will become unbearable after a period of time. Whereas the healthy person has the ability to assume any of a great variety of positions, the sick person's movements may be limited by disease, injury, or helplessness. It is the responsibility of the nursing worker to position the patient and to change his position frequently. Changing the patient's position accomplishes four things: (a) it contributes to the patient's comfort; (b) it relieves pressure on various parts of the body; (c) it helps prevent the formation of contractures or deformities; and (d) it improves circulation.

In this lesson, you will learn how proper body alignment of the patient contributes to his comfort and helps prevent decubiti and contractures from occurring. You will be introduced to the various aids that you can use to support the body part in good alignment or to immobilize a part when it is necessary to limit its movement. The importance of reducing pressure on parts of the body and preventing the formation of pressure areas will become an old familiar tune to you as it is emphasized over and over again.

Question 1. Four reasons for changing the position of the patient are:

a. _____   b. _____

c. _____   d. _____ .

Question 2. When the bed patient is positioned by the nurse, it is necessary to maintain

_____ .

Question 3. The patient may be limited in his ability to change his position owing to

_____ , _____ , or _____ .

ITEM 2. BODY ALIGNMENT

Before we discuss the subject of how to turn and position the bed patient, we will review body alignment briefly. You may remember that alignment refers to the relationship of the movable segments of the body to one another. Good alignment is achieved when there is no undue stress placed on the muscles or skeleton.

The *checkpoints of good body alignment* are shown in the accompanying sketch.

—Head up, eyes straight ahead.

—Neck and back straight.

—Arms relaxed at sides.

—Chest up and out.

—Abdomen tucked in.

—Knees slightly flexed.

—Feet slightly apart, toes pointing forward.

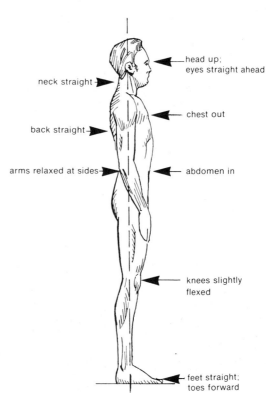

Good body alignment.

UNIT 8

PRINCIPLE I. GOOD BODY ALIGNMENT OF THE PATIENT IS MAINTAINED AT ALL TIMES.

Good body alignment of the patient should be maintained from side to side (laterally) as well as from front to back (anterior–posterior).

Problems of Poor Body Alignment. Examples of poor alignment of the bed patient are shown in the adjoining figures. In the first, the patient's neck and back are flexed so that his chest expansion is reduced in breathing, and his feet are hyperextended, which may lead to foot drop and interfere with later ambulation, or make ambulation impossible.

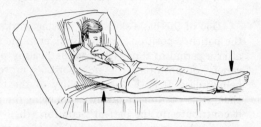

Poor body alignment: neck and back flexed, feet hyperextended.

The second sketch shows the patient lying on his arm while on his side. The blood circulation is impaired in that arm. The other arm and leg are lying unsupported behind the patient, causing strain on the shoulder joint, and inward rotation (turning) of the hip joint. The pull on the muscles makes this position very uncomfortable for the patient.

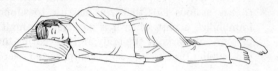

Poor body alignment: patient lying on arm, other arm unsupported.

Avoid Muscle Strain. When the patient is supine (lying on his back), the pull and weight of his extended arms and legs cause strain on the muscles of the back, the abdomen, and the extremities themselves. Muscle strain in the supine position is most commonly felt in the neck, small of the back, elbow, wrist, knee, and foot. These areas are shown in the next illustration. Even the top covers of the bed put strain on the foot and toes of the patient when bedding is tucked in tightly or is heavy with blankets, or when the patient is weak and unable to move by himself. Although modern mattresses used in hospitals may reduce the strain felt in the small of the back, some patients will still experience discomfort in this area.

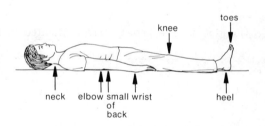

Supine Position: points of muscle strain.

Question 4. The discomfort felt by the patient when lying in one position for a long period of time is the result of _____.

Question 5. Name four of the areas where discomfort may be felt when a person is lying in the supine position.

     a. _____   b. _____

     c. _____   d. _____ .

ITEM 3. SUPPORTIVE AIDS

The patient's body alignment can be maintained, and his discomfort from muscle strain can be relieved, by your use of *supportive aids*. Pillows are most commonly used to support various parts of the body because they are soft and thus help reduce pressure; they can be folded over or rolled; and they can also be tucked firmly against the body to maintain its position. The footboard, sandbags, hand rolls, and trochanter rolls are also used to keep the body in alignment, to provide support for body parts, or to restrict movement of certain parts.

Pillows. Let us look at some of the ways that pillows may be used to support the patient's body. The helpless or weak patient who is turned onto his side may be unable to stay in this position, and tends to roll onto his back again. A pillow placed lengthwise along the patient's back with one edge tucked under his side, and the rest of the pillow rolled under (toward the surface of the bed) and tucked firmly against the back, will support the patient as he leans against it.

A pillow may also be used along the patient's abdomen when he is in Sims' position to prevent strain of sagging abdominal muscles. When a patient is lying on his side, a pillow placed between his knees helps reduce pressure on the knee joints and keeps the hip joint from rotating inward.

Pillows are used to support the neck, and should be placed under the patient's head and shoulders to prevent flexion of the neck that interferes with breathing and with swallowing. Strain on the muscles in the small of the back can be reduced by placing a small pillow or folded towel under the curve of the back. Avoid hyperextending the back. Hyperextension of the back causes strain on the abdominal muscles and some compression of the large blood vessels in the torso (trunk). Instead of using a pillow, which may be too large or bulky, it would be better to turn the patient to another position, if his condition permits.

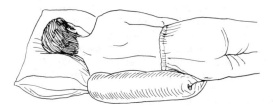

Pillow support of back.

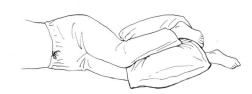

Pillow support of knee.

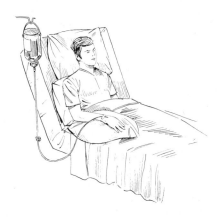

Pillow support with IV running.

U
N
I
T
8

You will often find it necessary to support the patient's upper extremities. When a patient's arm is immobilized because of an IV running in a vein or a cast applied for a fracture, the pulling strain on the shoulder muscles can be relieved with a folded towel placed under the upper arm and a pillow placed to support the forearm and hand. Patients who are totally helpless or who must avoid all exertion, should have their arms supported by pillows whenever they are in a sitting position. The positioning of pillows used to support the arm is shown.

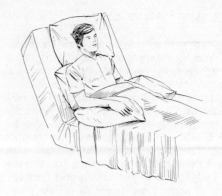

Pillow support of arms.

Question 6.   Two reasons for using aids in positioning the patient are:

a. _____   b. _____ .

Question 7.   Underline your answers in the following statement: A pillow placed between the knees of a patient lying on his side will (*increase*) (*decrease*) the pressure on the knee joint and keep the hip joint from turning (*inward*) (*outward*).

ITEM 4.   VARIOUS OTHER SUPPORTIVE AIDS

Hand Rolls. The hand roll is used to keep the fingers of the hand from being held in a tight fist, which could cause a flexion contraction. It provides some extension for the fingers and keeps the thumb in opposition to the fingers. It is used for the patient whose upper extremity is paralyzed, or who is unable to move his hand because of injury or disease.

The hand roll is a simple device and can be made by the patient's family or by volunteers if the hospital does not have an adequate supply. It is made of firmly woven cloth that is rolled into a cylinder about 4 to 5 inches long and 2 to 3 inches in diameter, and is then stuffed firmly. It should fit into the palm of the hand with the thumb curved on one side of the roll and the fingers flexed along the other side. A cloth loop or loose elastic band on one side for the fingers and on the other side for the thumb helps to hold them in position on the roll. (A rolled washcloth can be used temporarily.)

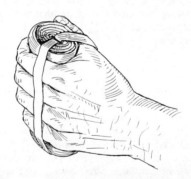

The hand-roll should be firm, not soft, and large enough in diameter to keep the fingers from curling into the palm of the hand.

Footboards. To help keep the bed patient's feet in good alignment, you should place a footboard between the end of the mattress and the foot of the bed. The common type of footboard is made of wood and is L-shaped so that one end can be slipped under the mattress to hold the board in a firm upright position; it should be covered with a cloth pad or sheet.

The patient should be lying in a supine position so that the bottoms of his feet rest flat against the surface of the footboard. The top bedding is brought over the top of the footboard so that it will not cause pressure on the toes. The position of the feet on the footboard and the top bedding over it are shown in the drawing.

Sandbags. Sandbags are just that—canvas, rubber, or plastic bags filled with sand so that they are heavy in weight, yet slightly flexible in use. Common sizes are 1 pound, 5 pounds, and 10 pounds. They are used to immobilize a part of the body by providing firm support that limits movement. You simply place the sandbag snugly next to the part that is to be supported. You will use sandbags on either side of the head following certain types of eye surgery when it is essential to prevent the patient from turning his head. Frequently, you will use sandbags to maintain the position of the feet on the footboard, especially when the foot tends to turn outward or inward. Sandbags are used as a temporary measure to immobilize a bone that has been fractured.

Trochanter Rolls. The trochanter roll should probably be used more often than it now is to support the hip joint and thigh. The trochanter roll prevents the hip and thigh from rotating outward and helps keep the foot in better alignment. Patients who have been paralyzed as a result of a stroke or other injury, those who have had a fracture of the femur, or those who have had surgery on the hip could benefit from the support given by the trochanter roll.

a. The roll is made by folding a light bath blanket or a sheet to the desired length of 2 or 3 feet.

b. It is then rolled into a tight cylinder.

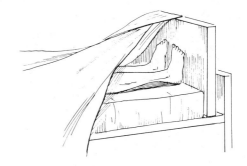

A footboard.

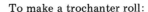

To make a trochanter roll:

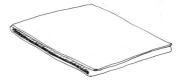

1. Fold in thirds.

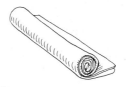

2. Roll up.

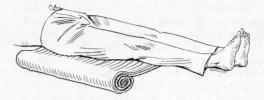

c. The loose end of the roll is placed under the patient's hip and thigh with the roll under the flap end.

3. Place flap under patient.

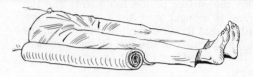

d. The roll is then tucked snugly along the hip and leg.

4. Roll in place.

The trochanter roll and its use are shown in the accompanying drawings.

This brings us to the second principle in positioning the patient.

PRINCIPLE II.   BODY PARTS ARE SUPPORTED IN GOOD ALIGNMENT TO PROMOTE COMFORT AND TO PREVENT UNDUE MUSCLE STRAIN.

ITEM 5.   USE OF FLEXION IN POSITIONING

A more comfortable position for the bed patient is produced by flexing (bending) segments of the body. The patient will feel better with some flexion of his elbows, hips, and knees while the alignment of the rest of his body is maintained. Those parts that are flexed may need to be supported to keep them in good alignment as well. Most of the positions in which you will place the bed patient will allow flexion of some part of the body.

Although the position with flexion is more comfortable for the patient, he must not be left in that position for more than two hours without extending (straightening out) the flexed body segment. A position of prolonged or habitual flexion by the helpless or weak patient may result in *contractures*.

Contractures are the result of muscles that are permanently contracted (shortened), which leads to "freezing" of the affected joint. The joints of the upper and lower extremities are most likely to be affected by contractures. Failure to move the patient or change his position regularly will cause even greater immobility. The patient who recovers from a serious disease or injury only to find that he is hopelessly crippled by contractures of his arms or legs represents a tragic result of inadequate nursing care.

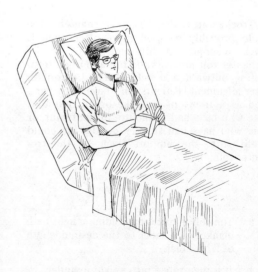

Positions of comfort involve alternating periods of flexion and extension of body parts.

Our third principle for positioning the patient is concerned with nursing diligence to prevent the formation of contractures.

PRINCIPLE III.   THE POSITION OF THE HELPLESS PATIENT MUST BE CHANGED AT LEAST EVERY 2 HOURS TO AVOID PROLONGED FLEXION OF ANY ONE BODY SEGMENT.

ITEM 6.   WHAT IS PRESSURE?

Perhaps the most important of all the reasons for changing the position of the patient is to reduce pressure on the various body parts and to prevent the formation of pressure areas. Now let us see why it is so important to reduce pressure by changing the patient's position frequently.

You already know that the body has weight, and that every part of the body also has weight. The arm has weight. The eyelid has weight. The liver, blood, hair, and nails all have weight. This weight exerts a force when it comes in contact with another body or object, and this force is called pressure.

The weight of the patient's body in contact with the bed causes pressure both on his body and on the bed. (We won't worry about the bed at this point.) The longer the patient remains in one position, the more the continued weight of the body presses down on the skin, blood vessels, and muscles on which the body rests. Since the skin, blood vessels, and muscles cannot exert an upward force, the pressure of the body weight makes them flatten out and become more compact.

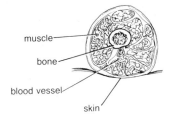

Initial Contact:
muscles, blood vessels, skin.

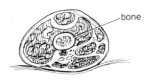

Continued Pressure:
muscles, skin, blood vessels.

Organs of the body are also affected by the force of pressure, and the lungs are extremely susceptible to it. The longer the patient's body remains in one position, the more the weight of the lung presses down on the rest of the lung beneath it and makes it more dense and compact. The air is squeezed out of the air sacs by the weight of the lung. The next two sketches show the lung changes produced by pressure.

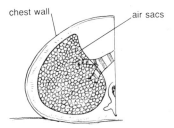

Initial Contact: lungs.

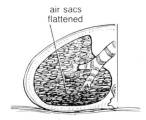

Continued Pressure: lungs.

The effects of pressure on the lungs can be very serious for the bedridden patient, even fatal. As a result of lying still, the person tends to take very shallow breaths and take in less air. The alveoli, or air sacs of the lung, do not expand fully and there is less oxygen available for the body to use. Decreased oxygen affects every body tissue and system, making them less efficient. With less air to expand the lungs, the alveoli are flattened, dark, warm, and moist — an ideal medium for the growth of bacteria. This often leads to pneumonia, a common complication of bed rest. Despite the use of antibiotic drugs, pneumonia is still the fifth leading cause of death in this country. Pneumonia due to lack of movement by the bed patient can be prevented by efficient nursing measures to (1) change the patient's position frequently, and (2) ask the patient to cough and breathe deeply every hour in order to give his lungs regular opportunities to expand fully.

Question 8. When a body comes in contact with another body or object, what causes the

force known as pressure?

Question 9. Prolonged pressure causes the skin, blood vessels, and muscles to become

_____ in shape.

Question 10. The effects of pressure on the lungs lead to the complication of

_____.

ITEM 7. PRESSURE ON THE SKIN

Although we cannot see the effect of pressure directly on the organs of the body (like the lungs), it can be observed in the skin. The skin areas most commonly affected by pressure are those located over bony prominences. They are the back of the head, the shoulder blades, the elbows, the sacrum, the trochanter of the femur, the knees, and the heels.

The continued weight of the body on these areas produces a reddening of the skin from the pressure. The blood circulation to the skin area is impaired because the blood vessels are flattened out and carry less blood. The skin and muscle tissues are also flattened, becoming more dense and compacted, further slowing down the flow of blood to the part. The slowdown of the blood flow away from the pressure area causes the redness of the skin. With continuing pressure, the skin and muscle tissues are deprived of the oxygen and foods carried by the blood cells, and so they begin to die. When this happens, the skin forms a pressure sore. Other names for a pressure sore are a bedsore or decubitus (plural, decubiti).

Pressure areas may develop within a period of a few hours on an undernourished patient and on the helpless or aged patient. Once a pressure area has broken down into a pressure sore it will take much time and effort to heal it. Some pressure sores take years of hospitalization to treat, cost thousands of dollars, and still never heal completely. *Prevention is the best cure*. Most often, pressure sores are the result of poor nursing care: not enough attention and care were given to turning the patient and preventing the development of pressure areas.

Question 11.   A pressure area that breaks down into a sore is called a _____

or a _____.

Question 12.   Pressure areas of the skin most often develop over _____ of bones.

Question 13.   The first sign of pressure usually noticed by the nurse is _____

of the skin.

ITEM 8.   PROTECTIVE AIDS TO
PREVENT PRESSURE

The primary method of preventing pressure areas is to change the patient's position at least every 2 hours. However, other aids are available for you to use to reduce pressure.

Antidecubitus Pads. The sacrum and the bony prominence of the hip joint (the trochanter of the femur) are frequent sites of pressure areas in the helpless bed patient. A synthetic lamb's wool pad, often referred to as decubitus pads, may be placed under the patient's hips from the waist to the knees to reduce the pressure. Patients generally find these pads comfortable. They have a deep pile which resists matting and traps air between the fibers, thus forming a soft support for the body. Most of these pads can be laundered and dried by machine, then fluffed by a gentle shake so that they can be used for more than a year. The pads can also be used to turn or lift the patient, thereby avoiding the friction of sliding the patient's tender skin areas on the bed linen.

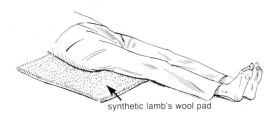

synthetic lamb's wool pad

Foam padding about 1/2-inch thick can be used to reduce pressure over any bony prominence. The sheet of padding can be cut to any size to fit under the body or protect the elbows, ankles, or heels. Specially designed heel pads are available, made of synthetic lamb's wool inside a sturdy cloth covering that is shaped to fit the heel.

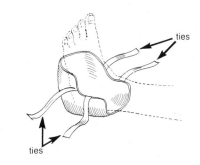

ties

ties

Heel protector

Flotation Pads. In recent years, new products have become available to help reduce pressure for people confined to bed, and for use in treating patients with decubitus ulcers. Some products with promise are the flotation-type mattresses and pads. All flotation devices are based on the principle of distributing the body weight over a larger area than the areas in contact with one another. The water-filled mattress of a waterbed is a flotation device that produces less pressure on the body than most other types in use today. However, the weight of water flotation pads and mattresses can be a disadvantage, as well as control of the water temperature and damage from possible flooding due to a punctured plastic pad.

Flotation devices that utilize air as a method of displacing part of the body weight include air cushions, alternating air-pressure pads, and air jets, which are all designed to reduce pressure on the body and prevent the formation of decubiti. Although air flotation is less efficient than water flotation in reducing pressure, it is more convenient and has fewer disadvantages. Silicone gel pads, developed to protect delicate instruments in space flights, have been effective in preventing pressure sores, but they are expensive and quite heavy to handle.

UNIT 8

Thick foam pads are available commercially that resemble the inside of an egg carton. The full-length pad is placed on the bed mattress with the projections extending upward, and is covered with a sheet. The weight of the patient's body flattens the projections somewhat, but the trapped air in the foam acts like a flotation pad to reduce pressure.

The Alternating Air-pressure Pad. The alternating air-pressure pad is currently a widely used flotation method for alleviating pressure in bedridden patients. The air pad is made of heavy vinyl plastic and has both an odd and an even set of vertical fingers or air chambers that alternately inflate and then deflate. The two sets of air chambers in the pad are connected by plastic tubes to a motor that cycles the air into the chamber. This produces a slight shifting motion that continually changes the pressure caused by the weight of the body.

To use the alternating air pad, place it on top of the bed mattress. Attach the tubes to the pump, plug the cord of the motor pump into an electric outlet, turn on the motor, and check to see that it is working. Cover the pad with the bottom sheet and then make the bed as usual, although you must not put thick pads under the patient that would reduce the kneading action of the alternating air pad. Even with the alternating air pad in use, the patient should be positioned in good body alignment and turned every 2 hours or more often, unless prohibited by the doctor's orders. When using the alternating air pad, you should (1) avoid kinking the tubes, and (2) avoid puncturing the plastic pad with pins or other sharp objects.

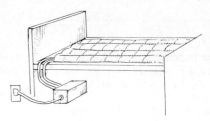

Alternating pressure mattress on bed, attached to electrical outlet.

25–watt
light bulb

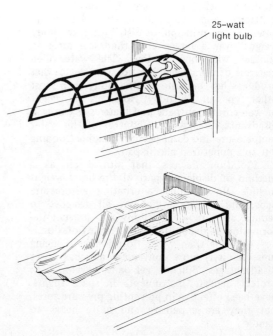

The Overbed Cradle. The overbed cradle is a device to prevent the weight of the top bedding from causing pressure on the patient's toes and feet. The cradle is placed over the bottom linen on the bed, and the top bedding is then brought over the cradle. Many overbed cradles are semicircular in shape. They may be made of wood and metal, or constructed entirely of metal tubing or slats, as shown.

A Word of Caution. The inflated rubber rings and round donuts, frequently used in the past by nurses to ease pressure areas on the sacrum or the heel, are not recommended for use. The donuts are made of absorbent cotton, shaped in a circle, and wrapped with gauze or other similar material. These devices tend to be too firm and cause additional pressure around their circumferences, which further decreases the blood flow to and away from the part already suffering from the effects of pressure.

Prevention of Pressure Areas. Although there are many devices to assist in preventing pressure sores, the key to their prevention is the nurse. Nothing can substitute for your personal, active attention and actions on the patient's behalf. Correct positioning of the patient, frequent change of position by turning, maintaining a clean and dry bed, and protecting body parts against pressure are important skills to use for the prevention of pressure areas and decubiti.

The final principle of positioning the patient can be stated as follows:

PRINCIPLE IV. PRESSURE CAUSED BY BODY WEIGHT ON ANOTHER BODY OR OBJECT CAN BE REDUCED BY CHANGING THE POSITION OF THE BODY OR BY USING PROTEC— TIVE AIDS.

Question 14. The primary method used by nursing workers to prevent the formation of pressure areas in the bed patient is _____ .

Question 15. In addition to the primary method, what other two methods might you use for the patient who shows signs of pressure on the skin over his sacrum?

a. _____ b. _____ .

ITEM 9. BASIC BODY POSITIONS AND THEIR VARIATIONS

We have now identified four principles to remember in the positioning of the helpless patient in bed. They are:

I. *Good body alignment of the patient is maintained at all times.*

II. *Body parts are supported in good alignment to promote comfort and to prevent undue muscle strain.*

III. *The helpless patient's position is changed at least every 2 hours to avoid prolonged flexion of any one body segment.*

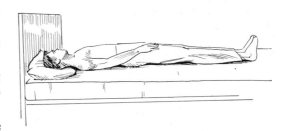

Supine position.

IV. Pressure caused by body weight on another object or body can be reduced by changing the position of the body or by using protective aids.

These principles form the guidelines for the skills you will use to position the bed patient.

There are three basic positions for the patient to assume while in bed. These are:

   a. the supine position with the patient lying on his back,

   b. the lateral position with the patient lying on one side, and

   c. the prone position, where the patient lies on his stomach.

These positions are shown in the accompanying sketches. All other positions that you will use for your patients are variations of these three.

The variations of the supine position include sitting with the head elevated. When only the patient's upper body and head are elevated 45°, the sitting position is called Fowler's position.

Semi-Fowler's position involves raising the head of the bed 45° and the knee rest of the bed 15°. The latter is more comfortable because it reduces strain on abdominal and leg muscles, and helps keep the patient from sliding down in the bed.

The other variation of the supine position has the patient's feet elevated and his head lowered in what is called Trendelenburg's position. This is used mainly for the patient who has gone into shock, or is in the operating room for certain types of surgery. There is a tendency for the patient to slide toward the head of the bed while in this position, and so you should pad the head of the bed with a pillow and place sandbags against the patient's shoulders.

The variation of the lateral position is Sims' position, in which the uppermost leg is sharply flexed so that it does not rest upon the lower leg.

Question 16. The four principles used in positioning the helpless bed patient are:

   a. _____

   b. _____

   c. _____

   d. _____

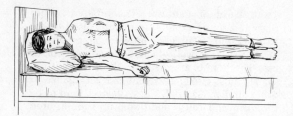

Lateral position.

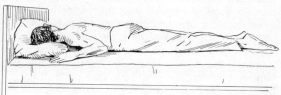

Prone position.

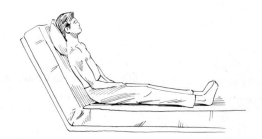

Fowler's position.

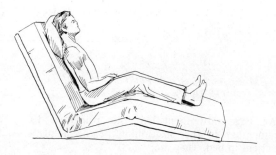

Semi-Fowler's position

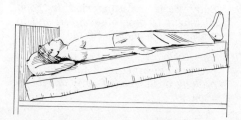

Trendelenburg's position

Question 17. Please place a check mark to indicate which of the following are *variations* of the basic positions of the bed patient.

 a. head elevated, hips and knees flexed.

 b. lying on one side with one leg resting on the other.

 c. lying with face and feet upward.

 d. lying with feet elevated and head lowered.

 e. lying with foot of bed level and head elevated.

ITEM 10. PLACING THE PATIENT IN THE SUPINE POSITION

 In the skill laboratory, practice placing the patient in each of the three basic positions and the four variations while using the principles of positioning to keep good body alignment, support parts of the body, and reduce pressure. One of the other students, or someone else, should play the part of the patient for your practice session. (Remember to use good body alignment principles for yourself.)

 Given a bed patient who became paralyzed on his right side two days ago, place him in a supine position using the principles of positioning as your guidelines, and the principles of good body movement to prevent injury or strain to yourself.

Important Steps	Key Points
1. Approach and identify the patient, explain what you are going to do, and enlist his cooperation.	The patient may be frightened by what has happened to him, as well as depressed or emotionally upset. You will have to reassure him of your ability to help him move. Explain the need to change his position frequently for his health and comfort. Wash your hands.
2. Provide privacy.	Pull the curtains around the bed, use screens, or close the door of the room.
3. Position the bed.	Place the bed in a flat or level position at working height, unless contraindicated. Common contraindications for bed position change may be severe cardiac (heart) or respiratory (lung) diseases or subarachnoid hemorrhage or some type of traction or cast that precludes changing the bed position. Be sure to obtain this information from your nurse when you receive your assignment, or refer to the patient's nursing care plan in the Kardex.
	Lower the siderails on the proximal side, if they are used. The proximal side should be the side on which the patient is paralyzed. It requires the most support from you, and working near it reduces the distance you need to stretch or reach.

Important Steps	Key Steps
4. Place the patient in the supine position.	If he is on his side, remove any supportive pillows, fold the top bedding back to his hips, and avoid any undue exposure of the patient's body, which may embarrass him or others. With one hand on his shoulder and one on the hip, roll his body in one piece (like a log) over onto his back. Always avoid twisting the back by moving the torso (trunk) of the body as a unit.
5. Use aids to reduce pressure on bony prominences, if indicated by the condition of the patient.	The paralyzed patient may not be aware of any discomfort caused by pressure, so you must be alert to prevent and reduce pressure, especially on any paralyzed parts. Place a synthetic lamb's wool pad under the patient's hips and thighs. With one hand on his shoulder and one hand on his distal hip, roll the patient toward you; continue to support his shoulder and chest with one hand, and place the pad along his hips and thigh with one half of the pad tucked close to his side and the bed. Roll the patient onto his back, reach under his proximal side, and pull the remainder of the pad into place. Be sure to reposition the patient's body parts. Place a piece of foam rubber padding under the patient's right heel, or use a protective heel of synthetic lamb's wool.
6. Align the patient's body in good position.	The head, neck, and spine should be in a straight line. The arms and legs should be parallel to the body. The hips, knees, and feet should be in good alignment.
7. Support the body parts in good alignment for comfort.	Place a pillow under the head and shoulders to prevent strain on neck muscles. Support the small of the back with a folded bath towel or small pillow. Since this patient is paralyzed on his right side, he will be unable to keep the right leg in good position. You should put a footboard at the foot of the bed and place him so that his feet are flat against it. Arrange a sandbag along the outer portion of the right foot to keep the foot upright. Now make a trochanter roll and arrange it along the right hip and thigh to keep the hip joint from rotating outward. Place a pillow under the right forearm

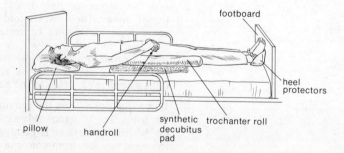

footboard

heel protectors

pillow   handroll   synthetic decubitus pad   trochanter roll

Patient in supine position with supportive
aids to maintain body alignment and protective
devices to reduce pressure.

Important Steps	Key Points

so that the arm is at least 6 inches from the body and place a hand roll in the paralyzed right hand. Use the loops of a slightly loose bandage to keep the fingers flexed and the thumb in opposition on the roll; otherwise the roll will slip out of place.

8. Provide for the patient's comfort.

Adjust the top bedding, leave the call bell where he can reach it with his unaffected hand, and raise the siderails. Place the bed in low position. Plan to change his position at least every 2 hours. Tell him when you expect to return.

9. Report and record as appropriate.

Report to the team leader or the nurse in charge that the patient has been positioned. Report and record any change in the patient's condition, such as reddened areas of the skin over bony prominences, decreased movement in his joints, pain on movement, or difficulty in breathing or swallowing. Charting example:

10:00 A.M. Turned to supine position; no reddened areas observed on back; moves easily without pain or dyspnea.   J. Jones, LVN

UNIT 8

ITEM 11. PLACING THE PATIENT IN FOWLER'S POSITION

Now that you have positioned the patient in a supine position, practice placing him in variations of that position. Given a patient with paralysis of his right side who is in a supine position in bed, place him in Fowler's position.

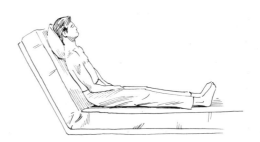

Fowler's position.

1. Approach and identify the patient, explain what you plan to do, and enlist his cooperation.

Whether the bed is an electrically operated or a manual Gatch-type, explain that you will raise the head of the bed slowly and ask him to tell you to stop if he becomes uncomfortable. Wash your hands.

2. Elevate the head of the bed.

Slowly raise the head of the bed. Ordinarily, it would be elevated between $15°$ and $60°$ (usually about $45°$) and would not be brought to the full upright position for any helpless patient because he may be unable to maintain his balance and could slip or fall.

3. Use aids to reduce pressure on bony prominences, if indicated by the condition of the patient.

You should prevent or reduce pressure, as you do for the supine position, by use of a synthetic lamb's wool pad or foam rubber pad under the hips, and a protective heel or pad on the right foot.

4. Place the patient in good body alignment.

See that the head, neck, and back are all straight. The weight of the body should be supported at the point where the hips are

Important Steps	Key Points
	flexed in the sitting position. See that the feet are straight and the toes are pointing in an upright position.
5. Support the body parts in good alignment for comfort.	The body parts should be supported in Fowler's position as they were in the supine position. Place the pillow under the head and shoulders, the trochanter roll along the right hip and thigh, the footboard at the foot of the bed, a sandbag along the outer part of the right foot, and a pillow under the right forearm to reduce the pulling drag on the shoulder joint. The hand and thumb should be supported on a hand roll.
6. Provide for the patient's comfort.	Adjust the top bedding, raise the siderails, and arrange drinking water or the call bell close at hand so that he can reach them easily. Place the bed in low position. Plan to change his position in 2 hours or less, to prevent prolonged flexion of the hips. Tell him when you expect to return.
7. Record and report as appropriate.	Be sure to notify other team members involved in the care of the patient about the time schedule for changing the patient's position. Charting example: 12:10 P.M. Position changed to Fowler's. Is in good spirits today, moving easily, without pain. J. Jones, LVN

ITEM 12. PLACING THE PATIENT IN SEMI-FOWLER'S POSITION

Given the same patient who has paralysis of his right side and who is lying in a supine position in bed, place him in semi-Fowler's position. Follow the same procedure as outlined in Item 11, except that you will add the following as part of Step 2.

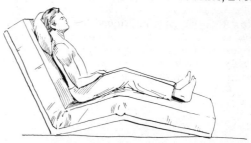

Semi-Fowler's position.

2. Elevate the knee rest of the bed approximately 15°.

Slight flexion of the knees gives more comfort by reducing strain on the patient's abdominal muscles and helps him maintain a sitting position without sliding down in bed. It also prevents hyperextension of the knees. Charting example:

12:10 P.M. Placed in semi-Fowler's position. Says this is the most comfortable.
J. Jones, LVN

ITEM 13. PLACING THE PATIENT IN TRENDELENBURG'S POSITION

Given a patient going into shock as a result of possible internal bleeding, immediately place him in Trendelenburg's position.

Important Steps	Key Points
1. Approach and identify the patient, explain what you plan to do, and enlist his cooperation if his condition permits.	The patient going into shock is likely to be quite apprehensive and know that something is wrong with him. As shock deepens, he will become more difficult to arouse and less alert. Wash your hands.
2. Position the bed.	If possible, place the head of the bed touching the wall. Lock the brakes on the wheels at both the head and the foot of the bed. Remove the pillow from under the patient's head and place it upright against the head of the bed. Lower the head of the bed.
3. Elevate the foot of the bed and place the patient in Trendelenburg's position. 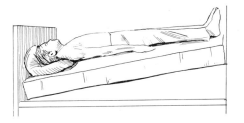 Trendelenburg's position.	If the bed is automatically adjustable (electric or manual), disengage the headrest hold, and raise the foot of the bed. This will also lower the head of the bed as the foot of the bed is elevated, so that the bed remains flat although on an incline. If the bed is a Gatch adjustable type, elevate the knee rest, then raise the footrest and engage the metal support in the ratchet on either side of the bed. Alternative methods of raising the foot of the bed: a hydraulic bed lifter is used to elevate the foot of the bed; two people lift the foot of the bed while a third person places wooden "shock blocks" under the wheels at the foot of the bed; or two people lift the bed and support the foot of it on the seats of two chairs.
4. Align the patient's body in good position.	The patient should always be in good alignment: head, neck, and back straight, legs and arms parallel to the body. (The weight of the arms on the chest or abdomen could restrict breathing movements.)
5. Support the body in good alignment for comfort.	Use small pillows or folded bath towels to support the neck and the small of the back in order to relieve muscle strain. Since the patient in this position will tend to slide toward the head of the bed, place a sandbag above the shoulders to help maintain his position.
6. Use aids to reduce pressure over bony prominences.	The initial use of Trendelenburg's position is generally required during a medical emergency, so other life-supporting treatment is carried out first. When time allows, you must reduce pressure because the patient's movements may be severely limited. Provide padding under the hips and heels as needed. The back of the head and the elbows may need to be padded as well.
7. Provide for the patient's comfort.	When the patient must remain in this position for more than 2 hours, you must turn him from side to back to side on a 2-hour schedule if his condition permits. Otherwise, make slight alterations in his position by propping the shoulder and arm on a pillow tucked partly under him, and other methods.

UNIT 8

Important Steps	Key Points
8. Report and record as appropriate.	Always report to the team leader or the nurse in charge *and* record on the patient's hospital chart that the patient has been placed in Trendelenburg's position, his condition at that time, and any changes in his condition thereafter. The patient must be observed closely during the emergency period and his early convalescence.

Charting example:
2:00 P.M. Placed in Trendelenburg's position, per order. Color remains pale, IV's running as ordered. Approximately 25 cc solution absorbed.   J. Jones, LVN

ITEM 14. PLACING THE PATIENT IN LATERAL AND SIMS' POSITION

Given an elderly patient who is extremely weak and unable to turn himself, position him in a lateral, and then in Sims', position using the principles of positioning.

Important Steps	Key Points
1. Approach and identify the patient, explain what you plan to do, and enlist his cooperation.	The patient may feel that it is too much work to turn, so explain how you will help him, provide support, and emphasize how necessary it is for his recovery and comfort. Other patients may resist turning because of fear or pain, especially those who have had surgery or an injury. Wash your hands.
2. Position the bed.	Lower the head and foot of the bed so that it is level or flat. Then lower the siderail on the proximal side where you are working, if it was in use.
3. Turn the patient onto his side toward you, or turn him onto the side away from you. (Obtain assistance, if needed.) 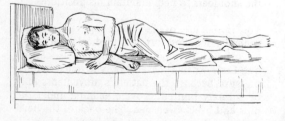	Fold the top bedding back to level of patient's hips, and avoid undue exposure of the patient's body, which may embarrass him or others.

To turn the patient onto his side toward you: Flex the patient's distal knee and cross his distal arm across his chest before moving him. Place one hand on his distal shoulder, the other on his distal hip, and draw his body toward you in one piece without twisting the back. Then slide both hands across the patient's back to his proximal hip and shoulder, lift slightly outward, and smoothly roll his body toward you. Remember to use good body movements so that your back is straight and your knees are flexed. Use large muscle groups for lifting movements.

To turn the patient onto his side away from you: This requires less effort, when the patient is large or extremely helpless, than to turn him toward you. With one hand on the proximal shoulder and the other on the hip, roll the patient's body away from you onto his distal side. Lower your hands to his distal shoulder |

Important Steps	Key Points
	and hip, and pull them toward you to stabilize the patient on his side. Again, you must use good body movement to avoid possible strain or injury to yourself.
4. Align the patient's body in good position.	Make sure that the patient is not lying on his arm. See that his head, neck, and back are in a straight line, that his legs are parallel, with the knees slightly flexed. The patient's uppermost arm may be flexed across his abdomen or supported on his body and hip.
5. Place the patient in Sims' position.	Flex the uppermost leg so that it does not rest upon the lower leg. The patient's lowermost arm may be at his back in this position. At the time he is turned, it should be parallel to his body, and when he is on his side, support and lift the shoulder slightly with one hand and with the other grasp his elbow and draw his arm smoothly from under him to his back.

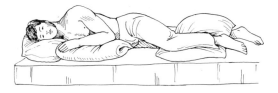

Sims' position.

Important Steps	Key Points
6. Support the body in good alignment for comfort.	Place a pillow under the patient's head and neck to prevent muscle strain and maintain alignment. Put a pillow under the uppermost leg so that it is supported from the knee to the foot. Another pillow may be placed firmly against the patient's abdomen to support the back and hip in better alignment.
7. Use aids to reduce pressure over bony prominences.	You may need to use a foam rubber pad or a protective heel to prevent pressure on the ankle of the lowermost leg. Also, a synthetic lamb's wool pad or foam rubber pad should be used under the patient's hip and thigh to reduce pressure on the trochanter at the hip joint. Many elderly patients who are thin tend to show signs of pressure in this area.
8. Provide for the patient's comfort.	Adjust the top bedding and siderails, if indicated. Leave the bed in "low" position. Place bedside articles so that the patient can reach them. Make sure his call button is within reach. Change his position in 2 hours or less. Tell him when you plan to return.
9. Report and record as appropriate.	Be sure to notify other team members involved in the care of the patient about the time schedule for changing the patient's position. Report and record any change in the patient's condition, such as reddened skin areas, pain on moving, fever, difficulty in breathing, or cough. Charting example:

4:00 P.M. Placed in left Sims' position. Seems more alert this P.M. No complaints.

J. Jones, LVN

UNIT 8

ITEM 15. PLACING THE PATIENT IN PRONE POSITION

Given a patient who is being treated for a draining wound of the sacral area, place the patient in a prone position using the principles related to positioning.

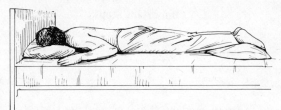

Prone position with foot positioned in good alignment to avoid hyperextension.

Important Steps	Key Points
1. Approach and identify the patient, explain what you plan to do, and enlist his cooperation.	If the patient is accustomed to sleeping on his abdomen, he would probably welcome the change. If not, he may resist, especially if he fears it would be painful. Some patients must be reassured that you will turn them back whenever the position becomes uncomfortable. Wash your hands.
2. Adjust the bed.	Lower the headrest and knee rest so that the bed is in a flat position. Raise the bed to working height. Lower the siderails on the side where you are working. Fold the top bedding down to the level of the patient's hips. Avoid undue exposure of the patient's body, which may cause embarrassment to him or to others.
3. Position the patient in bed.	When there is room between the mattress and the foot of the bed, the patient should be moved down in the bed so that his feet will extend over the edge of the mattress. Remove the footboard, if one is present.
4. Turn the patient onto his side and over onto his stomach (preferably roll him toward you so that you can observe him closely).	Turn the patient onto his side according to the procedure given in Item 14. Continue to roll the patient over until he is on his stomach. Be sure to turn his head to one side so that he can breathe easily.
5. Align the patient in good position.	The patient's head should be turned to one side; his neck and back should be in a straight line. The arms may be parallel to the body in a slightly flexed position, or the arm on the same side that the head is turned can be flexed sharply at the elbow so that the hand is near the head. The legs should be straight and the feet extended over the edge of the mattress to avoid hyperextension of the foot. If this is not possible, place a pillow under both ankles to prevent foot drop as a result of prolonged hyperextension.
6. Support the patient's body in good alignment.	A small pillow or folded towel under the head may be used if the patient requests it. Generally, it will not be needed for comfort.
7. Use aids to reduce pressure on any bony part.	For the woman patient in a prone position, pressure on the breasts is relieved by placing a

Important Steps	Key Points
	pillow under the chest and abdomen, below the breasts. A pillow placed under the lower abdomen of the male patient relieves pressure on his genital organs. Many infants and restless patients will develop reddened skin areas on the knees when in the prone position. The use of a synthetic lamb's wool pad or a foam rubber pad under the knees will reduce pressure and friction.
8. Provide for the patient's comfort.	Adjust the top bedding and raise the siderails. Put his call button within reach. Plan to change his position in 2 hours or less. Make sure his dressing is in place and dry. Tell him when you expect to return.
9. Report and record as appropriate.	Report and record any change in the patient's condition and the time schedule for changing his position. Charting example: 6:00 P.M. Placed in prone position. Dislikes this position — can't see what's going on! No redness noted on bony prominences. Back massaged. J. Jones, LVN 6:20 P.M. Sleeping quietly. J. Jones, LVN

UNIT 8

ITEM 16. MOVING THE PATIENT TOWARD THE HEAD OF THE BED

Given a patient who had abdominal surgery yesterday and who has slipped down toward the foot of the bed, move him toward the head of the bed, using the patient's own help, while following methods of good body movement.

Important Steps	Key Points
1. Approach and identify the patient, explain what you plan to do, and enlist his cooperation.	You will need to evaluate whether the patient can use his arms and legs to help move himself upward. If he is too large or heavy for one person to handle, or too weak, or unable to exert himself, you will need another person to assist you. Wash your hands.
2. Adjust the bed.	Place the bed in a flat or nearly flat position. Lower the siderail on the side where you are working.
3. Tell the patient how he can help move up in bed.	He should flex both knees, push down on the mattress with both feet in order to move the lower portion of his body upward in bed. If

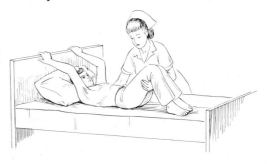

Important Steps	Key Points
	possible, he should reach and hold the head of the bed with one or both hands, and pull his body upward when he pushes with his feet. You will assist him to move the upper portion of his body and to avoid burning the skin of the lower trunk.
4. Move the patient toward the head of the bed.	When the patient is in position with his hands reaching the head of the bed and knees flexed, place one hand under his shoulder and across his back and support his head with the other hand. If there is no need to support the head, place the other hand under the hips to help move them. Upon your signal, both of you should move simultaneously toward the head of the bed.
5. Provide for the patient's comfort.	Place a pillow under his head and shoulders. Check to see that his body is in good alignment, and that the parts are well-supported. Use aids to reduce pressure when these are indicated. Raise the siderail, if required. Put the call button and other articles nearby so that the patient can reach them. Adjust the position of the bed so that it is comfortable or suitable for his activity. Tell him when you will return.

ITEM 17. CONCLUSION OF LESSON

You have now finished the lesson on positioning the bed patient. When you have practiced the procedures sufficiently to gain some skill in aligning the patient, moving him, and using the appropriate supportive and protective aids, arrange with your instructor to take the performance test.

VII. ADDITIONAL INFORMATION FOR ENRICHMENT

Positioning the bed patient is a basic skill that you will use daily in the care of all of your patients. Positioning is also an important part of the therapeutic treatment for many disease conditions. You may want to learn more about how positioning is used to meet a patient's special needs. Medical and surgical nursing textbooks are a rich source of information about the use of positioning in the treatment of various conditions. For example, the postoperative patient usually can be placed in Fowler's position, but not in semi-Fowler's position. The right lateral position is used to advance the Miller-Abbott intestinal tube, whereas the left lateral position is best for giving an enema. You will be better able to help the patient cooperate with the treatment if you understand the conditions for the use and purposes of positioning.

In view of the importance of this aspect of nursing care, you may wish to read further. Much has been written about the effect of pressure on the body. Two articles are listed below. The articles include references that will provide additional information and sources of material. Your instructor can give you still other references, if you wish.

Berecek, Kathleen: Treatment of Decubitus Ulcers, *Nursing Clinics of North America*, 10:171–210, March 1975. An overview of current measures used in the prevention and treatment of decubitus ulcers, including the use of mechanical devices, physical methods, ointments, and drugs. Many references are cited.

Pfaudler, Marjorie: Flotation Displacement and Decubitus Ulcers, *American Journal of Nursing*, 68:2351–2355, November 1968.

Carnevale, Doris, and Susan Brueckner: Immobilization — Reassessment of a Concept, *American Journal of Nursing*, 70:1502–1507, July 1970.
Harvin, J. Shand, and Thomas J. Hargest: The Air Fluidized Bed: A New Concept in the Treatment of Decubitus Ulcers, *Nursing Clinics of North America*, 5:181–187, March 1970. Describes an air flotation bed in which the air is pumped through a bed of glass spheres covered with a sheet on which the patient lies. The air bed promotes the healing of decubitus ulcers in paraplegic patients.

WORKBOOK ANSWER SHEET

Question 1. a. patient's comfort

  b. relieves pressure

  c. prevents contractures

  d. improves circulation

2. alignment of the body

3. disease, inability to move about, helplessness

4. strain on muscles

5. Any four of the following: neck, small of the back, elbow, wrist, knee, ankle; also (not mentioned in the text), shoulder, abdomen, hip

6. Any two of the following: to keep the body in alignment; to provide support for body segments; to immobilize or prevent movement in a part

7. decrease; inward

8. weight

9. flattened (dense, compacted, etc.)

10. pneumonia

11. bedsore; decubitus ulcer

12. prominences

13. redness

14. to turn frequently

15. Any two of the following: synthetic lamb's wool pad, foam rubber pad, alternating air-pressure pad

16. a. Good body alignment of patient is maintained at all times.

  b. Body parts are supported in good alignment to prevent undue muscle strain.

  c. Helpless patient's position is changed every 2 hours to avoid prolonged flexion of any part.

  d. Pressure caused by body weight on another object or body can be reduced by changing the position of the body or by the use of protective aids.

17. a., d., e.

UNIT 8

PERFORMANCE TEST

In the skill laboratory, your instructor will ask you to demonstrate your skill in carrying out two of the following procedures without reference to source material. For these activities, you will need another person to play the part of the patient.

1. Given a patient in a lateral position with paralysis of both legs, place the patient in a supine position using the principles of positioning to provide good alignment, support, and protection from pressure.

2. Given a patient in a supine position who has paralysis of both legs, place the patient (1) in Fowler's position, (2) in semi-Fowler's position, and (3) in Trendelenburg's position.

3. Given a patient who had abdominal surgery yesterday, place the patient in Sims' position, using the principles of positioning to provide good alignment, support, and protection from pressure.

4. Give an adult woman patient with a disease that limits her movement, place her in a prone position, utilizing the principles of positioning.

5. Given a patient with a high fever who has slipped down in bed while in a supine position, assist him to move toward the head of the bed, using principles of good body movement.

PERFORMANCE CHECKLIST

SUPINE POSITIONING OF PATIENT WHO HAS PARALYSIS OF LEGS

1. Wash your hands.

2. Approach and identify the patient.

3. Explain the procedure to the patient.

4. Provide privacy.

5. Place the bed in flat position, at working level.

6. Lower the siderails on the proximal side.

7. Remove supportive pillows from his back, and from between his knees.

8. Move the patient from his side to his back by placing your hands on his shoulder and hip, and moving his body as if it were a log.

9. Move and align his paralyzed legs with the hips, knees, and feet parallel.

10. Provide protection against pressure points:

    a. Place a decubitus pad under his hips, if one is not already being used.

    b. Use heel protectors for both feet.

    c. Use a bed board or a cradle to keep the bedding off his feet.

11. Use supportive aids to maintain good body alignment.

    a. Place a pillow under his head and shoulders.

    b. Place a small pillow or towel at the small curve of his back.

    c. Use a trochanter roll along the hip and thigh of both legs.

    d. Support the position of his feet with sandbags, if necessary.

12. Provide for the patient's safety and comfort. Leave the call signal and bedside stand within easy reach.

13. Chart the change of position and observations of the patient's condition.

POSITIONING THE SUPINE PATIENT WHO HAS PARALYSIS OF THE LEGS

— IN FOWLER'S POSITION

Steps 1 through 5: Same as for supine positioning above.

  6. Elevate the head of the bed to approximately $45°$.

  7. Check the alignment and support of the patient.

  8. Practice charting.

— IN SEMI-FOWLER'S POSITION

Steps 1 through 5: Same as for supine positioning.

  6. Elevate the head of the bed to approximately $45°$.

  7. Raise the knee gatch or the foot of the bed so that the knees are flexed approximately $15°$.

  8. Check the patient's alignment and support.

  9. Practice charting.

— IN TRENDELENBURG'S POSITION

1. Wash your hands.

2. Approach and identify the patient.

3. Explain the procedure.

4. Lower the head of the bed.

5. Elevate the foot of the bed by using the automatic controls or hydraulic lifter. Obtain assistance if the foot of the bed is to be placed on "shock blocks" or chairs.

6. Check the alignment and support of the patient.

7. Practice charting.

POSITIONING THE PATIENT IN SIMS' POSITION

1. Wash your hands.

2. Identify the patient.

3. Explain the procedure to him.

4. Adjust the bed to working height.

5. Prepare the patient for movement.

6. Place the patient in Sims' position.

    a. Place one hand on his distal shoulder, the other on his hip, draw the patient's body toward you, adjust his position when he is lying on his side.

    b. Flex his upper leg so that it does not rest on the lower leg.

    c. Position the lower arm to the rear.

7. Support his body for good alignment.

    a. Place a pillow under his head and neck.

    b. Place a pillow under the uppermost leg so it is supported.

    c. Put pillow against his abdomen to support the trunk and uppermost arm.

8. Use protective aids to reduce pressure, if required.

9. Provide for the patient's comfort.

    a. Adjust the bedding.

    b. Raise the siderails and leave the bed in low position.

    c. Place the call button in a convenient position.

    d. Inform the patient when you will return.

10. Chart the procedure.

POSITIONING THE PATIENT IN A PRONE POSITION

1. Wash your hands.

2. Identify the patient.

3. Explain the procedure to him.

4. Adjust the bed to working height.

5. Position the patient in bed with his feet extended over the edge of the mattress, if possible.

6. Turn the patient onto his stomach by placing one hand on the proximal shoulder and the other on the hip and rolling his body away from you.

7. Adjust the patient's body alignment.

    a. Turn the head to one side.

    b. Position the arms for comfort.

    c. Place a pillow under the abdomen to relieve pressure on the breasts.

    d. Align the feet and avoid hyperextension by (1) extending the feet over the mattress or (2) supporting the ankles with a pillow.

8. Use protective aids to reduce pressure, as required.

9. Provide for his comfort and safety; inform him when you will return.

10. Chart the procedure.

MOVING THE PATIENT TOWARD THE HEAD OF THE BED

1. Wash your hands.

2. Identify the patient.

3. Explain the procedure to the patient.

4. Adjust the bed to working height.

5. Instruct the patient as to how he can assist by:

   a. flexing both knees, placing the soles of his feet on the mattress;

   b. grasping the headboard with his arms;

   c. on command, pulling with his arms and pushing with his feet.

6. Initiate the procedure by:

   a. supporting his head;

   b. supporting his hips to assist in movement;

   c. coordinating the patient's efforts with your own.

7. Check his alignment and support.

8. Use protective aids to reduce pressure.

9. Provide for the patient's comfort; indicate when you will return.

10. Chart the procedure.

UNIT 8

POST-TEST

MULTIPLE CHOICE: Select the one best answer.

_____ 1. The force called pressure is the result of

     a. congestion with redness of the skin.

     b. having bony prominences.

     c. weight pressing down on another object.

     d. lack of friction when moving.

_____ 2. Prolonged pressure on the sacrum causes the skin, blood vessels, and muscles to

     a. become compact and flattened out.

     b. swell up and become larger.

     c. turn pale in color.

     d. receive too much oxygen and too many nutrients.

_____ 3. One organ of the body is quickly affected by pressure from lying in one position for a long period of time. This organ is

     a. the kidney.

     b. the stomach.

     c. the brain.

     d. the lung.

_____ 4. The nurse should see that the position of the bed patient is changed, at the minimum, how often?

     a. Once every shift.

     b. Every 2 hours.

     c. Every hour.

     d. Every ½ hour.

_____ 5. Jane has an injury to her arm and she has kept her elbow flexed continually for several days. This flexion could result in

     a. a decubitus.

     b. a contracture.

     c. pressure.

     d. swelling.

Mr. Rose had a stroke several days ago and is now paralyzed on the right side of his body. When positioning him in good alignment, you place a hand roll in his right hand.

_____ 6. The purpose of the hand roll is

     a. to encourage him to exercise his hand and fingers.

     b. to keep the palm of his hand warm and dry.

     c. to keep the fingers and the thumb flexed.

     d. to extend the fingers and keep the thumb in opposition.

_____7. A footboard is placed at the end of the mattress on Mr. Rose's bed. The purpose of the footboard is to

    a. keep the mattress from sliding toward the foot of the bed.

    b. support Mr. Rose's feet when lying in bed.

    c. keep the top bedding off the foot end of the mattress.

    d. prevent muscle strain in Mr. Rose's back.

_____8. All but one of the following are reasons for using aids in positioning the patient. Which one does not apply?

    a. To provide support of a body part.

    b. To improve elimination of wastes.

    c. To relieve pressure.

    d. To maintain the body in alignment.

POST-TEST ANNOTATED ANSWER SHEET

1.	c	(p. 107)	5.	b	(p. 106)
2.	a	(pp. 107–108)	6.	d	(p. 104)
3.	d	(p. 107)	7.	b	(p. 105)
4.	b	(p. 107)	8.	b	(p. 101)

UNIT 8

Unit 9

PATIENT MOVEMENT AND AMBULATION

I. DIRECTIONS TO THE STUDENT

Proceed through the lesson using this workbook as your guide. You must practice the procedures related to patient movements and ambulation in the skill laboratory with a student partner or other person. After the completion of the lesson and your practice of the procedures, arrange with your instructor to take the post-test for this lesson.

You will need the following items for your study and practice:

1. Projector and screen.

2. Film strip: Range of Motion, (BN-3 series, Trainex Corporation, Garden Grove, California 94642).

3. A robe.

4. Slippers or shoes.

5. The post-test.

Please read the following paragraphs carefully. They will tell you exactly what you will be expected to know and how you will be expected to assist the patient in his movements and ambulation. If you feel that you have the necessary skills, discuss this with your instructor. Then arrange to take the performance test consisting of a written test and demonstrations.

II. GENERAL PERFORMANCE OBJECTIVE

Upon completing this lesson, demonstrate your ability to assist the patient (or another person) to move his various joints through the range-of-motion exercises, to dangle his feet at the side of the bed, to stand, and to walk in a safe manner without causing additional pain or injury.

III. SPECIFIC PERFORMANCE OBJECTIVES

When this lesson is completed, you will be able to:

1. Assess the patient's physical and mental condition regarding aspects that may interfere with his ability to exercise his joints or to ambulate, and your own ability or limitations to carry out the procedures.

2. Explain to the patient who has limited or no motion in the joints on one side of his body the need for exercising all of the joints. Show him how to exercise the joints on his unaffected side, and carry out the range-of-motion exercises for the affected joints. In performing the range-of-motion exercises, you will:

    a. Provide support for the body part that is distal or away from the joint being exercised.

    b. Avoid forcing movement in the joint to the extent that it causes pain.

3. Assist the patient in bed to dangle his feet over the side of the bed by positioning him on the proximal side of the bed; bringing him to a sitting position; pivoting his

130

body; and swinging his feet over the side of the bed in smooth, flowing motions, using principles of good body alignment and movement.

4. Assist the patient to stand, to balance, and to walk safely, using principles of good body alignment, balance, and movement.

5. Assist the patient (whether a youth or an adult) who has lost his balance and begun to fall: grasp him firmly, slow the rate of descent, and ease him slowly to the floor or ground. This will prevent injury both to the patient and to yourself by utilizing the principles of gravity.

IV. VOCABULARY

Some words used in this lesson that may be unfamiliar to you are listed below. You will need to remember the meaning of these words for this and subsequent lessons.

active exercise—movement performed by the person himself without assistance from another.

axilla (plural is axillae)—armpit.

circumduction—the circular motion of a limb or body part in which the limb forms the side of a cone, and the joint nearest the body forms the apex or tip of the cone.

infiltration—seepage of fluid into the skin tissue that causes blanching (turning pale) and swelling.

pace—the distance covered in one step, or the number of steps per minute.

passive exercise—the moving of parts of a person's body by another person.

physiological changes—alterations in body function due to disease or injury.

pneumonia, hypostatic—an inflammation of the lungs caused by lack of movement, by remaining in the same position; a common complication of being in bed for a long period; can also occur rapidly following surgical operation.

pronation—the rotation of the palm of the hand so that it is facing downward (thumbs pointed medially).

rehabilitation—the process of restoring to a good condition, or an improvement in the state of one's efficiency or health.

rotation—the process of turning, or movement about an axis.

spasm—an involuntary, sudden movement or muscle contraction.

supination—the rotation of the palm of the hand so that it is facing upward toward the head (thumbs pointed laterally).

thrombus (plural is thrombi)—a blood clot that obstructs a blood vessel.

unconscious—the state of being insensible or without conscious experiences; in deep stupor; unresponding.

vertebra (plural is vertebrae)—the name for each of the 33 bones forming the spinal backbone in man.

Question 1.   If you have completed the lessons that were prerequisites for this one, you have already learned other important terms used here. As a review of these terms, please match the word and its meaning from the lists below.

_____ 1. proximal   a. toward the midline

_____ 2. abduction   b. a sudden circulatory accident

_____ 3. extension   c. on the near side

_____ 4. contracture   d. to bend

_____ 5. flexion   e. a sudden strong contraction

_____ 6. stroke   f. on the far side

_____ 7. distal   g. permanent shortening of a muscle

_____ 8. adduction   h. away from the midline

                             i. to straighten

U
N
I
T
9

ITEM 1.   IMPORTANCE OF MOVEMENT

Can you imagine what it would be like not to be able to move at all? Without movement, you would be a prisoner in your own body. How would you feel if you were unable to scratch your nose when it itched? Or unable to blink your eyelid when a speck of dirt irritated your eye? Or to walk, play, or participate in the many activities that make up your everyday life?

Movement is so important to the human being that most of our infancy and early childhood is devoted to learning and coordinating body movements. This task takes years to master. The infant must learn to focus his eyes, follow an object with his eyes, hold up his head, balance his body, and coordinate his hand and eye movements before he can learn the more complex movements involved in sitting, walking, grasping a cup, catching a ball, or dressing himself. As the child grows, he learns to perform progressively complex movements.

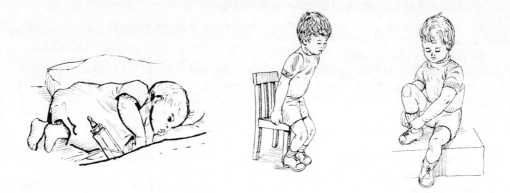

The health and well-being of a person is related to his ability to move his body and its various parts. Movement promotes more efficient functioning of all body parts. For example, movement enhances the firmness, tone, and elasticity of the muscles, and promotes the elimination of waste products from the body. It is essential for the strength and hardness of the bones, helps maintain the blood pressure and efficient blood circulation, stimulates the appetite, and reduces fatigue through good posture and change of position.

When he is injured or ill, the patient's ability to move part or all of his body may be impaired. In such situations, the patient must have exercise in order to regain his health. When he is unable to move by himself to get the exercise he needs, the nurse must move and exercise his body parts. It is only in recent years that emphasis has been placed on range-of-motion exercises as a basic nursing skill. You will meet experienced nurses who know the importance of exercise for patients with limited movement, but who may not know the range-of-motion exercises.

Question 2.   List at least four ways in which exercise promotes the functioning of the body.

a. _____   b. _____

c. _____   d. _____ .

Question 3.   _____ is essential to the well-being and health of the patient.

ITEM 2.   HOW DOES THE BODY MOVE?

The muscular and skeletal systems of the body provide support for the body structures, the means for movement and locomotion, and protection for the soft tissues of the body. The skeletal system is composed of a framework of bones. All movement of the body occurs through the action of the muscles on the skeletal bones. Muscles are attached to the bone by connective tissue, and usually work in pairs.

The movement of bones by the muscles occurs at the joints. A *joint* is a junction between (or an articulation of) two or more bones. Joints are classified according to the amount of movement they permit. A *fixed* or *immovable* joint allows no movement of the bones, e.g., the bones of the skull. A *slightly movable* joint allows limited movement; examples are the spinal vertebrae and the joints of the pelvis and sacrum. *Freely movable* joints are the most common and can be found in the extremities and the lower jaw.

Joints allow movements that are classified as flexion, extension, abduction, adduction, circumduction, and rotation. *Flexion* bends the part by decreasing the angle between the parts. *Extension* straightens the part by increasing the angle. In *abduction*, the body part moves away from the midline of the body, and in *adduction* the part moves toward the midline so that the distance from the midline is decreased. *Circumduction* occurs when a part is moved like the side of a cone in a circular manner, such as when you swing your arm in a circle. The circular or turning motion is called *rotation* and occurs when you turn your head from side to side. When the palm of the hand or the sole of the foot is rotated to an upward position, it is called *supination*. When the palm or the sole is in a downward position or toward the back of the body, it is called *pronation*. Supination of the foot may be referred to as dorsiflexion; pronation of the foot may be referred to as plantar flexion.

The amount of movement allowed at the joint is termed its range of motion. Forcing movement beyond this range of motion will cause pain.

Question 4. Movement is the result of action by _____ .

Question 5. Movement occurs at the _____ of the body.

Question 6. Please indicate in the adjoining sketches the type of movement allowed in the parts of the body, i.e., whether it is fixed, slightly movable, or freely movable.

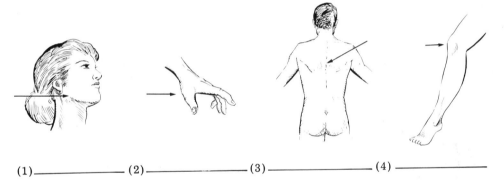

(1)_____ (2)_____ (3)_____ (4)_____

ITEM 3. HOW DO CONTRACTURES DEVELOP?

As stated before, muscles usually work in pairs. In the extremities (arms and legs), the flexor muscles are strong muscles that contract, or shorten, to move the part. The opposing muscle of the pair is the *extensor*, which is lengthened when the flexor muscle contracts, and which will straighten the part when it contracts.

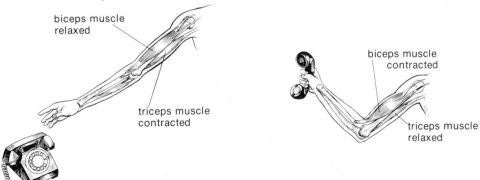

biceps muscle relaxed

triceps muscle contracted

biceps muscle contracted

triceps muscle relaxed

The prolonged flexion of muscles may result in common deformities that are painful and unattractive and that limit movement. These deformities are called *contractures*. A permanent contracture of the muscles "freezes" (or locks) the joint so that the part cannot be extended. This results from the inability of the extensor muscle to overcome the strength of its flexor partner.

Contractures can occur in a period of less than three weeks and result in permanent deformity of the joint. Those who develop contractures are people with a severe limitation of their movement involving one or more joints. Conditions that cause limited movement include fractures, severe burns, paralysis following a stroke, serious injuries, and states of coma. Contractures most frequently develop in the joints in the shoulder, elbow, wrist, hand, hip, knee, and ankle (where it causes foot drop).

Exercise and putting the joint through the range of motion several times daily can prevent contractures. If the patient is unable to do this, it is essential for the nurse to take over this activity. Once a contracture has occurred, the normal, full use of the joint will seldom, if ever, be completely regained. Even slight improvement in the extent of joint movement may require months or years of intensive, often painful treatment.

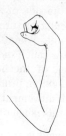

Contracture of the hand and elbow. The joints are rigid and can only be moved slightly.

Question 7.   The powerful muscles that contract and bend a part are called _____

_____ .

Question 8.   Contractures are caused by the muscular action of _____ .

Question 9.   Permanent "freezing" of a joint has been known to occur in _____ time.

ITEM 4.   PASSIVE AND ACTIVE EXERCISE

During illness, the patient needs some exercise. When he is unable to move a part of his body himself, it becomes the responsibility of the nurse worker to move it for him, unless there are medical orders not to do so. The movement performed by the nurse worker or therapist with no help from the patient is called *passive exercise*. However, the patient should be encouraged to perform the movement himself when at all possible; this is called *active exercise*.

Passive and active exercise should begin as soon as possible after onset of the patient's illness. Within a day or so of the time he becomes unable to move or exercise his joints himself, you should begin a program of passive exercises. As the patient improves, he should be involved in planning his own exercise program and be shown how to exercise his joints himself. The best time for the patient to exercise his joints through the *range of motion* is at bath time. Range-of-motion exercise should be done at least once every 8 hours, and some joints may need to be exercised every hour or so in order to keep them flexible.

The patient who has had IV's (intravenous injections) running in his arm for more than 4 to 6 hours will often have shoulder discomfort and soreness caused by the necessity of keeping his arm still. Range-of-motion exercise for the shoulder often relieves this discomfort, but must be performed with extreme care if the IV is still running.

You must take care to see that the tubing is long enough to permit movement, that the needle is not dislodged from the vein, and that the fluid does not infiltrate (seep into) the tissues. Notify your team leader immediately about any problem with the IV. The movement must be slow and smooth, and the arm must be supported. The movements of lateral and upward abduction and adduction are the most beneficial, followed with light massage to stimulate the circulation to the shoulder.

Question 10. An unconscious patient has been admitted to the hospital following a head injury in an accident. He is still unconscious the next day when you arrive to give him morning care and a bath. His vital signs have stabilized. What joints should be exercised? _____ . When should the exercises be started? _____ .

Question 11. When the patient needs the assistance of the nurse to exercise the joint, it is called _____exercise. When he is able to do it himself, it is called _____ exercise.

ITEM 5. ROLE OF THE REHABILITATION TEAM

The patient who has limited movement in one or more of his joints may have many emotional needs related to his inability to move. He may be concerned about his dependence on others for the help he needs; he may also be depressed about the nature of his disability, which could require a long convalescence; and he may have feelings of uncertainty or fears of being unable to resume his normal activities. You will need to show patience and understanding by accepting his right to feel as he does, but you must emphasize what can be done and encourage his cooperation in exercising, moving about, and using the abilities he still has.

Often the patient will receive care and services toward his rehabilitation from others, such as a physical therapist, occupational therapist, speech pathologist, his family, and, of course, his physician. The goal of all these experts is improvement in the patient's condition. The physical therapist provides treatment aimed at restoring the use of muscles and helping the disabled person to relearn how to perform essential activities such as walking or climbing stairs. Exercise, heat, water, and massage are commonly used in physical therapy. Occupational therapists concentrate on helping the patients regain the use of the upper extremities so that they can carry out their daily living and recreational activities. Speech and hearing therapists work with patients who have difficulties communicating as a result of physical or mental disorders. You should learn as much as possible about the therapy recommended for your patients, as well as the short and long-term goals of the therapy. Then you can better coordinate your care of this patient with that scheduled by other members of the rehabilitation team.

As a nurse worker, you are a very important member of the team because you will be with the patient for long periods of time during his illness.

Question 12. One of your patients is a man aged 49 who had a stroke several days ago. He is now conscious, but has slurred speech and is paralyzed on his left side. He had done plumbing work, and two of his five children are still in school. Now he seems irritable and upset. What might be some of the reasons for his feelings?

_____

_____ .

Question 13. Some of the persons who would be involved in the rehabilitation of the patient described above are:

a. _____ b. _____ c. _____

d. _____ e. _____ f. _____ .

ITEM 6. INSTRUCTIONS FOR VIEWING FILM

You are now ready to view the film, which shows how to put the various joints of the body through the range-of-motion exercises. You will note that several types of movements

UNIT 9

occur at a joint. For instance, the muscles acting on the shoulder joint allow for all types of movements — abduction, adduction, flexion, extension, hyperextension, circumduction, and rotation. The range-of-motion exercises for this joint include all of these movements.

Turn on the projector and the sound system. Watch the film and listen to the narrative description. When the film is ended, turn off the projector and the audio.

Question 14. Did you notice how the nurse supported the patient's arm while exercising the shoulder? How she supported the forearm when she put the shoulder and the elbow through the range of motion? The lower leg, when ranging the

ankle and foot? _____ . If your answer is no, turn on the projector and run the film again.

Question 15. The thumb joint is extremely important. According to the film, what essential movements occur in this joint?

_____

_____ .

ITEM 7.   RANGE–OF–MOTION EXERCISES FOR THE STUDENT (ACTIVE)

It is now time to see how well you understand how to do the range-of-motion exercises. Assume a standing position and carry out these movements. You will be performing active exercise.

1. Abduction and adduction of the shoulder: Raise your arm forward, up over your head, and return it to your side. Now, raise your arm to the side so it is straight with the shoulder, and return it to your side. Both exercises moved the arm away (abduction) from the midline and back again (adduction).

2. Flexion and extension of the elbow: Bend your elbow, touch your shoulder with your finger tips, and straighten your arm. Flexor muscles bring body parts closer together and extensors straighten out body segments.

3. Rotation of the shoulder: External (outward) rotation — flex your elbow, bring your elbow up to the level of your shoulder, and reach the back of your neck with your fingers. Internal (inward) rotation — flex your elbow, draw your arm across your chest, and place your hand on your distal shoulder.

4. Flexion and extension of the spine: Reach down, try to touch your toes without flexing your knees, and then straighten up. Can you feel the muscles working in your back? Put your hand against the small of your back as you bend over and straighten up. You will be able to feel the muscles move.

5. Abduction and adduction of the thumb and fingers: Spread your fingers and thumb far apart like a fan (abduction), then bring them together again (adduction).

6. Flexion and extension of the thumb and fingers: Flex your hand at the knuckles, keeping the fingers straight; then bend the fingers and thumb to make a fist, and straighten them again.

7. Rotation of the neck: Turn your head to the left side, then to the right side.

Lie down in a supine position (flat on your back) and practice these movements of the lower extremities.

1. Abduction and adduction of the hip: With your legs straight and toes pointed upward, move a leg to one side as far as possible (abduction), and return it to the original position (adduction).

2. Flexion and extension of hip and knee: Bend your knee (flexion) and bring it up toward your chest as far as possible, and then straighten your leg to the original position (extension).

3. Rotation of the hip: To rotate externally, or outward, flex your hip and knee so that your knee is parallel to the bed, and turn your foot outward. To rotate internally, flex your hip and knee so that your knee is elevated and parallel to the bed, and turn your foot inward.

4. Flexion and extension of ankles: Bend your toes upward as far as possible so that your foot is supinated (dorsiflexion), then extend your toes downward as far as possible so that your foot is pronated (plantar flexion).

Question 16. Which of these movements would you use to do the following?

        a. Brush your teeth? _____ .

        b. Wash the back of your neck and shoulders? _____ .

        c. Comb your hair? _____ .

ITEM 8. RANGE-OF-MOTION EXERCISES FOR THE PATIENT (PASSIVE)

In the skill laboratory with another student or someone else playing the part of a patient who is paralyzed on his left side, you will provide passive range-of-motion exercise to the joints of his neck, left shoulder, arm, hand, hip, knee, ankle, and foot while supporting the dependent part of the extremity, and avoiding range-of-motion exercise beyond the point of pain.

Important Steps	Key Points
1. Wash your hands, approach and identify the patient, explain the procedure, and enlist his cooperation.	One of the best times to do range-of-motion exercises is during the bath. Explain the need to exercise his joints to keep them flexible and prevent contractures, and how you will assist him. Encourage the patient to plan his exercise program — the time and the amount of exercise — and to learn to actively exercise the unaffected joints on his right side.
2. Prepare the patient.	If the bed is an adjustable high-low type, place it in the high position so you can assist the patient without stooping. Move the patient so that his paralyzed side is on the proximal side of the bed. This will keep you from straining when you reach to help him exercise. Use the bath blanket or top bedding to drape the patient. This leaves his arm and leg free for movement, prevents exposure of the rest of the body, and ensures the patient's modesty. If he is wearing pajamas, no drape may be needed except for added warmth.
3. Perform passive range-of-motion exercises of patient's neck and left upper extremity.	Use principles of good body alignment, balance, and movement while you carry out the procedure. Repeat each exercise a minimum of three times.

UNIT 9

Important Steps

Key Points

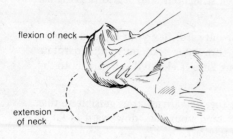

Flex and extend the patient's neck by supporting his head in your hands, bringing his head forward until the chin touches the chest, and returning his head to the pillow. Rotate his neck by supporting his head with your hands and turning it toward his right shoulder, then toward his left shoulder.

Exercise the patient's left shoulder and elbow by cupping his elbow with one hand and grasping his wrist with your other hand. Bring his arm up straight, flex his elbow, and move his arm up over his head. Move slowly and gently to avoid hurting the patient. This exercise involves the movements of flexion and extension of both the shoulder and elbow. Return his arm to his side.

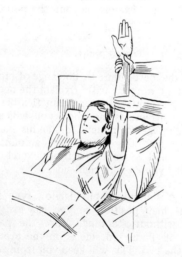

Extension of shoulder and elbow.

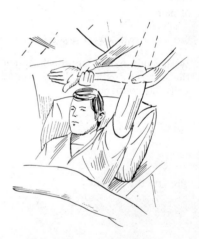

Flexion of elbow.

Rotate the patient's shoulder internally by placing one hand on his left arm above the elbow and holding his hand with your other hand. Lift his arm and move it across his chest toward the other arm. Then return his arm to its original position. To rotate the shoulder externally, place one hand on his arm above the elbow, and hold his hand with your other hand. Move his arm out from the side in abduction, flex his elbow, and move his arm over his head without causing him pain. Return his arm to the original position.

Important Steps	Key Points

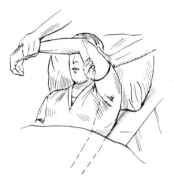

Internal rotation of shoulder.

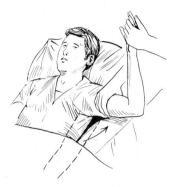

External rotation of shoulder.

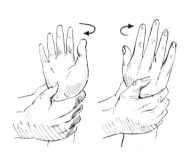

Rotation of wrist.

Rotate the wrist by grasping the patient's wrist in both of your hands and turning the palm of his hand toward his face for supination, and then toward his feet for pronation.

Hold the patient's wrist with one hand, and the palm of his hand with your other hand, keeping his fingers straight. Hyperextend his wrist by bending his hand backward; extend it by straightening his hand; and flex it by bending his hand forward and closing the fingers to make a fist. With one hand still holding the patient's hand, flex his thumb into the palm of his hand with your other hand, then extend his thumb away from his hand, and rotate the thumb in a circular movement.

Contractures of the upper extremities most often occur in flexion position (internal rotation of shoulder, flexion of elbow, wrist, and hand).

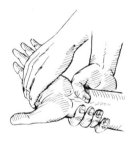

Hyperextension of wrist.

4. Perform passive exercises of the patient's lower left extremity.

Flex and extend the hip and knee by placing one hand under his left knee and cupping his heel in your other hand. Lift his leg up, bend his knee, and move his leg toward his chest as far as it will go without causing pain. Then straighten his leg by lifting his foot upward, and lower his leg to the bed.

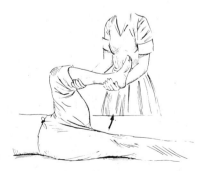

Flexion of knee and hip.

Important Steps   **Key Points**

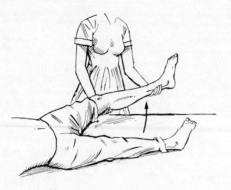

Abduction of hip.

To abduct and adduct the hip joint, place one hand under the patient's knee and the other hand under his heel. Keep his leg straight, and slowly move it toward you. Then return his leg to the original position.

The hip joint is rotated in the following manner: Place one hand under the patient's left knee, the other under his heel; lift his leg and flex the knee at right angles. Without moving the knee, pull his foot slowly toward you for external rotation, then move his foot away from you and over his other leg for internal rotation.

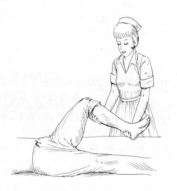

External rotation of hip.

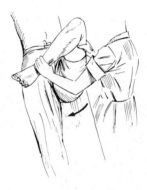

Internal rotation of hip.

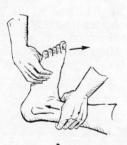

Dorsiflexion

To flex and extend the ankle, hold the patient's heel in one hand and place your other hand over his foot. Pull the foot forward and push down on the heel at the same time to flex the foot in supination (dorsiflexion). Then push on the foot to extend it in a "point-the-toes" position, and push up on the heel at the same time to hyperextend the foot in pronation (plantar flexion).

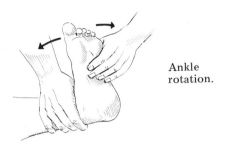

Ankle
rotation.

To rotate the ankle, hold his ankle with one hand; with the other hand, turn his whole foot outward, then turn it inward. The patient can be taught and should be encouraged to use his stronger extremity (arm or leg) to move the weaker extremity in the range-of-motion exercises to flex, extend, abduct, and rotate the part.

5. Provide for the patient's comfort.

Upon completing the range-of-motion exercises, adjust the patient's pillows and the bed as he may desire for comfort. Be sure that his body remains in proper alignment.

6. Report and record as appropriate.

Report to the team leader, or the nurse in charge, that the exercises have been carried out. Report and record how well the patient tolerated the range-of-motion exercises, and any changes in the amount of motion, or in the patient's condition, such as increased pain, spasms of muscles, difficulty in breathing, change of color of skin. Charting example:

7:10 A.M.   Range-of-motion exercises performed as part of A.M. care. Joints move more easily today, through the entire range. Experienced no pain. States he will try to do exercises by himself.   J. Jones, SN

UNIT 9

ITEM 9.   EFFECTS OF PROLONGED BED REST

The patient needs rest to facilitate the repair of damage by injury or disease. When at bed rest, the patient can use more of his energy to combat the causes of the damage and to rebuild his defenses. However, total rest or prolonged bed rest also produces harmful effects when the body does not receive enough exercise to promote good functioning of its systems. The patient's body at total rest undergoes physiological changes in body chemistry and sometimes develops hypostatic pneumonia, pressure sores, contractures, constipation, urinary retention, insomnia, diminished appetite, and tendency to form thrombi, or blood clots. Good nursing helps combat some of these changes, but the most important measure is early ambulation of the patient.

The patient who has been in bed for several days or more, or who may have had surgery just a few hours before, will need your assistance the first time he gets up. Even minor surgery produces circulatory, chemical, and emotional disturbances in the patient. When the physician has written an order allowing the patient to get up, the first step toward ambulation is for the patient to "dangle his feet" at the bedside. In dangling his feet, the patient has time to adjust to the change in position, recover from any dizziness, and adjust to a need for deeper breathing.

Question 17.   One advantage of bed rest for the patient with an injury or a disease is _____

_____ .

Question 18.   Which of the following are some of the hazards or dangers of bed rest? Place a check mark in front of your answers.

____a. Postoperative pain   ____b. Blood clots

____c. Dizziness   ____d. Pneumonia, hypostatic

____e. Altered body chemistries   ____f. Contractures

ITEM 10.   ASSISTING THE PATIENT TO DANGLE HIS LEGS

In the skill laboratory, practice the steps in the procedure of assisting a patient to dangle his legs at the side of the bed. One of your fellow students, or some other person, will be needed to play the part of the patient.

Important Steps	Key Points
1. Wash your hands, approach and identify the patient, explain the procedure, and enlist his cooperation.	The patient may be apprehensive or fearful about sitting up and dangling his feet. He may fear pain or weakness. Reassure him by explaining that you will assist and remain with him, and that dangling his feet is progress toward early ambulation, which will improve his circulation and breathing, and help him to regain his strength.
2. Position the patient.	Move the patient to the proximal (near) side of the bed. If the patient has limited movement in an arm or leg, you should work on that side so that it will be on the proximal side of the bed. You will not need to reach or strain as much since the patient may be able to help move his stronger extremity from the distal side of the bed.
3. Adjust the position of the bed.	If it is an adjustable high-low bed, place it in a low position. Elevate the head of the bed 45° or more, if possible. Raising the head of the bed allows the patient gradually to get used to the change in position, and makes it easier for you to bring him to a sitting position. Lower the siderail on the proximal side, if it is being used.
4. Assist the patient to sit at the side of the bed and dangle his feet. 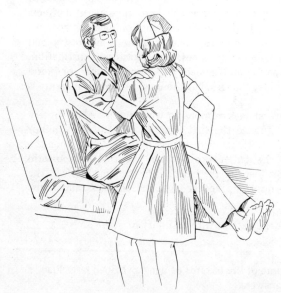	Place one hand on the patient's proximal shoulder, and the other hand under his distal axilla. Have him hold onto your shoulders with his hands, and pull him up to a sitting position. Continuing to support him with your hand on his shoulder, have him brace himself with his hands on the bed. Reach behind his distal knee with your other hand, and swing his legs off the bed while pivoting his body in that direction at the same time. Your movements should be smooth and flowing, not jerky. Be sure to use the principles of good movement by standing with your feet apart to provide a broad base, flexing your knees and hips, and keeping your back straight.
5. Provide for the patient's comfort.	Assist the patient to put on his robe, slippers, or shoes, or place a blanket over his lap to prevent exposure of his body and to provide

Important Steps	Key Points
	extra warmth. Many patients will feel chilly after getting out of a warm bed. The patient's feet should be flat on the floor, or on a footstool for proper support. Observe him closely to see how well he tolerates sitting up and dangling his feet. If the patient is doing well, you could fluff up his pillows and replace them.
6. Assist the patient to return to bed.	At the end of the specified period for dangling, or if the patient is unable to tolerate sitting up and dangling his feet, help him to get back into bed. Remove his robe, slippers or shoes, or the lap blanket. Support the patient at his shoulders with one hand, and with the other hand under both ankles, swing his legs up onto the bed while pivoting his body at the same time so that he is facing the foot of the bed. Ease the patient back onto the bed in a supine position.
7. Provide for the patient's comfort.	Adjust the top covers of the bed by pulling them up to the level of his axillae or over the shoulders. Adjust the pillows and the position of the bed as he may desire. Raise the siderails, if being used. Leave all signals nearby.
8. Report and record as appropriate.	Report to the team leader, or the nurse in charge, that the procedure has been carried out. Report and record how well the patient tolerated dangling his feet, and any such adverse effects as extreme weakness, dizziness, profuse perspiration (diaphoresis), cold or clammy skin, change in color, pain, and so forth. Charting example:
	9:30 A.M. Patient dangled for first time. Became cold, clammy, and pale. Returned to supine position. P88, R20.
	J. Jones, RN

U
N
I
T
9

ITEM 11. MECHANICS OF WALKING

How do you walk? Most of us would reply that you stand up and step forward on one foot, then on the other foot, and that is how you walk. We will now consider the mechanics of walking in more detail in order to assist the patient to walk.

Posture is important in walking. The body should be in good alignment with the head up, shoulders back, spine straight, buttocks tucked in, knees slightly flexed, and feet slightly apart with the toes pointed forward. Poor body alignment will produce strain on the muscles, loss of balance, poor coordination, and a jerky and jolting rhythm with unnecessary motion which wastes energy. Good posture in walking allows a more attractive and energetic appearance, as well as the more efficient functioning of the parts involved.

In the walking cycle, the person stands with both feet on the ground in the double stance position. The body weight is shifted to one foot in the single stance phase as the other foot moves forward in the swing phase. The swing phase is completed as the heel of the foot strikes the ground. In the swing phase, the body twists inward slightly. To counteract this twisting movement, the person swings his arm on the opposite side. The single stance phase includes shifting the body weight to the heel that is striking the ground, and moving the weight along the outer edge of the foot to the ball of the foot, and then to the toes, as they "push off" in the swing phase for the next step.

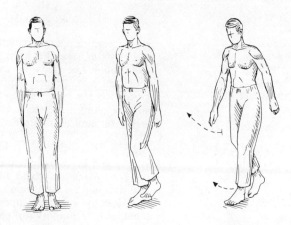

Double stance.   Single stance.   Swing.

The distance covered in each step is called a *pace*. "Pace" may also refer to the number of steps taken per minute. A normal pace for walking is 70 to 100 steps a minute, and a fast pace would be over 120 steps per minute. Most patients will walk at the slow pace of less then 70 steps per minute until they recover their physical strength.

In assisting the patient to walk, you should attempt to have him walk as normally as possible. In other words, he should stand and walk with his body in good alignment, or in the best alignment possible for him to maintain. If he has pain from a new operative site, he may be unable to stand erect; however, encourage him to stand and walk as erectly as possible. Patients are often fearful that their stitches will burst if they stand straight. Reassure him that this cannot happen because of the strong suture (surgical stitching material) that was used. When the patient steps forward in the swing and single stance phases, he may need your assistance to balance and support his body weight. He should be encouraged to step normally, striking the ground with the heel first, transferring his weight to the ball of his foot, and then "pushing off" with his toes, instead of shuffling, sliding forward, or letting his toes strike the ground first.

Question 19.   The most stable phase of the walking cycle is the _____ .

Question 20.   In walking, a person swings the arm that is opposite the forward-moving foot

in order to _____ .

Question 21.   Which portion of the foot should strike the ground first when walking?

_____ .

ITEM 12. ASSISTING THE PATIENT TO WALK

In the skill laboratory, practice helping the patient to walk and use the principles that are related to body alignment, balance, and movement. Ask another person to play the part of the patient for this practice session.

Important Steps	Key Points
1. Wash your hands, approach and identify the patient, explain the procedure, and enlist his cooperation.	If he has had prolonged bed rest, the patient may be apprehensive about walking because of weakness or fear of falling. If he has had recent surgery, he may fear pain or pulling his stitches loose. Reassure the patient that you will assist him and remain with him. Show how the incision can be supported by placing a hand along the side of it. Other patients may be so

Important Steps	Key Points
	eager to walk that they may overestimate their ability and strength. You will need to caution this person against overdoing; instruct him to walk slowly, and gradually to increase the distance in walking.
2. Position the bed.	If he is in an adjustable high-low bed, place the bed in the low position. Provide a footstool if it is a high bed. Elevate the head of the bed 30° or more to make it easier to bring the patient to a sitting position. Fold the top bedding back toward the foot of the bed.
3. Assist the patient to a dangling feet position at the side of the bed.	Follow the instructions for dangling given earlier in this lesson.
4. Prepare the patient.	Assist the patient to put on his robe and preferably hard-soled shoes. Bedroom slippers usually have soft soles, which provide little support for the foot and frequently cause slipping on waxed hospital floors.
5. Help the patient to stand.	Have him place his feet firmly on the floor or footstool and put his hands on the mattress to help push himself up. Place your hand under the patient's proximal axilla, and pull him up to a standing position. Stand at his side and hold on to his arm or shoulder to support him as he stands and balances himself before stepping down from the footstool or beginning to walk.
6. Assist the patient to walk.	Check his posture and encourage him to walk with his head up, eyes looking forward, and back straight. Help support him by walking at his side.
	a. For *minimal support*, the patient holds your elbow or hand with his hand;
	b. For *moderate support*, hold the patient's arm with your hand.
	c. To provide *more than moderate support* (to prevent the patient's loss of balance or falling), you should have another person help you so that support can be provided at each side.
7. Assist the patient to return to bed.	Have the patient walk to the side of the bed, pivot so that his back is to the edge of the bed, and reach for the mattress with his hands for support. With your hand under his axilla, help him to a sitting position. Remove his robe and

UNIT 9

Important Steps	Key Points
	shoes. Help him swing his feet onto the bed as in the .instructions given for dangling. Use a footstool as necessary.
8. Provide for the patient's comfort.	Adjust the top bedding and pull it up to his axillae or over his shoulders. Adjust the pillows and the position of the bed as the patient may desire. Make sure his body is in good alignment.
9. Report and record as appropriate.	Report to the team leader or the nurse in charge that the patient has been helped to walk. Record the length of time the patient walked, how well he tolerated ambulation, and any changes in the patient's condition, such as complaints of pain, profuse perspiration, dizziness, headache, or difficulty in breathing. Charting example:
	10:15 A.M. Patient ambulated the full length of the hall. Tolerated well. Returned to bed quite tired. J. Jones, RN

ITEM 13.   PREVENTION OF PATIENT FALLS

Patient falls are the most common accidents that occur in the hospital, the extended-care facility, or the home. A frequent question that occurs when the health worker assists patients to ambulate is "What do you do when the patient starts to fall?" *What* should you do?

The physical and environmental hazards that contribute to falls should be eliminated as much as possible. Anything spilled on the floor should be wiped up promptly, and foreign objects should be picked up. During the mopping or waxing of floors, the area should be posted with a warning sign, and preferably, roped off so that no one walks on the wet surface. Floor wax should be of the non-slip type. Electric cords should be shortened and not allowed to lie loose on the floors. Small objects or equipment should be removed from areas where patients walk. To assure additional safety for patients, siderails should be used on the bed for restless, aged, confused, or sedated patients. The patient's ability to balance and support his weight when ambulating should be evaluated, and adequate assistance or mechanical aids provided.

In spite of all these precautions, the patient may lose his balance when walking, and begin to fall. The help that you can provide will depend on the size of the patient, whether his center of gravity is still within his base of support, and also on your own size.

Question 22.   The most common type of accident among patients in the hospital is _____

_____ .

ITEM 14.   WHY PATIENTS FALL AND WHAT TO DO WHEN THEY FALL

Basically, there are two reasons why a standing person will fall: (1) as the result of the *collapse* of his lower extremities, or (2) through the *loss of his balance*. In the collapse type of fall, the muscles of the legs lack the strength needed to support the body weight. The extensor muscles of the knees give way to gravitational pull so that the knees "buckle under" the person, and he falls. In the collapsing fall, the safest method of assistance is to try to "break the fall" and ease the patient slowly to the floor. You should be walking at the patient's side or slightly behind him when helping him to walk, so that you can grasp him firmly at the wrist or under his axilla and ease him down to the floor if he begins to fall. It is necessary for you to keep your body in good alignment, with your line of gravity within your base of support, and to lower your own body by stooping correctly.

Remember that stability is maintained when one's line of gravity and center of gravity are within the base of support. When the patient loses his balance and begins to fall, his line of gravity and center of gravity are outside his base of support.

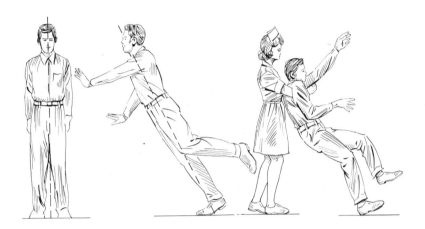

Stable balance.   Loss of balance.   Breaking patient's fall.

Unless you can bring the patient's line of gravity and center of gravity within his base of support, he will continue to fall. In order to help him to regain his balance, you need to be large enough and strong enough to overcome the force of the patient's body weight moving downward. With an adult patient, once he has started to fall, the amount of force that is needed is more than you can safely provide. You should then attempt to break his fall, slow his rate of descent, and ease him to the floor in order to avoid possible injury to him or to yourself. Remember, it is easier to guide the patient slowly down to the floor than it is to lift him up.

You may have an urge to try to hold up or to lift the falling patient. If you act on this impulse, you risk losing your own balance and falling, or straining or injuring your muscles. The most common disabling injury of hospital workers is muscle strain, usually of the lower back. Many of these injuries could be prevented by the use of good body alignment, proper movement, and safer methods of work.

Any patient who has fallen, or who has been eased to the floor, should be examined by a doctor or a nurse for possible injury before being moved. You should stay with the patient, comfort and reassure him, and have someone go for additional help to get the patient up or return him to bed after he has been examined. (Remember to protect the patient's modesty.)

Question 23.   When a person loses his balance and begins to fall, his center of gravity is: (Select the best answer.)

    a.   too high from his base of support.

    b.   too close to his base of support.

    c.   inside his base of support.

    d.   outside his base of support.

Question 24.   Once a patient has started to fall, the best method of helping him is to _____

_____.

Why would you use this method? Explain. _____

_____ .

Question 25.   You are helping a patient to walk who weighs about 200 pounds. He has begun to fall. If you try to prevent his falling further, what possible effect might this action have on you?

_____ .

ITEM 15. COMPLETION OF THE LESSON

You have now completed the lesson on patient movement and ambulation, which has included range-of-motion exercise, dangling, walking, and patient falls. Please make an appointment with your instructor to take the post-test.

V. INFORMATION FOR ENRICHMENT

Since exercise and ambulation are so important to the patient, you may be interested in reading more about the role of movement in nursing care. Patients with orthopedic, neurological, or cardiovascular problems may have limited movement and special needs related to their diseases. You will add more skill to your care of these patients as you learn more about their special needs. So much has been written about nursing care of specific diseases that to start you off, only a few articles will be listed. Many of the articles have references at the end that you can use to find other related articles and books.

Carnevali, Doris, and Susan Brueckner: Immobilization — Reassessment of a Concept, *American Journal of Nursing*, 70:1502–07, July 1970. The many types of immobilization (physical, emotional, intellectual, social) and their causes are illustrated in a case study of a patient with cardiovascular accident.

Ellis, Rosemary: After Stroke: Sitting Problems, *American Journal of Nursing*, 73:1898–99, November 1973.

Elwood, Evelyn: Nursing the Patient with Cerebrovascular Accident, *Nursing Clinics of North America*, March 1970, pp. 47–53. Describes basic nursing care, including support of paralyzed limbs, and some major considerations in acute and long-term-care cases.

Haber, Martha E.: Parkinson's Disease: Challenge to the Health Professions, *Nursing Clinics of North America*, June 1969, pp. 263–273. The challenge posed by this neurological disease that causes muscular rigidity and flexion contractures is described, and a plan for nursing care is outlined.

Pfaudler, Marjorie: After Stroke: Motor Skill Rehabilitation for Hemiplegic Patients, *American Journal of Nursing*, 73:1892–96, November 1973.

Snyder, Mariah, and Rebecca Baum: Assessing Station and Gait, *American Journal of Nursing*, 74:1256, July 1974.

Stone, Virginia: Give the Older Person Time, *American Journal of Nursing*, 69:2124–27, October 1969. Explains why the older person requires more time to perceive, to learn, and to move.

Tooley, Patricia, and Corrine W. Larson: Range-of-Motion Exercise: Key to Joint Mobility, American Rehabilitation Foundation, Minneapolis, Minnesota, 1968.

WORKBOOK ANSWER SHEET

Question 1.   The best answers for the meaning of the words are:

      1. c

      2. h

3. i

4. g

5. d

6. b

7. f

8. a

2. Any four of the following (among others): promotes firmness, tone, and elasticity of muscles; promotes elimination of waste products; strengthens and hardens bones; maintains blood pressure; promotes blood circulation; stimulates the appetite; reduces fatigue; promotes respiratory action

3. movement or exercise

4. muscles

5. joints

6. a. freely movable

   b. freely movable

   c. slightly movable

   d. freely movable

7. flexors

8. flexion

9. less than three weeks

10. All of his joints should be exercised.

    Exercises should start as soon as possible and you could give them during the bath.

11. passive; active

12. Some of the feelings the patient may have are related to his inability to speak clearly, inability to move his left side, worry about his role as a father and husband, concern about his ability to return to work and provide for his family, and so forth.

13. The rehabilitation team could be:

    a. nurse

    b. physician

    c. speech and hearing therapist

    d. physical therapist

    e. occupational therapist

    f. family

14. yes

15. adduction, abduction, extension, flexion, and opposition or grasping

16. a. internal rotation

    b. external rotation

    c. internal and external rotation

UNIT 9

17. repair the damage, or rebuild defenses

18. b, d, e, and f

19. double stance

20. counteract the twist of the body

21. the heel

22. patient falls

23. d.

24. Ease him to the floor. This method provides more safety for the patient and the worker by breaking the force of the fall and working with gravity rather than trying to lift against gravity; prevents possible injury to patient and worker.

25. You may lose your balance and fall, strain your muscles, or injure yourself.

PERFORMANCE TEST

In the skill laboratory, you will be asked to perform the following activities for your instructor without reference to any source material. You will need another person to take the part of the patient.

1. Given a patient with limited or no motion in the joints on one side of his body, explain the need for exercising all of his joints and put his affected joints through range-of-motion exercises. In ranging the joint, support the part distal to the joint and avoid movement to the extent that it causes pain.

2. Given a patient who has been on bed rest and must be gotten up to dangle his feet at the side of the bed, assist him to a sitting position, pivot his body, and swing his feet off the bed, using smooth flowing motions and principles of good body alignment and movement.

3. Given a patient who has been on bed rest and is to get up to walk, assist him to dangle his feet at the side of the bed, help him stand and balance at the bedside, and then walk, using principles of good body alignment, balance, and movement.

4. Given a patient who has begun to fall, assist him by grasping him firmly, slowing his rate of descent, and easing him slowly to the floor, using principles related to gravity to avoid possible injury to the patient or yourself.

UNIT 9

PERFORMANCE CHECKLIST

PATIENT MOVEMENT AND AMBULATION

RANGE OF MOTION EXERCISES

1. Wash your hands.
2. Identify the patient.
3. Explain the procedure to the patient.
4. Move the patient to the proximal side of the bed (on the affected side).
5. Orient the patient to the need for exercise.
6. Exercise the joints on the affected side through the range of motion where applicable.
   a. Abduction
   b. Adduction
   c. Flexion
   d. Extension
   e. Internal rotation
   f. External rotation
   g. Circumduction
   h. Hyperextension
7. Throughout the procedure be careful not to cause pain to the patient.
8. Support the distal and proximal ends of the limbs during the exercise.

G

1. Wash your hands.

2. Identify the patient.

3. Explain the procedure to the patient.

4. Move the patient to the proximal side of the bed.

5. Adjust the bed to the low position. Raise the headrest to approximately 45°.

6. Raise the patient to a sitting position with one hand on his proximal shoulder and the other under his distal axilla.

7. Continue supporting his shoulder and place your other hand under his distal knee, swinging his legs off the bed while pivoting his body.

8. Maintain principles of good body alignment while completing the motion. Patient movement should be slow, smooth, and steady.

9. Dress the patient in his robe and slippers for comfort and modesty.

10. Fluff his pillow while the patient is dangling his feet.

11. Remove his slippers and robe when he is ready to lie down.

12. Return the patient to the supine position, using one hand on his proximal shoulder and the other under his distal axilla.

13. Support the patient's shoulders with one hand, with your other hand under both of his ankles.

14. Swing his legs up onto the bed while pivoting his body.

15. Maintain principles of good body alignment while completing the motion. Patient movement should be slow, smooth, and steady.

ASSIST PATIENT TO WALK

1. Wash your hands.

2. Identify the patient.

3. Explain the procedure to the patient.

4. Move the patient to the proximal side of the bed.

5. Adjust the bed to the low position.

6. Raise the patient to a sitting position, with one hand on his proximal shoulder and the other under his distal axilla.

7. Continue supporting his shoulder and place your other hand under his distal knee, slipping his legs off the bed while pivoting his body.

8. Assist the patient to stand at his bedside.

9. Align him in good body position, correcting his posture.

10. Walk with the patient:

    a. To give minimal support: hold his arm or hand.

    b. To give moderate support: hold his left arm with your hand.

    c. To give maximal support: obtain assistance by having another health worker walk on the other side of the patient.

11. The health worker must maintain good body alignment and balance throughout th[e] procedure.

SAFEGUARDING THE FALLING PATIENT

1. Explain the rationale for breaking the patient's fall rather than catching and trying to raise him.

   a. Injury to the patient.

   b. Injury to yourself.

   c. Abrupt change in movement.

2. As the patient begins to fall, the worker positions herself to the rear of patient, attempting to break his fall by grasping him under the armpits.

3. Once contact is made, the health worker flexes her legs to lower the patient gently to the ground.

4. Maintain the patient in a sitting or lying position on the floor.

5. Remain with the patient, reassuring him and providing warmth until required help arrives.

6. Examine the patient for possible injury.

7. Prepare an accident report.

U
N
I
T
9

POST-TEST

in the blanks in the following statements. The statements encompass the
s used in this lesson. Your answer should be the word(s) that the
bes.

1. ıne triangular bone of the lower posterior torso is the _____ .

2. _____ is the turning upward of the sole of the foot.

3. In the walking cycle, a _____ is the distance covered from one single stance to the next single stance.

4. The _____ is the bony basinlike cavity of the lower torso.

5. The movement of turning outward on an axis is called _____ .

6. The movement of turning the palm of the hand downward is _____ .

7. Movement of one person's joint or limb by another person is _____ .

Section B. The following diagrams show different types of movement. Please fill in the name of the movement and then circle the best answer of the choices given in the accompanying statement.

8. The movement is _____ .
The movement that occurs is (circular) (decrement).

9. The movement is _____ . The distance from the midline is (increased) (decreased).

10. The movement is _____ .
The angle between the two parts is (increased) (decreased).

11. The movement is _____. The arm forms the (apex) (base) (side) of the cone.

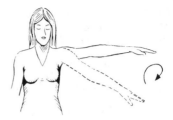

12. The movement is _____. The distance from the midline is (increased) (decreased).

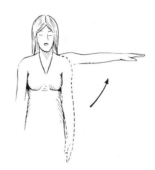

13. The movement is _____. The angle between the two parts is (increased) (decreased).

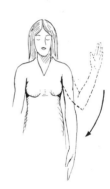

UNIT 9

Section C. In the situation described below, several multiple choice questions are asked. Select the best answer(s). More than one answer may be right.

Mr. Bond is a 67-year-old man in Bigtown University Hospital who had a stroke three days ago. He has been in the Intensive Care Unit until 1 hour ago when he was transferred to the Medical floor. He is one of the patients assigned to you for care. When you first meet Mr. Bond, you notice that his mouth droops on one side, that his speech at this time is limited to "boler," "soup," and "no," and that his left arm and leg are paralyzed. He is conscious, but seems quite depressed.

1. Later that morning, you return to Mr. Bond's bedside and explain that you will give him his bath and exercise his paralyzed arm and leg. He sobs and says "Boler, boler, boler." You don't understand what he is trying to say. What would you do now?

____a. Report to the team leader that he is crying, that he keeps saying "boler," and that you wonder if he is having pain or discomfort.

____b. Ask the patient to nod his head for "yes" and shake his head for "no," then explain again and ask questions to see if he understands what you mean.

____c. Go ahead and carry out the bath and exercises. He must be confused since he isn't making sense, and you know that he needs the exercises.

____d. Tell Mr. Bond that he shouldn't cry, reassure him that everything will be all right, and give him his bath.

tray arrives with his lunch. As you feed him, you hand him a piece of bread,
...lds in his unaffected hand. As he moves his hand to his mouth to eat, what
...es he use?

...n of the wrist

...l rotation of the shoulder

...ternal rotation of the shoulder

_____d. pronation of the wrist

3. When feeding Mr. Bond from a position on the left side of his bed, you notice that he doesn't seem to be able to see your hand and the food until it is near his mouth. In order to see more on his left side, he raises his head slightly from the pillow and turns his head in order to look straight at you. The movements of his neck are:

_____a. flexion and abduction

_____b. flexion and rotation

_____c. hyperextension and rotation

_____d. extension and adduction

_____e. none of these

4. The exercise program you have planned with Mr. Bond includes the range-of-motion exercises during his bath time. He has become interested in exercising the joints of his right side, but needs you to exercise his affected side. When performing the range-of-motion exercises, you know that you must:

_____a. place several pillows under the affected knee to support it.

_____b. support the part distal to the joint being ranged.

_____c. avoid moving the paralyzed joints.

_____d. avoid moving beyond the point of pain.

5. Mr. Bond's rehabilitation includes physical therapy and speech therapy. He has been making a lot of progress since his stroke. His speech has improved greatly and he has been learning to balance, stand, and use the parallel bars in physical therapy. Although other patients would go to an extended-care facility, Mr. Bond is being kept in the hospital. His doctor has written an order allowing Mr. Bond to get up and walk with assistance. Before you assist him to walk for the first time, you help him to dangle his legs. The reason(s) for this could be:

_____a. to strengthen his leg muscles before he stands.

_____b. to see how well he maintains his balance with one side paralyzed.

_____c. to help him adjust to the change of position and recover from any dizziness.

_____d. to prevent contractures of his paralyzed arm and leg.

6. When helping a patient like Mr. Bond who is paralyzed on his left side, you would have him dangle his feet on the left side of the bed because:

_____a. he should avoid turning to his unaffected right side.

_____b. if he loses his balance, his paralyzed side is closer to the bed.

_____c. it would be easier for him to move his stronger right side from the distal side of the bed.

_____d. you don't have to reach so far to support his weaker left side.

7. The weak or unsteady patient, like Mr. Bond, will require most of your assistance when walking during the

____a. swing phase

____b. single stance phase

____c. double stance phase

8. Let us assume that Mr. Bond is now ready to walk with assistance. You and Miss Jones will help him walk in his room for the first time. Which of the following will you do?

____a. Provide support with one person on each side of the patient.

____b. Make sure his bedroom slippers have a soft sole so his left foot will bend it easier.

____c. Have him hold his head up, look forward, and walk at a pace of about 80 steps per minute.

____d. Encourage him to walk as normally as possible and have his right heel strike the ground first.

9. Suppose that Mr. Bond has made progress in walking. You later assist him by yourself to walk to the bathroom. He has taken about ten steps when suddenly his left knee buckles and he begins to fall. You have been walking on his left side. What should you do?

____a. Grasp him firmly at the waist and chest to keep him from falling to the floor.

____b. Use your right thigh and foot to brace his buckling knee and foot to help him regain his balance.

____c. Hold onto him to slow his rate of descent, and ease him to the floor.

____d. Brace your feet firmly to overcome the force of his fall and call for help.

10. If Mr. Bond should fall, the probable reason for this would be:

____a. His line of gravity and center of gravity are outside his base of support.

____b. His line of gravity and center of gravity are inside his base of support.

____c. His unaffected right leg is unable to support the weight of his body.

____d. His affected left leg is unable to support the weight of his body.

POST-TEST ANNOTATED ANSWER SHEET

Section A.

1. sacrum (pp. 100, 133)

2. supination (pp. 131, 133)

3. pace (pp. 131, 144)

4. pelvis (pp. 60, 133)

5. external rotation (p. 136)

6. pronation (pp. 131, 133)

7. passive exercise (pp. 131, 134)

UNIT 9

cular (p. 133)

ecreased (p. 133)

ased (p. 133)

...ion; side (p. 133)‾

12. abduction; increased (p. 133)

13. extension increased (p. 133)

Section C.

1. b (pp 134, 135)

2. c (p. 136)

3. b (pp. 137–138)

4. b and d (p. 137)

5. b and c (p. 141)

6. c and d (p. 142)

7. b (p. 144)

8. a and d (p. 145)

9. c (pp. 146, 147)

10. d (p. 146)

MECHANICAL AIDS FOR AMBULATION AND MOVEMENT

I. DIRECTIONS TO THE STUDENT

Proceed through the lesson using this workbook as your guide. You will need to practice the procedures related to the use of mechanical aids for ambulation and movement with student partners in the skill laboratory, or with other persons. After you have completed the lesson and your practice of the procedures, arrange with your instructor to take the post-test.

For this lesson you will need the following items:

1. A stretcher.
2. A walker.
3. A pair of crutches.
4. A wheelchair.
5. A mechanical lifter.
6. A walking belt or drawsheet.
7. A back brace.
8. A short leg brace if available.
9. A robe.
10. Slippers or shoes.

Please read the following paragraphs carefully. They will indicate what you will be expected to know and how you will be expected to assist the patient to use such mechanical aids as a *walker, wheelchair, crutches,* and *braces.* If you feel that you have the necessary skills and could better use your time studying other material, discuss this with your instructor, and then arrange to take the performance test. All students are expected to accurately demonstrate the required skills in the performance test.

II. GENERAL PERFORMANCE OBJECTIVE

Upon completion of this lesson, you will demonstrate your ability to assist the patient (or another person) to use the common mechanical aids for ambulation or movement in a safe and effective manner.

III. SPECIFIC PERFORMANCE OBJECTIVES

When this lesson is completed, you will be able to:

1. Assess any physical or mental condition that may interfere with the patient's ability to use the mechanical aids in his ambulation or movement; assess your own ability

itations in carrying out the required procedure; when needed, obtain
al help.

icate patience, gentleness, and concern for the patient verbally as well as
lly through your behavior and actions.

stance, transfer a helpless patient from the bed to a stretcher by
...oning the stretcher, using a sheet to lift and move the patient, and using safety
belts or siderails to protect the patient from falling.

4. Assist the patient (one who is able to stand) to transfer from the bed to a
   wheelchair: position the chair; set the brakes, then have him dangle his legs from
   the bed; ask him to stand, pivot his body, and sit in the wheelchair; then transfer
   him out of the wheelchair.

5. With assistance or the use of a mechanical lifter, transfer a patient (one who is
   unable to stand) from the bed to a wheelchair by positioning the chair, setting the
   brakes, positioning the patient, lifting on signal, placing him in the wheelchair, and
   adjusting the leg and foot rests.

6. Instruct the patient in the use of a wheelchair when he requires one as a means of
   locomotion.

7. Assist the patient in bed to transfer into and out of a walker safely, so as to prevent
   slipping or falling, and adjust the walker to the height best suited to his use.

8. Measure and adjust a pair of crutches to the proper length needed by the patient,
   and adjust the hand-bar.

9. Demonstrate two-point, three-point, and four-point crutch-walking, and explain the
   conditions related to each type.

10. Explain the principles of crutch-walking and the cause of "crutch palsy."

11. Apply a strap-on type of back brace for the patient, and explain how to check for
    proper fit and possible pressure areas.

12. Apply a short leg brace to the patient's leg, and explain the care of the brace and
    how to check for proper fit and possible pressure areas.

IV. VOCABULARY

Some of the new words introduced in this lesson are listed below.

axillary bar—the upper crosspiece of a crutch, fitting under the armpit.

bony prominence—a jutting or protruding portion of a bone, e.g., the shoulder blade
(scapula).

brace—an appliance made of fabric, leather, plastic, or metal that supports a specific portion of the body.

crutch—a staff or support used in walking, usually with a crosspiece to fit under the armpit
(axilla).

crutch palsy—a condition caused by pressure on nerves in the axilla that results in weakness
of the forearm, wrist, and hand.

four-point, three-point, two-point gaits—methods of walking with crutches.

irritation—a stimulation that causes a physical reaction of the skin or organ, such as redness
or itching.

locomotion—the process of moving from place to place.

mechanical lifter—a device utilizing hydraulic principles so that a small force can lift a heavy
weight.

Naugahyde—a tough and sturdy synthetic upholstering material.

pallor—lack of color, paleness.

self-esteem—the respect and value with which a person regards himself.

therapeutic—pertaining to the treatment or cure of a disease.

walker—a metal rectangular frame with wheels used to assist a person to walk.

wing screws—adjustment screws, used on walkers, crutches, and other devices, that have two thumbpieces, or wings, for easier use.

ITEM 1. WHY DO YOU NEED TO KNOW ABOUT MECHANICAL AIDS?

Movement is one of the primary functions of the body. The heart pumps and moves the blood through the body, the chest wall moves to allow the lungs to draw in and expel air, the eyelids blink to protect and lubricate the eyes, the jaws move so that the teeth may chew food, and so forth. The muscles, bones, and joints work together so that a person may move himself from one position to another. For the patient, the ability to move about or to walk during his illness or convalescence decreases his dependence on others, and increases his self-esteem. It also improves his mental outlook and widens his world beyond his bed or the four walls of his room. The general functioning of all of his body systems is enhanced through movement.

In order to move about or to walk, the patient may need to use a mechanical aid, such as a wheelchair, walker, crutches, or braces, either temporarily or permanently. In general, when such an aid is needed permanently by the patient, he is taught how to use it by a physician, a physical therapist, or a member of the rehabilitation team. However, when the patient requires the use of a wheelchair, walker, or crutches on a temporary basis, teaching the patient how to use the device often becomes the responsibility of the nursing worker. As the nursing worker, you must know how to use the mechanical aid safely and effectively before you can teach the paitent how to use it.

Please complete the following statements:

Question 1. The use of a mechanical aid by the patient for walking or moving about may be

on a _____ or a _____ basis.

Question 2. The nursing worker may be responsible for teaching the patient how to use a

pair of crutches when these are to be uses on a _____ basis.

ITEM 2. WHAT KINDS OF MECHANICAL AIDS ARE USED IN
AMBULATION?

The type of mechanical aid that is selected for the patient's use will depend on his physical condition and the degree of support that he needs. General support for the body is provided by the wheelchair, walker, and crutches, with the wheelchair furnishing the greatest support. Braces support specific portions of the body. Some patients with orthopedic (bone) problems may progress from one aid to the next, whereas most patients may need the general support of a wheelchair for a short time until they can walk unassisted. The pictures on the next page show how a patient may progress toward walking unaided.

Not all patients regain the strength and ability needed to walk unaided. Certain patients, like some of the elderly, become weaker and need progressively more support until the only way they can get about may be in a wheelchair. It is important that you remember to encourage the patient to do what he can for himself and to provide support for the motor abilities that he lacks.

The support provided by mechanical aids allows for a *progression* by the patient toward walking without assistance. The levels in the progression toward ambulation are shown in the following illustrations.

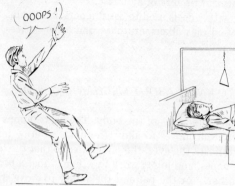

Person falling.

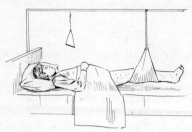

Patient in bed — maximum support.

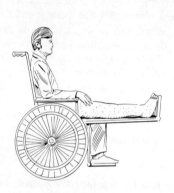

In wheelchair —
intermediate support.

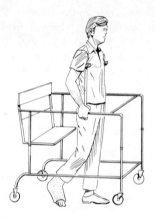

Use of walker —
intermediate support.

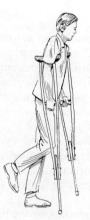

Patient
with
crutches.

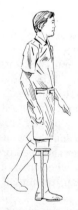

Support
with
leg
brace.

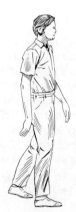

Walking
unassisted.

Progressive levels of patient movement and ambulation, from the total support provided by
bed or stretcher, to the level of walking without assistance.

The patient's physician orders the level or the degree of ambulation desired for the patient. This level of ambulation may be the goal for the patient to achieve or the limitation of the amount of freedom allowed because of his condition. Generally, you may use the mechanical aids for the patient that are *below* the level ordered by the doctor, but *not those above* this level. As an example: The doctor said, "Use crutches for walking." The patient should be encouraged to use crutches for some or most of his walking, but you may provide a wheelchair or a walker for his use when he is tired, becomes weak, or has to travel a longer distance than usual. However, you should not allow the patient to walk without his crutches, because this would be ambulation at a higher level than allowed by the doctor's order.

From the information given, you should be able to answer these questions:

Question 3. Mrs. Jay had an abdominal operation three days ago and now must be taken to X-ray. The doctor has written an order for Mrs. Jay to be up in a chair four times a day. Which of the mechanical aids would you use to take Mrs. Jay to X-ray?

_____ .

Question 4. Mr. Zee came to the hospital several days ago for various tests. He is 68 years old, and the doctor has prescribed ambulation as desired. He feels weak today following extensive laboratory tests, but would like to go to the patients' solarium to visit with his wife. What kind of supportive aid would you provide for Mr. Zee, and why?

_____ .

ITEM 3. TRANSFERRING A HELPLESS PATIENT ONTO A STRETCHER

Frequently, you will be asked to help move a patient onto or off a stretcher. The stretcher is used to transport the bed patient to another area or department in the hospital, such as surgery or X-ray. Patients who are moved in this manner are usually more seriously ill, more limited in their movements, and consequently, in greater need of support and assistance. Although some may be able to move freely from the bed to a stretcher, most of these patients will require help.

The stretcher is a type of bed that is made of metal; it is lightweight, with wheels that make it easy to roll. It is equipped with a pad for comfort, and a safety belt or siderails to protect the patient from falling off.

In the skill laboratory, practice the procedure of assisting the transfer of a helpless patient from the bed to a stretcher. Ask one of your classmates to serve as a patient, and others to help you move the patient.

Important Steps	Key Points
1. Obtain the stretcher from storage.	Make sure that the pad of the stretcher is covered neatly with a clean sheet. Take along a bath blanket or sheet with which to cover the patient. If he has an IV running, you will need a standard to fit the stretcher or to roll along with it. Wash your hands.
2. Approach and identify the patient, explain what you are going to do, and secure his cooperation.	Be particularly careful to identify the patient; he may be so ill or affected by medications that he may not understand what you say.
3. Provide for privacy.	Pull the curtains of the cubicle, use screens, or close the door. Avoid exposing the patient unnecessarily.

4. Position and prepare the patient.

Bring him to the proximal side of the bed. Adjust the bed to the high position (flush with the height of the stretcher). Loosen the top bedding from the foot of the bed, remove the overbed cradles, excess pillows, and other things that might be in the way. Check all tubes that might be attached to the patient; make sure that they are free of the bedding and long enough to permit you to move him. Loosen the drawsheet and use it as a "lifting" sheet.

5. Position the stretcher next to the bed and transfer the patient onto it.

Two workers station themselves next to the stretcher and lean across to reach the patient. The worker on the far side of the bed may have to get up and kneel on the side of the bed in order to avoid stretching so far as to be off balance. All three then grasp the "lift" sheet, and on signal, move the helpless patient onto the stretcher. Cover him with the bath blanket or sheet and remove the top bedding; which you leave on the bed. Place a pillow under his head, and raise the siderails or fasten the safety belt.

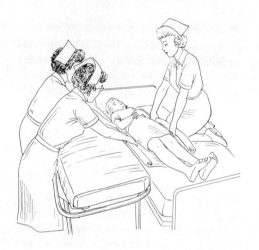

Workers transferring helpless patient from bed to stretcher. Those leaning over stretcher use body weight to help them pull patient over onto stretcher as they straighten up.

6. Transfer the patient from the stretcher to his bed.

Reverse the procedure. Have the top bedding fan-folded to the side or the foot of the bed so that it is out of the way when moving the patient. You may find that it is easier to pull the patient onto the bed by having two workers on the distal side of the bed and one worker on the stretcher side.

7. Provide for the patient's comfort.

Place the patient in good alignment and support his body parts with pillows. Check IV's and any tubing to make sure that the tubes are draining and not kinked. Straighten the bedding, raise the siderails, leave the bed in low position, and put the call signal within the patient's reach.

8. Return the stretcher to storage.

Remove the soiled sheet and replace it with a clean sheet.

9. Report and record as appropriate.

Charting should include the time and destination of the patient. Any changes in the patient's condition should also be included in the notation. Charting example:

9:30 A.M. To X-ray per stretcher.

L. Smith, NA

10:35 A.M. Returned from X-ray per stretcher.
Complains of pain in incision. IV running well.

L. Smith, NA

ITEM 4.   THE WHEELCHAIR

Now we will examine the wheelchair. It is the
most commonly used aid to move the patient
safely from one place to another, and provides
a great degree of general support for him when
he is out of bed.

A wheelchair consists of a seat on a frame
suspended between two large rear wheels and
two small front wheels. It has a turning rim on
the large wheels, pushing handles on the rear of
the seat, footrest pedals, and brakes. Most
wheelchairs are constructed so that they can be
folded for storage and transportation. The seat
and back are usually made of a plastic or
Naugahyde material, which is easily cleaned
with a damp cloth.

In order to be moved in a wheelchair by
another person, the patient must have the
ability to sit in an upright position. For the
patient to move himself about in a wheelchair,
he must be able to sit upright, support his
upper body and head, and have the use of at
least one of his arms in order to turn the wheel
or set the brakes. The patient who must propel
himself should be instructed in the techniques
of using the chair. This consists of teaching him
how to set the hand brakes, transfer into and
out of the chair, raise or lower the footrests
with his foot, and propel the chair.

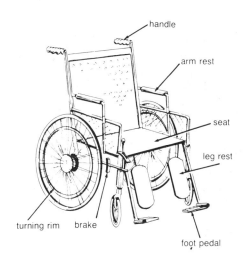

handle

arm rest

seat

leg rest

turning rim   brake

foot pedal

Question 5.   In order to propel himself in a wheelchair, a patient needs to be able to:

a. _____

b. _____

c. _____

ITEM 5.   WHEELCHAIR TECHNIQUES

Let us now consider some of the elements of
wheelchair technique. Before instructing a patient in this technique, you must first learn to
do it yourself.

Set Brakes. The wheelchair should be
equipped on each large wheel with a brake that
is operated by a hand lever. The accompanying
figures show the hand brake in a "set" or
locked position and in a released or unlocked

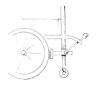
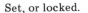

Set, or locked.   Released, or unlocked.

position. Locate the hand brake levers on your wheelchair and set the brakes on both wheels.

Adjust Foot Pedals. With the brakes in the set or locked position, locate the footrest pedals. Notice that each pedal can be swung upward to provide a clear entry to the chair and can be swung downward to serve as a footrest for the person in the wheelchair.

Now raise the foot pedals and sit in the wheelchair. Raise one foot and use it to swing the foot pedal down for that foot; repeat, using the other foot. Now remove one foot from the footrest, use the toe to swing the footrest pedal upward, and place your foot on the floor. Repeat, using the other foot. You should practice lowering and raising the foot pedals, using both feet. Now try lowering and raising the pedals by using only one foot.

Pushing and Turning. Pushing a patient in a wheelchair requires equal pressure on both handles for straight-ahead motion. To make a left turn with the wheelchair, your left hand on the handle should move just slightly or not at all, and you must exert more push on the right handle as the right portion of the chair moves a greater distance to make the turn. To make a right turn, the pressures would be reversed.

Passing Through Doorways. When approaching a closed door, turn the wheelchair around so that you approach the door backwards. You can then use one hand to open the door; pull the chair through as your body continues to force the door to open wider. Turn the wheelchair around to a forward direction after you have cleared the door. This method prevents possible injury to the patient's feet or arms, damage to the finish of the door, and awkward or jerky movements of your body that may cause injury. You should practice pushing another person in the wheelchair, making several left and right turns, and going through a door.

Propelling Yourself. To propel yourself in a wheelchair, sit in the chair, place your feet on the footrests, and release the brakes on both wheels. Place your hands on the turn rim of the large wheels. For a straight-ahead movement, roll the rims forward with equal force on both rims. Turns to the left or to the right are made in the same manner as when you push the wheelchair by the handles, only now you use the turning rim. Practice propelling yourself in a wheelchair and making right and left turns.

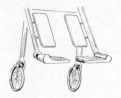

Footrest pedals in down position

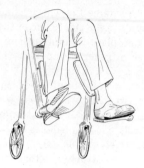

Raising footrest pedal with foot.

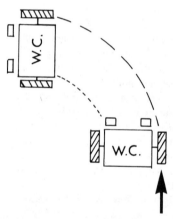

To make left turn, apply more force at point of arrow.

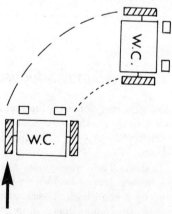

To make right hand turn, apply force in direction of arrow.

You have practiced those steps of wheelchair technique that relate to the use of the hand brakes and the footrest pedals, and to the propelling or pushing of the chair. Now we will go on to the procedure of transferring the patient into and out of the wheelchair.

ITEM 6.   WHEELCHAIR PROCEDURAL SKILLS

In the skill laboratory you are to practice the procedure of transferring a patient (who can stand) into and out of a wheelchair. Have one of your fellow students play the role of the patient. A bed should be available for use by the "patient."

Important Steps	Key Points
1. Obtain the wheelchair.	Attempt to select a wheelchair appropriate to the *size* and *condition of the patient*. Use a small size for children, standard size for the average adult, and large size with reinforced frame for very heavy adults. A chair with a *high back* or an extension back will provide support for the shoulders and head of the very weak patient. Check the working order of the brakes, wheels, arm and leg rests, foot pedals, and seat (safety) belts if used in your agency. Safety belts work in the same manner as seat belts in your car. Wash your hands.
2. Approach and identify the patient, explain the procedure, and enlist his cooperation.	The patient may be apprehensive about getting into a wheelchair, or may feel that its use is a sign of weakness and that he can walk unaided. Accept the patient's right to his feelings and explain that the wheelchair is a safe method of moving, provides a measure of independence, or is a sign of progress.
3. Position the wheelchair at the side of the bed near the patient.	Position the chair parallel to the side of the bed. Place the back of the chair even with the foot of the bed; the seat will be facing the head of the bed. Set the brakes on both wheels. Raise both footrest pedals.
4. Assist the patient to a "dangling-feet" position at the side of the bed.	If patient is in an adjustable high-low bed place the bed in the low position. Assist the patient to dangle according to instructions in "Patient Movement." Dress patient in robe and slippers.
5. Help the patient to stand up.	Ask him to push his body up from the bed, or have him clasp your hands, arms, or shoulders and rise to a standing position. Use principles of good body alignment and movement to prevent injury to yourself.
6. Assist the patient into the wheelchair.	Have him pivot so that his back is toward the seat of the chair, then reach down to grasp the arms of the chair, and have him lower himself to a sitting position. Or you may step to the side of the wheelchair, facing the patient. Support him at the armpit nearest you with your left hand. Help him to lower himself

Important Steps	Key Points
	gently into the wheelchair. Then place both his feet on the footrests. Disengage, or release, the brakes.
7. Transfer the patient out of the wheelchair.	Reverse the procedure used to transfer him into the wheelchair. Position the side of the wheel chair parallel to the side of the bed and facing the foot of the bed. Set both brakes, raise the footrest pedals, and have him push up from the armrests to a standing position. Have the patient pivot so that his back is toward the bed and ease him into a sitting position on the side of the bed. Remove his robe and slippers, and swing both of his feet onto the bed.
8. Provide for the patient's comfort.	See that he is lying in good body alignment. Adjust the bed and the pillows as he may request. Straighten the top bedding. Place the bedside stand and call signal within easy reach.
9. Remove the wheelchair.	Release the brakes and return the chair to storage.
10. Report and record as appropriate.	Report to the team leader or the nurse in charge that the procedure has been carried out. Report any changes in the patient's condition or any complaints that he may have had, such as discomfort caused by moving, change in the color of skin, pallor, flushing, profuse perspiration, distress in breathing, or headache. Charting example:
	2:10 P.M. Up in wheelchair for 20 minutes. Condition remained good throughout activity. Returned to bed. Complained of being extremely weak. Vital signs remained stable.
	J. Jones, SN

ITEM 7.   USE OF A MECHANICAL LIFTER TO TRANSFER A HELPLESS PATIENT

A mechanical lifter should be used whenever a helpless or very heavy patient is to be transferred out of bed and into a chair, a wheelchair, or a tub. It is the safest method for handling the patient and avoiding injuries to health workers. Although not every nursing unit is equipped with a mechanical lifter, most hospitals have at least one. There is a variety of lifters on the market; some of them, such as the Hoyer lift, are operated with hydraulic pressure.

Two workers are needed to transfer the patient safely from the bed to a wheelchair when using the mechanical lifter. One worker guides the patient into the sling while the other operates and rolls the lifter.

In the skill lab, practice transferring a helpless patient from the bed to a wheelchair, using a mechanical lifter similar to the Hoyer. One of your fellow students can play the role of the patient. Ask how it feels to be suspended by the lift, and find out how you can reassure the patient.

Important Steps	Key Points
1. With another worker, obtain the lifter and wheelchair from storage.	Check the mechanical lifter to make sure you have the necessary chain hooks and the canvas belts or slings that support the patient's body.
2. Approach and identify the patient, explain the procedure, and enlist his cooperation.	Reassure him that you and the other worker, when using the mechanical lifter, will provide for his safety.
3. Position the wheelchair and set the brakes.	Allow enough space so that you can maneuver the mechanical lifter between the bed and the chair.
4. Position the mechanical lifter.	Place it with the base wheels under the bed and at right angles to it. Adjust the level of the lifting bar over the bed and close the hydraulic pressure valve.
5. Place the patient in the sling of the lifter.	With a worker on each side of the bed, pass a sling strap under the patient's shoulders and another under the thighs. Fasten the strap to the corresponding hooks on the lifting bar.
6. Operate the lifter, and with assistance, move the patient to the wheelchair.	Release the pressure valve and pump the handle to raise the lifting bar with the patient in the sling straps so that his body clears the bed. Close the hydraulic pressure valve, and roll the lifter to the wheelchair while the other worker guides the patient into position over the chair seat. Release the pressure valve to lower the sling. Unhook the straps after the patient is in the chair, leaving them in place; then move the lifter out of the way.

U
N
I
T
10

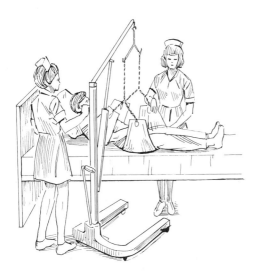

Transfer of patient from bed . . .

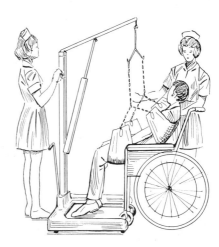

to wheelchair using
mechanical lift.

Important Steps	Key Points
7. Return the patient to bed.	Reverse the procedure when getting the patient back into bed.

Follow steps 8, 9, and 10 of the wheelchair procedure, Item 6.

ITEM 8. TRANSFERRING A HELPLESS PATIENT TO A CHAIR WITHOUT A MECHANICAL LIFTER

Often you will be called upon to get a helpless patient out of bed and into a chair. It is possible to lift some patients with the assistance of one or more workers when a mechanical lifter is not available for the transfer. Avoid the method of lifting or swinging the patient, from the bed to a wheelchair placed parallel to the side of the bed. Although this method is frequently used, many workers are injured by twisting and bending their backs, and lifting while off-balance.

You will need another person to assist you to transfer the helpless patient from the bed to a wheelchair. In the skill laboratory, practice the procedure until you feel at ease with it, and confident of of your ability to perform with an actual patient.

Important Steps	Key Points
Follow steps 1 through 3 in the wheelchair procedure, Item 6.	
3. Position the wheelchair and set the brakes.	Place the chair at right angles to the bed and about the level of the patient's hips. Put the bed in a low position — or even with the seat of the wheelchair.
4. Position and prepare the patient.	Move him to the proximal side of the bed. Dress him in his robe and slippers, if appropriate, and bring him to an upright sitting position.
5. With assistance, transfer the patient into the wheelchair.	With one worker on each side of the patient, place one arm around his shoulders and one under his hips. Some patients may be able to sit erect and put their arms around the workers' necks and help support their weight, but weaker patients cannot do this. On signal, the workers slide the patient back into the seat of the wheelchair. One worker then releases the brakes and moves the chair slowly away from the bed. The other worker supports the patient's feet, and lowers them onto the foot pedals.

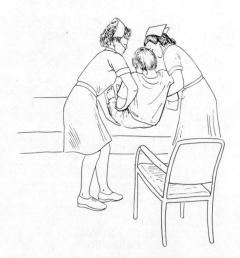

Using form of chair carry to transfer patient to wheelchair or chair.

Important Steps	Key Points
6. Return the patient to his bed.	Reverse the procedure. The use of a trapeze for the patient to grasp is especially helpful for moving him back onto the bed.

Then follow steps 8, 9, and 10 of the wheel-chair procedure, Item 6.

ITEM 9.   WHAT IS A WALKER?

Another mechanical aid that provides support for the patient in moving about from place to place is the *walker*, a waist-high tubular metal frame constructed in a rectangular shape with wheels attached to its legs. The preferred model has a movable swing-up seat and removable backrest that allows for easy entry and exit to and from the frame. The seat can be put down for use when the patient becomes tired.

The walker should be adjustable in height because it is used to provide support and stability for the patient who is learning to walk again. Any patient who has been confined to bed for a long period of time, and those who have had fractures of the hip or bones in the lower extremity and must restrict weight bearing on the affected part can use a walker. It is also employed to prepare the patient for the use of crutches or braces.

In order to use a walker, the patient must be able to bear weight on one foot, balance in an upright position, and have the use of his hands and arms. The walker should be adjusted to a height in which the upper rail fits the palm of the patient's hand with his elbow flexed or bent at a 30° angle.

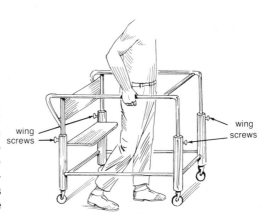

Wing screws —
for adjusting height.

Question 6.   In order to use a walker, the patient must be able to do three things. These are:

a. _____ b. _____

c. _____ .

Question 7.   When using the walker, you noted that the patient's elbows were flexed (or bent) at a 90° angle and were resting on the upper rail of the walker. This

would indicate that the height of the walker was too _____ .

Question 8.   Another patient was observed using a walker with his upper back and shoulders flexed and his arms extended straight down to reach the upper rail. The height

of the walker was too _____ .

Question 9.   The recommended degree of flexion, or bend, of the elbow is _____ when using a walker.

ITEM 10. WALKER PROCEDURAL SKILLS

In the skill laboratory, practice the following steps in the procedure of assisting a patient into and out of a walker. Have someone play the part of the patient.

Important Steps	Key Points
1. Obtain a walker from storage.	Check the walker to see that it is adjustable and has a seat and back attachment. Take it to the patient's room. Wash your hands.
2. Approach and identify the patient, explain the procedure, and enlist his cooperation.	Most patients seem to accept a walker quite well because it lessens their fear of falling and fatigue, and increases their mobility. It often signifies progress to more independence.
3. Assist the patient to a sitting position.	If he is in an adjustable high-low bed, place the bed in the low position. Assist him to a dangling position at the side of the bed (see "Patient Movement and Ambulation") and help him to dress in robe and slippers.
4. Position the walker at the bedside.	Raise the seat; remove the back support, or move it to one side of the walker, and place the open back end of the walker in front of the patient. Securely hold the walker in place with one hand and use one foot to block one of the rear wheels.
5. Assist the patient into the walker. 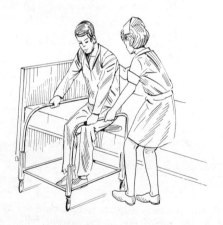 Assisting patient in and out of walker.	Ask the patient to grasp the upper frame of the walker on each side and rise to a standing position. Have him flex his elbows about 30° and measure the height needed to bring the upper rail of the walker to the level of the palm of his hands. If adjustment is needed, have the patient sit on the side of the bed while you loosen the screws and bolts on each of the four legs of the walker, and refasten them at the adjusted height. Steady the walker with your hand to prevent it from slipping away from the patient and causing him to fall. Use your foot in front of the rear wheel to assist in holding the walker steady. After adjustment, have the patient stand and step forward into the walker. Then lower the seat and replace the back support. Caution the patient to take small steps and to avoid going too fast or bumping into the front frame of the walker.
6. Assist the patient out of walker.	While he is still using his walker tell him to approach the side of the bed, turning the walker around so that the back end is against the bed or chair. Remove the backrest or move it to one side and swing the seat up out of the way. Hold the walker securely with one hand, use one foot to block one of the rear wheels, and instruct the patient to keep his hands on the upper rail while stepping back one or two

Important Steps	Key Points
	steps to the edge of the bed. Have him then reach for the bed with his hand and ease himself to a sitting position. Remove his robe and slippers after pushing the walker to one side and help him to swing his legs onto the bed.
7. Provide for the patient's comfort.	See that he is lying in good body alignment. Adjust the bed and pillows as he may request. Straighten the top bedding. Place the bedside stand and call signal within easy reach. Ask if there is anything else you can do before leaving. Tell him when you expect to return.
8. Remove the walker.	If the patient is to continue using the walker, it may be left at the bedside in an area out of the line of traffic. Otherwise, return it to storage.
9. Report and record as appropriate.	Report to the team leader or to the nurse in charge that the procedure was carried out, the way in which the patient tolerated the use of the walker, and any changes in his condition such as those mentioned in the wheelchair procedure. Charting example:
	10:10 A.M. Ambulated for first time in walker. Tolerated procedure well. Returned to bed in good condition in 15 minutes. Seems pleased with his progress. J. Jones, SN

U
N
I
T
10

ITEM 11.   CRUTCH–WALKING

The patient must have various abilities in order to use crutches. For some patients, crutch-walking is a difficult skill that requires careful supervision and practice. Crutch-walking is literally learning to walk with your hands. To use crutches, the patient must be able to balance his body in an upright position, have adequate strength in the arm and shoulder muscles to support much of his weight with his hands, have control of hip and knee joints to keep them from buckling under him, and be able to bear partial weight on both legs or full weight on one leg.

The physical preparation for crutch-walking can be started early, when the patient is still confined to the bed or in a wheelchair. He should be encouraged to perform exercises that will help strengthen the muscles he will use, particularly those of the arm and shoulder. Some of the exercises include: lifting sandbags while lying flat in bed, grasping the head of the bed with his hands and pushing his body down in the bed, and alternately "setting" or con-

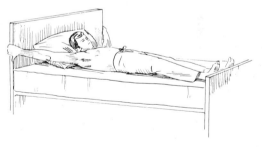

Arm exercises.

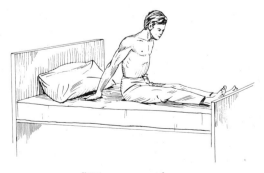

Sitting-up exercises.

tracting the muscles of the arm and leg without moving the joint, then relaxing them. When the patient is able, he should practice using his hands to push himself up to a sitting position in bed. While sitting in a chair or in bed, he should place his hands on the seat and push his body upward so that his buttocks clear the seat. Some of these exercises are illustrated on this page.

Question 10.   In crutch-walking, much of the patient's weight is supported by his _____.

Question 11.   It is essential that the patient have at least _____ weight bearing on both legs or _____ weight bearing on one leg in order to learn crutch-walking.

Question 12.   "Set" the muscles in your arm without bending your elbow. Can you feel the muscles contract? _____.

ITEM 12.   TYPES AND MEASUREMENT OF CRUTCHES

Types of Crutches. There are many types of crutches, several of which are illustrated below. The most commonly used is the first one shown; it is adjustable in length, has a movable hand-bar, and may be constructed of wood or aluminum. All types should have heavy rubber suction tips to decrease the danger of slipping. The top of the crutch has a crossbar, called the "axillary bar", which may or may not be padded. Some doctors believe that padding reduces the pressure on the rib cage or the axillae.

Crutch Palsy. The pressure of bearing the body weight on the axillae (armpits) may cause weakness of the forearm muscles, wrist, and hand, a condition called "crutch palsy." Crutch palsy has been known to occur within a period of 4 hours of leaning on the axillary bar in order to totally support the weight of the body (without using the hands to bear any of the weight). Some doctors therefore feel that not padding the axillary bar will discourage the patient from leaning so heavily on it and thus bearing his body weight solely from the axillae.

Adjustment of Crutches. Crutches must be measured and adjusted to the proper length for the individual patient. An easy method of measuring for crutches is to have the patient lie in bed, place a crutch next to him on the bed, and measure from the axilla to a point 6 to 8 inches out from the side of his heel. Adjust the crutches to this length, using the wing nuts and bolts. The hand-bar should be located at a point equivalent to the distance from the axilla to the middle of the palm of the hand with the wrist slightly hyperextended and the elbow flexed

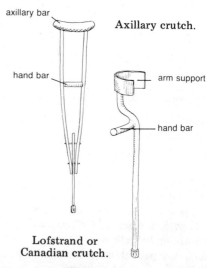

Axillary crutch.

Lofstrand or Canadian crutch.

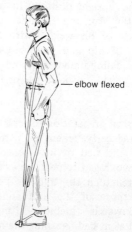

Crutch-walking — standing position.

30°. Adjust the hand-bar as needed; this allows the arms, and hands to bear more of the body weight, by lifting the body slightly by straightening the arms.

Crutches can be checked for proper fit by passing two fingers between the axillary bar and the axilla when the patient is in a standing position. The elbow should be bent about 30°, with the hand gripping the hand-bar and the axillary bar resting firmly against the patient's chest wall.

Using Crutches. The principles of crutch-walking include the following:

a. The head is held up and the eyes look ahead, as in normal walking.

b. The crutches are placed slightly ahead of the patient's feet and to the outside of each foot.

c. The hands, not the axillae, are used to support the body weight.

d. The back should be kept in straight alignment and the patient should bend at the ankles or at the hips.

e. A smooth, easy rhythm should be achieved in shifting the weight from the crutches to the good or unaffected leg and then to the crutches again.

f. The crutches should be of proper length and equipped with heavy rubber suction tips to prevent slipping.

g. The gait used will depend on the weight bearing status of the lower extremities and the patient's ability.

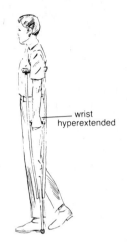

wrist hyperextended

Crutch-walking —
weight-bearing
position.

Question 13. You should be able to answer these questions about crutches.

a. Why is the elbow flexed about 30° when measuring or fitting crutches?

_____.

b. In the figures shown in the text, in which position is the elbow extended?

_____.

In which position is the wrist hyperextended? _____.

c. In crutch-walking, the patient should keep his back straight and bend

from the _____ or _____.

d. The patient should look _____ when walking on crutches.

U
N
I
T
10

ITEM 13. GAITS USED IN CRUTCH–WALKING

The type of gait that the patient will use in crutch-walking depends upon the amount of weight he is able to support with one or both legs. The three-point gait is used more often in temporary crutch situations by patients with one affected leg, such as those with a fracture of the bones of one leg, knee or hip surgery, or paralysis of one leg. The four-point and two-point gaits are used by patients who can bear partial weight on both legs, e.g., those with cerebral palsy or arthritis.

In the skill laboratory, measure a pair of crutches and adjust them to the length you need for a good fit. Then practice the three-point, four-point, and two-point gaits of crutch-walking until you are familar with each one. Remember to keep your head up, look forward (not down), keep your back straight, and bear your weight on your hands, not on your armpits.

A. Three-point Gait

Full weight bearing on one leg and partial or no weight bearing on the other.

Sequence of the gait: advance with both crutches forward, shift weight to crutches, then advance the unaffected leg and shift the weight onto it. (The affected leg may be advanced with the crutches or with the unaffected leg.)

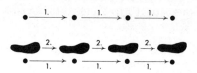

Three-point gait with the two crutches advanced first and then followed by the unaffected leg.

Advantage of the three-point gait: it allows the affected leg to be partially or completely free of weight bearing.

B. Four-point Gait

Partial weight bearing on both legs is necessary.

Sequence of the gait: in standing position: (1) advance the left crutch, (2) then advance the right foot, (3) the right crutch, and then (4) the left foot.

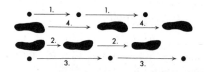

Four-point gait.

Advantage of the four-point gait: it is the most stable.

C. Two-point Gait

Partial weight bearing on both legs is necessary.

Sequence of the gait: in standing position: (1) advance left crutch and right foot, and
(2) then the right crutch and the left foot.

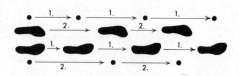

Two-point gait most nearly resembles the normal walking pattern.

Advantages of the two-point gait: it is a faster version of the four-point gait and is a more normal walking pattern with opposing arm and leg traveling forward at the same time.

Many patients are taught a swing-to and swing-through gait for rapid walking. However, you are not required to learn this gait in this lesson.

ITEM 14. ASSISTING WITH THE USE OF CRUTCHES

In the skill laboratory, practice the steps of the procedure for assisting a patient with crutch-walking, with another person playing the role of the patient.

Important Steps	Key Points
1. Wash your hands, approach and identify the patient, explain the procedure, and enlist his cooperation.	He may be apprehensive about using crutches, have a fear of falling, or doubt his ability to learn to use crutches. Accept his right to have these feelings and explain the manner in which you will demonstrate the use of crutches. Assist him to use them, and stay with him as he practices. Encourage him to regard the use of crutches as a sign of progress toward greater independence.
2. Obtain the crutches.	Secure crutches from the storage or supply room. Select the size most appropriate for the patient: child, youth, adult, or tall adult. Make sure that the crutches are an adjustable type with a good pair of rubber suction tips. Worn tips should be replaced with new ones to prevent slipping. Take the crutches to the patient's bedside. Wash your hands.
3. Measure the patient and adjust the crutches to the proper length.	Have the patient lie supine in bed, in good body alignment. Measure the distance from the patient's axilla to a point 6 to 8 inches from the side of his heel. Loosen the wing screws and bolts of the crutches, adjust the length, and refasten. Measure the distance from his axilla to the palm of his hand with his elbow flexed at a 30° angle and the wrist slightly hyperextended; then adjust the hand-bar. It is better to have the crutches an inch or so too short than to have them too long; this insures weight bearing on the hands rather than on the axillae.
4. Prepare the patient.	Assist him to dress in pajamas, robe, and shoes, or in street clothing. Pajamas are preferred for the beginner because they cover the legs, prevent exposure in case of a fall, and may be grasped at the waist by the nurse worker to guide or give support. When possible, use a walking belt or a folded drawsheet around the waist of the beginner to provide support and help prevent him from falling.
5. Position the patient.	If patient is in an adjustable high-low bed, place the bed in the low position. Assist him to sit at the side of the bed with his feet dangling. (See lesson on "Patient Movement and Ambulation.")

UNIT 10

Important Steps	Key Points
6. Demonstrate the crutch-walking gait the patient is to use.	The demonstration and explanation will show the patient how to use the crutches to walk. He will be better able to watch the demonstration in the sitting position, and will have more support of his body, than if he were standing.
7. Assist the patient to use the crutches and learn the crutch gait.	Help him to stand at the side of the bed and hand him both crutches. Check the fit of the crutches and have him balance on them while standing. If the patient is unsteady in balancing, report this to your team leader before proceeding any further. When the patient is learning crutch-walking, walk behind him and hold the walking belt, the pajama waistband, or the ties of the drawsheet in order to provide support in case he becomes unsteady or begins to fall. Have another person walk at the side or in front of the beginner to help give additional support when needed.
8. Help the patient return to bed.	Keep practice sessions short to avoid strain and muscle fatigue. Ask the patient to walk, using his crutches, to the side of the bed and then turn so that his back is to the bed. Have him hand you one crutch or set it aside, and with his free hand reach down for the side of the bed. He will then set the other crutch aside and lower himself to a sitting position. If the patient is able to use crutches without assistance, place them where he can reach them later. Help him to remove his robe and slippers, take off the walking belt or drawsheet if used, and swing his legs onto the bed.
9. Provide for the patient's comfort.	Adjust the bed and pillows as he may desire. Straighten the top bedding. Place the bedside stand and call signal within easy reach.
10. Report and record as appropriate.	Report to the team leader or the nurse in charge that the procedure has been carried out. Report and record any change in the patient's condition as suggested for other parts of this lesson, including the patient's tolerance for crutch-walking and his progress in learning. Charting example: 3:10 P.M. Ambulated first time on crutches. Walked easily in his room. Became tired quickly. Returned to bed. Vital signs remained stable. J. Jones, SN

Some patients will need to learn how to go up and down stairs using crutches. Although you will not be required to know this information for the performance test, you will find it included in the workbook as information for enrichment.

The procedure for assisting the patient in and out of bed with crutches is easily adapted to instructions for using crutches to sit in and rise from a chair. This is shown in the accompanying sketches.

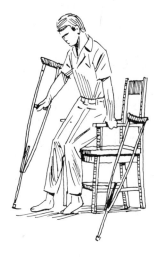

Sitting down in chair.

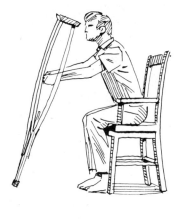

Getting up from chair.

ITEM 15.   WHAT ARE BRACES?

Braces provide specific support for weakened muscles and joints or provide immobilization of the injured part. Braces are ordered by the physician, and the cost of the brace is charged to the patient. Almost all braces are custom-made and fitted to the individual patient. The most common types of braces are those for the neck, the back, the arm, and the leg.

The well-made and well-fitted brace should not cause pressure at any point on the patient's body. However, time is required for the patient to adapt to the support of the brace, and even the best-fitting brace may cause slight pressure or soreness on the bony prominences or at the upper and lower cuffs of the brace. When there is irritation at these areas, thin layers of sponge rubber or folded layers of soft linen may be used to pad the area. Cotton batting should not be used because it has a tendency to become compacted and uneven. The most common cause of poorly-fitting braces is putting them on wrong. No brace will fit properly or be effective if it is put on backwards or upside-down.

There are many types of braces, and it would be impossible to describe them all. Most are made of various combinations of metal, leather, and cloth. Some braces, especially those for the arm or leg, have a hinge to allow movement at the joint. The hinges should be oiled every six weeks, and the metal lubricated to prevent rust. Lubricate hinges slightly with

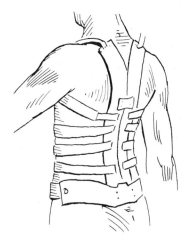

Back brace.

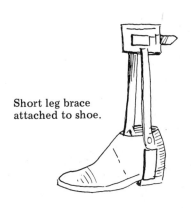

Short leg brace attached to shoe.

Important Steps   Key Points

cup grease or silicone grease. The use of vaseline
or light household oils is not advised because
they are too thin, tend to run, and could stain
clothing. Cloth braces should be hand-washed,
and the leather portions cleaned periodically.
Almost all leg braces are attached to the
patient's shoe.

Question 14. After reading this section on braces, you should be able to answer the
following questions.

 a. A brace is used to provide _____ or _____ for weakened
     muscles or joints.

 b. The most frequent cause of poor fitting braces is putting the brace on

     _____ or _____ .

 c. The moving metal parts and hinges of braces should be oiled every

     _____ weeks.

 d. The patient who is wearing a brace may develop pressure areas or soreness

     over _____ or _____ .

ITEM 16. ASSISTING WITH BACK BRACE

In the skill laboratory, you are to practice the procedure of assisting to put on a back
brace. Ask another person to play the part of the patient for your practice period.

Important Steps	Key Points
1. Approach and identify the patient, explain the procedure, and enlist his cooperation.	Most patients are cooperative because they have already been fitted for the brace and have also had to pay for it. However, a patient may resist wearing the brace if it causes pain, pressure, or more discomfort.
2. Obtain the back brace.	Since it is the patient's property, it is generally kept at the bedside or with his belongings. Wash your hands.
3. Position the patient.	Have him lying flat (supine position) in bed. Help him to move to the proximal, or near, side of the bed by using good body alignment and movement.
4. Put the back brace on the patient.	Keep his back and neck in straight alignment and roll his body toward you. Place the top of the brace over the upper back and the bottom cuff or edge of the brace over the hips and lower back. The brace should slip readily into place and follow the contour of the patient's back. Gently roll him and his brace from the side position to his back. Reach under the proximal, or near, side of the patient and draw the straps of the brace through. Bring the straps over from the distal, or far, side of the brace and fasten them together snugly in the front.

Important Steps	Key Points
5. Check for pressure points caused by the brace.	With the brace snugly fastened, assist the patient to a dangling or sitting position at the side of the bed. Check for possible pressure areas over the bony prominences of the hips, over the ribs, over the breastbone (sternum), and at the upper and lower edges of the brace. You should be able to slip your finger between the brace and the flesh at these points. If the brace fits properly and still causes some soreness in these areas, pad them with sponge rubber or soft cloth.
6. Assist the patient as needed for his comfort and safety.	Help him to put on his robe and slippers or to dress in street clothing. Generally, the patient may walk or sit in a chair with his back brace on. Some patients who have had recent surgery on the spine may begin wearing a brace while still on bed rest and would not be allowed in a sitting position to undergo a check for pressure areas.
7. Remove the back brace from the patient.	Assist the patient to lie flat in bed. Unfasten the straps in the front of the brace and push the proximal side straps down close to his side. Keep his back and neck in straight alignment and roll his body toward you. Grasp the brace and remove it. Then return the patient to his original position.
8. Store the brace in the proper place.	Usually the brace will be kept at the patient's bedside. Inspect the brace and clean it if necessary before storing it.
9. Report and record as appropriate.	Report to the team leader or the nurse in charge that the procedure has been carried out. Also report and record any complaints of discomfort caused by the brace. Any area of pressure, redness, or irritation of the skin should be described fully. Charting example: 6:10 P.M. Back brace applied for first time. Brace fits well, no pressure areas noted. Remained in chair throughout evening meal. In good spirits.　　　　J. Jones, SN or 6:10 P.M. Back brace applied for first time. Brace fits well except for excessive rubbing over right iliac crest. Area padded with foam rubber, with no relief. Brace removed. Reported to doctor.　　　　J. Jones, SN

UNIT 10

ITEM 17.   ASSISTING WITH LONG LEG BRACE (AK, ABOVE THE KNEE)

A long leg brace, one that extends from the foot to the upper thigh, is also put on the patient while he is lying in bed. For the post-test on this lesson you will not be required to demonstrate assisting the patient to put on a long leg brace.

ITEM 18.   ASSISTING WITH SHORT LEG BRACE (BK, BELOW THE KNEE)

You should now practice assisting the patient to put on a short leg brace, if one is available for your use.

Important Steps	Key Points
1. Approach and identify the patient, explain the procedure, and enlist his cooperation. Wash your hands.	Some patients will object to wearing leg braces because of the weight of the brace and the strain on muscles that are weak or in poor alignment. However, most leg braces should be worn consistently for support or immobilization.
2. Obtain the brace.	The brace is made and fitted for the patient; as his property, it would normally be kept at his bedside or with his belongings. Check to see that it is clean and in good working order.
3. Position the patient.	Assist him to a dangling or sitting position at the side of the bed. Most short leg braces are attached to a shoe and are easier to put on in a sitting position.
4. Put the leg brace on the patient.	Loosen the laces of the shoe if it is a laced type. Make sure the cuff of the brace is untied or unfastened. Slip the patient's foot (of the affected leg) into the shoe attached to the brace. Make sure that the toes are not curled under the foot. Tie the laces of the shoe. Slip the upper cuff of the brace around the calf of the affected leg and tie or fasten it snugly, but do not fasten so tightly that it interferes with the blood circulation.
5. Check the brace for pressure areas.	Have the patient stand at the bedside and check the areas around the upper cuff of the brace, and the bony prominences just below the knee and around the ankle. You should be able to slip your finger between the brace and the flesh underneath it. Check the function of the hinge at the ankle (if the brace has one) by having the patient take one step on it. It should keep the toe of the shoe slightly upward to prevent the toe from dragging.

Important Steps	Key Points
6. Provide for the patient's comfort.	Assist the patient to put on his robe and other slipper or to dress in street clothing. Most patients are permitted to be up in a chair or walk with a brace on. Stay near him to give assistance if this is his first trial.
7. Assist the patient to remove the short leg brace.	Have him sit at the side of his bed. Untie or unfasten the upper cuff of the brace and then untie the laces of the shoe. Slip the shoe and the brace off the affected leg. Assist him to swing his legs onto the bed, to undress, and to put on pajamas or a gown. Leave the bedside stand and call signal within easy reach. Ask if there is anything else you can do for him, and tell him when you expect to return.
8. Report and record as appropriate.	Report to the team leader or the nurse in charge that the procedure has been carried out. Also, report and record any complaints the patient may have of discomfort, and be sure to describe any areas of pressure or irritation caused by the brace. Charting example:

4:30 P.M. Applied short leg brace to left leg for first time. Tolerated well. No pressure areas observed or reported.   J. Jones, SN

6 P.M. Short leg brace removed. Tolerated well.
J. Jones, SN

U
N
I
T
10

ITEM 19. ASSISTING WITH THE NECK BRACE

Neck braces are used frequently to support and to immobilize the neck following an injury. Generally, the neck brace is applied while the patient is in a sitting position. It is slipped under the chin and fastened at the back of the neck. You will not be expected to demonstrate the application of a neck brace in the performance test for this lesson.

ITEM 20. CONCLUSION OF THE LESSON

You have now completed the lesson on assisting the patient to use mechanical aids for ambulation and movement. When you have had sufficient practice in using these aids correctly, make an appointment with your instructor to take the post-test.

V. ADDITIONAL INFORMATION FOR ENRICHMENT

Those of you who have a special interest or who wish to learn more about the use of mechanical aids to assist the patient in ambulation and movement may want to read further. Some special items are included in this section, but you will not be required to learn them or to demonstrate the skills in the performance test for this lesson.

SPECIAL SKILLS FOR CRUTCH-WALKING

Patients who use crutches to walk must learn the skills of opening doors and going up or down steps. To open a door, the patient on crutches approaches the door, reaches out with one hand to unlatch the door, and pushes it open. He then holds the door open with the tip of his crutch and proceeds through the door.

The rule to remember when instructing the patient in going up and down steps is "angels go up and devils go down." When going up steps, the good or unaffected leg is advanced to the next step because it will support the weight. It is followed by the crutches and the affected leg. In going down steps, the crutches and the affected leg lead off to the next step as the good leg again supports the weight until it can be shifted to the crutches.

In going up or down a flight of stairs some patients may use only one crutch — but take the other along — and rely on the handrail or bannister for support. Caution the patient to take both crutches with him — he will need them after negotiating the stairs.

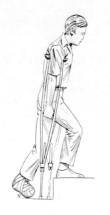 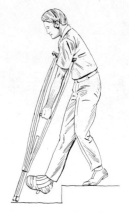

"Angels" go up . . .   "devils" go down.

The unsteady patient or the one who may be too weak to lift his body weight up or down steps on crutches could manage steps in this manner, sitting on step after step and dragging the affected leg along, if it were necessary. But don't forget the crutches.

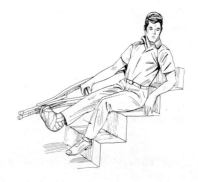

Even this works!

USE OF CANE

Canes are another form of mechanical aid for patient ambulation. Most people need little or no instruction in how to use a cane. However, the cane should be of proper height for the patient; with his elbow flexed at a $30°$ angle, the curve or handle of the cane should fit the palm of his hand and extend to the floor at a point about 6 inches out from his foot. The cane should have a good rubber suction tip to prevent slipping. There are many varieties such as crab canes, tripod canes, and others.

WORKBOOK ANSWER SHEET

1. Temporary; permanent

2. Temporary

3. Wheelchair or stretcher

4. Wheelchair or walker — to provide support

5. a. sit upright

   b. support his neck and head

   c. use at least one of his arms

6. a. balance in upright position

   b. bear weight on one foot

   c. have use of arms and hands

7. High

8. Low

9. 30°

10. Hands

11. Partial; full

12. Yes

13. a. when arm is straightened using the crutch, it will lift the body slightly

    b. weight bearing; weight bearing

    c. ankles; hips

    d. straight ahead

14. a. support; immobilization

    b. backwards; upside down

    c. six

    d. bony prominences; around edges or cuffs of the brace

U
N
I
T
10

PERFORMANCE TEST

In the skill laboratory, your instructor will ask you to perform four out of the seven activities listed below without reference to any source material. For several of the activities you will need another person to take the part of the patient.

1. Given a patient sedated for surgery, you will obtain assistance from other workers, and transfer the patient from the bed to a stretcher without causing discomfort or injury.

2. Given a patient who can stand on one or both feet, you will transfer the patient from the bed to a wheelchair.

3. Given a patient who cannot stand, you will use a mechanical lifter or obtain assistance from other workers to transfer the patient from the bed to a wheelchair, using good body alignment and movement to prevent strain, and observing the principles of balance and lifting to prevent the patient from slipping or falling.

4. Given a patient who will use the wheelchair himself as a method of locomotion, you will demonstrate and explain the wheelchair technique for operating the brakes, using the footrest pedals, propelling the chair, and making a turn.

5. Given a patient in bed who needs support while walking, you will adjust a walker to the proper height and transfer the patient into the walker in a safe manner to prevent slipping or falling.

6. Given a patient who needs the support of crutches for walking, you will measure the crutches to the proper length for the patient, adjust them to this length, and adjust the hand-bar.

7. Given a patient who is beginning to learn crutch-walking, you will demonstrate one of the following gaits and state the weight-bearing condition related to that gait: (a) four-point gait, (b) two-point gait, or (c) three-point gait.

8. Given a patient who needs a brace for support of a specific portion of the body, you will apply one of the following braces and state the possible areas of pressure that could result from wearing the brace.

   a. Back brace

   b. Long leg brace

   c. Short leg brace

   d. Neck brace

PERFORMANCE CHECKLIST

MECHANICAL AIDS FOR AMBULATION AND MOVEMENT

TRANSFERRING THE PATIENT FROM THE BED TO THE STRETCHER.

1. Obtain a stretcher.

2. Wash your hands.

3. Identify the patient and explain the procedure.

4. Provide for privacy.

5. Position and prepare the patient.

    a. Put his bed in high position.

    b. Loosen the top bedding.

    c. Check all tubing.

    d. Loosen the drawsheet for use as a "lifting" sheet.

6. Position the stretcher next to the bed.

7. Transfer the patient onto the stretcher by using the "lifting" sheet.

8. Make the patient comfortable.

    a. Place a pillow under his head.

    b. Cover him with a blanket or sheet.

    c. Remove the top bedding.

    d. Raise the siderails or fasten the safety belt.

    e. Check and provide for tubes and tubing.

9. Report and record the procedure as appropriate.

TRANSFERRING THE PATIENT FROM THE BED TO THE WHEELCHAIR

1. Obtain the proper equipment.

2. Wash your hands.

3. Identify the patient and explain the procedure.

4. Position the wheelchair and set the brakes.

5. Position and prepare the patient.

    a. Place his bed in the low position.

    b. Assist him to sit on the side of the bed and dangle his feet.

    c. Help him to put on his robe and slippers.

6. Assist him into the wheelchair.

    a. Have him stand and walk to the chair.

    b. Have him pivot and sit down in the chair.

    c. Place his feet on the footrest pedals.

    d. Release the brakes and transport the patient to his destination.

7. Record and report as necessary.

TRANSFERRING A HELPLESS PATIENT BY USING A MECHANICAL LIFTER.

1. Obtain the mechanical lifter and wheelchair.

2. Wash your hands.

3. Identify the patient and explain the procedure.

4. Position the wheelchair and set the brakes.

UNIT 10

5. Position the mechanical lifter.

6. Place the patient in the slings.

   a. Put one sling under his shoulders at the level of the axillae and the other under the thighs.

   b. Attach the hooks of the slings to the lifting bar.

7. Operate the mechanical lifter.

   a. Release, or open, the hydraulic pressure valve to raise or lower the lifting bar and the patient in the sling.

   b. Close the hydraulic pressure valve to stabilize the position of the lifting bar.

   c. Use the handle pump to increase hydraulic pressure when the valve is open.

   d. With assistance in guiding the patient in the sling, roll the mechanical lifter to the wheelchair.

8. Place the patient in the wheelchair by lowering the lifting bar.

   a. Position him in good alignment.

   b. Support him with a pillow and safety belt, as needed.

   c. Put his feet on the footrest pedals.

   d. Release the brakes and transport him to his destination.

9. Record and report as appropriate.

INSTRUCTING THE PATIENT IN THE PROPER TECHNIQUES FOR USING A WHEELCHAIR

1. Obtain the appropriate equipment.

2. Check the equipment for proper working condition.

   a. Brakes.

   b. Wheels and tires.

   c. Upholstery.

3. Wash your hands.

4. Identify the patient and explain the procedure.

5. Demonstrate and describe the correct techniques for using the wheelchair to the patient.

   a. Proper use of brakes (setting and releasing).

   b. Positioning the footrest.

   c. Propelling the chair in a straight line.

   d. Turning corners.

   e. Passing through an ordinary doorway or one equipped with an automatic closing device.

6. Provide the patient with an opportunity to practice under supervision the techniques of propelling his wheelchair.

7. Encourage him to utilize the proper method of manipulating the wheelchair.

8. Chart the procedure.

TRANSFERRING THE PATIENT FROM THE BED TO THE WALKER — ADJUSTMENT OF THE WALKER

1. Obtain the proper equipment.

2. Wash your hands.

3. Identify the patient and explain the procedure.

4. Adjust the bed to the low position, if required.

5. Assist the patient to dangle his feet and dress in his robe and slippers.

6. Prepare the walker for occupancy and position it in front of the patient.

    a. Raise the seat.

    b. Remove the back support.

7. Secure the walker in place with one hand and use a foot to block a rear wheel.

8. Help him to stand and step into the walker frame.

    a. Check and adjust the height of the walker as required.

    b. Have his elbows flexed approximately $30°$.

    c. Lower the seat and replace the back support in the walker.

    d. Caution him to take small steps and to avoid going too fast.

9. Chart the procedure.

ADJUSTING CRUTCHES TO THE REQUIRED LENGTH

1. Obtain the proper equipment.

    a. Crutches should have no splinters, breaks, or bends.

    b. The crutch tip must be in good condition.

    c. The axillary pad bar should be installed, if required.

2. Wash your hands.

3. Identify the patient and explain the procedure.

4. Ask the patient to lie flat on the bed.

5. Measure to determine the length of crutch required.

6. a. The crutch tip should be approximately 6 to 8 inches from the side of the heel.

    b. There should be approximately two fingers' distance between the axillary bar and the axilla.

    c. The elbows should be flexed approximately $30°$.

7. Adjust the position of the hand-bar and the height of the shaft as required.

8. Tell the patient when he will have his crutch-walking lesson.

9. Chart the procedure.

CRUTCH-WALKING — GAIT USED FOR CRUTCH-WALKING

1. Identify two-, three-, and four-point gaits.

2. Perform the three-point gait.

    a. Conditions for use — full weight bearing on one leg, partial or no weight bearing on the other.

3. Perform the four-point gait.

    a. Conditions for use — partial weight bearing on both legs.

4. Perform the two-point gait.

    a. Conditions for use — partial weight bearing on both legs.

APPLYING A BRACE

1. Wash your hands.

2. Identify the patient.

3. Review the procedure with him.

4. Obtain the proper brace.

5. Position the patient appropriately.

6. Apply the brace correctly.

    a. Observe the principles of body alignment when manipulating the patient.

    b. Prepare the brace for application.

    c. Position the brace on the patient's body.

    d. Secure the brace correctly.

7. Adjust the brace for correct support and fit.

8. Check for pressure points.

9. Provide for the patient's comfort by assisting him in dressing or moving to a chair, and so forth.

10. Report and record the procedure.

HOSPITAL BEDS

I. DIRECTIONS TO THE STUDENT

Please read the following paragraphs carefully. They will tell you what you will be expected to do and know at the end of this lesson. After you have read the unit and have seen a film or demonstration on bedmaking, practice operating the hospital bed and the procedures of making a hospital bed in your classroom or skill laboratory. Use the principles of body alignment, balance, and movement that you learned earlier; if you are not sure of them, review the units on Body Alignment, Balance, and Movement and Using Body Movement.

When you have completed the unit and practiced the procedures, arrange with your instructor to take the performance test and demonstrate your skills in operating a hospital bed and making a hospital bed for various purposes.

II. GENERAL PERFORMANCE OBJECTIVE

Upon completion of this unit, you will be able to prepare the unoccupied (closed), occupied, and anesthetic hospital bed in a way that presents a neat appearance, remains intact with use, and provides a safe and comfortable environment for the patient. You will also be able to operate the controls of the bed in order to adjust the position of the bed as may be required.

III. SPECIFIC PERFORMANCE OBJECTIVES

When you have completed this lesson, you will be able to:

1. Adjust both manually operated and electrically operated beds to the positions used during bedmaking as well as the positions appropriate for completed beds, raising or lowering sections of the bed in the proper sequences, without errors in the selection and operation of the controls.

2. Make an unoccupied bed starting from the bare mattress by selecting the required bed linens, placing them correctly and securely on the bed, and adjusting the bed to the appropriate position. This must be accomplished in *6 minutes or less.*

3. Make an occupied bed, which has a patient in it who is able to move without assistance, by selecting the required bed linens to change all but the top linen, by giving the patient the correct directions for moving, and by adjusting the bed to the proper position for your work. This should take from 10 to 12 minutes to accomplish.

4. Make an anesthetic or surgical bed by selecting and using the appropriate items of bed linen, with the top bedding pie-folded or fan-folded on one side of the bed to permit easier transfer of a helpless patient into the bed, and by then adjusting the position of the bed appropriately, in *6 minutes or less.*

IV. VOCABULARY

anesthetic bed (postoperative, recovery, or surgical)—a bed made with top linens folded in such a way as to permit easy, rapid transfer of a patient from a stretcher to his own bed.

closed bed—a clean bed with linens on it that is ready for a newly admitted patient; the top spread covers the entire bed and protects the bottom linens from dust until occupied by a patient.

contour bed—the head, knee, and foot sections of the bed are elevated.

drawsheet—a special sheet (rubber, plastic, or cotton) that is about one-half the size of a regular sheet and is placed across the middle third of the bed to protect the bottom sheet from soiling; may be used to assist in moving heavy patients.

foundation sheet—the bottom (lower) sheet placed directly over the mattress pad or the mattress.

Gatch—the notch that fits into a ratchet on the underframe of the bed to maintain it in a sitting position; the Gatch bed was named after Dr. William Gatch, an American surgeon, who invented it in the late 1800's.

hyperextension—the head and foot of the bed lowered so that the middle section is at an angle of *not more than 15°*.

miter—a method of making equal angles so that sheets, blankets, and bedspreads fit corners properly and hold firmly.

occupied bed—the complete linen change with a patient lying in the bed.

pleat (tuck)—folded or double layer of material; a method of providing additional room in the top linens on a bed to prevent pressure on the patient's feet and toes.

reverse Trendelenburg's—the head elevated and the foot section of the bed lowered.

taut—tense, or pulled tightly.

Trendelenburg's—the head of the bed lowered and the foot of the bed elevated.

V. INTRODUCTION

Patients in a hospital spend a great part of their time in bed and the condition of the bed will influence the way the patient feels and behaves. Wrinkles and bumps in the foundation part of the bed or improperly placed top covers may cause the patient to feel uncomfortable and to become irritable. Hospital beds can be made skillfully so that wrinkles are reduced and the bed is comfortable.

A hospital bed must be made so that it is easy for the patient to get into it despite the physical disabilities he may have. It must also be easier for hospital workers to put a helpless patient into bed. This may require adjusting the position of the bed and making the bed in special ways. The patient's condition and the usual procedure of the hospital are considered when determining the method for making the bed.

Many of the patient's activities are carried on while he is in bed, e.g., various medical treatments, eating, elimination, bathing, and diversional activities. A comfortable and relatively wrinkle-free bed contributes to the patient's feeling of well-being.

In this unit, you will learn how to operate manually or electrically controlled beds and to put the bed into various positions. There are routine ways of making beds in hospitals efficiently, uniformly and neatly so that they meet the needs of most patients. You will learn how to make an unoccupied and a closed bed, an occupied bed, and an anesthetic or surgical bed.

ITEM 1. SCIENTIFIC PRINCIPLES RELATED TO BEDMAKING

These underlying principles drawn from biological science are relevant to bedmaking and the patient who is resting in bed:

Anatomy and Physiology.

1. The body exerts uneven points of pressure against different areas of the mattress. The sacrum may become the site for a pressure sore because of the weight of the patient's body and a reduced blood supply to the tissues over bony prominences.

2. Oxygen in combination with hemoglobin is carried to the body cells by the blood. Pressure reduces the blood supply of oxygen to the tissue and causes damage in the form of a pressure sore or decubitus.

3. Bed linen must be kept free from wrinkles or food crumbs that may act as irritants to the body and thus encourage possible breaks in the skin.

4. Perceptions, which are influenced by the person's physiological and psychological states, and past experiences, affect his behavior. The patient should be able to perceive the bed as a comfortable and safe place.

Chemistry.

1. Woolen blanket fibers may cause irritation to the patient's skin; there must always be a sheet to separate the blanket from the patient.

2. Strong detergents, soaps, and bleaches used in commercial laundries may cause skin irritation if bed linens are not thoroughly rinsed.

Microbiology.

1. Pathogenic microorganisms may be transferred from the source to a new host directly by contaminated linen. You should wash your hands before and after making a bed.

2. Bed linen should be folded away from your body to minimize the transfer of microorganisms to your clothing.

3. Fanning bed clothing stirs up bacteria in the air, and air motion is a method of transfer. Linen should therefore be changed with as little motion as possible.

U
N
I
T
11

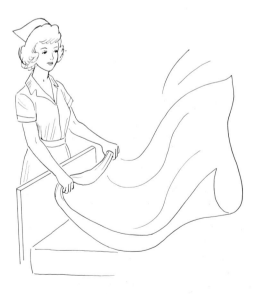

Never fan linen.

Physics.

1. Good posture should be maintained when changing bed linen. These points reduce strain on your body:

   a. Always keep your back straight; bend from your hips.

   b. Bend your knees to exert the force of work on the big, strong leg muscles rather than on your back muscles.

   c. Articles of linen should be placed on the edge of the bed rather than be held above the shoulder-level or with arms outstretched.

   d. The stability of the body is maintained by keeping the center of gravity over its base, the feet. Assume a broad stance, and bend at the knees and hips; keep your back straight.

Psychology.

1. Explain how the patient may cooperate with the bedmaking procedure if he is confined to bed. This allays his anxiety.

2. Use skill and efficiency in making the bed to minimize undue exertion and fatigue for the patient. If the procedure brings comfort and relaxation, his attitude will improve.

Sociology.

1. Suitable conversation enables you to learn about the patient and alleviates the stress of the bedmaking procedure.

2. Learn to listen as well as to talk; open a subject, then allow the patient to talk.

3. Subjects of interest to the patient usually involve his condition, his family, his work, his recreational hobby, or noncontroversial national events.

ITEM 2. THE FUNCTIONS AND STRUCTURES OF HOSPITAL BEDS

Manually Operated Bed. The hand-cranked bed requires effort and muscle power. When you operate this bed, it is essential that you use good body alignment and movements.

The manually operated bed has hand-cranks at its foot that are used to adjust the position of the bed.

To raise and lower the entire bed, pull out the hand-crank at the center of the bed and turn it clockwise to *raise* the bed. Turn it counterclockwise to *lower* the bed.

To place the bed in Fowler's and semi-Fowler's positions, pull out the hand-crank at the left foot side of the bed and turn it clockwise to *raise* the head of the bed. Turn it counterclockwise to *lower* the head of the bed. (Semi-Fowler's position is raised to approximately a 45° angle. Fowler's position is raised to approximately a 90° angle.)

To raise and lower the knees, pull out the hand-crank at the right foot side of the bed, and turn it clockwise to *raise* the knee portion of the bed. Turn it counterclockwise to *lower* the knee portion of the bed.

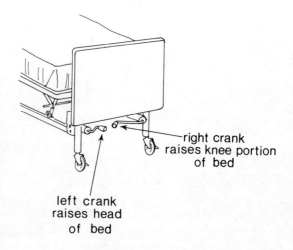

right crank raises knee portion of bed

left crank raises head of bed

Manually operated bed.

The most common positions used with this bed are the flat, Fowler's, and semi-Fowler's positions.

Siderails. Siderails are used to provide for the safety of the patient and are in no way to be considered a restraint. Siderails range in size from half the length of the bed side to the full length. Each type of siderail has special levers for raising or lowering; check with your agency for proper instructions.

Siderails are used to:

1. Prevent patients from falling out of bed.

2. Protect the restless patient.

3. Remind the patient that he is near the side of the bed, and may be in danger of falling off the edge.

4. Help the patient to lift or turn himself.

5. Provide security to the patient without causing him to feel penned in.

6. Assist ambulatory patients to get into and out of bed safely.

7. Give the patient support to grasp and hold when moving about.

Below are some examples of single safety siderails and double safety siderails:

Safety Sides in Three Positions:

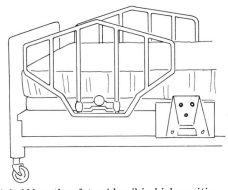

High Position. Used by the patient to turn or move about in bed. Helps the ambulatory patient to get in or out of bed. In high position the Safety Side offers needed protection to the hospital patient day and night.

A half-length safety siderail in high position.

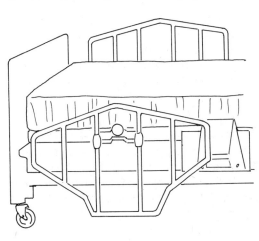

Intermediate Position. Needed when the Safety Side is not in use to provide adequate toe room for the nurse standing beside a bed in low position. Used during treatment or nursing care procedures.

U
N
I
T
11

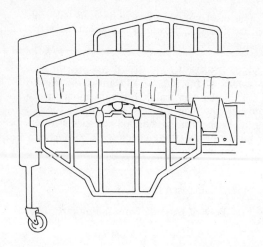

Low Position. Used only when the bed is being made or the linen changed. In this position the Safety Side does not interfere with bedmaking.

Before placing the Safety Side in low position, the bed should always be raised to high position. Damage to the Safety Side can thus be prevented.

When Two Pairs of Safety Sides Are Needed:

Two pairs of Safety Sides may be used in the few cases where a full-length guard is needed.

Electrically Operated Bed. The electric bed was first introduced in 1956. Before that time, manually operated beds were used. The electric bed is operated by a motor that adjusts the bed to the desired position for treatment or for comfort. The patient may operate the bed controls by touch, unless the controls have been purposely locked to insure a prescribed position.

Electric beds are made by a number of manufacturers who produce different types of adjustment controls used to operate the bed. Generally, the controls are sliding levers attached to a panel on the side of the bed, or push-buttons located on a moveable device connected to the bed by a cable. The controls enable the patient or the nurse to change the position of the bed with little effort.

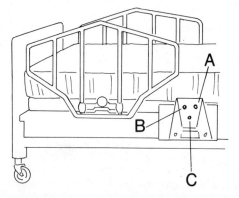

Electric controls are located at side of bed.

To raise the backrest, Push the "Head Up" button, or move control lever "A" toward the foot of the bed. *To lower the backrest,* Push the "Head Down" button, or move control lever "A" toward the head of the bed.

To raise the knee rest, Push the "Foot Up" button, or move control lever "B" toward the foot of the bed. *To lower the knee rest,* Push the "Foot Down" button, or move control lever "B" toward the head of the bed.

To raise the bed to the high position, Push the "Bed Up" button, or move control lever "C" vertically to its highest setting. *To lower the bed to the low position,* Push the "Bed Down" button, or move control lever "C" downward to its lowest setting.

There are other minor variations among electric bed control systems, depending on which manufacturer produces them. These controls may be located in various places on the bed, and may consist of levers or push-buttons that raise or lower the bed. You should check with your agency for the specific method and procedure to adjust the position of the electric bed used.

ITEM 3. BED POSITIONS

Most hospital beds can be adjusted to meet various needs of the patient for treatment or comfort. Some of the common positions are: *Fowler's.* The backrest is raised 18 to 20 inches above the bed level. This is used for patients with certain respiratory or cardiac diseases to permit better chest expansion.

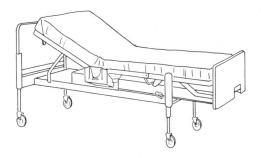

Fowler's Position (head of bed 18 to 2 inches above bed level).

Semi-Fowler's. The backrest is raised 45°. Knees may be raised 15°. This is used for the general comfort of the patient; it may prevent his sliding down in bed. Raising the knee rest may impair circulation in the lower extremities. Check with the charge nurse before elevating the knee rest.

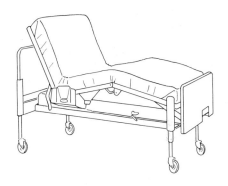

Semi-Fowler's Position (knee position may be raised 15°.)

Trendelenburg's. The head section of the bed is lowered; foot section is elevated. (Sometimes the foot of the bed is placed on "shock blocks," raised by a mechanical jack or lifter, or placed on a chair if the foot section cannot be elevated by mechanical means.) This position may be used for patients in shock from severe blood loss or other causes.

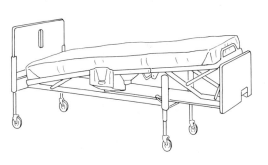

Trendelenburg's (shock).

Reverse Trendelenburg's. The head section of the bed is elevated; foot section is lowered. (The head of the bed can be raised on "shock blocks" or by a mechanical jack or lifter, or placed on a chair if the head section cannot be mechanically placed in this position.) This position is used for patients with certain circulatory diseases.

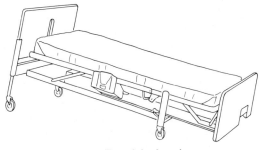

Reverse Trendelenburg's.

U
N
I
T
11

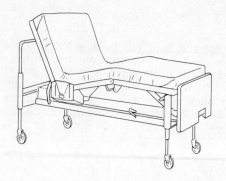

Contour. The head section is elevated; the knee and foot sections are elevated. The contour position is used for certain injuries or diseases of the lower extremities.

Contour (head section elevated and knee and foot section elevated).

Hyperextension. The head section and foot section are lowered. This position may be used for spinal fractures. *Caution:* The angle of the "break" should be no more than 15°. This is a dangerous position for a patient lying on his back. It can cause pressure on large veins in the body, for example, the vena cava, and result in decreased circulation, blood clots and other ill effects. Patients have died following slight movement after lying in this position for six hours or more. You should not put patients into this position without supervision. If you are caring for patients in this position, keep this warning constantly in mind.

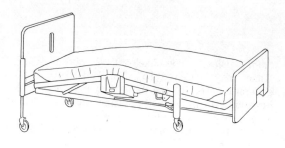

Hyperextension (head section and foot section lowered).

ITEM 4. PRACTICE IN THE OPERATION AND ADJUSTMENT OF HOSPITAL BEDS

In your classroom or skill laboratory, practice operating the hospital bed, whether manual, electrical, or both types.

1. Check the siderails of the bed. Locate the button or lever to release the siderail so that you can raise and lower the siderail several times. Notice how the siderail is attached to the bed.

2. On the manually operated bed, locate the hand-cranks at the foot of the bed. Pull the crank out and engage it so that you can raise or lower that portion of the bed. Notice how you disengage the hand-crank and replace it so that it is out of the way when you work around the bed. Notice the gatches under the head and foot of the mattress, which can be engaged in ratchets to keep those parts of the bed elevated.

   Practice raising and lowering the parts of the bed into all possible positions: Fowler's, semi-Fowler's, Trendelenburg's, reverse Trendelenburg's, contour, and hyperextension.

3. On the electrically operated bed, locate the controls. Check the levers or buttons that raise or lower portions of the bed, or the entire bed.

   Practice raising and lowering the bed into the various positions: Fowler's, semi-Fowler's, Trendelenburg's, reverse Trendelenburg's, contour, and hyperextension.

ITEM 5. PROCEDURE FOR MAKING AN UNOCCUPIED BED

There are certain principles in making a bed that should be followed to make the work easier:

Principle 1. Always stand facing the direction in which you are working, and avoid twisting your body.

Principle 2. Make one-half of a bed entirely before going to the other side, and complete the head part of the bed before going to the foot, or vice versa. An efficiency expert has said that a bed can be made taking less than 50 steps or foot movements from start to finish.

Principle 3. Most hospital linen is folded in half horizontally, then folded again. The main center fold may be from top to bottom, or from side to side. In either case, half of the sheet can be placed on the bed and the other half unfolded to cover the remaining portion of the bed. By using the center fold as a guide, you can position the sheet on half of the bed, and need not go around the bed to check whether you have half of the sheet to cover that side.

Principle 4. Wash your hands before you begin bedmaking.

In your classroom or skill laboratory, practice the following procedure for making an unoccupied bed. There should be a bed frame with mattress available for your practice use, and linen to make the bed.

Important Steps	Key Points
A. *Prepare for Bedmaking*	
1. Wash your hands.	Hands are washed before any procedure.
2. Assemble the linen supplies needed.	You will need a mattress pad, two large sheets, a plastic or rubber drawsheet, a cloth drawsheet, a blanket, a spread, two pillows, and two pillowcases. In addition, you should have a bath towel, washcloth, and patient gown in the linen pack for the patient's use. In most general hospitals, the patient is supplied with these clean items each day, or as needed throughout the day when the items become soiled.
3. Place the bed in a high position.	Having the bed in a high position puts your work at a comfortable level and helps to reduce or prevent back strain.
4. Move the mattress to the head of the bed.	Mattresses slip down when the head of the bed is raised. Stand at one side of the bed facing the head and grasp the mattress about the center and at the bottom edge. Move it toward the head of the bed, using good body alignment and movements.
B. *Make the Foundation of the Bed on One Side*	
1. Place the mattress pad on the mattress.	(Omit this step if mattress pads are not used in your agency.) Smooth the pad free of wrinkles and secure it to the mattress with elastic, ties, or zipper if any of these are used. Some pads simply lie over the mattress and are not secured.

Important Steps	Key Points
2. Place the large bottom sheet over the mattress and pad.	Place the *center fold* at the *center of the bed*, working from the foot of the bed to the head. Then unfold the top layer onto the distal half of the bed. The lower hem of the sheet should be even with the edge of the mattress at the foot. The seam should be facing toward the mattress. Tuck the excess length of sheet under the mattress at the head of the bed.
3. At the head of the bed, miter the corner where the sheet has been tucked under the mattress.	Pick up the side edge of the sheet so that it forms a triangle to the head of the bed, and the side edge is perpendicular to the bed.

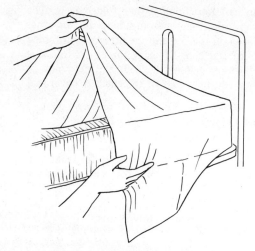

Stand facing head of bed.

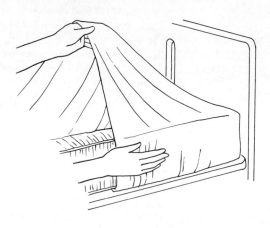

Tuck sheet under mattress.

Use the palm of your hand to hold the sheet against the side of the mattress, and tuck the excess sheet under the mattress.

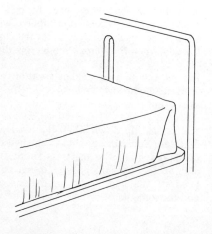

Completed square corner.

Drop the sheet over your hand, then withdraw your hand, and tuck the rest of the sheet under the mattress.

4. Tuck the sheet under the side of the mattress all the way to the foot of the bed.

Important Steps	Key Points
5. Place a plastic or rubber drawsheet over the middle section of the bed.	(This step is optional; drawsheets may not be used in your agency.) Place the center fold of the drawsheet at the center of the bed and unfold the top layer toward the distal side of bed. The drawsheet should be 12 to 15 inches from the top of the bed. Tuck the proximal edge neatly under the mattress.
6. Place the cloth drawsheet over the rubber drawsheet.	(Some agencies use a cloth-covered plastic drawsheet, so a separate cloth drawsheet is not needed. This step may also be eliminated if your agency does not use drawsheets.) Place the center fold of the drawsheet at the center of the bed and unfold the top layer toward the distal side of the bed. Tuck the proximal edge neatly under the mattress.

C. Make the Top Bedding Portion of the Bed on One Side

1. Place the top sheet on the bed.	Start at the head of the bed with the edge of the sheet even with the mattress, seam side up. Place the center fold of the top sheet along the center of the bed, and unfold the upper layer over on the distal half of the bed.
2. Make a toe pleat in either of two ways: Method A—At the center of the foot of the mattress, make a 6-inch lengthwise pleat in the sheet. Tuck the end of the sheet under the mattress; *or* Method B—About 6 to 8 inches from foot of bed, fold a 2-inch pleat across the sheet. Tuck the end of the sheet under the mattress.	The toe pleat provides room for the feet to move in bed, and prevents pressure and strain on the toes or ankles. *Note:* The toe pleat is optional — follow your agency procedure. In some agencies, the top linens over the toes are simply elevated slightly to provide additional toe space if you should draw the top linens too tightly when securing them under the bottom edge of the mattress.

U
N
I
T
11

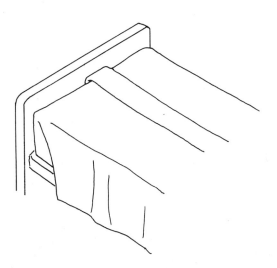

Method A
Longitudinal toe pleat.

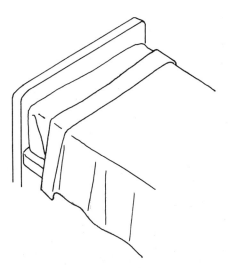

Method B
Horizontal toe pleat.

Important Steps	Key Points
3. Place the blanket on the bed.	Start at the head of the bed, about 4 inches from the top of the mattress, and place the center fold of the blanket along the center of the bed. Unfold the remaining half toward the distal side of the bed. Tuck the remaining portion of the blanket under the foot of the mattress. Make a toe pleat if used. In warm weather or if the room is warm, a blanket may be optional.
4. Put the bedspread on the bed.	Start at the head of the bed, about 4 inches from the top of the mattress, and place the center fold of the spread along the center of the bed. Unfold the remaining half of the spread toward the distal side of the bed. Make a toe pleat if used. Tuck the remaining portion of the spread under the edge of the mattress.
5. Miter the corner of the top linens at the foot of the bed.	Pick up the edges of the sheet, the blanket, and the spread, and smooth around the corner so that the side edge is perpendicular to the bed. Use the palm of your hand to hold the sheet, blanket, and spread against the mattress. Tuck the hanging portion under the mattress. Bring down the upper portion, which had been picked up, and smooth it into a neat line.

D. Move to the Other Side of the Bed and Complete Making the Bed

1. Fan-fold top linen back toward the center of the bed while you complete the foundation.	
2. With the bottom sheet, miter the corner at the head of the bed.	See steps listed in Section B. Grasp the edges of the sheet tightly in both hands with your knuckles on top, pull them tightly and smoothly down over the side of the mattress and tuck them under the mattress. Repeat the pulling and tucking all along the side, working toward the foot of the bed.
3. Grasp the bottom edge of the sheet and pull it tightly in a *diagonal direction* to remove the last wrinkles and looseness.	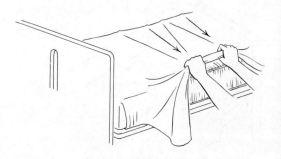 Grasp sheet; pull tight.
4. Grasp the edge of the plastic or rubber drawsheet in both hands with your knuckles on top, pull it down tightly over the side of the mattress, and tuck it in under the mattress. In situations where no drawsheet is available, fold a large sheet in half and use it as a drawsheet. Place the folded edge toward the head of the bed.	
5. Straighten and grasp the drawsheet in both hands with your knuckles on top, pull it down tightly over the side of the mattress, and tuck it in.	

Important Steps   Key Points

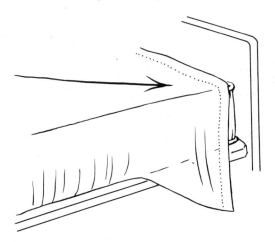 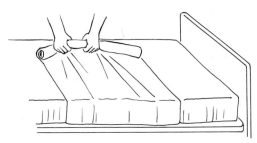

Pull sheet diagonally to remove wrinkles.   Grasp drawsheet and pull tight over mattress.

6. Move to the foot of the bed, and take the edge of the top sheet, and tuck it under the bottom edge of the mattress.

7. Straighten the blanket, and tuck the remaining portion under the bottom edge of the mattress.

8. Straighten the spread, and tuck the remaining portion under the bottom edge of the mattress.

9. At the foot of the bed, miter the corner of the top linens, using the top sheet, blanket, and spread as one unit.

10. Move to the head of the bed, and fold back the top sheet over the top edge of the blanket and spread.

         This makes a cuff over the spread and blanket, and protects them from becoming soiled when drawn up under the patient's chin. It also prevents irritation to the patient's chin by covering the rough blanket with the smooth sheet.

E. Dress the Pillows

1. Open the pillowcase.

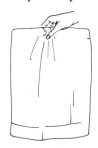 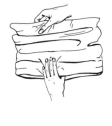

         With one hand, grasp the center of the closed end of the case. With your other hand, gather the open pillowcase (as you would a stocking before putting it on) up over the hand at the closed end.

(1) Grasp center.   (2) Gather open pillowcase.

U
N
I
T
11

Important Steps   **Key Points**

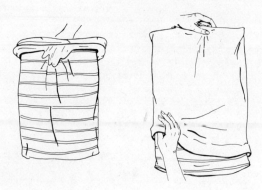

Grasp the pillow with your covered hand while holding it away from your body. With the other hand on an open edge, pull the open edges down over the pillow. Do this until the pillow is completely covered. Adjust the pillow inside the case, keeping it from contaminating your uniform.

(3) Grasp pillow.   (4) Pull pillowcase over pillow.

2. Place the dressed pillows on the bed.

Put them at the center of the head of the bed one on top of the other. Position them so that the open ends of the cases are away from the door of the room. This gives the bed a neater appearance.

F. Prepare an Unoccupied Bed for the Patient to Get into Easily

1. Fan-fold the top covers toward the foot of the bed,

or

Bring the top edge of the covers to the foot of the bed, then fold them back toward the center of the bed. The top covers will be near the middle of the bed.

2. pie-fold the covers.

Place one finger at the center of the top covers facing the head of the bed. Lift the edge of the top covers and fold it back toward the center of the bed making a triangle.

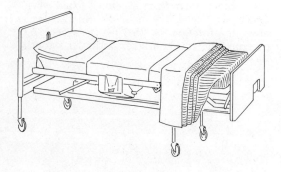

Fan-fold covers.

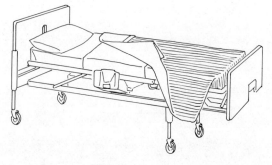

The pie-fold.

G. Prepare the Bed and Unit for the Patient

1. Lower the bed to its bottom position.

This is most convenient for newly admitted, ambulatory, and semiambulatory patients to get into bed Apply the brakes at the foot of

Important Steps	Key Points
	the bed. The brakes should be in the locked position to prevent the bed from moving when the patient attempts to get into bed.
2. Attach the signal cord to the bed in a place where the patient can reach it easily.	Many cords have a special clip that clamps onto the pillowcase or foundation sheet.
3. Put the linens for the patient in the proper places.	Put towels and washcloth in the bathroom or in the bedside stand; put the hospital gown on the bed or in the bedside stand. (Use your agency procedure.)
4. Tidy the unit.	Neatly arrange the furnishings in the room, and remove linen and other items not needed for the patient's use.

ITEM 6.   THE CLOSED BED

The designation "closed bed" indicates that no patient occupies the bed. It is made so that the top covers and spread cover the bed completely to protect the linen beneath from soil or dust.

The procedure for making the closed bed is identical to that followed in making the unoccupied bed except for the spread. In the closed bed, the bedspread is put on as follows:

1. Place the center fold of the spread on the bed, seam side toward the mattress. Begin at the head of the bed, and place the top edge of the spread even with the edge of the mattress.

2. Unfold the spread over the other half of the bed.

3. Tuck the spread under the bottom edge of the mattress.

4. Miter the corner on each side of the foot of the bed, making a smooth, neat corner.

5. Place the dressed pillows in the correct position with the open end of the case away from the door, and carry out the procedure in Section G to prepare the unoccupied bed and unit for the arrival of a new patient.

ITEM 7.   THE ANESTHETIC OR SURGICAL BED

The anesthetic bed is also called the postoperative bed (post-op), the recovery bed, or the surgical bed. The object is to make the bed with all top bedding folded out of the way so the patient can be transferred from a stretcher to the bed with a minimum of time and movement, and then covered with the top bedding. This type of bed can be made for use when the patient undergoes medical treatments or has severe physical limitations of movement due to his condition or his disease. It is not restricted to patients who undergo surgery.

Basically, the bed is made in the same manner as the "unoccupied bed." There are some minor changes, which you should practice in the classroom or skill laboratory.

Important Steps	Key Points
1. Prepare the foundation of the bed as described in Item 5.	
2. Place a cotton bath blanket over half of the foundation bed, and tuck it under the mattress on the side where you are working. (This is optional.)	In some colder climates, the cotton bath blanket provides additional warmth for the patient. (Follow your agency procedure.)

U
N
I
T
11

Important Steps	Key Points
3. Make the top of the bed according to Item 5, except that the top sheet, blanket, and spread *are not tucked* under the mattress at the foot of the bed, nor are the corners mitered.	Instead of tucking the top linens under the mattress, fold the covers back toward the head of the bed to make a 6- to 8-inch cuff that is even with the edge of the mattress at the foot of the bed.
4. Fold the top covers to the side or to the foot of the bed.	
a. Fan-fold the top covers lengthwise to the side of the bed,	Fold the overhang of the covers up onto the bed, even with the side of the bed. Lift the covers with both hands and make a 6- to 8-inch fold; repeat once more so that all covers are folded lengthwise on the far side of the bed.

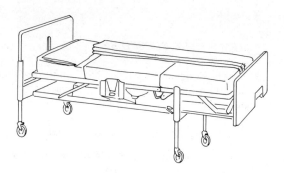

Fan-fold lengthwise.

b. or fan-fold them widthwise to the bottom of the bed.	Fold accordion-type pleats 6 to 8 inches wide from the head of the bed to the foot, *or* fold half of the top cover toward the foot of the bed, and accordion pleat once or twice so that all covers are at the foot of the bed.
5. Place a towel or disposable pad at the head of the foundation bed.	This is intended to protect the sheet if the patient should vomit (have an emesis).
6. Place the pillows.	Put pillow either on a chair near the bed or in an upright position at the head of the bed.
7. Prepare the unit for the arrival of the patient.	
a. Check to see that siderails are attached to the bed, are in working order, and are in the lowered position.	
b. Attach the signal cord to the bed.	
c. Leave the bed in a high position.	The high level of the bed is approximately the same level as a stretcher in order to make it easier to transfer the patient from one to another.
d. Lock the brakes of the bed.	This prevents it from moving when the patient is being transferred into it.
e. Move furniture away from the bed.	Clear a space to allow room for the easy passage of the stretcher and for workers to transfer the patient from the stretcher to the bed.

Important Steps	Key Points
f. Tidy the unit, and remove linen and other items not needed for the postoperative care of the patient.	Other items that are required for the care of a patient returning from surgery will be discussed in the unit on postoperative care.

ITEM 8.   PROCEDURE FOR MAKING AN OCCUPIED BED

In the day-by-day care of patients, it is often necessary to change some of the linen on the patient's bed while he is still lying in his bed. Not all patients are able to get out of bed while it is being made up with fresh linen. In most hospitals, some of the linen on the bed is changed daily or as needed throughout the day and night, and some linen is used again unless it has been soiled or is wet.

Practice the procedure of making a bed with a patient in it by having one of your classmates play the part of a patient while you make the bed in the classroom or skill laboratory. Remember to use good body alignment and movements as you work. When you instruct the patient where to move, you should be concerned with his alignment as well. Use smooth, coordinated movements in your work to avoid jarring the patient or causing him discomfort. Explain what you are doing as you go along so that he will be better able to cooperate and to understand what is expected of him.

This must be accomplished in 10 to 12 minutes.

Important Steps	Key Points
1. Wash your hands, identify the patient, explain what you plan to do, and enlist his cooperation.	While doing so, you can check the condition of the linens on his bed, and estimate what you will need to change it.
2. Provide for the patient's privacy.	Close the door of the room, pull the bedside curtains, or use screens to provide privacy.
3. Obtain the articles of linen you will need.	You should have a large sheet, drawsheet, spread, patient gown, towel, washcloth, and linen hamper for soiled linen. You should plan to change the bottom sheet and use the cleaner top sheet as the bottom sheet. However, some agencies may use entirely clean linen each day. Follow your agency procedure. In most hospitals, you may not be able to take a linen hamper to the unit, but may have to share it with other workers who are also making beds. In other hospitals, all soiled linen is carried to a central area and put in hampers that are kept there. Place the clean linen on the seat of a chair or on a dresser near your work area.
4. Remove the used linen from the bed.	Work on one side of the bed and complete your work there before going to the other side.
a. Lower the siderail on the side of the bed where you will begin work.	
b. Unfold and place the bath blanket over the patient and the top covers.	The bath blanket may be kept in the patient's bedside stand or issued with his daily linen pack. It provides additional warmth during the procedure. Have the patient hold the top edge of the bath blanket, or tuck it under his shoulders to secure it. Reach under the bath blanket, grasp the top bedding (sheet, blanket, and spread), and fan-fold them to the bottom of the bed. The patient is now covered by the bath blanket, and the top covers are at the foot of

UNIT 11

Important Steps	Key Points

the bed. This provides privacy and prevents exposure of the patient.

c. Loosen the top covers at the foot of the bed.

Move around to the foot of the bed, and remove the covers that were tucked under the mattress.

d. Remove the spread.

You are to use a fresh spread in this practice procedure, so the soiled spread should be discarded into the laundry hamper. If the spread were to be used again on the bed, you would fold it in eighths and hang it over the back of the chair.

e. Remove the blanket, and fold it for reuse.

Fold the blanket and keep it from touching the floor during the procedure. Fold it in half—top edge to bottom edge or side edge to side edge. Grasp the center of the folded blanket, and fold it in half again. Fold it in half once more. Place it over the back of a chair for reuse.

f. Remove the top sheet and fold it for reuse as described above.

Place it over the back of a chair.

5. Move the mattress to the top of the bed.

a. If the patient is able, ask him to grasp the head of the bed with his hands, and pull when you give the word.

b. Grasp the side edge of the mattress with both hands and move it toward the top of the bed as in Item 5, Making an Unoccupied Bed.

Tell the patient when you are ready to move so that he can help pull himself toward the head of the bed. Be sure to use good body alignment and movements. If he is unable to help, you may need to obtain help to move the mattress with the patient on it.

c. When moving a mattress with a helper, one person should stand at each side of the bed, grasp the mattress with both hands, and on your cue, slide it toward the head of the bed.

6. Move the patient to the distal side of the bed.

Turn him away from you and on his side according to the instructions in the unit on positioning the bed patient. He may hold onto the siderail on the far side of the bed for support. If he is unable to hold on, he may need a pillow at his back for support.

7. Make the foundation of the bed on one side.

a. Loosen the foundation linens (sheet, drawsheet, and plastic drawsheet) from the top and side of the bed.

b. Fold or roll the drawsheet toward the patient, then the plastic drawsheet, then the bottom sheet; tuck the soiled linen rolls as close to the patient's back as possible.

c. Straighten the mattress pad to remove wrinkles.

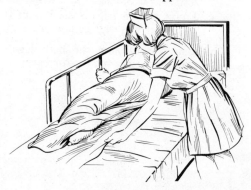

Fold or roll linen as close to patient as possible.

Important Steps	Key Points

d. Take the used large top sheet from the back of the chair and put it on the bed as a bottom sheet.

Proceed to tuck in and miter the corner as in Item 5, Making an Unoccupied Bed. (Tuck it under the mattress, and miter the corner.) Fan-fold the other half of the sheet toward the patient, and tuck it *under* the soiled bottom sheet that is to be removed.

e. Unfold or unroll the plastic drawsheet, bringing it over both rolled bottom sheets; smooth it free of wrinkles, and tuck it firmly under the mattress.

f. Place a clean cloth drawsheet on the bed.

Open it halfway and lay the center fold at the middle of the bed, and fan-fold the far half and tuck it under the patient's back. Tuck the side nearest you under the mattress.

g. Place the clean sheet, blanket, and clean spread on the bed according to Item 5, Making an Unoccupied Bed.

Make the toe pleat if used, and miter the corner.

8. Move the patient to the clean side of the bed.

 a. Reach under the top covers, and hold them up as you assist the patient to roll himself over the folded linen and onto the clean side of the bed.

 b. Position the clean top covers over the patient, and remove his bath blanket.

Hold onto the top covers with one hand, and remove the bath blanket with the other. Avoid exposing the patient. Fold the bath blanket for reuse and put it away in the bedside stand or closet, or discard it if a new one is supplied with the daily linen pack.

 c. Raise the nearest siderail and ask patient to hold on to it for support.

 d. Dress the pillow, and place it under the patient's head. (See Item 5, Making an Unoccupied Bed.)

9. Move to the other side of the bed, and complete making the other side.

 a. Lower the siderail so that you can reach your work without straining.

 b. Loosen the foundation linen on this side of the bed, and remove the soiled drawsheet and large bottom sheet.

Place the soiled linen in the laundry hamper or bag.

 c. Straighten the mattress cover, and remove wrinkles.

 d. Pull and straighten the bottom sheet, tuck it under the head of the bed, miter the corner, and pull the sheet tightly along the side of the bed to remove wrinkles as you tuck it under the mattress.

 e. Bring the plastic drawsheet toward you over the bottom sheet, pull it tightly to remove wrinkles, and tuck it under the mattress.

UNIT 11

Important Steps	Key Points
f. Bring the cloth drawsheet over the plastic drawsheet, pull it tightly to remove wrinkles, and tuck it under the mattress.	When the foundation of the bed is completed the patient can return to the center of his bed in a dorsal recumbent position (flat on his back). *Note:* Steps e and f are optional. Follow your agency procedure.
g. Straighten the top sheet, blanket, and spread on the proximal side of the bed.	Tuck top linens under the mattress at the foot of the bed. Miter the corner and complete the cuff at the top of the bed (see Item 5, Making an Unoccupied Bed).
10. Attach the patient's signal cord within his reach.	Never leave your patient without some means of summoning help when he needs it.
11. Provide for the patient's safety.	
a. Adjust the siderails according to the agency regulations.	
b. Place the bed in the low position.	Most patients are not accustomed to a high bed. They are less likely to fall if the bed is in a low position.
12. Provide for the patient's comfort.	
a. Place the patient in a Fowler's or semi-Fowler's position if this is allowed for his condition.	
b. Position the pillows under his head for good alignment and comfort.	
c. Place the bedside stand and table nearby or within the patient's reach. Put items the patient may need or wish to use within his reach.	
13. Tidy the room.	
a. Remove the soiled linen and the linen hamper if used.	Follow the procedure of your agency for the handling of soiled linen. Some hospitals object to having linen placed in a pillowcase, but require a laundry bag. Others may use laundry chutes, or other methods.
b. Put clean towels, a washcloth, and the patient's gown in the proper place, (bathroom, bedside stand), then neatly arrange the top of the bedside stand.	
c. Remove from the room other equipment that is no longer being used, and return it to its proper place.	
d. Tell the patient when you expect to return.	

ITEM 9. CONCLUSION OF THE LESSON

You have completed the unit on making the hospital bed. After you have practiced operating the hospital bed, placing it in the various positions, and making the unoccupied bed, the anesthetic bed, and the occupied bed, you should arrange with your instructor to take the performance test. You will be expected to demonstrate your skill in performing these activities.

VI. ADDITIONAL INFORMATION FOR ENRICHMENT

The bed is the most important part of a patient's environment because he occupies it during much of his hospital stay. There are many different types of beds, and variations of bedmaking. One kind is achieved by adding boards under the mattress; this makes a firm bed. It is used for orthopedic patients, or those with bone problems, or for patients with injuries to the spinal cord. The firmness provides support and thus contributes to a better recovery. Various types of traction may be attached to ordinary hospital beds to apply a steady pull on some part of the patient's body. Traction pulls a bone so that it is properly aligned during healing. Traction can also be used to release strain on a part of the body. Adding traction equipment to the ordinary hospital bed does not interfere with making the bed.

Modern beds have a storage space for the IV rod. This may be a metal troughlike container, or it may be an empty rod-shaped container. In either case, the IV rod is placed in it. This provides access when there is a need for intravenous therapy.

There are six convenient receptacles for placement of the IV rod. Two are placed on the head panel, two on the root panel, and two are placed in the center frame of the bed. There is a locking-type notch to lock the rod in place when it is inserted in the receptacle. Turn it clockwise to lock it in place. Turn it counterclockwise to unlock it and to remove it.

It should be noted that bed linen and blankets may be a source of staphylococcal infection. This type of infection is recognized as an enormous problem throughout the world. Therefore, you must keep soiled linen from touching your uniform. (Be sure to refer to the unit on handwashing.) Boils, abscesses, carbuncles, impetigo, pus formation, or superficial infections may be signs of staphylococcal infection. When the staphylococcal infection reaches the blood stream, it causes septicemia (blood poisoning). It may localize in the kidneys, liver, joints, lungs, or other body parts, or it may be found in some inflammatory conditions of the urinary tract, middle ear infections, meningitis, pneumonia, and osteomyelitis. *Prevention* of infections is the best practice.

Remember, wash your hands and keep soiled linen away from your uniform.

U
N
I
T
11

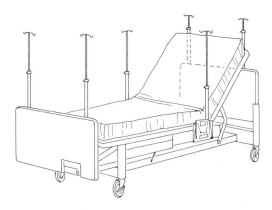

The six locations where
IV rod may be used.

PERFORMANCE TEST

In the classroom or skill laboratory, your instructor will ask you to demonstrate the following activities and procedures. You are to perform these without reference to the instruction book, notes, or other source materials.

1. Given a hospital bed set in a low horizontal position, you are to adjust the bed to a number of different positions. Your instructor will tell you what position to adjust the bed to. When you have completed the adjustment, step back from the bed, and the instructor will tell you the next position from among the following:

   a. Adjust the bed to Fowler's position.

   b. Adjust the bed to semi-Fowler's position.

   c. Adjust the bed to the position you would use when moving the bed.

   d. Adjust the bed to the contour position.

   e. Adjust the bed to the position in which you would leave a completed *unoccupied* bed.

   f. Adjust the bed to the hyperextension position.

   g. Adjust the bed to the position in which you would leave a completed anesthetic bed.

   h. Adjust the bed to Trendelenburg's position.

   i. Adjust the bed to reverse Trendelenburg's position.

2. Given a hospital bed adjusted to a low position with the brakes off and the siderails down, make an unoccupied bed in 6 minutes or less. Obtain the following supplies before beginning:

Mattress cover or pad.	Blanket.
Large sheets.	Bedspread.
Plastic or rubber drawsheet.	Bath blanket.
Cloth drawsheet.	Patient gown.
Pillow.	Towels and washcloth.
Pillowcase.	Laundry bag or hamper.

   Notify your instructor when you are ready to begin.

3. Given a hospital bed without any linen on it, and with siderails down, brakes off, and signal cord unattached, obtain the linens listed above, and make an anesthetic bed. Inform your instructor when you have collected your supplies and are ready to begin.

4. Given a hospital bed occupied by a patient (simulated, or played, by another student), with the bed adjusted to a low position, siderails up, brakes off, and signal cord unattached, make the bed and change all linen except for the spread, blanket, and top sheet, which you will use again. Collect the linen you will need to change the bed: a large sheet, a cloth drawsheet, and a pillowcase. Inform your instructor when you are ready to begin.

PERFORMANCE CHECKLIST

MAKING HOSPITAL BEDS

ADJUSTMENT OF BEDS

The student will show the proper procedures for adjusting the hospital bed.

Adjust the bed correctly in the following positions without errors in selection and movement of controls:

1. Fowler's position.
2. Semi-Fowler's position.
3. Bedmaking position.
4. Contour position.

5. Unoccupied bed position.
6. Hyperextension position.
7. Reverse Trendelenburg's position.
8. Trendelenburg's position.

MAKING AN UNOCCUPIED BED

1. Select and assemble all materials required before beginning to make the bed.

2. Adjust the bed to the highest position without errors in selection and use of controls.

3. Place the mattress pad on the bed, smooth it free of wrinkles, and position it properly.

4. Place the sheets, drawsheets, and blankets, and spread them in the proper sequence; position each item correctly.

5. Tuck each piece of bedding under the mattress neatly, and make sure that each is smooth and taut.

6. Form all required mitered corners smoothly and neatly.

7. Form a toe-pleat correctly at the foot of the top linens.

8. Fold back the top sheet and adjust the spread correctly in relation to the top sheet. Fold the covers correctly to open the bed; or pie-fold the covers correctly to open the bed.

9. Handle and dress the pillow correctly, keeping it from contact with your body and clothing.

10. Position the pillow correctly with the open end away from the door.

11. Attach the signal cord within the patient's reach.

12. Lower the bed to its lowest position, and set the brakes.

13. Adjust the siderails to the "up" position.

14. Observe good body alignment principles at all times.

15. Be cognizant of and minimize contact between materials, and reduce or eliminate sources of contamination as much as possible.

16. Proceed smoothly from one step to another without hesitation, false starts, or wasted motions.

17. Complete a neat and correctly made bed within 6 minutes.

UNIT 11

MAKING AN ANESTHETIC BED

1. Select and assemble all materials needed before beginning to make the bed.

2. Wash your hands.

3. Raise the bed to working height.

4. Place the mattress pad on the bed, smoothing it free of wrinkles, and securing or placing it in the proper position.

5. Place the sheets, drawsheets, blankets, and other materials in the proper sequence, positioning each piece correctly.

6. Tuck each piece under the mattress correctly, making sure that each is smooth and taut.

7. Form all required mitered corners smoothly and neatly.

8. Fan-fold the top bedding to the side of the bed or to the foot of the bed, or pie-fold the top bedding to one side of the bed.

9. Place the pillows correctly, either on a chair or at the head of the bed in a horizontal position.

10. Handle and place the pillow slip on the pillow while keeping the pillow from contacting your uniform.

11. Attach the signal cord within the patient's reach.

12. Place the bed in the correct position with the siderails down, and set the brake.

13. Move furniture to make room for the stretcher.

14. Observe the principles of body alignment and proper movement at all times.

15. Reduce or eliminate contact and contamination as far as possible.

16. Proceed smoothly from one step to another in the procedure, working on one side before going to the other.

MAKING AN OCCUPIED BED

1. Assemble and select all materials before beginning to make the bed.

2. Identify the patient.

3. Wash your hands.

4. Stack the materials on a chair in order of use.

5. Raise the bed to its highest position.

6. Place the bath blanket correctly to cover the patient.

7. Pull the top covers to the foot of the bed without exposing the patient.

8. Remove the top covers and fold them correctly.

9. Move the mattress toward the top of the bed and straighten the mattress cover.

10. Remove the bottom sheet and drawsheets on each side of bed, and fold and secure the new linen, performing all operations in the correct sequence.

11. Move the patient to the correct position for each step of the procedure.

12. Give appropriate explanations, directions, and assistance to the patient each time he is moved. Observe techniques of good body alignment when moving patients.

13. Remove the bath blanket from under the top sheet without exposing the patient.

14. Place sheets, drawsheets, blanket, and spread in the proper sequence, positioning each piece correctly.

15. Tuck each piece under the mattress neatly, and make sure that each is smooth, free of wrinkles, and taut.

16. Form all required mitered corners smoothly and neatly.

17. Form a toe-pleat correctly at the foot of the top linens.

18. Fold back the top sheet and adjust the spread correctly in relation to the top sheet.

19. Remove the soiled pillowcase, and dress the pillow with a new case, handling the pillow correctly.

20. Position the pillow correctly with the open end away from the door.

21. Place the soiled linen in a laundry bag.

22. Attach the signal cord within reach of the patient.

23. Lower the bed to the lowest position, and set the brake.

24. Adjust the siderails to the "up" position.

25. Adjust the bed to a comfortable position as requested by the patient.

26. Arrange the furniture in the proper position.

27. Examine the patient in bed to see that he is comfortable and everything is in order.

28. Proceed smoothly from one step to another, without hesitations, false starts, or wasted motion.

29. Complete a neat and correctly made bed within 10 to 12 minutes.

Unit 12

DRESSING AND
UNDRESSING

I. DIRECTIONS TO THE STUDENT

Please read these paragraphs carefully. They will tell you exactly what you will be expected to know and what you will be expected to do at the end of the lesson. Proceed through this lesson unit using this workbook; practice the procedure in the skill laboratory with a student partner or some other person, and prepare to perform the post-test demonstrations for your instructor.

You will need the following items for this lesson: this workbook, a pen or pencil, a hospital gown, a robe and slippers, and the performance test for this lesson.

If you believe that you already have the necessary skills, discuss this with your instructor, and if she agrees, take the performance test. All students are expected to demonstrate the required skills accurately during the performance test.

II. GENERAL PERFORMANCE OBJECTIVE

You will be able to provide partial or total assistance, when needed by the patient, in putting on or removing articles of clothing. The assistance may be needed by a patient of any age, ranging from the newborn to the elderly. You will provide assistance regardless of the physical or mental condition of the patient, and without causing him additional discomfort or distress.

III. SPECIFIC PERFORMANCE OBJECTIVES

You will be able to:

1. Explain the biological and physical principles concerned with body movement and function that may be used in assisting the patient to dress and undress without further injury, discomfort, or distress.

2. Assess the factors in the patient's physical condition and ability to cooperate that may interfere with his competence to dress or undress, and your own ability or limitations in carrying out the procedures. *Note:* When needed, secure additional help.

3. Demonstrate your regard for articles of clothing as the property of others (belonging to the patient or to the hospital) by carefully and neatly storing items not in use, and by not cutting, tearing, or causing other damage to clothing.

4. Provide total assistance in removing the soiled gown of an adult bed patient, and put a clean gown or pajamas on him in 5 minutes or less.

5. Provide partial assistance to the patient when he is removing his gown, and assist him to dress in undergarments, street clothing, and shoes in 10 minutes or less.

6. Assist the patient to put on and remove his robe and slippers.

7. Remove soiled gown from a patient who has an IV running, and put on a clean gown.

216

IV. VOCABULARY

You will need to learn or review the meaning of the following words, which are used in the lesson.

brain impairment—decreased function of the brain, damage to all or a part of the brain from any cause, e.g., mental retardation, tumor, injury, stroke.

distal—further away; the most distant.

maturation—the gradual process of growth and development that includes the integration of the body structures, such as the infant who must grow sufficiently to integrate the bony and muscular structures with the sensory organs of vision and balance before he can learn to walk.

mental retardation—the slower than normal development and maturation rate of the brain's intellectual functions.

monitoring device—a mechanical appliance that detects or measures one or more of the body functions, such as the vital signs of the heart action, respiratory rate, blood pressure, and temperature.

postoperative—the condition of the patient following a surgical operation; commonly called "post-op."

preoperative—the condition of the patient immediately before surgery.

proximal—the near side; closest.

stroke—a sudden, severe attack; usually refers to an accident in the circulatory system in the brain; also may be called apoplexy or cerebral hemorrhage.

ITEM 1.   WHY PATIENTS NEED HELP WITH DRESSING AND UNDRESSING

Does it seem a little unusual to have a lesson on helping the patient to dress and undress? Didn't everyone learn how to put on and take off clothing as a young child? You have been doing this for so many years that it may seem like a simple procedure. However, as a young child learning to dress yourself, you had to have practice to learn how to get your arms into sleeves, how to fasten buttons, and how to tie your shoelaces. You had to learn all of the body movements that are involved in the process of dressing or undressing. You no longer consciously think of the movements that you perform in the process of dressing *except* when there is interference or restriction of your freedom of movement. Then dressing or undressing becomes complicated for you. And so it is with the patient.

The patient who is an infant or young child will need your help to dress or undress because he has not reached the maturation level necessary to know and coordinate all the movements required in dressing. The older child or adult patient may need your assistance when his movements are restricted as a result of his illness or the type of treatment he is receiving.

Your knowledge of how to help the patient dress or undress and your skill in performance will have an effect on the patient. The manner in which you assist him may increase or decrease his feelings of comfort, pain, trust, fear, confidence, acceptance, or rejection. By the time you complete this lesson, you should be able to recognize ways of helping the patient emotionally as well as assisting him to change clothing.

ITEM 2.   LIMITATION OF BODY MOVEMENT

Physical Factors.   Various conditions tend to limit movement. The patient's ability to perform movements required in dressing or undressing may be limited by one or more of the following conditions:

1. Lack of maturation, as in the case of infants and small children.

2. Brain impairment, as in mental retardation, injury, or coma.

U
N
I
T
12

3. Weakness.

4. Pain from any cause, such as disease or surgery.

5. Fractures.

6. Contractures.

7. Paralysis.

8. Special appliances or equipment, such as IV's, casts, braces, or monitoring devices.

9. Absence of a portion of a limb.

10. Lack of vision.

Psychological Factors. Some people may refuse to move or help themselves even when there seems to be no physical reason to limit their movement. Those who are unable or unwilling to move or dress and undress themselves will also need help and assistance from the health worker.

Psychological factors that may restrict movement include the fear of pain, discomfort, or possible harm resulting from the movement. The post-op patient is often afraid that moving will tear loose the sutures in the incision or dislodge the IV needle from a vein. Others may dislike being told what to do or being required to do something they feel is unnecessary. People who feel depressed or "blue," grief-stricken, worried, or tense often find it difficult to make decisions, even one as simple as to get out of bed and dress in street clothing.

You should accept the person's right to express his feelings. However, as the health worker, you must reassure, encourage, and explain how you will help him to dress.

ITEM 3. CLASSIFICATION OF ARTICLES OF CLOTHING

Most of the clothing that we wear can be classified into several basic types. Although the styles may differ, each type requires similar movements in order to put on or remove the garment. The clothing you will be handling while assisting patients to dress and undress falls into these basic groups:

• cardigan-type — completely open from the neck to the lower edge in front or in back of the garment; examples are hospital gown, shirt, blouse, sweater, coat, jacket, vest, robe, pajama coat, and bra.

• pullover-type — has a short or incomplete opening in the front, side, or back of the garment; examples include placket style of shirt, sweater, blouse, dress, skirt, slip, undershirt, and pajama top.

• pants-type — pulled up over the lower extremities and the hips, for example, trousers, slacks, shorts, pajama bottoms, panty girdle, and panty hose.

• diapers — similar to pants, but pinned or adjusted to fit around the hips.

• shoes and stockings — includes elastic hose.

• accessories — items such as belts, ties, hats, suspenders, purses, etc.

Loose-fitting clothing of the cardigan type is the easiest to put on the person who needs help in dressing.

ITEM 4. SOME GENERAL GUIDELINES

Clothing as Personal Property. The health worker should regard all clothing as the property of others, whether it belongs to the patient or to the hospital. Avoid cutting, tearing, or otherwise damaging it unless absolutely necessary. Even when the clothing appears worn and out of style, it should not be discarded because its replacement may cause a financial hardship to the owner.

Care of Clothing. Hospitals provide gowns and pajamas as part of the linen supply. These items can be obtained from the linen room or the linen cart. When soiled, they must be put into the soiled linen hampers; they are then laundered with the rest of the hospital linens.

Personal clothing belonging to the patient is usually stored in the patient unit. It should be neatly folded, or hung on hangers in the closet. Soiled clothing should be set aside to be cleaned by the family. Soiled garments belonging to patients are not usually laundered by health workers. However, when the hospital provides for the cleaning of patients' clothing, follow the procedure for handling this responsibility.

Dressing an Affected Extremity. The patient who has limited movement in one or more extremities (either arms or legs) generally needs help to dress and undress. Select cardigan-type clothing, or a pull-on garment with the largest possible opening. Pants-type clothing should be loose and easy to pull on.

When assisting the person to dress, start by putting the garment on the affected arm or leg; then slip on the rest of the garment. When undressing the patient, remove clothing from the unaffected limbs first, and then from the immobilized extremity. As described, the rule for the affected limb is to dress it first and to undress it last.

Adults and Diapers. Many unthinking health workers have made it a practice to put diapers on adult or elderly patients who have lost control of their bowels or bladder. This is a deplorable practice and should not be done. It does not remedy the patient's loss of control, but only serves to create more complex problems. Treating the older patient as an infant lowers his self-esteem, the urine or feces in the diaper irritate the skin, and the diaper itself indicates lack of a rehabilitative outlook on the part of the health worker.

You will learn more about the rehabilitative aspects of this problem in the units on elimination. Meanwhile, we must resolve that diapers are to be used solely for infants and young children who have not yet achieved control of bowel and bladder.

ITEM 5. CHANGING THE HOSPITAL GOWN (CARDIGAN-TYPE, WITH BACK OPENING)

In the skill laboratory, practice dressing and undressing the patient. One of your fellow students can play the role of the patient who needs help in dressing.

Given a helpless patient whose hospital gown has become wet, remove the soiled gown and replace it with a clean one in 5 minutes or less.

Important Steps	Key Points
1. Wash your hands and obtain a clean hospital gown.	Gowns are usually kept in the nursing unit's linen room or on the linen cart.
2. Approach and identify the patient.	Explain what is to be done and the assistance you will give, and enlist his cooperation.
3. Provide for privacy.	Pull the cubicle curtain around the bed, place screens, or close the door of the room. This protects the patient's modesty and avoids causing embarrassment to others in the area. Wash your hands.
4. Position the patient.	Move him to the proximal (near) side of the bed and especially protect the patient who may have a fear of falling by using your body as a barrier (block). If the bed is an adjustable high-low type, it should be in the high position with the siderail lowered on the side of the bed where you are working.

Important Steps	Key Points
5. Avoid undue exposure of the patient's body.	Fold the top covers of the bed back to the patient's waist. Exposure of more of the body may cause chilling, or may offend the patient's sense of modesty.

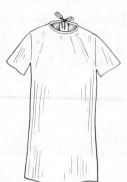

Typical hospital gown is cardigan-type garment with back opening. Gown is between knee and mid-thigh in length.

Important Steps	Key Points
6. Untie or unfasten the gown and slip it off the patient's body.	Place one of your hands under the patient's head to support it; with the other hand, reach under his neck, pull the neck fastening to one side, and unfasten. Free the sides of the gown from under the patient, and slip his arms out of the sleeves. Fold the top portion of the gown down to cover his chest.
7. Clean or dry the patient's body as needed.	Use a washcloth and towel to clean and dry him before putting on a clean gown.
8. Put a clean hospital gown on the patient.	Slip the patient's arms into the sleeves, one at a time, and pull the gown up over the shoulders. Reach under the patient's neck, grasp the other edge of the gown and tie, draw the tie through, and fasten or tie at the side of the neck. Smooth the gown over the shoulders, and down over the body.
9. Remove the used or soiled gown.	Reach under the clean gown and remove the soiled gown from the patient's chest. Place it in the linen hamper.
10. Provide for the patient's comfort.	Position him in a supine position (on his back) or on his side, using principles of good body alignment. With one hand under the patient's head to raise and support the head, use the other hand to remove the pillow(s). Fluff them with several shaking motions. Remember to keep the pillows away from your uniform. While supporting the head with one hand, use the other hand to position the pillow(s) under the patient's head and neck. If the patient is lying on his side, support and comfort for the back may be provided by placing a pillow lengthwise along his back, firmly rolled under, and tucked along his side. Smooth the top coverings of the bed to the patient's *axilla* or armpit, or up to his shoulders. Return the bed to a low position unless contraindicated.
11. Record and report.	Report any changes in the patient's condition to the team leader or the nurse in charge.

Important Steps	Key Points
	Conditions to be reported include change in color, difficulty in breathing, fever, chills, nausea, vomiting, reddened or broken skin areas, drainage, pain, and so forth. Record as may be appropriate. Charting example:
	8:30 A.M. Complete bed bath given. Gown changed; was able to put on gown with limited assistance. Is proud of progress toward doing for himself. J. Jones, SN

ITEM 6.   CHANGING A GOWN WITH AN IV RUNNING

You will find that many patients have restricted movement in one or both arms due to an IV running in a vein of the arm, to paralysis of the arm following a stroke, or to a cast applied to immobilize a fractured bone. Some hospitals provide a special IV gown for such patients, a cardigan-type with a back opening, and sleeves open from the neckline to the lower edge. Each sleeve can be closed with Velcro fasteners or ties. It is a simple matter to remove this type of gown and replace it with a clean one. However, it is frequently necessary to change the regular style of hospital gown or pajama top for a patient who is receiving an IV; this garment should be removed from the unaffected arm first, thereby allowing the patient more freedom of movement and better manipulation of the garment, which makes it easier to remove from the affected arm.

In the skill laboratory, given a patient with an IV running in one arm, remove the soiled hospital gown and put a clean one on, using a regular gown.

Important Steps	Key Points
Follow steps 1 through 5 of Item 5.	
6. Untie or unfasten the soiled gown and slip it off the patient's unaffected arm.	Pull up the sheet or use a towel to cover his body and avoid undue exposure.
7. Remove the gown from the affected arm.	Slide the sleeve down the affected arm, past the needle, and onto the tubing. Support the arm and tubing to avoid dislodging the IV needle. Now, slide the gown along the tubing, remove the bottle of fluids from the IV stand (holding it higher than the level of the arm to keep the blood in the vein from running into the tubing), and slip the gown over the bottle. Hang the bottle on the IV stand. Put the soiled gown in the linen hamper.

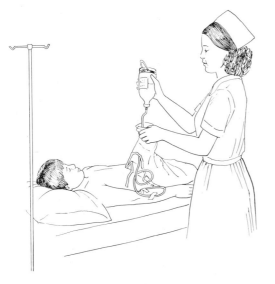

IV bottle and tubing are passed through the sleeve to remove soiled gown and to put on clean gown.

U
N
I
T
12

Important Steps	Key Points
8. Put a clean gown on the patient.	Slip the gown on the affected arm first. Slide the gown and the proper sleeve over the IV bottle, the tubing, and the affected arm (using the same procedure in reverse as in Step 7, and observing the same precautions). Then put the gown on the unaffected arm, fasten it at the neck, and smooth it down over the body.

Conclude with steps 9 and 10 from Item 5.

ITEM 7.   ASSISTING THE PATIENT WITH SLIPPERS AND ROBE (CARDIGAN–TYPE WITH FRONT OPENING)

In the skill laboratory, practice dressing and undressing a partner with items of clothing representing various types of garments in order to increase your skills.

Assist the patient to put on his robe and slippers before getting out of bed to sit in a chair, and later, to remove the garments when he returns to bed.

Important Steps	Key Points
1. Approach and identify the patient.	Explain what you plan to do, how you will help, and enlist his cooperation.
2. Obtain the robe and slippers to be used.	The patient's own robe and slippers are kept in the room. When these items are supplied by the hospital, pick them up from the linen room and keep them in the patient's room for continued use.
3. Provide for privacy.	Even though the patient is wearing a gown or pajamas, it is better to pull the cubicle curtain, use screens, or close the door to assure privacy.
4. Position the patient.	Adjust the bed to the low position for the patient's safety. Help him to sit on the side of the bed and dangle his legs. (For the helpless patient, keep the bed in a high position and the patient lying supine.)
5. Help the patient put on his robe.	Ask him to slip one arm into the sleeve, place the robe around his back, and guide his other arm into the other sleeve. Fasten the buttons and tie the belt if needed. (For a helpless patient or a small child, run your hand through the proper sleeve of the garment, clasp the patient's wrist and pull his arm through the sleeve. Put the robe over his back, roll him to the other side, and then pull the garment toward you. (Repeat the above procedure to put his other arm into the remaining sleeve.)

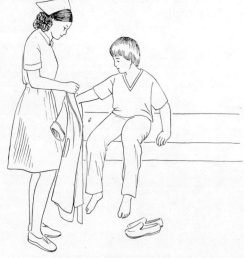

Assisting patient with slippers and robe.

Important Steps	Key Points
6. Assist the patient to put on his slippers.	As he dangles his feet on the side of the bed, stoop down, using good body movements. Support the patient's ankle, and slide the slipper over the toes, foot, and heel. Make sure that his toes are not curled under the foot inside the shoe, especially when the patient is a small child or an aged person. Finally, have the patient stand in order to position the foot better in the slipper or shoe.
7. Provide for the patient's comfort.	Help him to stand up and straighten his robe. When he is sitting in a chair, give him a pillow, personal articles such as a comb or brush, or diversional items such as a newspaper or book.
8. Remove the patient's robe and slippers when helping him back to bed.	Have him stand at the side of the bed, if he is able to do so. Loosen the belt and unfasten the buttons. Pull the sleeve off one arm, slip the robe off his back, and then remove it from the other arm. While he sits on the side of the bed, remove both slippers. Use good body alignment when stooping.
9. Put the robe and slippers away in the proper place.	Hang the robe in the wardrobe or closet in the patient's room. Slippers may be kept at the bedside, in the bedside stand, or in the closet.
10. Record or report as appropriate.	When dressing the patient in robe and slippers to get him up, it is seldom necessary to chart this specific procedure. However, report any changes in the patient's condition to the team leader or the nurse in charge. Conditions to be reported include weakness, complaints of dizziness, shortness of breath, faintness, or pain.

UNIT 12

ITEM 8. ASSISTING WITH PULLOVER GARMENTS

Pull-on garments include undershirts, sweaters, blouses, dresses, and skirts, many of which are pulled on or off over the head. The key points for assisting with a pull-on garment is described for the neck-opening placket-type.

Important Steps	Key Points
Undressing	Unbutton or spread open the neck opening if there is one. Gather the body of the garment up to the patient's arms, and ease it down over his distal shoulder. Grasp the sleeve at the lower edge, support the patient's arm, and remove the sleeve from it. Repeat this step to remove the sleeve from the proximal arm. Gather the front of the garment from hem to neckline, and slip it smoothly over the head, reassuring the patient during the time his head is covered. Support the patient's head and neck with one hand, reach under his neck with the other hand, grasp the garment, and pull it toward you. Remove the garment.

Important Steps	Key Points
Dressing	Put your hand through the proper sleeve of the garment, clasp the patient's distal wrist, and pull it through the sleeve. Repeat this step for the patient's proximal arm. Pull the garment up toward his shoulders. Gather the back of the garment from hem to neck in your hand, and with the other hand, stretch or shape the neck opening. Have the patient raise his arms — or assist him by pulling the garment up — and slide the neck opening smoothly over his head. Reassure the patient during the short time his head is covered. Smooth the garment down over his shoulders and body. Roll the patient on his side toward you, support him in this position, and smooth down the back of the garment. Return him to a supine position and button or fasten the neck opening, if there is one.

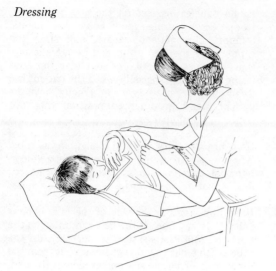

Assisting patient to remove a
pullover type of garment.

ITEM 9.   ASSISTING WITH PANTS–TYPE GARMENTS

Both males and females wear a variety of pants-type garments, and pajamas are especially popular apparel for hospital patients. As a health worker, you need to know how to assist the patient with this type of garment. This section describes how to dress and undress the male patient in pajama pants.

Important Steps	Key Points
Undressing	Unfasten the pants closing. Place a sheet or drape over the patient's lower abdomen and thighs. If he is able to lift his buttocks, have him do so, and with your hand at each side of the pants, slip them down over the buttocks to the thighs. If the patient is unable to lift his buttocks, roll him on his side toward you, support him in this position, and ease the pants down over the buttocks. Return the patient to a supine position, reach under the proximal side, and pull the pants down over the buttocks on that side. Continue to pull each pant leg down over his thighs and legs toward the ankles. Supporting the ankle with one hand, pull the pant leg off the foot, and repeat this step for the other foot. Remove the pants.
Dressing	Free the top coverings from the foot of the bed and fold them back to the patient's knees. Position the patient on the proximal side of the bed so that his feet and legs can be reached without stretching. Gather most of the pant leg of the garment in one hand, clasp the patient's distal ankle with the other hand, and guide the foot through the pant leg. Repeat this step with the proximal foot. Ease the pants up over the patient's knees and thighs. If the patient is able

Important Steps   Key Points

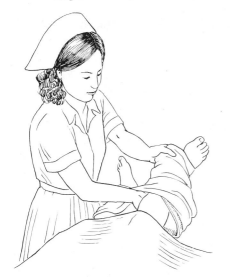

to raise his buttocks, have him do so while you reach under the top coverings, grasp the pants on each side, and pull them up to his waist. If the patient is unable to raise his buttocks, roll him on his side toward you and pull the pants up over the buttocks to the waist. Return the patient to a supine position, reach under his proximal side, and pull the pants up to his waist. Fasten the pants closing.

Top sheet or blanket serves to drape patient and avoid undue exposure when putting on garments such as pajama pants.

ITEM 10.   CHANGING DIAPERS

Diapers are used to collect the urine and stool eliminated by infants and small children who have not established control of their bowels or bladders. The diaper should be changed promptly when it is soiled. Prolonged contact of the wet, soiled diaper with the baby's tender skin can cause an irritation, or diaper rash.

Many mothers today use a rubber or plastic panty over the baby's diaper to protect other clothing and the bed linen from getting wet or soiled. However, you will recall that bacteria thrive in warm, damp places, so it is important to keep the baby clean and dry when the plastic panties are worn.

The use of disposable diapers has become increasingly popular in recent years. These diapers are prefolded, absorbent, and are thrown away following use. Many have an adhesive tape fastening, which eliminates the need for safety pins. However, the reusable cloth diapers are the most economical type. Large squares or rectangles of soft, absorbent material such as flannel or muslin are used to make the diapers. The material is then folded to fit the baby. In this section, the process of folding, removing, and putting a diaper on an infant is described.

Important Steps   Key Points

Folding the diaper properly.

The purpose is to arrange layers of absorbent material to fit the baby's lower trunk, which are usually in the shape of a rectangle or a modified triangle where the front tip is folded inward to provide extra absorbency. When using rectangular diapers, fold over excess material in the front for boys (and all infants who are placed on their stomachs to sleep). For baby girls, fold down the extra length in the back of the diaper. To adjust the fit and decrease the width of the diaper between the legs, fold the sides under or inward.

U
N
I
T
12

Important Steps	Key Points

a. Disposable diaper with sealing tabs.

b. Modified triangular diaper.

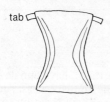

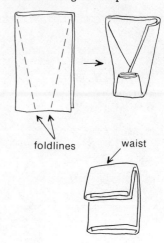

foldlines   waist

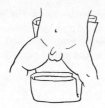

c. Extra-absorbent layers in front of diaper.

d. Folding diaper to provide extra layers at the back.

Methods of folding baby diapers.

Remove the soiled diaper.

When providing general care for infants, such as dressing, undressing, or bathing, there are several guidelines to follow:

Do Not Leave Baby Unattended. Raise the sides of the crib, or carry the baby with you if you need to get some article.

Close Safety Pins and Keep Out of Reach of Baby. Obtain a supply of clean diapers, cleaning materials, and powder if used. Place the baby on a flat, padded surface such as a bed or bassinet. Unfasten the diaper at each side and draw the front downward. Grasp the baby's ankles with one hand and raise the buttocks or roll the baby to one side. With the other hand, use the dry, clean portion of the diaper to gently wipe the urine and feces from the skin. Then clean the skin with a moistened piece of cotton or washcloth, and pat dry. Fold the diaper inward, and remove.

Put on the clean diaper.

Lay a fresh folded diaper on a smooth surface. Place the baby on the diaper with the back edge at his waist level. Draw the front portion of the diaper between the baby's legs and up to the waist. (An alternative method is to grasp the baby's ankles with one hand, raise his buttocks, and with the other hand position the diaper under him.) Fasten or pin the diaper securely at each side so that it fits snugly at the waist and thigh. When using safety pins, place your hand under the area being pinned so that baby will not be pricked or jabbed.

ITEM 11.   ASSISTING WITH ELASTIC STOCKINGS

Many patients in the hospital who have medical or surgical conditions are required to wear elastic stockings to prevent circulatory complications. Such stockings are generally removed during the bath so that the patient's legs and feet can be washed; they are reapplied before he gets out of bed or has the bed made. The following method will help you avoid unnecessary struggling when putting elastic stockings on the patient. In fact, this method can be used for all types of hose.

Important Steps	Key Points
Remove the stockings.	Unfasten them from the garters if used. Roll or pull the stocking down the leg to the ankle. Support the ankle with your hand and pull the stocking down over the heel and foot, and off the toes. Repeat this procedure to remove the other stocking.
Put on the stockings.	Turn the leg part of the stocking inside out to the ankle portion just above the heel. Slip the foot portion of the stocking over the toes, foot, and onto the heel. Pull the everted leg portion of the stocking smoothly over the leg, avoiding wrinkles or folds in the elastic stockings. Ordinarily, garters are not used with elastic stockings, but may be necessary with women's midthigh-length stockings.

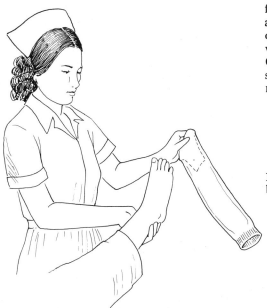

Elastic stocking is slipped on foot more easily by everting (turning inside out) leg of stocking down to foot part.

U
N
I
T
12

ITEM 12.   CONCLUSION OF THE LESSON

You have completed the lesson on dressing and undressing the patient. After you have practiced the procedures to gain initial skills in assisting the patient to dress and undress, make an appointment with your instructor to take the performance test and demonstrate these skills. The performance test instructions follow.

PERFORMANCE TEST

In a performance testing situation in the skill laboratory, demonstrate your knowledge of body movement and the procedure for dressing or undressing the patient by performing the following activities without reference to any source material.

1. In 5 minutes or less, give total assistance to a helpless patient by removing a hospital gown and replacing it with a clean one. Identify the conditions that limit the patient's movement. Standards to be used in this activity include:

   a. Use of principles of body alignment, balance, and motion for yourself and your patient.

   b. Carrying out of procedure without injury, discomfort, or distress to the patient.

2. Remove the soiled hospital gown from a patient receiving an IV and put a clean gown on him without disturbing the IV.

3. Give assistance as needed to the patient in putting on a robe and shoes or slippers preparatory to his getting out of bed. Standards to be used in this activity include a. and b. above.

4. In 10 minutes or less, assist a newly admitted patient to remove his street clothing and dress in a hospital gown or pajamas. Identify the conditions that limit the patient's movement. Standards to be used in this activity include a. and b. above.

DRESSING AND UNDRESSING

CHANGING THE HOSPITAL GOWN (CARDIGAN–TYPE WITH BACK OPENING) IN 5 MINUTES

1. Wash your hands.

2. Obtain the clean gown.

3. Approach and identify the patient.

4. Explain the procedure to the patient.

5. Place the patient on the proximal side of the bed in supine position, with the bed in the high position.

6. Fold back the top bed covers to the patient's waist.

7. Untie the gown, slip his arms out of gown, and fold it down over his chest.

8. Clean and dry the patient's body as needed.

9. Take the clean gown and slip the patient's arms into the sleeves.

10. Pull the gown over his shoulders and tie at the side of his neck.

11. Smooth the gown over his shoulders and down his body.

12. Remove the soiled gown and put it into the linen hamper.

13. Provide for the patient's comfort by adjusting the linen, positioning him in good alignment, and placing the bed in the low position.

14. Record and report as appropriate.

CHANGING THE HOSPITAL GOWN OF THE PATIENT RECEIVING AN IV

1. Wash your hands.

2. Obtain the clean gown.

3. Approach and identify the patient.

4. Explain the procedure to the patient.

5. Place the patient on the proximal side of the bed in a supine position, with the bed in the high position.

6. Fold back the top bed covers to the level of the patient's waist.

7. Untie the gown and slip the sleeve off the unaffected arm.

8. Remove the garment from the arm with IV running in it (affected extremity).

   a. Carefully slide the sleeve of the gown down the arm onto the tubing.

   b. Support the arm and tubing while removing the gown.

   c. Slide the gown along tubing and remove the IV bottle from the holder.

   d. Keep IV bottle above the level of the needle and slip the gown over the bottle; remove gown.

   e. Replace the bottle on the IV stand.

9. Put a clean gown on the patient by starting with the affected extremity.

   a. Remove the bottle from the IV stand.

   b. Slide the gown and the proper sleeve over the bottle.

   c. Replace the bottle on the IV stand and slide the gown over the IV tubing and the affected arm.

   d. Carefully support the arm and tubing during this step.

10. Slip unaffected arm into the other sleeve, pull the gown over the shoulders, and tie it at the neck.

11. Smooth the gown over the shoulders and down over the body.

12. Put the soiled gown into the linen hamper.

13. Provide for the patient's comfort by adjusting the linen, positioning him in good alignment, and placing the bed in the low position.

14. Record and report as appropriate.

ASSISTING THE PATIENT TO PUT ON A ROBE AND SLIPPERS

1. Approach and identify the patient.

2. Get the patient's robe and slippers.

3. Provide for privacy.

4. Position the patient; put the bed in the low position, and assist him to dangle his legs at the side of the bed.

5. Assist patient to put on his robe by slipping his arm into the proper sleeve, placing the robe over his back, and guiding his other arm into the other sleeve.

UNIT 12

6. Stoop down and assist the patient to put on his slippers.

7. Assist the patient to stand; adjust his robe, tie the belt, and button it.

8. Provide for the patient's comfort while he is sitting in a chair.

9. Help him return to the bed by removing his robe and slippers.

   a. Have him stand at the side of the bed if he is able.

   b. Unfasten and untie the belt of the robe.

   c. Slip the sleeve off one arm, slide the robe off his back, and remove the other arm from its sleeve.

   d. Have the patient sit on the side of the bed; remove his slippers.

10. Put the robe and slippers away in the proper place.

11. Record or report as appropriate.

ASSISTING THE SICK PATIENT TO REMOVE STREET CLOTHING AND PUT ON HOSPITAL GOWN IN 10 MINUTES OR LESS.

1. Approach and identify the patient.

2. Explain the procedure.

3. Obtain a hospital gown if not supplied in his admission pack.

4. Provide privacy.

5. Identify the conditions that limit the patient's movement.

6. Position the patient, either sitting on the side of the bed or lying down.

7. Remove his shoes and stockings.

   a. Untie any shoelaces, supporting the ankle with one hand, and with the other hand slide the shoe off the heel, foot, and toes.

   b. Unfasten the stockings from their garters (if used), slide the stocking down the leg, and over the heel, foot, and toes; remove.

8. Remove cardigan-type garments like coats, jackets, shirts, sweaters, blouses, dresses, or bras.

   a. Unbutton or open any fastenings.

   b. Slip the patient's arms out of the garment and remove it. If the patient is in the supine position, remove the garment from one arm, roll the patient to the distal side, tuck the freed portion of the garment along his side, roll the patient back, reach under his side for the garment, and remove it from the patient's other arm.

9. Take off pullover garments such as shirts, sweaters, blouses, skirts, or dresses. (Skirts are usually removed like pants.)

   a. Unbutton or open the neck or side fastenings.

   b. Gather the body of the garment up to the patient's arms.

   c. Remove the sleeve from one arm, then take off the other sleeve.

   d. Gather the front of the garment from the hem to the neckline and slip it smoothly over the patient's head.

   e. Remove the garment.

10. Put the hospital gown on the patient, avoiding unnecessary exposure of the body.

   a. Slip the patient's arms into the sleeves.

   b. Pull the gown over the shoulders and tie at the neck.

   c. Smooth the gown down over the body.

11. Remove the pants-type garments such as trousers, shorts, and panties.

   a. Loosen or open any fastenings.

   b. Have the patient raise his buttocks, if able, and slide the pants down over his hips.

   c. Pull the pants down over the patient's thighs and legs.

   d. Support the patient's ankle and slip his pants off the foot. Repeat for the other leg.

12. Provide for the patient's comfort. Place him in good body alignment, adjust the bedding, and leave the call light within reach.

13. Put the patient's personal clothing away in the proper place.

14. Report and record as appropriate.

BATHS

I. DIRECTIONS TO THE STUDENT

Proceed through the various kinds of baths and become familiar with the differences between them and the effects desired of each bath. Practice giving a bed bath. Correct your mistakes, then be prepared to demonstrate the proper method of giving a bed bath.

II. GENERAL PERFORMANCE OBJECTIVE

You will be prepared to meet the patients's comfort requirements related to his physical, emotional, and mental well-being by giving the appropriate baths.

III. SPECIFIC PERFORMANCE OBJECTIVES

You will be able to prepare and give at least one of the following baths for the performance test:

1. A partial bath.

2. A cleansing bath.

3. A medicated bath.

4. A therapeutic bath.

5. A sitz bath.

You will also gain knowledge of the scientific principles of bathing.

IV. VOCABULARY

anatomy—the study of the form or structure of the body.
chemistry—the science dealing with the composition of substances, elements, and compounds.
microbiology—the study of microorganisms.
necrotic tissue—dead tissue.
perineal region—the area between the thighs at the lower end of the trunk of the body, including the rectum and the genitals.
perineum—the area between the anus and vulva in the female and between the anus and scrotum in the male.
pharmacology—the science dealing with drugs and their nature, action, and properties.
physics—the science dealing with matter and energy.
physiology—the study of the organic processes of the body.
psychology—the science dealing with the mind and behavior.
sociology—the study of the development and organization of human groups.
sordes—a collection of brown, crusty material on the mouth and teeth of persons having fevers.
stomatitis—inflammation of the mouth.

suppuration—the formation of pus.

vaginal—relating to the genital canal in the female, extending from the uterus (womb) to the vulva (the external genitourinary opening).

V. INTRODUCTION

Care of the person includes certain health measures whether or not there is acute medical or surgical illness, chronic disease, or mental deterioration. The extent to which these health measures can be carried out depends on the patient's anatomical and physical condition as well as his psychological state. The age of the patient is an important factor related to these health needs; for example, the older patient may not need a complete bath every day. A daily bath may result in excessively dry skin, with scaling and itching caused by loss of natural oils and decreased perspiration.

The following factors, grouped under subject classification, support the reasons for certain health measures related to the bath:

Anatomy and Physiology. These require adjustment through the bath.

1. Waste products from glands need to be removed from the skin.

2. Dust and bacteria accumulate on the skin and must be removed.

3. Oils secreted from the glands have a protective function in preventing dryness, but excessive amounts provide a base for bacteria and must be removed through washing.

4. Bathing produces a soothing, relaxing effect in prepared situations due to the function of numerous nerve endings in the skin.

5. The mouth is lined with mucous membrane (skin covering) and must be kept clean through mouth care, which is considered a part of the bath.

Chemistry. This is directly relevant in selecting materials used in the bath.

1. Hard water is not suitable for the bath because it does not combine with soap to produce a lather.

2. Soap that is strongly alkaline may remove protective oils from the skin and have an irritating effect.

3. Perspiration of the skin is slightly acid; it is clear in appearance but contains some of the body's sodium (salt). It contains urea, a body substance that is excreted as waste.

4. Rubbing alcohol toughens the skin because it hardens the skin's protein. It is said to make the skin resistant to pressure sores.

5. Body powder provides some antiseptic effect and is soothing. It does have the disadvantage of "caking" and with much perspiration can have an abrasive effect.

Pharmacology.

1. Alcohol acts as follows:

   a. Toughens and strengthens the skin and helps prevent pressure sores.

   b. Evaporates quickly and is cooling to the skin. It may be used in sponge baths to reduce the temperature of the body.

2. Salt (sodium) solution may be used in these ways:

   a. As an effective mouthwash and gargle, and as a means of cleaning the teeth.

   b. To make a stimulating bath solution or to produce a protective action and decrease irritation.

3. Cornstarch, which is smooth and without grit, serves as:

    a. Dusting powder for the skin.

    b. A soothing bath to irritated skin (by emulsifying oils and allaying irritation of skin and mucous membranes).

4. Sodium bicarbonate has two uses in the bath procedure:

    a. It serves as a tooth powder. (Salt and soda mixed together serve as an excellent tooth-cleaning agent because they dissolve mucus).

    b. In bath solution, it dissolves dead tissues and secretions; it also has a soothing effect in some skin diseases.

    c. Soda may be added to the oatmeal preparation for a soothing bath. It has an adhesive and coating action and serves as a protective coating on the skin and mucous membrane.

5. Vinegar may be used in rinsing soap from the hair. It reduces the alkaline action of soap and dissolves adhesive substances at the hair shaft.

Microbiology.

1. Bacteria, which are ever-present on the skin, enter the body through the skin only if there is a broken area of the skin. Skin should be washed as a protective measure.

2. A bath is necessary to remove dirt, oil, and the cells of the skin that shed from the outer surface. Dirt, oil, and dead cells can harbor pathogenic organisms.

3. Soap used in bathing acts by lowering the surface tension of the grease and dirt on the skin surface therefore permitting easier removal. If soap is not rinsed from the skin, it may become irritating.

4. Hands transport bacteria to and from the patient and must be washed before and after each care given.

5. Mouth care helps in these ways:

    a. It prevents dental caries (decay).

    b. It prevents sordes, stomatitis, and the feeling of uncleanliness.

    c. It protects the body from bacteria traveling to the digestive tract and other parts of the body.

    d. It prevents lips from becoming unduly dry and cracked. Cracked lips provide an entry for bacteria to the body.

6. Bacteria (microorganisms) need moisture for growth and reproduction. Keeping the skin dry and preventing breaks in the skin provides a line of defense.

Physics.   These facts provide additional appreciation of the bath process.

1. Water is a conductor of heat. The bath water should be warmer than the skin temperature to prevent the patient from feeling cold.

2. Water tends to evaporate. Water is used to sponge a patient who has an elevated temperature. Alcohol may be added to water; this decreases the time required for evaporation to take place.

3. The human body, when put into water, displaces an equal amount of volume. This should be taken into consideration in filling the bathtub or foot tub.

4. Heat produced by activated water in a whirlpool bath relaxes muscles and stimulates circulation.

UNIT
13

5. Continuous pressure on bony prominences causes decreased circulation of blood to an area and may result in a pressure sore. Pressure from an object such as a cast may cause a pressure sore because the decreased circulation to the area fails to bring food and nourishment and carry away waste products. Sheepskin under a bony area may reduce pressure since wool is resilient.

6. Friction from rubbing produces heat at the skin surface and causes blood vessels to dilate, thus bringing more blood to the area.

Psychology. The impact of a bath on human behavior.

1. Provide privacy for the patient at all times. Certain persons are extremely modest and resent even minor exposure. The patient's attitude toward treatment and other hospital measures depends on the protection of his privacy at all times.

2. Listen to complaints the patient may offer during the bath. Observe his attitude toward his illness and hospital environment, and his response to health workers. Govern your conversation by the patient's condition and desires. Allow the patient to relieve his mental strain through talking.

3. Expected benefits of therapeutic or medicated baths should be explained for the patient's benefit. It will enhance cooperation and benefits.

4. Special care of the mouth makes the patient feel better and prevents possible additional health problems.

5. Special care of the toenails, fingernails, and hair bolsters the morale of a patient and improves his self-image. This is especially true for women. The very ill male patient should be shaved regularly to keep up his morale.

6. Resentment by a patient toward close supervision of a tub bath or sitz bath may be overcome by explaining the need for safety measures. The health worker should speak in well-modulated tones free from anxiety.

7. Irritating procedures should be done first, soothing ones last.

8. Answer all questions in a professional way that shows interest in the patient without becoming "familiar."

9. Anticipate the needs of the patient and render service in a manner that instills confidence.

Sociology. Functions carried out during the bath affect the patient.

1. Wash your hands before and after treatment. Patients notice. Failure to do this may destroy the patient's confidence in you.

2. Work methodically and quietly. Plan your work; then work your plan.

3. If a patient must remain in bed at home after treatment at a health facility, refer to your team leader. She will arrange for a visiting nurse to call on him. Teach the family what is needed and the functions of caring for the patient.

4. Keep the patient under constant observation when he is in a tub of water, to prevent drowning or injury.

5. Treat the patient as a guest.

6. Introduce yourself to the patient and introduce him to the environment.

7. Explain hospital routine in order to allay his fears.

8. Shield the patient from annoyances.

9. Care for his personal belongings carefully.

10. Be prepared to provide reassurance, understanding, protection, and service as a general confidante to the patient and his family.

ITEM 1. TYPES OF BATHS

1. Cleansing bath

A bath performed to:

(1) cleanse the skin

(2) increase elimination through the skin

(3) stimulate circulation of blood

(4) refresh the patient

The entire body is washed; water temperature: 105°F.

Note: Include the backrub.

2. Medicated bath

May be administered as a tub bath or sponge bath; it is intended to serve as soothing sedation or provide relief of a skin disorder. Skin is patted dry following the bath; it is never rubbed because this produces friction, which increases itching.

a. Soothing bath

Keep conversation at a minimum; water temperature: 100–105°F.

(1) *Oatmeal.* The new instant oatmeal can be added directly to the bath water. Stir in the amount needed to make desired consistency. Proceed as with a regular tub bath. To use regular oatmeal in a bath, add *3 cups* of regular oatmeal to *2 quarts* of water and cook until it is similar to paste. Place the cooked oatmeal in a cheesecloth bag and tie it securely. Twirl the bag in the bathtub of water until a desired consistency of mucilaginous material appears in the water. Fill the tub 1/3 to 1/2 full, continuing to use the 3:2 ratio.

(2) *Sodium bicarbonate.* A 5 per cent solution is prepared by adding *1 teaspoon of soda* to *500 cc of water* (1 pint). Pour this into the tub bath. Fill tub 1/2 full by continuing to pour in a mixture of this 1:500 ratio.

(3) *Starch.* Mix *1 pound of cornstarch* with *cold water.* Add boiling water to make a thin solution. Boil this solution 1 or 2 minutes and add to half-filled tub. Proceed with the regular tub bath.

b. Stimulating bath

(1) *Saline.* A solution of sodium chloride (NaCl), such as artificial sea water, is prepared. This is saltwater — *1 teaspoon of salt* to *500 cc of water.* Fill tub half full by continuing to add a mixture of this 1:500 ratio. Proceed to

give the tub bath. This has a stimulating effect on the skin. Water temperature: 95–108°F.

(2) *Mustard*. Preparation for
Adult: 1 tablespoon dry mustard per
        gallon of water.
Child: 1/2 teaspoon of dry mustard
        per gallon of water.
Dissolve mustard in tepid water and
add to the tub of bath water. This has
a stimulating effect on the skin and
relieves muscle spasms and convulsions. Water temperature: 98–100°F.

3. Partial bath

For the convalescent or for the person not in
need of a full bath. This includes the face,
hands, armpits, back, and perineal area. Water
temperature: 105°F.
Note: Include the backrub.

4. Self-administered bath (also called "self-
help")

Performed by the patient, except for the back
and possibly the feet. The health worker washes
the back, gives the backrub, and may do the
feet. Water temperature: 105°F.

5. Therapeutic bath

Performed for a desired physical reaction.

   a. Relaxing bath

The patient assumes a horizontal position in a
bathtub. Water is provided to cover the entire
body. Only the head is above water. The
patient remains 15 to 20 minutes. Water temperature: 105°F.

   b. Hot water bath

Given to remove muscle soreness and strain.
Water temperature: 110°F.

   c. Sponge bath

Given to reduce temperature, nervousness, and
tension. Range for water temperature may be
from room temperature to warm.

(1) A sponge bath is given to aid the skin
    in elimination or to reduce nervousness
    and tension by washing the entire
    body. Water temperature: 105°F.

(2) A sponge bath given *to reduce tem-
    perature requires an order from the
    physician.* The patient's temperature is
    taken before the procedure and again
    30 minutes after it is completed. Body
    temperature is decreased by the trans-
    fer of heat that takes place when
    evaporation occurs. When air comes
    into contact with water, some water is
    absorbed into the air in the form of
    vapor; as a result, the body feels cool.
    Plain water may be used or alcohol
    may be added to it. Alcohol evaporates
    much faster than water and hastens the
    cooling process. This procedure will be
    discussed in detail later.

   d. Whirlpool

A mechanism is attached to the bathtub or a
specially prepared tub is used. The motor of the
mechanism causes a whirling movement of the

water that gives the skin a gentle massage and has a generally soothing effect. Tension and discomfort are relieved.

e. Soaks

Certain soaks may be ordered as a part of the bath. The soak has therapeutic value because it loosens diseased or necrotic tissue. The soak promotes suppuration (pus formation) of a wound. *The solution, temperature, and frequency of the soak will be prescribed by the physician.* Burned patients may be placed in normal saline (saltwater) for a stated time of soaking in order to ease removal of "dead" tissue. Preparation for a soak includes thorough cleaning of the tub before and after the soak.

f. Sitz bath

Brings moist heat to the perineum or anal area for the promotion of healing a wound and to relieve discomfort. Commonly used following rectal or vaginal surgery and following the birth of a baby (delivery).

ITEM 2. EARLY A.M. CARE

This routine is usually performed early each morning before the activities of the day begin and breakfast is served. It generally consists of:

1. Offering the patient a bedpan or urinal.

2. Pulling the overbed tray across the bed.

3. Supplying a basin of warm water, soap, washcloth, and towel.

4. Permitting the patient to wash his face and hands, and get ready for breakfast.

5. Giving the patient oral hygiene care (completing this for him if he is unable to wash himself).

6. Straightening the bed linen, fluffing the pillow.

7. Positioning the bed in Fowler's position for breakfast.

8. Removing the washbasin and supplies, cleaning and returning them to storage, and leaving the room neat and tidy.

9. Charting.
   Charting example: 6:30 A.M.   Early A.M. care given.   J. Jones, NA

ITEM 3. H.S. ("HOUR OF SLEEP") CARE OR P.M. CARE

This routine is performed at bedtime:

1. Offering the patient the bedpan or urinal.

2. Providing a basin of warm water, soap, washcloth, and towel; permitting the patient to wash face and hands (doing this for him if he is unable).

3. Washing and drying his back; giving him a backrub. (Follow step 16 in bath procedure.)

4. Removing the washbasin and supplies, cleaning and returning them to storage, and leaving the room neat and tidy.

5. Placing the call signal and bedside stand nearby.

U
N
I
T
13

6. Straightening the bed linens and fluffing the pillow.

7. Positioning the bed to the low position and adjusting the siderails to the *up* position.

8. Charting.
   Charting example: 8:30 P.M. h.s. care given early. Patient very sleepy tonight, states he needs no sedative.   J. Jones, NA

ITEM 4. OFFERING THE BEDPAN

Important Steps	Key Points
1. Obtain the equipment.	You will need a bedpan, bedpan cover, toilet tissue, basin of water, soap, and towel.
2. Approach the patient.	Wash your hands. Provide privacy by pulling the curtains around the unit or closing the door of a private room. Warm the bedpan by running water inside the pan and along the rim. Dry the outside of the pan. Anticipate the patient's needs and render service.

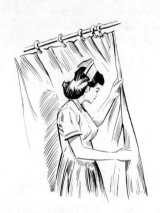

Screening the patient.

3. Place the patient on the bedpan.

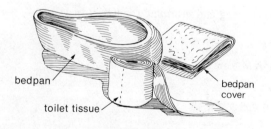

bedpan

toilet tissue

bedpan cover

Equipment to offer a bed pan.

Fold back the bed covers, and cover the patient with the top sheet or blanket. Raise the patient's gown. Ask the patient to flex his knees. Slide your hand under his lower back and direct the patient to lift his hips. Slide the pan into place and adjust it for the patient's comfort. The edge of the pan is placed at the end of the sacrum so that the buttocks form a seal along the rim of pan. Raise the head of the bed if allowed. Place the toilet tissue and signal cord within reach of the patient and step away.

4. Ask the patient to signal when finished.

Return after a reasonable time or when the patient signals.

5. Remove the bedpan.

Have the patient flex his knees and raise his hips. Cover the bedpan immediately and place it on a chair. Assist the patient if he is unable to clean himself.

Important Steps	Key Points
6. Assist the patient if he is unable to clean himself.	Turn him on his side. Wipe the anal area with toilet tissue and wash it as needed. Dry the parts of the patient's anal area. Position the patient for comfort, and replace the bed covers.
7. Take the bedpan to the bathroom or utility room.	Check the bowel contents for any abnormal condition. Obtain a specimen if one is needed.
8. Empty the bedpan. Clean and store it in the appropriate place.	
9. Wash your hands and those of your patient. Remove screening or open the door.	
10. Report and record.	Chart the time, whether the patient had a bowel movement, and the color, consistency, and amount of the waste in the bedpan.

ITEM 5. POSITIONING THE BEDPAN FOR THE HELPLESS PATIENT

Important Steps	Key Points
Follow steps 1 and 2 of Item 4.	
3. Assist the patient onto his side; position the bedpan.	Stand facing the patient's back. Place the bedpan firmly against the patient's back region at the level of his sacrum, or the top of the fold of his buttocks. Hold his hip with one hand and the bedpan with the other hand. Roll the patient onto the bedpan and check its position for comfort.

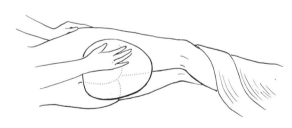 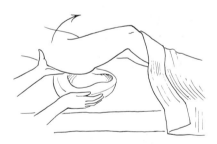

4. Remove the bedpan when the patient is finished.	Hold the bedpan securely with one hand. Place the other hand on the patient's hip and roll him off the bedpan. Cover the bedpan.
5. Wash the anal area and dry the skin. Position the patient for comfort.	
6. Empty and rinse the bedpan. Store it in the proper place.	
7. Wash your hands.	

ITEM 6.   GIVING THE URINAL

Important Steps	Key Points
1. Obtain the equipment.	You will need a urinal, urinal cover, basin of water, soap, and towel.

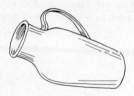

Male urinal.

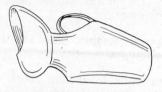

Female urinal.

2. Approach the patient.	Assist the patient to place the urinal properly. Put the toilet tissue within reach and leave the room.
3. Return to the room after a reasonable time, or when the patient signals.	
4. Remove the urinal and cover it.	Note any unusual color or odor. Take a urine specimen if required.
5. Empty the urinal.	Measure its contents if the patient is on "Intake and Output." Rinse the urinal and return it to its storage place.
6. Adjust the patient and the unit for comfort, and remove the screening.	Offer the washbasin and towel to the patient. Wash your hands.
7. Chart any unusual condition of the urine.	Charting example: Voided 500 cc pale yellow urine. Patient shows no discomfort. J. Jones, NA

ITEM 7.   MOUTH CARE FOR THE CONSCIOUS PATIENT

Important Steps	Key Points
1. Obtain the necessary equipment.	You will need a toothbrush or applicators; mouthwash solution if available; and toothpaste, toothpowder, or mixture of (1) salt and soda, or (2) ½ milk of magnesia and ½ hydrogen peroxide. (Salt and soda may be used instead of toothpaste or toothpowder; milk of magnesia and hydrogen peroxide may be used with an applicator.)

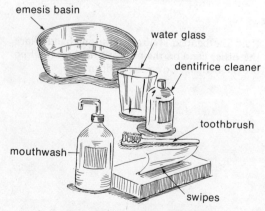

emesis basin
water glass
dentifrice cleaner
toothbrush
mouthwash
swipes

Equipment for mouth care.

You should also have a water glass with water, an emesis or curved basin, a face towel, and a denture container if one is needed.

Important Steps	Key Points
2. Remove any items from the overbed table, and place mouth care equipment on the table.	
3. Position the patient.	If allowed, raise the head of the bed to Fowler's position. If the patient is unable to sit up, turn him to the side facing you. Place the towel and curved basin under his chin. Moisten the toothbrush with water or mouthwash and spread toothpaste or toothpowder on it. Hand the toothbrush to the patient.
4. Assist the patient to brush his teeth as needed.	Teeth should be brushed in this manner: downward on upper teeth and upward on lower teeth. This applies to both front and back teeth. Allow the patient to rinse his mouth into the curved basin. Rinsing may be done as many times as the patient desires. (Use water or mouthwash.) Wipe the patient's mouth with a towel when rinsing is completed.
5. Clean the equipment and put the materials away.	Rinse the toothbrush and return it to its assigned place. Rinse the curved basin and place it with items to be cleaned later. Wash your hands. Caution: Sodium bicarbonate is not used as a dentifrice for the "heart patient." Check with the nurse for a suitable cleaning agent if toothpaste or toothpowder is not available.

ITEM 8. MOUTH CARE FOR THE UNCONSCIOUS PATIENT

Mouth care is a must for this person.

Important Steps	Key Points
Follow steps 1 and 2 of Item 7.	
3. Position the patient.	Turn the patient's head to the side facing you, and place the towel and curved basin under his chin.
4. Cleanse his teeth and mouth.	Using an applicator (commercial applicators are prepared with glycerin and lemon), thoroughly clean the inside of the mouth, the cheek sides, the roof of the mouth, the teeth, and the tongue. A 4X4-inch gauze wrapped around the index finger may be effectively used instead of an applicator. Half-strength hydrogen peroxide and milk of magnesia make a good agent for cleaning the mouth. Discard the applicators into the trash, and wash the patient's mouth with mouthwash and rinse it with water. Very small amounts of liquid are used since the patient is not able to spit it out. However, you must keep the teeth and tissues of the mouth clean and moist. Keep the patient's head in such a position that fluid drains out of the mouth by gravity.

UNIT 13

Important Steps

Key Points

Dry the patient's mouth and lubricate the lips to prevent cracking. Sterile Vaseline may be used. Do not use mineral oil since it may drain down into the lungs and cause lipid pneumonia.

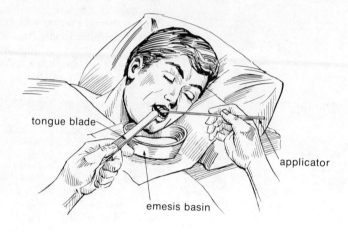

Oral hygiene.

5. Clean the equipment and return it to its assigned place.

ITEM 9. CARE OF DENTURES

Comatose patients' dentures should be removed from their mouths and placed in containers.

Important Steps

Key Points

1. Assemble the equipment for denture care.

You will need a toothbrush or denture brush, denture container, denture cleaner, and 4X4 gauze (if needed to clean the mouth).

Dentures must be handled with care; dropping may cause breakage. When not in the mouth, they should be kept in a labeled denture box with water or normal saline to keep them moist.

2. Remove the dentures and put them into their container.

If the patient cannot remove his dentures, you must do it. To remove the upper denture (it is held in place by a vacuum), grasp the front teeth with the thumb and index finger. Move the denture up and down slightly to break the vacuum seal. Slip it out of the mouth.

The lower denture may be picked out of the mouth; exercise care to turn it slightly to prevent the discomfort of stretching the lips.

Important Steps	Key Points

Place the dentures in a basin and take them to the sink to wash. *Use caution not to drop them.*

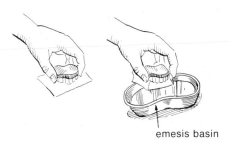

emesis basin

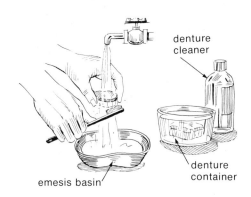

denture cleaner

emesis basin

denture container

Care of dentures.

3. Clean the dentures.

Use a toothbrush, and toothpaste or toothpowder to clean by brushing motions. Brush down on the upper teeth and brush upward on the lower teeth. (A commercially prepared material may be used for soaking the dentures.)

Rinse them with running water, exercising care not to allow the wet dentures to slip from your fingers.

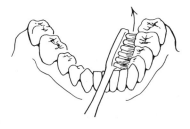

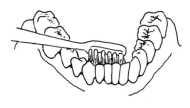

Brush dentures from gum-line up to edge of teeth.

4. Replace the dentures in the patient's mouth.

Return to the bedside and allow the patient to put the dentures in his mouth, or do it for him. Dry the patient's mouth and hands.

ITEM 10.   THE BED BATH

Important Steps	Key Points
1. Obtain the equipment.	You will need the following items:

a. Basin of warm water: $110°-115°$F.

b. Desired soap.

c. Clean linen stacked in order of use.

d. Bath blanket.

e. Two towels and washcloths as needed (provide for extra towels to remain at bedside).

f. Clean gown.

g. Laundry bag for soiled linen.

h. Patient's toilet articles from the bedside stand.

i. Toilet tissue at bedside.

2. Approach the patient.

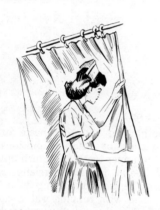

Wash your hands. Introduce yourself if you are new to the patient. Check his identification band. Explain the treatment to be done. Pull the curtains around the unit, provide privacy in the manner available, or shut the door in a private room.

3. Offer the bedpan or urinal.

See Items 4 and 5 of this unit.

4. Arrange the bath equipment.

Check the temperature of the room; allow no draft. A room temperature of $75°-78°$F is desirable. (Aged persons need warmer temperatures.)

Remove any items from the bedside table and place the bath articles on the table top. Loosen the bedding around the bed.

5. Provide for the patient's mouth care.

See Items 6 and 7 of this unit.

6. Assemble the equipment on the bedside table.

Prepare the bath water at $110°-115°$F (water cools rapidly). Place the soap dish near the basin of water. Do not leave the soap in the

Important Steps	Key Points

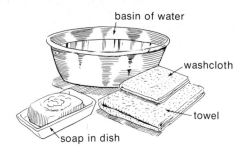

basin of water

washcloth

towel

soap in dish

Bath equipment.

bath water; the water becomes excessively soapy.

Raise the bed to working level.

7. Replace the top linen with the bath blanket.

Fan-fold the bath blanket and place it across the patient's chest. Ask the patient to hold the top edge of the bath blanket.

Grasp the bottom edge of the bath blanket and the top of the covers, and pull the covers and bottom edge of the blanket to the foot of the bed. (The patient maintains privacy.)

8. Remove the top bedding.

Inspect the spread for soiled areas. If it appears clean, fold it in this manner:

a. Bring the top edge to the bottom edge. The spread is now in half.

b. Fold this side to the other side edge. The spread is now in quarters.

c. Fold it again in half. Place it over the back of the chair.

If the blanket is on the bed, remove it and fold as above.

Discard the top sheet into the laundry bag. (In some settings the top sheet, if clean, may be reused as the bottom sheet. In this case, fold the sheet as above and hang it on the back of the chair.)

9. Prepare the patient.

Lower the siderail on the side near the bedside table. Remove the gown, being careful to keep patient covered with a blanket. If an IV is in place, see Assisting the Patient to Dress and Undress, page 221.

Remove the pillow unless the patient is more comfortable with it. Spread a towel across patient's chest.

10. Make a bath mitt.

Grasp the washcloth at an edge and fold 1/3 over the palm of your hand. Bring the opposite edge across the palm of your hand and hold it with your thumb. Bring the extreme end of the cloth up to your palm and tuck the edge under

U
N
I
T
13

Important Steps

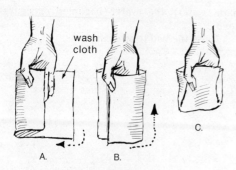

wash cloth

A.   B.   C.

How to make a bath mitt.

11. Wash the patient's face and neck.

12. Wash the arms.

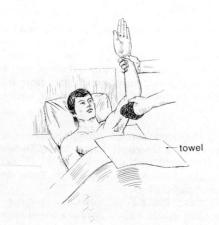

towel

Wash arm with long, sweeping strokes.

13. Wash the chest and abdomen.

Key Points

the upper edge. You now have a bath mitt. This prevents loose ends of the washcloth from dragging across the patient. These tails become cool quickly and chill the patient.

The patient may wash his face if he is able. Use soap only if the patient desires. If patient is unable to do this, moisten the bath mitt with water and wash one eye from the inner lid to the outer side near the ear. Rinse the cloth before washing the other eye. Dry well. Wash the forehead from center to side. Rinse and dry it well.

Wash the cheeks from the nose to the side of face. Wash the bridge and tip of the nose. Wash the mouth area with a circular motion. Wash the neck. Rinse and dry the face and neck well.

Place a towel under the distal arm and place the basin of water convenient for soaking the hand. Soap may be used. If an IV is in place, take care not to disturb the needle.

Make a bath mitt and wash the entire arm with long, sweeping strokes. Give special care to the armpit with extra soaping. Rinse and dry it well. Wash the hands and fingers, rinse, and dry. Dry well between the fingers. Wash the proximal arm and hand in the same manner and dry them well.

Place a towel over the patient's chest. Fold the bath blanket to his waistline. Make a bath mitt and wash under the towel to include the entire chest. Wash the breast with circular movements. Rinse and dry it well. Fold the blanket to the top of the pubic bone and wash the lower abdomen. Dry well.

Important Steps	Key Points
14. Wash the feet and legs.	Expose only the leg being washed. Tuck the blanket around the patient to prevent draft. Flex one leg and place a towel lengthwise on the bed. Place the bath basin on the towel. Lift the patient's foot, placing your hand under the heel, and put it into the water. This is very refreshing for the patient. Wash from the hip to the knee with long, sweeping strokes. Wash from the knee to the foot in the same manner. Rinse and dry the leg well. Wash the foot and dry it. Dry each toe separately and place the leg and foot under the blanket. Wash the remaining foot and leg in the same manner.

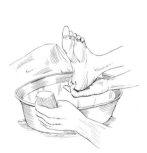
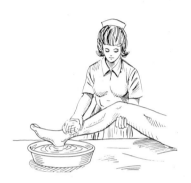

Place foot in water.

15. Change the bath water.	Remove the bath water and obtain fresh bath water 110° to 115°F. Return to the patient, and prepare to complete the bath.
16. Wash the patient's back.	Turn the patient to his side. Wash the back with long, sweeping motions. Rinse and dry it well.
17. Give a backrub.	Stand with your feet about 12 inches apart and put lotion in the palms of your hands. Place your hands at the patient's shoulders, and with the fingers of each hand, rub his neck with circular motions to the hairline. Place your hands at the sacral area, and rub with your fingers in circular motions. Begin at the sacral area and rub toward the neckline with long, smooth strokes. Proceed down toward the sacrum with broad circular motions. Complete the backrub by long, smooth strokes over the entire back from the shoulders to the sacrum.

   A backrub tones muscles and stimulates circulation. Bed confinement limits activity and the backrub is very important to relieve tension and produce a relaxing affect for the patient. If the backrub is administered properly, the patient will feel relaxed but invigorated. Often the backrub provides an alternative to giving the patient a pain medication or sedative. *A backrub can be given at any time of the day or night as indicated by patient need.* |

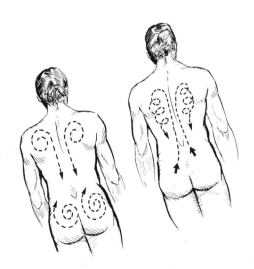

Circular motions for back rub.

UNIT 13

Important Steps	Key Points
18. Wash the genital area.	If the patient is able, he may wash himself. It is the duty of the health worker to prepare the washcloth and place the bath equipment so that the patient can reach it. While the patient washes his genitals, the health worker may walk outside the unit but remain within hearing distance. If the patient is unable to wash his genitals, the health worker is obliged to do so. An important point to remember is to use a washcloth or towel to hold body tissue while washing between the folds of the body with another cloth. The genitals are washed thoroughly, rinsed well, and dried carefully. If the patient has a catheter in place, attention is given to washing around the catheter with soap and water to remove body secretions. Rinsing follows. Check with your health facility for catheter care used.
19. Put a clean gown on the patient.	If the patient is able, he may put on his gown. If the patient is unable to put on his gown, or has an IV in place, proceed as described in Unit 12, Dressing and Undressing.
20. Complete the personal care.	Comb the patient's hair. Refer to Unit 30 for information on Special Hair Care. Care for the fingernails and toenails. Take care not to break skin when doing the nails. Some agencies do not permit cutting nails. Check with your agency procedure. *Caution:* A diabetic patient should have an order from his physician for nail care. An accidental break in the skin of a diabetic patient may be hazardous to him. Permit the patient to shave. Assemble an electric shaver, a mirror, and the shaving lotion of patient's choice. Provide warm water and shaving cream if the patient uses a safety razor. This helps improve the male patient's morale. If he needs help, follow the hospital policy for shaving patients or calling the barber. Many agencies do not permit staff to shave patients with a straight edge or safety razor. Remove the bath basin. Clean, rinse, and return it to storage.
21. Make an occupied bed.	See the unit on Hospital Beds and follow the directions given there.
22. Tidy the room.	Return supplies to the storage area. Dispose of soiled linen. Place the call signal and bedside stand near the patient. Tidy the bedside stand and leave items arranged in an orderly fashion. Empty ashtrays. Replace the wastepaper bag on the bed. Obtain fresh water for the patient. Ask if there is anything else you can do. Raise the siderails if indicated. Tell the patient approximately when you will return (15 or 30 minutes, or an hour).

Important Steps	Key Points
23. Report and record.	Report any unusual occurrences to the charge nurse. Charting example: 8:00 A.M. Complete bed bath given. Special attention given to mouth. Mouth was dry and crusty. Carefully cleansed with glycerin applicator. Became very tired with the exertion. Promptly took nap following bath. J. Jones, NA

ITEM 11.   THE PARTIAL BATH

Partial baths may be given to convalescent patients who wash as much as they can reach but need help to complete the bath, or to those not in need of a complete bath. Such patients include those scheduled for physical therapy, or others for specified reasons. The partial bath includes the face, hands, armpits, back, genital area, and feet.

Use the equipment used for the bed bath. Refer to these steps in the section on bed baths:

1. Approach the patient.
2. Offer the bedpan or urinal.
3. Arrange the bath equipment.
4. Do mouth care.
5. Position the patient for the bed bath.
6. Assemble the equipment on the bedside table.
7. Replace the top linen with the bath blanket.
8. Prepare the patient.
9. Make a bath mitt.
10. Wash the patient's face and neck.
11. Wash the arms.
12. Wash the back.
13. Give a backrub
14. Wash the genital area.
15. Put a clean gown on the patient.
16. Complete personal care.
17. Make an occupied bed.
18. Chart.
   Charting example: 9:30 A.M. Partial bath given. Is very restless and talkative. Complained of severe pain in upper right quadrant.   J. Jones. NA

ITEM 12.   TUB BATH

This may be used for cleansing, medicated, or therapeutic baths.

Important Steps	Key Points
1. Assemble the bath materials.	Before the patient leaves his bed, clean and prepare the bathtub and assemble equipment.

Important Steps	Key Points

Place a bath mat by the tub. Wash your hands, identify the patient, and explain the procedure.

Accompany the patient to the bathtub. Seat your patient comfortably nearby, and fill the bathtub ½ full. Check the temperature and adjust it to read 100°–115°F. If you must add warm water during the procedure, avoid direct contact with the patient's skin to avoid burns.

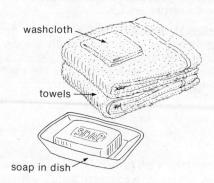

washcloth

towels

soap in dish

Tub bath equipment.

2. Assist the patient to the tub.

Assist the patient into tub. Explain the system to signal for help if needed. Hang the "occupied" sign on the door, and return within a few minutes to see if the patient is satisfactory. Do not lock the door.

If the patient appears weak, remain with him, and assist with the bath. (The male patient may use a towel for a sarong to provide privacy for himself when a female health worker cares for him.) Remain near the patient at all times. Ill patients frequently become weak and may faint.

3. Wash the patient's back.

4. Assist the patient to get out of the tub.

Support the patient with hands under armpits. Have him use the side of the tub, and the grab bars to pull himself up to a standing position. Provide a bath mat outside the tub to stand on.

5. Dry the patient and return him to his room.

Assist the patient in drying himself and putting on a clean gown. Escort the patient back into bed. Give him his backrub. Change the linens.

6. Restore the equipment for another use.

Return to the bathroom and wash the bathtub. (Use the scouring powder and disinfectant prescribed by your agency.) Remove the towels and soiled linen, and prepare the facility for another to use. Remove the "occupied" sign.

If the patient does not require complete assistance, the bed may be changed while he bathes. The bath should not exceed 15 to 20 minutes. Close observation of the patient during the bath is very important.

7. Chart the procedure on the nurses' notes or check-off sheet.

ITEM 13. SITZ BATH

There may be a specially designed tub used for the sitz bath, or the common bathtub may be used. The principle is the same, which is to provide moist heat to the perineal or rectal area to promote healing and relieve discomfort.

Plastic sitz bath kits are now available, which are more convenient to use. The basin fits over the toilet and a bag with tubing is used to supply additional warm water to the basin during the procedure. The patient sits on the seat and the excess water in the basin drains down the toilet. Equipment for the sitz bath is the same as for the tub bath.

Important Steps	Key Points
1. Prepare the equipment.	Wash your hands. Fill the tub about 1/3 full. Water temperature should be 100°–110°F. Place a towel or folded bath blanket in the bottom of the tub. Hang "occupied" sign on the door.

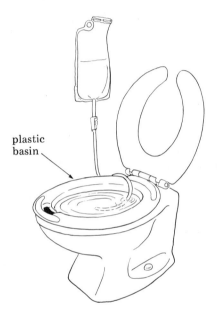

plastic basin

Sitz bath basin placed on toilet.

2. Assist the patient to the tub.	Check the patient's identification band and explain the procedure. Assist the patient to remove his robe and sit in the tub with the hospital gown on. Allow the patient to remain 20 to 30 minutes as ordered. *Check frequently* on the patient's condition, and keep the temperature of the water even. When adding hot water, avoid burning the patient.
3. Remove the patient from the tub.	Help the patient to remove the gown if wet, and stand up and step out of the tub. Assist him to dry himself and put on his hospital attire. Loosen the drain plug of the sitz bath so that the water may drain out.
4. Return the patient to his room.	Assist the patient to return to his room. (This may be on foot, or by wheelchair if needed. The bed may have been made while the patient was in the sitz bath. If not, make up a clean bed at this time.

U
N
I
T
13

Important Steps	Key Points
5. Restore the equipment for use.	Clean the sitz bath with the scouring powder or disinfectant used in your agency and return the equipment to the proper place. Remove the "occupied" sign from the door. Leave the bathroom clean, neat, and dry.
6. Record.	Enter on the patient's chart the time, the temperature of the water, and any observation of the patient. This includes how he tolerated the bath, his skin color, his pulse, his respiration, and his general reaction. Charting example:
	11:00 A.M. Sitz bath taken for 30 minutes. Stated that procedure was very comforting. Tolerated procedure well today. Vital signs remained stable. J. Jones, NA

PERFORMANCE TEST

In the laboratory setting, with a student partner, you will give a complete bed bath, tub bath, or sitz bath following the procedure outlined in the student manual. Keep in mind the supplies you will need, the major steps of the procedure, and the comfort and modesty of the patient.

You should be prepared to explain to your instructor the indications and procedure for the partial bath, the medicated bath, A.M. care, and h.s. care.

PERFORMANCE CHECKLIST

THE BED BATH

1. Wash your hands.

2. Select and assemble all needed materials before beginning the bed bath.

3. Identify the patient and explain the procedure to the patient.

4. Raise the bed to working height. Use good body alignment procedures.

5. Offer the bedpan or urinal to the patient.

6. Permit the patient to give himself mouth care. Remove, clean, and return the equipment to storage.

7. Describe the procedure for giving mouth care to an unconscious patient; include the head position. Using a glycerin and lemon applicator, clean the interior of the oral cavity completely; rinse the mouth with water or mouthwash, and dry the patient's mouth.

8. Apply the bath blanket correctly.

9. Remove and dispose of the linen correctly (either fold clean linen and hang it over the back of the chair, or dispose of soiled linen in the proper container, being careful not to let it touch your uniform).

10. Remove the patient's gown correctly, being careful not to expose the patient. Keep the patient covered with the bath blanket.

11. Wash and dry his face using a correctly folded bath mitt.

12. Wash and dry his arms correctly.

    a. Protect the bedding with a towel under the patient's arm.

    b. Put the basin of water on the bed.

    c. Soak his hand.

    d. Dry the patient's arms and hands carefully.

    e. Remove the basin to the bedside stand without spilling.

13. Put a towel across his upper chest; fold the bath blanket to his waist. Wash and dry the chest using circular motions.

14. Fold the bath blanket to the pubis, with a towel across the chest.

15. Wash and dry the abdomen.

UNIT
13

16. Expose the leg.

    a. Flex the leg.

    b. Put the towel lengthwise under the leg.

    c. Place the bath basin on the towel.

    d. Place the foot in the basin.

17. Wash his legs with long, firm strokes, and dry them well.

18. Wash and dry his feet, and remove the basin.

19. Change the water when cool; water temperature should be 110° to 115°F.

20. Wash and dry his back.

21. Give him a backrub using strong friction and rotary movements. Give special attention to bony prominences, scapula, and sacrum.

    a. Observe principles of body alignment.

22. Wash or permit the patient to wash the genital area.

23. Help the patient to put on his gown.

24. Comb his hair or provide assistance to the patient as needed (mirror, comb, brush, towel, covering, etc.).

25. Check his nails; clean or cut them as needed.

26. Remove the soiled items, and clean the equipment and return it to storage.

27. Make the occupied bed using good body movement, and without raising dust by shaking the linens. Carry the linens away from your uniform.

28. Leave the unit neat and tidy with the bedside stand and call signal within easy reach of the patient.

29. Chart the procedure.

THE TUB BATH

1. Wash your hands.

2. Assemble the supplies and equipment for use.

3. Check the tub and clean it if necessary.

4. Identify the patient and explain the procedure to him.

5. Assist the patient to the bathroom using principles of body alignment, movement, and balance for the patient and yourself.

6. Fill the tub half full with water at 100° to 105°F.

7. Assist the patient into the tub.

    a. Observe principles of body alignment.

8. Hang the "occupied" sign on the door.

9. Check on the patient frequently.

10. Wash and dry patient's back.

11. Assist the patient as needed to get out of the tub and dry his body.

12. Put a clean gown on the patient.

13. Return the patient to bed.

14. Give him a backrub.

15. Change the linen and dispose of the soiled linen in the designated manner.

16. Leave the room neat and tidy.

17. Return to the bathroom.

  a. Remove the soiled linen and equipment.

  b. Clean the tub.

  c. Remove the "occupied" sign from door.

18. Chart the procedure.

THE SITZ BATH

1. Wash your hands.

2. Prepare the equipment: fill the tub one-third full of water ($100°$ to $110°$ F). Hang an "occupied" sign on the door.

3. Explain the procedure to the patient and check his identification band.

4. Assist the patient to the tub, allow him to remain there for 20 to 30 minutes. Check him frequently. Keep the water warm throughout the procedure.

5. Assist the patient out of the tub, and in drying himself.

6. Drain the water from the tub.

7. Help the patient back to bed.

8. Change the bed linens.

9. Leave the room neat and tidy.

10. Return to the bathroom.

  a. Remove the soiled linens and equipment.

  b. Clean the tub.

  c. Remove the "occupied" sign from the door.

11. Chart the procedure.

Unit 14

THE VITAL SIGNS: TEMPERATURE, PULSE, RESPIRATION, AND BLOOD PRESSURE

I. DIRECTIONS TO THE STUDENT

Proceed through this lesson When you have finished, practice taking temperature, pulse, respiration, and blood pressure with other students in the skill laboratory and in the presence of your instructor.

You will need the following equipment:

1. Graphic chart.

2. Pen and ruler.

3. Watch with a second hand.

4. Thermometer (glass or electric).

5. Sphygmomanometer (blood pressure cuff).

6. Stethoscope.

When you believe you can demonstrate taking the vital signs accurately. arrange with your instructor to take the performance test.

II. GENERAL PERFORMANCE OBJECTIVE

After completing this lesson, you will be able to obtain an accurate temperature, pulse, respiration, and blood pressure on adults and children, and record readings correctly on the patients' charts.

III. SPECIFIC PERFORMANCE OBJECTIVES

Following this lesson you will be able within stated time limits to accurately:

1. Take and record the body temperature of an adult and a child by the oral, rectal or axillary use of a glass or electric thermometer.

2. Take and record an apical and radial pulse.

3. Count and record the patient's respirations.

4. Take and record blood pressure.

5. Recognize deviations from normal vital sign patterns.

IV VOCABULARY

1. Temperature

axilla—the armpit.

centigrade—a thermometer scale used to measure heat; it is divided into 100 degrees (°) from the freezing point of water at 0°C at the bottom, to the boiling point at 100°C at the top; used mainly in Europe and Latin America; scale recorded as 100°C, or 100 degrees centigrade.

enzyme—a complex substance produced by living cells that acts on other substances, causing them to split up into simpler substances; they are found for example, in the digestive juices.

Fahrenheit—a thermometer scale used to measure heat; the freezing point of water is 32°F, and the boiling point is 212°F; and used chiefly in the U. S. (Medically, a thermometer is a glass or electric instrument used to measure the body temperature.)

febrile—feverish, pertaining to fever.

fever—pyrexia, or elevation of temperature above normal, which is 98.6°F (98.6 degrees Fahrenheit) for the average person.

metabolism—all the chemical reactions needed to keep the body tissues living and functioning.

mucosa—mucous membrane, which lines body passages and cavities communicating with the air, and which secretes mucous.

2. Pulse

arrhythmia—irregular heart beat.

bradycardia—slow heart action; generally a rate below 60 beats per minute for an adult and below 70 per minute for a child; seen in cases of uremia, jaundice, fractured skulls, and stroke.

bounding—a full, strong pulse.

tachycardia—abnormal rapidity of heart action, usually over 100 beats per minute for adults at rest, and over 200 in infants; seen in patients with heart diseases or goiter, or those in shock.

thready—a pulse that feels weak and feeble; it can hardly be felt.

3. Respiration

apnea—absence of respirations.

Cheyne-Stokes—a type of irregular or arrhythmic breathing; at first it is slow and shallow; then it increases in rapidity and depth until it reaches a maximum, after which it decreases gradually until it stops for 10 to 20 seconds, then repeats the irregular rhythm.

deep breathing—large amount of air taken in.

diaphragm—a musculomembranous wall separating the abdominal cavity from the thoracic (chest) cavity.

dyspnea—difficult breathing, breathing hard as though one had just climbed a stairway; it is usually rapid, labored, and noisy; long periods of dyspnea are very tiring for the patient.

hyperpnea—increased respiratory rate or breathing that is deeper than usual while resting; frequently occurs after exercise.

hyperventilation—to increase (hyper) ventilation by breathing excessively fast.

orthopnea—respiratory condition in which breathing is possible only when person sits or stands in an erect position; seen in some severe cardiac or pulmonary diseases.

shallow breathing—small amount of air taken in.

4. Blood Pressure

sphygmomanometer—device used to measure blood pressure
stethoscope—instrument used to listen to sounds within the body.

V. INTRODUCTION

The vital signs provide the first means of assessing a patient's condition. Mechanisms in the body that govern these signs are so finely adjusted that departure from normal rates is looked upon as a symptom of disease. The variations of certain vital signs are typical of certain diseases or stages of a disease; therefore, the medical care plan and diagnosis can entirely depend on these signals, which include the body temperature, pulse, respirations, and blood pressure.

ITEM 1. BODY TEMPERATURE

A. The Importance of Taking Body Temperature

We are concerned with body temperature because a definite temperature range is required for efficient cellular functioning. The body temperature represents a balance between heat produced in the tissues and the external environment, and the heat lost to the environment. Fevers (high temperatures) indicate a disturbance of the heat-regulating centers.

In the human being (a warm-blooded animal), when the balance between heat produced and heat lost is in equilibrium (balance), the average body temperature reading on a thermometer is 98.6 degrees Fahrenheit (98.6°F) or 37 degrees centigrade (37°C); 1° centigrade equals 1.8° Fahrenheit; 36.9°C equals 98.5°F. Changes in the temperature range between 36° to 38°C (97.6 to 99°F) are within normal or average range. Heat is lost by the body through feces, urine, expired air, and perspiration.

Whether the patient's temperature is taken orally (by mouth) or rectally (by rectum) usually depends on the patient's condition and his physician's order. Rectal temperatures should be taken when oral measurements are contraindicated because of questionable accuracy or discomfort due to mouth breathing, nasal congestion, nasal surgery, or nasal tubes, or when the patient will not keep his mouth closed over the thermometer. Oral temperatures should be taken when there is a chance of inaccuracy or discomfort, as with rectal or perineal surgery. Axillary temperatures are taken when oral or rectal temperatures are contraindicated, or when agency procedure requires.

Oral temperatures *should not* be measured within 30 minutes following the intake of hot or cold foods or fluids, or when the patient has been smoking or chewing gum, because these actions will produce a temporary incorrect reading. In other words, you would be getting a temperature recording of the mouth, not the body temprature.

Body temperature should be evaluated in relation to:

1. The patient's usual body temperature. Some people run a "low-normal" or a "high-normal" temperature consistently. This then is the normal body temperature for those people; for example, some individuals' normal temperature may be recorded as 97.6°F.

2. The time of day. The body temperature upon awakening is generally in the low-normal range due to the inactivity of muscles. Conversely, the afternoon temperature may be high-normal due to metabolic processes, activity, and the temperature of the atmosphere.

3. Environmental temperature. As you might expect, the body temperature is lower in cold weather and warmer in hot weather.

4. The phase of the patient's menstrual cycle and pregnancy. Body temperature drops slightly just before ovulation (the normal monthly ripening and rupture of the mature Graafian follicle which releases an ovum), and then may rise to one whole degree above normal during ovulation. Within a day or two preceding the onset of the next menstrual period, the temperature drops again. During pregnancy, the body temperature may consistently stay at high-normal due to an increase in the patient's metabolic rate.

5. The amount of physical exercise the patient performs. Physical exercise calls for the use of large muscles, which create greater body heat by burning up the glucose and fat in the tissues. Muscle action generates heat. You know that when you are cold, you exercise to warm up. Also, chattering or shivering are ways in which the body tries to keep its temperature balanced. The reverse is true in hot weather; we tend to become inactive since muscle exercise generates heat.

6. The age of the patient. In old age, the loss of subcutaneous tissue (tissue directly under the skin) and decrease of blood flow due to arterial changes may cause the temperature to be lower and may cause less tolerance for cold weather. The muscle activity of older patients is limited, and therefore less heat is produced. At birth, heat-regulating mechanisms are generally not fully developed, so there may be marked fluctuations in body temperature occurring during the first year of life.

7. The emotional status of the patient. Highly emotional states cause an elevation in body temperature. The emotions increase the activity of secreting glands and thereby increase the heat production.

8. The diseased condition of the patient. Toxins from some infective agents, pathogenic diseases, or chemical reactions may produce elevated body temperatures or fevers. The fever is a protective defense mechanism that the body employs to fight germs and their toxins.

9. The method of measuring body temperature. A rectal temperature usually measures slightly higher than oral, and an axillary temperature measures lower than oral.

The course of a fever can be observed on the recorded temperature graph in the patient's chart. There are three distinct stages in a fever:

1. The *onset*, when temperature begins to rise. It can be sudden and violent as in pneumonia or it can be slow and gradual as in typhoid fever.

2. The *fastigium* or *stadium*. (Fastigium is a Latin word for roof; stadium is a Greek word for the distances in a race.) This is the period when the temperature remains at a high, constant level.

3. The *subsiding* stage, or the period during which the temperature returns to normal. It can fall slowly over a period of days or abruptly; in the latter case it is called the *crisis*. The crisis used to be a very significant point in the recovery or death of a pneumonia patient. However, with the advent of powerful drugs to combat pneumonia, the temperature now drops more gradually.

Fevers are classed according to certain characteristics:

1. During *constant fever* the temperature is continuously elevated; usually there is less than one degree of variation within a 24-hour period.

2. *Intermittent fever* is the alternate rise and fall of the temperature, e.g., low in the morning, high in the afternoon, or low for 2 to 3 days followed by a high temperature for 2 to 3 days.

3. *Remittent fever* is the falling of a high temperature, usually in the morning, rising later in the day. The significant fact is that the temperature never falls to normal in this type of fever until recovery occurs.

U
N
I
T
14

B.   Equipment Used in Measuring Body Temperature

Clinical Thermometers. The self-registering Fahrenheit clinical thermometer is the instrument used in the United States. The clinical thermometer is a glass bulb containing mercury and a stem in which the mercury can rise. On the stem there is a graduated scale representing degrees of temperature, the lowest registered being 95°F and the highest 110°F because body temperatures below and above these points are rare. In other words, the range registered on a Fahrenheit thermometer scale is 95° to 110°F. (The range on a centigrade thermometer scale is 35° to 43.3°C.) An arrow on the scale marks normal temperature at 98.6°F. The long lines on the scale represent full degrees, but only the *even numbers are written*. The short lines on the scale represent two-tenths (2/10) of a degree. Temperatures are recorded using an even number to represent tenths, for example, 99.2°F or 99.4°F, but never 99.3°F or 99.5°F.

Oral thermometers with long, slender bulbs register more rapidly than rectal thermometers with short, fat bulbs because there is a greater glass surface surrounding the mercury; therefore, the heat expands this mercury more rapidly. In the short bulb, there is less glass surface over the mercury and it takes longer to heat the mercury to make it rise in its column. The slender bulb must *not* be used in the rectum because it is likely to puncture and injure the mucosa. However, both mouth and rectal thermometers are made with short, fat bulbs and are less easily broken than the slender type. The oral thermometer is used to take either an oral or axillary temperature.

The portable battery-operated electric thermometers register body temperature in 10 seconds or less. They usually have an "on-off" button or an area to be pressed in order to activate the battery. They require a warming-up period, which consists of activating the battery and placing the tip of the probe against your finger to activate the gauge. The gauges come in two types: digital, on which you press the "on" button to register the degree on a scale with a needle, much as a weight scale indicates pounds; and numerical, which has a scale like that on the clinical glass thermometer. The probe, oral or rectal, consists of a totally disposable unit or is covered with a plastic sheath that is changed and then discarded after each use.

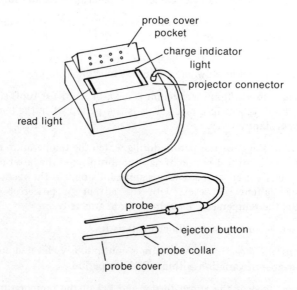

Electric thermometer.

Measuring the Oral Temperature

<table>
<tr><td align="center">Important Steps</td><td align="center">Key Points</td></tr>
</table>

1. Wash your hands. Approach the patient and explain what you are going to do.

   Identify the patient by checking his identification band. Determine his condition: can he cooperate and safely use an oral thermometer? If not, you may need to take a rectal or axillary temperature (these procedures will be described later).

2. Obtain the equipment.

   In some agencies the patient is issued his own thermometer on admission. It is usually stored somewhere in the patient's room. In other agencies the thermometers come on a tray daily from the supply room. Remove the thermometer from the container. If it is stored in an antiseptic solution, you must *always rinse* it under cold water to remove the solution before placing the thermometer in the patient's mouth. Remember, do not use hot water to rinse because it will cause the mercury to expand, which could break your thermometer. If you are using an electric thermometer, assemble the monitoring kit and the supply of disposable covers for the probe. Place a clean cover on the probe and push the "on" button to warm up the machine.

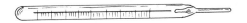

Glass oral thermometer.

3. Check the level of the mercury in the thermometer.

   If the mercury is above the 96°F mark, it will need to be shaken down.

4. Shake the mercury down.

   Hold the thermometer securely at the top end between your right thumb and index finger (reverse if you are left-handed). Shake the thermometer in a quick downward flip and with a twisting motion of the wrist. (See the diagram.) Usually this will take some practice. Shake down to 96°F or lower.

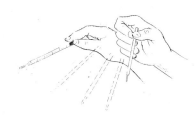

Shake mercury down.

5. Place the thermometer in the patient's mouth.

   Ask him to open his mouth, then put the thermometer slightly to one side of his mouth under his tongue. By placing the thermometer deep in the mouth it will be surrounded by tissue that is rich in blood supply, thus enabling an accurate temperature reading. Remind him to keep his lips closed tightly; this will prevent the cooler outside air from influencing the temperature recording.

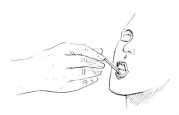

Place thermometer in patient's mouth.

U
N
I
T
14

Important Steps	Key Points
6. Leave the thermometer in place for an accurate recording.	When using the glass thermometer, leave it in place for 3 to 5 minutes. Be sure to warn the patient not to bite down on the glass thermometer; it might break and he could swallow the broken glass or mercury.

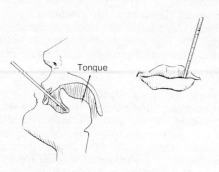

Tonque

Ask patient to close lips.

7. Remove the thermometer.	Again, hold the top end of the thermometer between your thumb and index finger. Wipe the thermometer off with tissue. Wipe from the top end to the bottom to avoid taking the patient's germs up to your fingers.
8. Read the thermometer.	Hold the thermometer at your eye-level. Rotate it toward you until you can clearly see the column of mercury. Observe the marking (calibrations) on the scale that is even with the top of the mercury column. Remember, each of the long lines represents a full degree and only the even-numbered degrees are numbered, 96°, 98°, etc. The four short lines alternating with the long lines represent 2/10 of a degree.

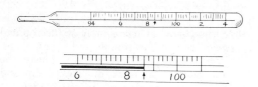

Hold thermometer at eye-level and read.

If the mercury column ends at one of the small lines, look to see which long line is immediately below it (nearer the patient's mouth); that will tell you the degree, e.g., 98°F. If the mercury level is at the second small line above the 98°F mark, the patient's temperature is 98.4°F.

9. Replace the thermometer in its holder.	Check to see that the thermometer is not broken. If it is, replace it immediately, using your agency procedure. Shake the mercury down to 96°F. Return it to the holder. Holders without antiseptic solution (dry method) are recommended. Wash your hands.
10. Record the patient's temperature.	Note it immediately on your work sheet; since you will be taking several readings, you will forget it if you don't record it immediately. This information must be transferred to the patient's chart when you have time to do your charting.

The method of cleansing of the thermometers is determined by agency procedure. If you are using an individually issued thermometer, the cleansing you give it after taking it out of the patient's mouth will be sufficient inasmuch as he is the only one using it. If the agency returns thermometers to the processing area after each use, you will need to wash it in *cold* running water and soap before returning it to the stock tray for reprocessing. Follow your agency procedure.

Do not store oral and rectal thermometers together; they can easily be confused. It would be totally unsanitary to place a rectal thermometer in a patient's mouth by error!

Taking the Rectal Temperature

Important Steps	Key Points
1. Wash your hands; approach and identify the patient.	Generally you will take rectal temperatures in special cases, such as patients who are confused, comatose adults, children, or those with an oral injury or disease. Always explain the procedure if the patient is conscious.

2. Obtain the equipment.

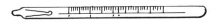

Rectal thermometer.

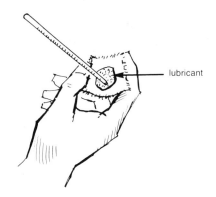

lubricant

Apply lubricant to tip of rectal thermometer.

Rectal thermometers will also probably be stored in the patient's room. Shake the mercury down to 96°F or below. Lubricate the bulb end of thermometer with K–Y jelly or mineral oil for smooth, comfortable insertion into the rectum. If it is not lubricated well, it may be irritating to the mucous lining of the muscles and stimulate the rectum to expel (push out) the thermometer. Do not dip the thermometer into a jar of lubricant because you will contaminate the contents of the jar. Instead, use a tongue depressor to take the amount of lubricant you need and place it on a piece of gauze. Then put the tip of the thermometer in the lubricant. Use the gauze to spread it over the entire tip. Hold the thermometer at the top end as described in the previous section.

3. Place the patient in Sims' position.

This will make the anal opening clearly visible for ease of insertion. Drape the upper bed covers to expose only the rectal area. Do not expose the patient unnecessarily.

4. Insert the thermometer in the patient's rectum.

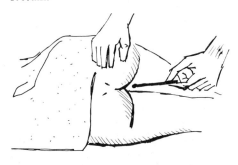

Insert rectal thermometer in rectum.

With your left hand, lift his upper buttock slightly so that you can see the anus clearly. Holding the thermometer in your right hand (reverse if you are left-handed), insert the lubricated bulb end into the rectum about 1½ inches. Ask the patient to take a deep breath; this will relax the rectal sphincter and make for easier insertion of the thermometer.

Important Steps	Key Points
5. Hold the thermometer in place.	If the patient is restless and you are not holding the thermometer securely, it could easily move inside the patient. Removal of a thermometer after it has gone inside the patient's rectum may even necessitate taking the patient to surgery. You must prevent this from happening.
6. Leave the thermometer in for the required length of time to obtain an accurate reading.	Leave the glass thermometer in for 3 to 5 minutes, as in the previous procedure.
7. Remove the thermometer and read it.	Wipe it clean with gauze or tissue. Read it in the same manner as you would an oral thermometer. The rectal temperature is usually ½ to 1 degree higher than the oral temperature because it is in a closed cavity and not exposed to outside air, which could lower the temperature (for example, when the patient opens his mouth while having his oral temperature taken). Wash your hands.
8. Record the temperature.	Note it immediately on the work sheet. Chart the temperature on a graphic sheet. All temperature recording on the graphic sheet are oral temperatures unless otherwise designated. Therefore, when recording a rectal temperature, you chart this sign ® over the temperature reading to designate that it was taken rectally, as shown here:

®
98.6°F

Using an Electric Thermometer

Important Steps	Key Points
(Wash your hands before proceeding)	
1. Remove the probe from its stored position in the face of the thermometer.	This automatically turns the thermometer on and a digital display of 94.0°F or 34.0°C appears on the lighted panel.
2. Insert the probe into the probe cover while the cover is still in the box.	Be sure to hold the probe by its collar near the ring of the top.

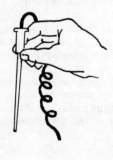

Grasp probe by probe collar.

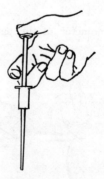

Eject the probe cover.

Important Steps	Key Points
3. Press the probe firmly into its cover.	Do not push on the probe top, which is the ejection button to remove the probe cover. *Note:* Color coding is used for oral and rectal thermometer probes. *The thermometer is ready to use.*
For Oral Temperatures:	*Use the probe color code designated for oral temperature.*
1. Hold the probe between thumb and index finger while sliding it back under the front of the patient's tongue.	Place it along the gum line to the back of his mouth, i.e., the sublingual area at base of the tongue.
2. Hold the probe steady and in constant contact with body tissue until an audible signal is heard.	This should take about 10 to 20 seconds, after which the read light will appear.
3. Read the temperature and record it.	
4. Discard the probe cover.	Press on the top of the probe with your thumb while holding the probe collar between your index and middle fingers.
5. Return the probe to its stored position in the face of the thermometer machine.	This will automatically turn off and reset the thermometer so that it is ready for the next reading.
6. Store the thermometer in its charging base when not in use.	When storing, make sure that the probe is in its storage position; the temperature display must be off and the charging indicator light must be on to indicate the proper charging of the rechargeable battery. (The temperature light will not go on when the battery is discharged.)
For rectal temperatures:	*Use the probe color code designated for rectal temperature.*
Repeat the steps for Electric Oral Temperatures.	*Caution:* Take care that the depth of insertion in the rectum does *not* bed the tip of the probe in feces.

Measuring the Axillary Temperature

Important Steps	Key Points
Steps 1 through 4: Use the same procedure as for taking oral temperatures.	
5. Place the thermometer in the patient's axilla (armpit).	Be sure that the axilla is dry. If wet, pat it dry gently—excessive rubbing will generate heat. Place the thermometer in the center of the armpit. Have the patient hold his arm tightly against his chest; the arm can rest on his chest.

U
N
I
T
14

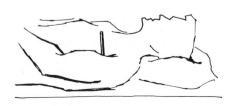

Axillary temperature.

Important Steps	Key Points
6. Leave the thermometer in place for *10 minutes*.	This is the least satisfactory way to take the temperature and is done when the temperature cannot be taken orally or rectally. The axillary temperature is about one degree lower than the oral temperature. This is true because the arm cannot be held tight enough to avoid air contact, which produces some cooling effect.
Steps 7 through 10.	These are the same as in the oral temperature procedure, except that when charting an axillary temperature on the graphic record, write Ⓐ over the temperature reading to indicate that it was taken by the axillary method: Ⓐ 97.6°F

ENRICHMENT FOR TEMPERATURES OF THE BODY

Human beings maintain body temperature independently of the environment. The body keeps its temperature through the activity of special cells in the hypothalamus, a part of the brain, which is located in the cranium. Control of body heat is thought to be activated by the temperature of the blood when it reaches the brain and spinal cord.

The body temperature depends on a balance between heat production and heat loss. Heat is produced by the metabolic processes of the body, and it is lost by the processes of conduction, convection, radiation, and vaporization. When the balance between heat production and heat loss is disturbed, as in the case of illness, body temperature may rise or fall in comparison to the normal registration.

Heat Production	Heat Loss
1. Increased metabolic rate.	1. Increased perspiration.
2. Specific action of foods.	2. Air movement.
3. Vital physiological processes.	3. Cooler environment.
4. Basal heat production from: 　a. carbohydrates ⎫ 　b. proteins　　　⎬ foods 　c. fats　　　　　⎭	4. Basal heat loss from: 　a. conduction 　b. radiation 　c. vaporization
5. Shivering or muscular activity.	

INTERVENTION FOR BODY TEMPERATURES

Subnormal	Elevated
1. Adjust the room temperature to 72.0° or above.	1. Adjust room temperature so that it is cooler.
2. Eliminate drafts.	2. Increase the rate of circulating air.
3. Give warm fluids if permitted.	3. Reduce the amount of clothing or bed covers.
4. Provide additional clothing, or covers on the bed.	4. Control the amount of body activity.

5. Implement the physician's plan for therapy.

6. Increase muscular activity if allowed.

5. Implement the physician's plan for therapy re:
   a. fluids
   b. diet
   c. medications

ITEM 2. PULSE

Every time the heart beats, it contracts the left ventricle and sends blood through the arteries. The pulse is the resulting throb of the heartbeat in the artery. The pulse can be felt wherever a superficial (beneath the skin) artery can be held against firm tissue, such as a bone. The pulse is felt most strongly over the following areas:

1. Radial artery in the wrist at the base of the thumb.

2. Temporal artery just anterior to, or in front of, the ear.

3. Carotid artery on the front side of the neck.

4. Femoral artery in the groin.

5. Apical pulse over the apex of the heart.

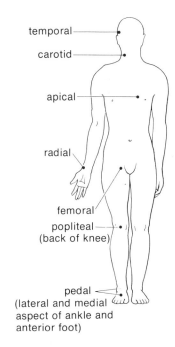

Locations where pulse can be taken.

If the pulse is difficult to find in these areas (for example, in infants and the obese, or in the case of some cardiovascular diseases), the physician may order an apical pulse, which is one that is taken by the use of a stethoscope over the apex (tip) of the heart.

You may also be requested to take *both* a radial and an apical pulse to see if there is a difference in the rates. If there is a significant difference, it may indicate some disease of the blood vessels.

In general, the heart rate has an inverse relationship to the blood pressure and to the size of the individual, e.g., a rapid pulse usually accompanies a low blood pressure. The average pulse rate for a newborn is 130 to 140 beats per minute, while the average pulse rate for an adult at rest is 70 to 80 beats per minute. Exercise, fever, and digestion are some of the factors that may cause an accelerated (faster) pulse rate. Because of the increase in the metabolic rate during pregnancy, the pulse rate may be up to 100 beats per minute, which is generally considered the upper limit of normal when a woman is pregnant.

A temporary increase in pulse rate may be due to fear, anger, physical exercise, anxiety, or elevated body temperature. A prolonged rapid rate may be indicative of hemorrhage or heart disease. A rapid pulse rate is called *tachycardia.* Some drugs, brain disorders, and cardiac diseases cause a slow pulse rate called *bradycardia.*

The strength of the pulse is equally as important as the rate of the pulse. With moderate pressure of the first two or three fingers on the vessels, a strong pulse would beat regularly and with good force. There are several means of describing the strength of a pulse. Most of the common ways are:

1. Strong and regular—even beats with good force.

2. Weak and regular—even beats with poor force.

3. Irregular—both strong and weak beats occur within a minute.

4. Thready—generally indicates that it is weak and irregular.

Each time the heart contracts to force blood into an already full aorta (artery leading from heart), the arterial walls in the blood system must expand to accept the increase in pressure. This expansion is called the *pulse.* By counting *each* expansion of the arterial wall, the *pulse rate* can be determined.

When the pulse is being counted, the rate, rhythm, and volume should be noted. According to the following graphs, the pulse rate and rhythm may be:

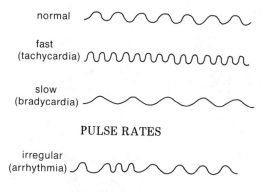

PULSE RATES

PULSE RHYTHM

PULSE VOLUME

The volume of the pulse cannot be correctly measured, but a good indication of volume may be likened to a faucet:

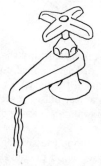

This volume indication is described as *feeble, weak,* or *thready.*

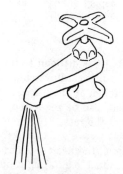

This volume indication is described as *full and bounding.*

In taking a pulse, you are interested in the *rate* of the beats (the number per minute), the *force* of the pulse beat (strong or weak, and regular or irregular), and the *rhythm* of the beats (normal rhythm has the same interval between the beats).

What does your own pulse feel like? Place your first two fingers over your radial artery with enough pressure to feel your pulse. How does it feel?

Equipment Used in Measuring Pulse

For taking all pulses you will need a watch with a second hand, a pad, and a pen. For taking an apical pulse, you will need a stethoscope in addition to the other items. A stethoscope is an instrument used to detect and convey the sounds produced in the body (i.e., by the heart, lung, and so forth). Ordinarily it consists of Y-shaped rubber tubing connected to a plastic or metal earpiece at the top of the Y, and either a flat disc or cone diaphragm at the bottom of the Y. The earpieces fit snugly into the outer ear (or the external auditory meatus). The earpiece is usually bent slightly forward; this part goes toward the front of the ear. When using the cone-shaped body piece, the free end goes against the patient's skin.

In the disc-type instrument the free, flat diaphragm side lies against the patient's skin, and is placed over the apex of the heart near the midline of the chest to the left of the sternum (breastbone).

Alcohol, aqueous Zephiran, or a similar antiseptic solution should be used to cleanse the earpieces before and after you place them in your ears, and to cleanse the disc or cone diaphragm to prevent the spread of infection. *Never* place a stethoscope back in the equipment area unless you have cleansed both the disc and earpieces. You could transmit an ear infection to the next user, or contract an ear infection from a stethoscope that has not been correctly cleaned after use.

Measuring the Radial Pulse Rate

Important Steps	Key Points
1. Wash your hands, approach and identify the patient, and explain what you are going to do.	Of course, this is a part of taking the vital signs, so you will probably already have explained what you are doing. The pulse can be taken separately, however. See that the patient is settled in a comfortable supine position.
2. Place your three middle fingertips over the radial artery in the patient's wrist at the base of the thumb.	Sometimes it is helpful to place the patient's arm comfortably across his chest while you are counting his pulse. Do not start counting immediately, since the movement of the arm creates some exertion. Place your fingertips flatly and lightly on the radial artery. (Do not use the end of your fingers because you might poke or scratch the patient with your fingernails.) If you press too hard, you will obliterate (close off) the artery and you will feel no pulse. Do not use your thumb to take the pulse; you will probably feel your own pulse in your thumb and not the patient's.

U
N
I
T
14

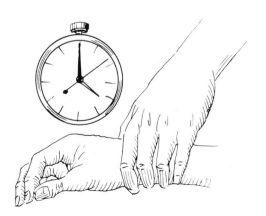

Radial pulse.

Important Steps	Key Points
3. Count the pulsations.	Count beats for one full minute. (Use the second hand of your watch to observe the 60 seconds.) As you count, note the regularity or irregularity and the strength of the beat. You may need to count for the second minute to be sure you counted correctly. Average pulse rates are:

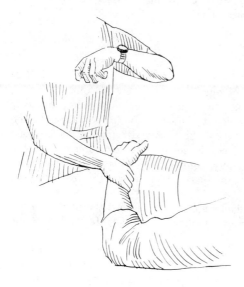

You may place patient's arm comfortably across his chest.

For infants: 115–130 beats/minute.

For adults: 70–80 beats/minute.

For the adult females: 76–80 beats/minute.

For the adult males: 72 beats/minute.

Measuring an Apical Pulse Rate

1. Wash your hands, approach and identify the patient, and explain what you are going to do.	Gain his confidence. Explain that you can hear the pulse beat more accurately through the stethoscope than you can feel it with your finger.
2. Position the patient and obtain the stethoscope.	The supine position is best for taking the apical pulse. (The head of the bed may be slightly elevated if it is more comfortable for the patient.) Obtain a stethoscope from the storage area. Wipe the earpieces and diaphragm clean with antiseptic gauze (some are prepackaged).
3. Drape the patient.	Expose the chest just enough to see the area over the apex of the heart. Fold the top bedding to the bottom of the patient's rib cage. Fold this gown up toward his head, exposing an area of about 12 square inches.
4. Warm the diaphragm in your hand for a moment.	The metal is cold, and you must avoid startling the patient by placing a cold object on his chest (this would momentarily increase the heart rate). Place the diaphragm over the apex of the heart just to the left of the sternum (breastbone).
5. Insert the earpieces into your ears.	If the earpieces bend forward a bit, they should be placed so that the forward bend is anterior (in front of) the ear. (Some of the newer disposable stethoscopes have straight ear-

Important Steps	Key Points

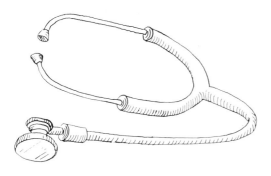

A stethoscope is used to hear and
record an apical response.

6. Listen for the heartbeat.	If you are unable to hear a beat, move the diaphragm around on the anterior, lower left quadrant of the left chest until you pick up the sound. Count the beats for a full minute (observe the second hand on your watch for the correct time). Note the rate, rhythm, and strength of the beat for the purpose of recording it later on the chart.
7. Remove the stethoscope.	Straighten the patient's gown and bed linen.
8. Wipe the earpieces and diaphragm with an antiseptic.	This will help prevent the spread of infection from worker to worker, or patient to patient. Replace the stethoscope in the storage area. Leave the patient comfortable.
9. Record on patient's chart.	The apical pulse is usually recorded in the nurses' notes; for example, 8 A.M. apical pulse rate was 60. Pulse was strong and regular. J. Jones, S.N.

Measuring an Apical/Radial Pulse Rate

This procedure is ordered by the physician for patients with cardiac impairment or for those who are receiving medications to improve heart action.

Important Steps	Key Points
(Refer to "Important Steps" for measuring radial pulse rate and measuring apical pulse rate. Follow the steps for each.)	Two nurses are required for this procedure. One nurse uses a stethoscope to measure the apical rate while another simultaneously measures the radial rate.
1. Place a watch conveniently so that both nurses can see it.	Each nurse listens to or feels the pulse beat for the best possible count.
2. The nurse taking the apical pulse rate gives the signal to begin counting.	A time is decided upon to begin counting, for example, when the second hand is on the 15 or 30 position.

U
N
I
T
14

Important Steps	Key Points
3. Count one full minute; end by saying "stop."	Return the patient to a comfortable position. Compare the pulse rate count with the other nurse later *out* of the patient's hearing.
4. Record the information on the patient's chart.	

ENRICHMENT FOR PULSES OF THE BODY

Pulse Rate. Women have a slightly faster pulse rate than men, and the range may vary from seven to eight beats per minute. Other factors that affect the pulse rate are:

Age:	The pulse rate gradually diminishes from birth to adulthood, then increases with old age.
Body Build and Size:	Tall, slender persons may have a slower rate than short, stout persons.
Blood Pressure:	When the blood pressure rises, it causes a decrease in the pulse rate. When the blood pressure is lower, there is an increase in the pulse rate because the heart is attempting to increase the output of blood.
Drugs:	Stimulants increase the pulse rate. Depressants decrease the pulse rate.
Exercise:	Increases the pulse rate as the heart pumps faster to meet circulatory needs.
Foods:	Increase the pulse rate slightly as a result of metabolic processes.
Increased Body Temperature:	The pulse rate increases at the rate of 7 to 10 beats for each degree of temperature.
Pain:	Increases the pulse rate.

Pulse Rhythm. An intermittent pulse is one that has a period of normal rhythm broken by periods of irregularity or skipped beats. This can occur as a temporary condition of emotional stress or fright. Prolonged intermittent pulse is indicative of heart disease and should be considered a serious sign.

ITEM 3.   RESPIRATIONS

The respiratory system in the human body provides for the exchange of oxygen and carbon dioxide between the atmosphere and the circulating blood. During inspiration (inhalation of air), the diaphragm (large flat muscle separating the chest and abdominal cavity) descends (or lowers) as it contracts, and the rib cage is lifted upward and outward; the lungs therefore have room to expand. During expiration (exhalation of air), the diaphragm ascends (rises) as it relaxes and the rib cage is drawn downward and inward.

To some degree, an individual can control the rate and depth of his respirations. Emotional stress, exercise, and cardiorespiratory diseases all affect the respiratory rate. For example, when a person cries, his respiratory rate becomes rapid and shallow.

The average respiratory rate for infants is 30 to 50 respirations per minute, while in an adult the average rate is 16 to 20 per minute. If an adult does not breathe at a minimal rate of 10 respirations per minute *and* in sufficient depth, you may note some of the following symptoms as a result of low oxygen supply in the blood:

1. Cyanosis or skin color changes, particularly around the mouth and in the nailbeds.

2. Confusion, dizziness, and a change in the level of consciousness.

3. Apprehension and restlessness.

Respirations are generally described as follows:

1. Rapid, shallow.

2. Very slow or very deep.

3. Regular, both in rate and depth.

4. Irregular (Cheyne-Stokes), which is hyperpnea (deeper than usual) followed by a period of no breathing or apnea.

5. Dyspnea, which is labored or difficult breathing, usually with pain.

6. Orthopnea, in which breathing is possible only when the person sits or stands in an erect position.

Equipment Used in Measuring Respirations

A watch with a second hand, a pad, and a pencil are the only necessary equipment for this procedure.

Measuring the Respirations

For an accurate accounting of the respirations, the patient should be at rest and unaware of the counting process. Since this is difficult to do with children who are hospitalized, their respiration rates are generally taken when they are sleeping. If an adult patient is aware that you are counting his respiration, he may voluntarily breathe faster or slower.

The most satisfactory time to count respirations is after the patient's pulse count. When you have taken his pulse, continue to hold his wrist as though taking the pulse and count or feel the times his chest or abdomen rises. You can also see the rise and fall of the chest. Remember to count the rise and fall of the chest and abdomen as one respiration. Respiration includes both the inspiration and expiration. Check your wristwatch for accurate timing. Counts for 30 seconds are acceptable but then you must multiply by two to obtain a full minute's rate. Respirations are recorded as the number in a full minute. If there appears to be an abnormality in the rate or depth, count for a full minute.

ENRICHMENT FOR MEASURING RESPIRATIONS

Respiration is the process by which oxygen and carbon dioxide are interchanged. External respiration refers to the delivery of oxygen to the lungs so that it can be taken into the blood stream. Internal respiration is the process by which oxygen from the blood is taken to the cells in the body, and carbon dioxide is removed from tissues and carried into the blood.

Exhalation is the process of expelling air from the lungs. Inhalation is the process of taking air into the lungs. Note that the chest circumference is greater during inhalation than it is during exhalation.

U
N
I
T
14

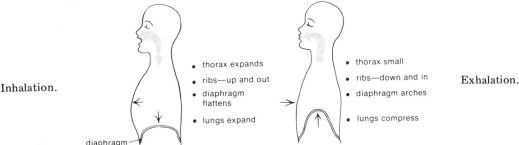

Inhalation.

- thorax expands
- ribs—up and out
- diaphragm flattens
- lungs expand

diaphragm

- thorax small
- ribs—down and in
- diaphragm arches
- lungs compress

Exhalation.

Rate and depth of respiration are controlled by the
respiratory center in the brain.

Age is a factor in respiratory rate. Infants breathe rapidly (30 to 50), but the rate diminishes through childhood (22 to 28), adolescence (18 to 22), and adulthood (16 to 20); finally the elderly (14 to 16) breathe more slowly than any age group. The relationship between the respiratory rate and heartbeat rate is fairly consistent: one respiration to four heartbeats.

Normal respirations are deep enough to that there is a satisfactory exchange of oxygen for carbon dioxide. Shallow breathing results in anoxia, and as a result, the skin and mucous membranes will appear dusky and bluish. This skin coloring is called cyanosis, and it appears more prominently where numerous small blood vessels lie close to skin surfaces (e.g., the nailbeds, the lips, the lobes of the ear, and the cheeks). When taking respirations, it is essential to observe the patient for evidence of this condition.

The body temperature is likewise related to the rate of respiration. When the temperature is elevated, the respiration rate increases because the body attempts to rid itself of excess heat. Shallow breathing may lead to an accumulation of carbon dioxide and a decrease of oxygen, but the body compensates by speeding the respiration rate in an attempt to "blow off" the carbon dioxide.

Head injury or any incidence of increased intracranial pressure will depress the respiratory center and result in shallow or slow breathing. Certain drugs also tend to depress the respiratory rate.

ITEM 4.   BLOOD PRESSURE (BP)

Blood pressure may be defined as the pressure exerted by the blood on the walls of the vessels. The blood pressure is registered by two numbers on the sphygmomanometer (blood pressure apparatus) representing the *systolic pressure* or the highest point reached by the contraction of the heart, and the *diastolic pressure*, which is the lowest point to which it drops between beats. Blood pressure varies with age, sex, altitude, muscular development, and fatigue. Generally it is lower in women than in men, and lower in childhood and higher in advancing age.

Normal systolic pressure in adults ranges from 110 to 146 mm of mercury. The normal diastolic pressure range for adults is from 60 to 90 mm of mercury (mm is the abbreviation for millimeter). The average systolic and diastolic pressures for infants are 80/50 mm systolic to 58/40 mm diastolic.

Blood pressure is best measured by checking a large artery. The most commonly used is the brachial artery, which runs from the shoulder to the elbow. A patient's position, emotional state, heart condition, vessel condition, and amount of circulating blood, and the muscular strength of his heart are some factors that affect his blood pressure.

Whenever possible, try to get some information about the person's blood pressure range and what is a usual reading for him. The reason for knowing the range is to prevent discomfort to the patient caused by pumping up the cuff higher than is necessary to obtain an accurate reading. There are several ways to get this data:

1.   Ask the patient if his usual BP is in the high, normal, or low range.

2.   Look at the previous record of BP on the chart.

3.   Palpate the radial pulse at the wrist, pump up the sphygmomanometer, and note the point on the scale when the pulse disappears. Release all the air from the cuff before proceeding.

Equipment Used in Measuring Blood Pressure

A stethoscope, a sphygmomanometer, a pad, and a pencil are required for this procedure. The sphygmomanometer is a broad rubber bag or cuff about 6 inches wide and 24 inches long, covered with cloth. It has two rubber tubes extending from the rubber bag (or bladder): one tube connects to the rubber tubing extending from the base of the mercury column on the sphygmomanometer, and the other connects to a rubber bulb air pump. The cuff may be snapped, secured with Velcro fastening, or tucked in to stay in place, depending on the kind your agency uses.

Measuring Blood Pressure

<table>
<tr><td>Important Steps</td><td>Key Points</td></tr>
<tr><td>1. Wash your hands, approach and identify the patient, and explain what you are going to do.</td><td>Bring the stethoscope, sphygmomanometer, paper, and pencil with you.</td></tr>
<tr><td>2. Position the patient and equipment.</td><td>The patient is usually more relaxed when lying in the supine position, but the sitting position can also be used. Place his arm in a comfortable outstretched position on the bed or chair arm. Put the BP equipment on the bedside stand near him or on a BP standard at the bedside. Some agencies supply a wall-mounted BP apparatus just above the head of the bed. Positioning is important for accurate measuring.</td></tr>
<tr><td>3. Wrap the BP cuff around the patient's arm.</td><td>Either arm can be used. Place the top edge of the cuff 2 inches above his elbow. Wrap the cuff neatly around the arm so that each layer is directly on top. If there is a gauge attached to the cuff, be sure that it faces you so you can easily read it. Otherwise, place the gauge on a flat surface where you can clearly read the scale. Secure the distal cuff end. No more than $^5/_6$ of the upper arm should be covered by the width of the cuff. Use the pediatric size for small, thin persons and children.</td></tr>
</table>

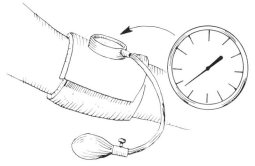

The aneroid sphygmomanometer gives blood pressure reading on dial indicator.

4. Attach the tubes from the BP cuff.

One tube goes to the air pump bulb, the other to the gauge tubing.

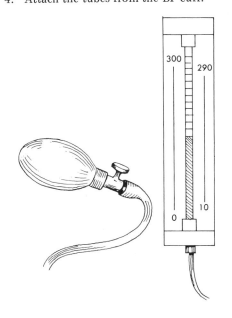

The mercury column sphygmomanometer
gives blood pressure reading
on mercury column.

Important Steps	Key Points
5. Place the stethoscope earpieces in your ears, and the diaphragm over the brachial artery.	With your left fingertips, feel for the pulse of the brachial artery. The brachial artery is usually easy to find; it is located in the center of the anterior elbow area.

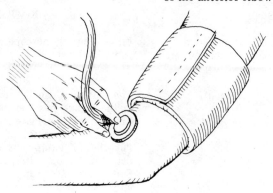

Place stethoscope diaphragm in
antecubital space.

6. Close the valve on the air pump.	With your right thumb and index finger, turn the thumbscrew on the air pump bulb in a clockwise direction until it is tight.

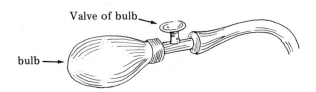

Valve of bulb

bulb →

Bulb and valve that control air pumped
into blood pressure cuff.

7. Pump the air bulb with your right hand.	The rubber bag on the BP cuff will inflate. As you pump, the column of mercury will rise in the sphygmomanometer. Pump the cuff up to 140 mm, or at least 10 mm higher than the usual range for the patient. Tell the patient that his hand might tingle a bit because the BP cuff is temporarily constricting the flow of blood in the arm.
8. Open the valve on the air bulb. Release the pressure slowly to let the mercury column descend.	When taking the BP you will have to *watch* the mercury column very carefully while you also *listen* to the sounds through the stethoscope.
9. Note the line on the sphygmomanometer gauge at which the first beat is heard.	As the mercury column descends (because air is released from the BP cuff which constricted the blood vessels in the arm), note the exact numerical line on the scale where you first hear a clear beat—this is the *systolic reading*. It is the point at which the greatest force is exerted by the heart and the greatest resistance put forth by the arterial walls.

Important Steps   Key Points

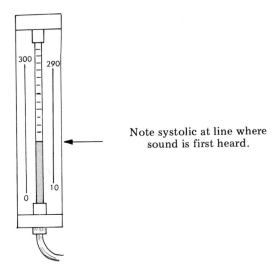

Note systolic at line where sound is first heard.

10. Continue to open the valve slowly until all air is removed.

As the mercury descends, the heartbeat becomes louder and clearer, then almost immediately becomes softer and quieter. Note the number on the gauge as the last clear sound is heard—this is the *diastolic reading*. This is the point of greatest cardiac relaxation. Agencies differ as to whether it is the last clear beat or the last beat heard that is recorded as the diastolic beat (check your agency procedure).

11. Repeat the process to check your accuracy.

Pump air into the BP cuff until the mercury is at least 10 mm higher than the patient's usual systolic pressure, as in Step 7. Proceed through succeeding steps, carefully checking the level on the BP scale at which you hear the first and last pulse beats. They should be the same as your first reading; if not, remove all air from the BP cuff and inflate it again for the third reading. You must open the valve slowly, observe the mercury column closely, and listen to the pulse beats carefully. This part of the procedure is difficult and will take considerable practice. The systolic pressure, or the first sound you hear, is written as 130/ ; the diastolic pressure, or the last sound you hear is recorded as /80. Thus the final and complete BP would be recorded on the patient's chart as "BP 130/80."

12. Remove the cuff from the patient's arm.

Remove the stethoscope earpieces from your ears. Be sure that all the air is removed from the BP cuff before taking it off.

13. Fold the BP cuff and return it to storage.

Return the folded cuff, stethoscope, and sphygmomanometer to the storage area. Remember to clean the stethoscope pieces and diaphragm with an antiseptic wipe before returning it to storage, as an infection control precaution.

UNIT 14

Important Steps   Key Points

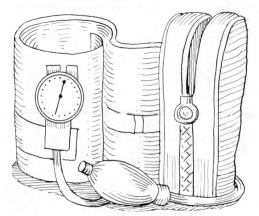

Replace aneroid equipment in case.

14. Record on the patient's chart.

Describe any unusual aspects of the BP (extremely strong, weak or faint, high, or low readings). If the BP is abnormal, report this at once to the charge nurse; she will relay the information to the physician, if indicated.

Note: It is difficult to obtain blood pressure readings on some people. When you have trouble, *do not hesitate* to ask for assistance or confirmation of your reading. Even after you have been in the business many years, you may still find the need to have assistance occasionally. It is more important to get a correct reading to ensure that the patient can be correctly treated than for you to be embarrassed about asking for assistance.

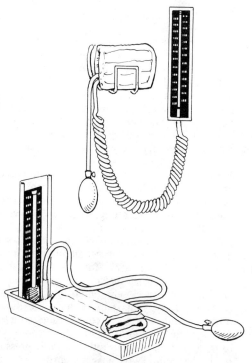

Replace cuff and bulb, and snap down mercury manometer part to cover case.

ENRICHMENT FOR BLOOD PRESSURE

Pressure in blood depends on the contraction force of the ventricles, the output from the heart, and the resistance to the blood's flow through the vessels. Under resting conditions, the heart normally pumps 4 liters (approximately 4 quarts) of blood each minute. Strenuous exercise increases the amount of blood pumped out of the heart. Likewise, transfusion increases the volume of blood and also increases blood pressure. When arteries become inelastic, as in patients who have arteriosclerosis, greater resistance is offered to the blood flow, and the pressure thus becomes higher. To summarize, blood pressure depends upon (1) the force of the heartbeat, (2) the volume of blood in the circulatory system, and (3) the resistance in the blood vessels.

Certain physiological factors affect blood pressure. They are:

1. Age. Blood pressure is lower in children; it may be elevated in adults.

2. Sex. Blood pressure is higher for men than women of the same age level.

3. Body build. Obese persons usually have higher blood pressure than those who are normal in size.

4. Exercise. Muscular exertion temporarily increases pressure.

5. Physiological conditions such as the following:
    a. Pain — moderate and severe pain will usually elevate pressure.
    b. Emotion — fear, worry, or excitement will increase pressure.
    c. Disease — any disorder affecting the circulatory or renal system may increase the blood pressure.
        Disease that weakens the heart may lower the blood pressure.
    d. Drugs — vasoconstrictors elevate blood pressure.
        Vasodilators decrease blood pressure.
        Certain narcotics decrease blood pressure.
    e. Hemorrhage — decrease of volume lowers pressure and may lead to shock.
    f. Intracranial Pressure— elevates blood pressure.

A noisy environment and crowded conditions in the room may cause a temporary elevation of blood pressure. Take a person's blood pressure in a quiet room with a relaxed environment.

Gravity affects arterial blood pressure. When a person is standing, greater pressure is exerted on the femoral artery of the leg than on the brachial artery of the arm. This is the reason for having the person either sitting or lying down when you take his blood pressure.

The time for taking the blood pressure should be midway between meals, in order to avoid the increased pressure brought about by food consumption and increased body heat.

Drugs such as digitalis are often given to strengthen the heart muscle, which in turn strengthens the cardiac output.

An accurate blood pressure reading depends upon the width of the blood pressure cuff. If the cuff is too small, the pressure could be higher than that recorded on the instrument. If the cuff is too large, such as when an adult cuff is used on a child, the reading may be less than the pressure in the artery. A safe rule to follow is to make sure that the width of the cuff is no more than $5/6$ of the upper arm, or 1.2 times the diameter of the limb.

ITEM 5.   CHARTING VITAL SIGNS

Refer to the blank graphic sheet (Sample A). The graphic sheet has space for recordings for 9 days. Each space is ruled into A.M. and P.M. columns, each of which is divided into three hourly columns for recording purposes. They are numbered for:

12 midnight (2400)	4 A.M. (0400)	8 A.M. (0800)
12 noon	4 P.M. (1600)	8 P.M. (2000)

How to Record Temperature. The top half of the graphic sheet is for recording the temperature. Note that the temperature range of degrees is $95°$ to $106°$ F.

1. Record in even numbers. The graphic sheet is scored so that each line equals $2/10$ of a degree. Do not use odd numbers unless you used an electric thermometer with measurements accurate to $1/10$ of a degree.

2. Place a dot on the center of the appropriate line; the dot should be at the intersection of the appropriate hour and temperature reading.

3. Using a ruler, connect the dots with a straight, accurate line.

4. If the temperature is rectal, indicate above the dot with ®.

5. If the temperature is axillary, indicate above the dot with Ⓐ.

U
N
I
T
14

How to Record Pulse. The pulse is charted on the same graph as the temperature, except that the pulse scale is used to locate the placement of the dot. Note that the pulse range is from 50 to 160. Each line between the bold lines represents 2 pulse beats.

Record the pulse in even numbers, such as 80, 86, 102. Using a ruler, connect the dots with a straight, accurate line.

How to Record Respiration. The lower portion of the graphic sheet is used for recording the respiratory rate. Note that the respiration scale is from 10 to 50. When the respiratory rate to be recorded is one of the numbers indicated on the sheet (such as 20 or 40), then place the dot in the center of the appropriate line. Otherwise the dot is centered at the correct vertical distance between two lines.

Example: Respiration 48 is recorded as
$$\begin{array}{l} \underline{\qquad}\ 50 \\ \cdot \\ \underline{\qquad}\ 40 \end{array}$$

Record in even numbers such as 22, 46. Using a ruler, connect the dots with a straight, accurate line.

How to Record Blood Pressure. In the section of the graphic sheet labeled "blood pressure," write the systolic pressure above the slanted line and the diastolic pressure below the line.

On Sample A of the Graphic Record, practice charting the following vital signs. Be sure to enter the dates and connect the dots for one temperature reading with the dot for the next temperature reading, and do the same for the pulse and respiration values.

Day	8 A.M.	12 noon	4 P.M.	8 P.M.
1	100.2—88—20 160/88	100.8—92—22	102.4—108—24 156/86	103.2—112—24
2	99.6—96—20 148/88	100.6—100—22	100.8—102—22 134/70	98.8—80—18
3	98—76—20 130/80		98.6—72—18 144/88	
4	96.8—66—16 110/70		98.4—84—18 114/64	

Check your work for accuracy with your instructor or another student.

Now refer to Graphic Sheet Sample B. The form differs from the one you've used to practice charting. The temperatures are charted in a separate section from the pulse. Notice that in the pulse and respiration sections the interval between the lines equals ten. If the pulse were 76, the dot would be placed about two-thirds of the distance above the line representing 70.

GRAPHIC CHART

Sample "A"

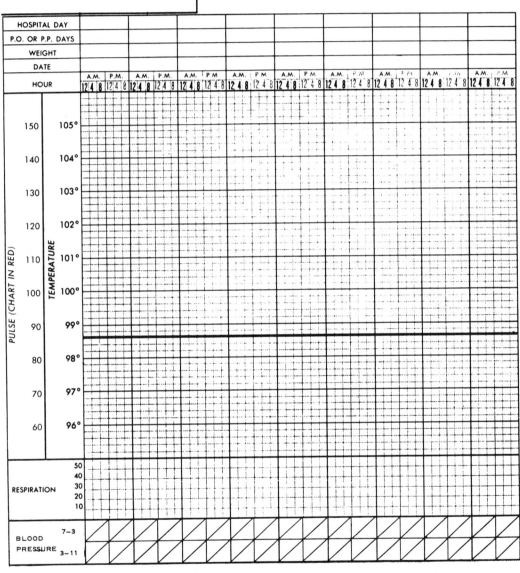

		A.M.	P.M.	A.M.	P.M.	A.M.	P M	A.M.	P M	A.M.	P M	A.M.	P M	A.M.	P M	A.M.	P M
HOSPITAL DAY																	
P.O. OR P.P. DAYS																	
WEIGHT																	
DATE																	
HOUR		12 4 8	12 4 8	12 4 8	12 4 8	12 4 8	12 4 8	12 4 8	12 4 8	12 4 8	12 4 8	12 4 8	12 4 8	12 4 8	12 4 8	12 4 8	12 4 8

PULSE (CHART IN RED) — TEMPERATURE

150	105°
140	104°
130	103°
120	102°
110	101°
100	100°
90	99°
80	98°
70	97°
60	96°

RESPIRATION 50 40 30 20 10

BLOOD PRESSURE 7-3   3-11

U N I T 14

GRAPHIC CHART

Sample "B"

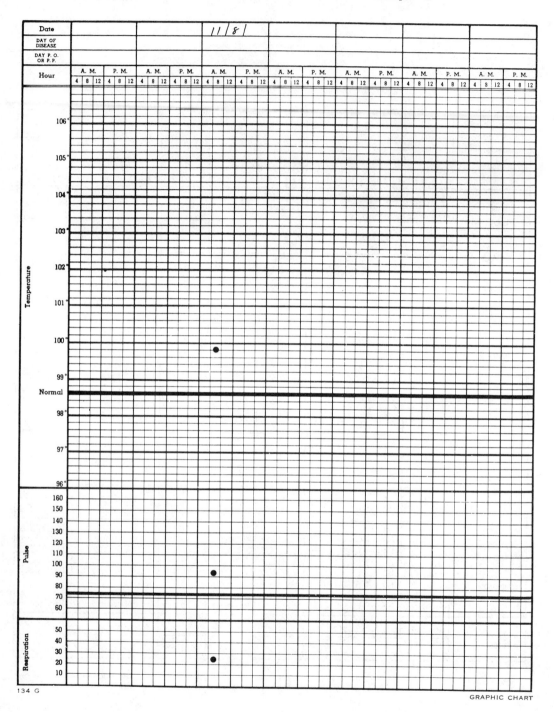

Now see if you can read the vital signs on this Graphic Sheet. Record the TPR's in the space provided.

Dates	Temperature	Pulse	Respiration	Time
12/1				

GRAPHIC CHART

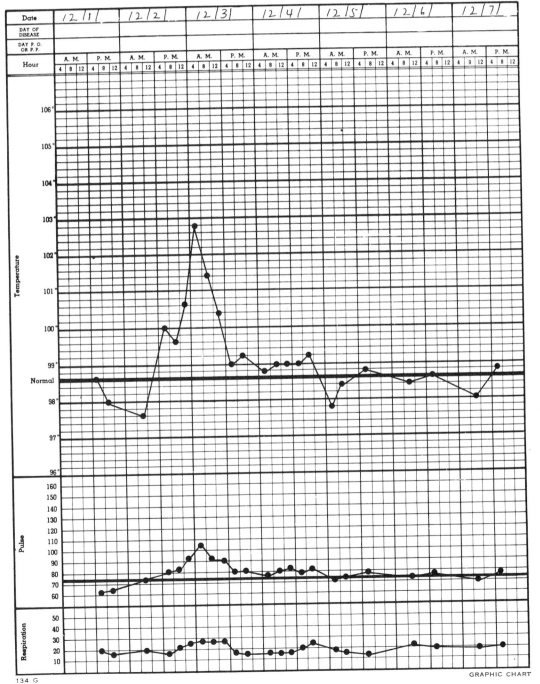

GRAPHIC CHART

134 G

PERFORMANCE TEST

1. In the skill laboratory, correctly and accurately take the vital signs (T, P, R, and BP) of your partner, using the procedures presented in class, e.g., oral, rectal, and axillary temperatures, and radial, femoral, temporal, carotid, and apical pulse.

2. In addition, accurately chart the vital signs you took on your lab partner on a practice nurses' notes and graphic record.

3. Complete the attached Vital Signs Worksheets.

PERFORMANCE CHECKLIST

VITAL SIGNS

ORAL TEMPERATURE WITH GLASS THERMOMETER

Demonstrate the correct method of taking an oral temperature with a glass thermometer.

1. Wash your hands.

2. Approach the patient and explain the procedure.

3. Obtain the equipment.

4. Prepare the equipment for use: clean the thermometer according to your agency regulations; rinse the thermometer in cold water if necessary.

5. Check the level of the mercury in the thermometer; if it is above 96° Fahrenheit, the level must be lowered by shaking the thermometer.

6. Place the thermometer in the patient's mouth:

   a. Place it under the tongue.

   b. Place it deep into the area.

   c. Ask the patient to keep his mouth closed.

7. Leave the thermometer in place from 3 to 5 minutes.

8. Remove the thermometer, holding the top end between your thumb and index finger.

9. Wipe the thermometer with tissue, making sure to wipe from top to bottom.

10. Read the thermometer.

11. Place the thermometer in its holder.

12. Record the reading appropriately on the patient's chart.

ORAL TEMPERATURE WITH ELECTRIC THERMOMETER

Demonstrate the correct way to take an oral temperature with an electric thermometer.

1. Wash your hands.

2. Approach the patient and explain the procedure.

3. Obtain the equipment.

4. Prepare an electric thermometer for use: place a clean cover on the probe and warm up the machine.

5. Insert the probe under the patient's tongue.

    a. Ask the patient to keep his mouth closed.

    b. Make sure to insert the probe into the rear of the patient's oral cavity.

6. Leave the thermometer in place from 10 to 20 seconds.

7. Remove the thermometer.

    a. Wipe it with tissue from top to bottom.

    b. Remove the disposable cover.

8. Read the scale.

9. Record the temperature on the patient's chart or appropriate worksheet.

OBTAINING RECTAL TEMPERATURE WITH A GLASS THERMOMETER

Demonstrate the correct procedure for obtaining a rectal temperature with a glass thermometer.

1. Wash your hands.

2. Identify and approach the patient.

3. Obtain the thermometer and K–Y jelly.

4. Position the patient in Sims' position, being careful to maintain his privacy and warmth.

5. Insert the thermometer into his rectum: lift his upper buttock slightly; insert the lubricated end of the thermometer about 1½ inches into his rectum.

6. Leave the thermometer in the cavity from 3 to 5 minutes. Make sure to hold the thermometer during the entire time because it could slip into the rectum.

7. Remove the thermometer and wipe it clean with gauze or tissue, wiping from top to bottom.

8. Read the temperature.

9. Record the temperature on the patient's chart.

10. Make sure to indicate that the temperature was taken rectally ®.

OBTAINING RECTAL TEMPERATURE WITH AN ELECTRIC THERMOMETER

Demonstrate the correct method to obtain a rectal temperature using an electric thermometer.

1. Wash your hands.

2. Approach and identify the patient, and explain the procedure.

3. Obtain the equipment.

4. Prepare the equipment for use: insert a probe into the thermistor; warm up the machine; coat the probe with lubricant.

U
N
I
T
14

5. Position the patient in Sims' position, being careful to maintain his privacy and warmth.

6. Insert the thermometer into his rectum: lift his upper buttock slightly; insert the lubricated end of the thermometer about 1½ inches into his rectum.

7. Leave the thermometer in the cavity from 10 to 20 seconds. Make sure to hold the thermometer during the entire time because it could slip into the rectum.

8. Read the temperature on the dial indicator.

9. Record the temperature on the patient's chart.

10. Indicate the temperature as having been taken rectally ®.

TAKING TEMPERATURE BY AXILLARY METHOD

Demonstrate the correct method used to obtain axillary temperature.

1. Wash your hands.

2. Identify the patient and explain the procedure.

3. Obtain the equipment—a glassblown thermometer.

4. Prepare the equipment for use: shake down the thermometer if necessary; rinse and wipe it dry if necessary.

5. Place the thermometer in the patient's axilla—make sure it is dry.

6. Leave the thermometer in, holding the top end between your thumb and index finger for 10 minutes.

7. Remove the thermometer, holding the top end between your thumb and index finger.

8. Wipe the thermometer with a tissue, making sure to wipe from top to bottom.

9. Read the thermometer.

10. Place the thermometer in its holder.

11. Record the reading on the patient's chart, indicating that it is an axillary temperature Ⓐ.

TAKING RADIAL PULSE AND OBSERVING RESPIRATORY RATE

Show the correct procedure for taking a radial, femoral, and temporal pulse, and observing respiratory rate.

Taking a pulse.

1. Wash your hands.

2. Identify and approach the patient.

3. Explain the procedure to the patient.

4. Place your three middle fingertips over the appropriate artery.

5. Count the pulsations for a specific period of time—usually 60 seconds.

6. Note the rate, force, and rhythm of the beats.

7. Record the reading appropriately.

Observing respiration rate.

1. Identify the patient.

2. *Remember that the patient must not be aware of the procedure.*

3. Observe the rate, depth, and rhythm of respiration.

4. Record the procedure appropriately on the chart.

TAKING AN APICAL PULSE RATE

Demonstrate the correct procedure for determining an apical pulse rate.

1. Wash your hands.

2. Identify the patient and explain the procedure.

3. Obtain the equipment.

4. Position the patient and provide for his privacy, warmth, and comfort.

5. Warm the stethoscope with your hands.

6. Place the diaphragm of the stethoscope over the apex of the patient's heart.

7. Insert the earpieces into your ears; the bend should be forward in the ears.

8. Listen for the heart sound, and relocate the diaphragm if necessary.

9. Record the apical pulse, noting the rate, force, and rhythm.

10. Remove the stethoscope from your ears and chest.

11. Record the information on the patient's chart.

12. Clean and replace the equipment in the proper area.

BLOOD PRESSURE

Demonstrate the correct procedure for taking a patient's blood pressure.

1. Wash your hands.

2. Identify the patient and explain the procedure.

3. Obtain the equipment.

4. Position the patient.

5. Attach the equipment to the patient appropriately: place the cuff at approximately heart level, 2 inches above the elbow; wrap the cuff neatly around his arm; secure the cuff end with tape or adhesive.

6. Attach the tubes from the blood pressure cuff to the air pump and sphygmomanometer.

7. Adjust the stethoscope position: arrange the ear pieces; place the diaphragm over the brachial artery.

8. Close the valve on the air pump.

9. Inflate the cuff to at least 140 mm or 10 mm higher than the person's usual range, and inform the patient that this may cause some tingling.

10. Open the valve of the air bulb—release the pressure slowly.

11. Observe the mercury column and listen to the pulse sounds carefully. Record the value when the first sound is heard.

12. Continue to decrease the pressure slowly.

13. Record the value when you hear the last sound.

14. Repeat the process to check your recording.

15. Remove the equipment from the patient's arm.

16. Return the materials and equipment to storage.

17. Record the readings on the patient's chart.

18. Clean the stethoscope and return it to storage.

POST-TEST

Define the following:

1. febrile: _____

2. bradycardia: _____

3. tachycardia: _____

4. apnea: _____

5. hyperventilation: _____

6. orthopnea: _____

7. apical pulse: _____

8. Fahrenheit: _____

9. stethoscope: _____

10. diastolic pressure: _____

Complete the following:

1. Temperature, pulse, respiration, and blood pressure are known as _____ signs.

2. _____°F or _____°C are the average adult body temperatures.

3. List three circumstances that can either raise or lower body temperature.

    a. _____

    b. _____

    c. _____

4. List two conditions that make it necessary to take ® temperature in adults.

    a. _____

    b. _____

5. After drinking hot or cold fluids, chewing gum, or smoking, an oral temperature should not be taken for _____ (period of time).

6. The clinical glass thermometer with the _____ bulb is the only one used for rectal temperatures.

7. A thermometer is kept in a patient's mouth for a minimum of _____ minutes.

8. Rectal thermometers are always well-lubricated to prevent _____

9. _____ temperatures are always taken on small children.

10. _____ , _____ , and _____ are three arteries that may be used to take a pulse.

11. _____ pulse is the only one recommended to take for children under two years of age.

12. The heart rate has a/an _____ relationship to the blood pressure.

13. _____ , _____ , and _____ may cause an accelerated pulse rate.

14. The correct placement of the stethoscope's earpieces is _____ .

15. Which digit is *never* used to take a pulse? _____ .

16. Pressing too hard on a vessel _____ it.

17. _____ position is used to take an apical pulse.

18. _____ per minute is the average respiration rate for infants, and_____ per minute is the average respiration for adults.

19. Cyanosis, confusion, and rapid, thready pulse may be symptoms of low_____ supply in the blood.

20. The highest point caused by the contraction of the heart is called the_____ _____ pressure.

21. The average blood pressure for an adult is _____ .

22. The instruments needed to take a blood pressure are _____ and _____ .

POST-TEST ANNOTATED ANSWER SHEET

1. feverish, pertaining to fever. (p. 259)

2. slow heart action, a rate usually less than 60 beats per minute in adult, less than 70 per minute in child. (p. 259)

3. abnormally rapid heart action, usually over 100 per minute in an adult and over 200 per minute in an infant. (p. 259)

4. absence of respirations. (p. 259)

5. a state caused by an increased amount of air due to excessively rapid breathing. (p. 259)

6. condition in which the patient can breathe only in a sitting or standing position. (p. 259)

7. pulse rate that is taken by means of a stethoscope placed over the apex of the heart. (p. 269)

8. a thermometer scale for measuring heat (freezing point is $32°F$; boiling point is $212°F$). (p. 259)

9. an instrument used to detect, convey, and study the sounds produced by the body, i.e., heart, lung, and so forth. (p. 271)

10. the last sound that is heard as the mercury drops in the blood pressure apparatus; it is the point of greatest cardiac relaxation. (p. 279)

1. vital signs (p. 260)

2. $98.6°F$ or $37°C$ (p. 260)

3. time of day, environmental temperature, phase of menstrual cycle or pregnancy, exercise, age, emotions, disease (pp. 260 and 261)

4. mouth breathing due to nasal congestion, nasal surgery, and nasal tubes; patients who won't keep their mouths closed (pp. 260 and 265)

5. 30 minutes (p. 260)

6. short, fat (p. 262)

7. 3 to 5 (p. 264)

8. irritation to the rectal mucosa (p. 265)

9. rectal (p. 265)

10. radial, temporal, carotid, femoral (p. 269)

11. apical (p. 269)

12. inverse (p. 269)

13. exercise, fever, digestion (pp. 269–270)

14. with the tips bent forward to the front of the ear, or as comfortable as possible with straight earpieces (p. 271)

15. thumb (p. 271)

16. obliterates (p. 271)

17. supine (p. 272)

18. 30 to 50; 16 to 20 (p. 276)

19. oxygen (p. 276)

20. systolic (p. 276)

21. $\dfrac{110 \text{ to } 146}{60 \text{ to } 90}$ (p. 276)

22. stethoscope; blood pressure apparatus or sphygmomanometer (p. 276)

Unit 15

URINE ELIMINATION

I. DIRECTIONS TO THE STUDENT

You are to proceed through the lesson using this workbook as your guide. You will need to practice the tasks using the different kinds of equipment with the mannequin (Mrs. Chase), with student partners in the skill laboratory, or with other persons. After you have completed the lesson and practiced the tasks, arrange with your instructor to take the post-test.

For this lesson you will need the following items:

1. Pen or pencil.

2. Bedpan.

3. Fracture pan.

4. Female urinal.

5. Male urinal.

6. Washbasin.

7. Washcloth.

8. Towel.

9. Bedside stand.

10. Mannequin (Mrs. Chase).

11. Toilet tissue.

Please read the following paragraphs carefully. They will tell you what you will be expected to know and how you will be expected to assist the patient to use such equipment as a bedpan, female urinal, fracture pan, and male urinal. If you feel that you already have the necessary skills, discuss this with your instructor. You would then arrange to take the post-test, during which you must correctly demonstrate the skills you have acquired in this lesson.

II. GENERAL PERFORMANCE OBJECTIVE

You will achieve the capability to assist the patient (or another person) in using the designated equipment to void in a safe and effective manner, to collect specific urine specimens, and to test urine for sugar and acetone content by following the prescribed procedure.

III. SPECIFIC PERFORMANCE OBJECTIVES

Upon completion of this lesson you will be able to:

1. Assist the patient to safely and modestly use the equipment to void in such a way that the urine can be measured with 100 per cent accuracy.

294

2. Obtain a specified urine specimen (routine, clean-catch, timed), correctly label it, provide for its immediate transfer to the laboratory for analysis, and record the appropriate information on the patient's chart.

3. Record significant observations about the urinary output, such as the amount, color, odor, and time.

4. Enter accurate intake and output measurements on the Intake and Output Record.

5. Remove, clean, dry, and return to storage the designated equipment used in urinary elimination and the testing of diabetic urine.

6. Provide an opportunity for the patient to wash and dry his hands following elimination.

7. Obtain and test a specimen of diabetic urine for sugar and acetone, and record the appropriate information on the patient's record.

IV. VOCABULARY

catamenia—the menses, the periodic menstrual discharge of blood from the uterus.

fracture pan—a specific type of shallow bedpan used by bed patients who have difficulty raising their hips in order to use the regular bedpan.

frequency—the condition of having to urinate often.

incontinence—the inability to retain feces or urine; lack of voluntary control over the sphincters.

micturition (urination, voiding)—the act by which urine is expelled.

preservative—an agent having the power to keep a substance from decaying or spoiling.

rectum—the distal portion of the large intestine located between the sigmoid and the anal canal.

retention—failure to expel the urine from the bladder.

urgency—the immediate need to urinate.

vagina—the mucomembranous tube that joins the passageway between the uterus and the external opening (vaginal—related to the vagina).

vulva—the external female genitalia.

V. INTRODUCTION

The urinary system plays a vital role in body excretion; it is one of the most important systems of elimination. Urination is normally accomplished without discomfort and is essential to the well-being of the patient. The amount of urine excreted depends on the amount of liquids ingested into the body. Adequate intake of liquids dilutes the toxins (poisons) in the body and aids in their elimination.

The tasks and skills carried out by the health workers that are described in this unit are directly related to urinary elimination. You will thus acquire the basic information necessary to understand the importance of accurately and safely performing the tasks related to urinary elimination.

Urination is a natural function that is not usually discussed openly and frankly in public. It is for this reason that you can expect the patient to be ill at ease, or to indicate verbally (by speaking) or nonverbally (by facial expressions, body posture) his embarrassment when asking for assistance with the bedpan. Your behavior, verbal and nonverbal, should convey an attitude that is helpful and nonjudgmental. Utilize your skills confidently, efficiently, and effectively to give the patient a feeling of modesty, security, and dignity at all times.

UNIT
15

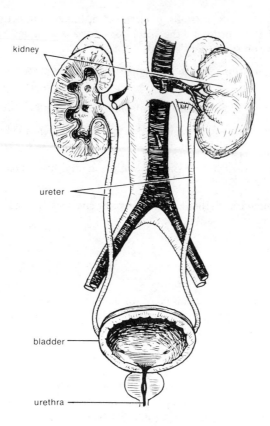

kidney

ureter

Urinary system.

bladder

urethra

A. Organs of the Urinary Tract

There are two kidneys, which are glandular organs that secrete urine. Urine is composed of the waste products that are filtered through an elaborate system of coiled tubes (nephrons) within the kidney. As the blood flows through these tiny tubules, the liquid waste products are filtered out of the blood and diluted with water; this then becomes urine.

The two ureters are ducts (tubes) that carry the urine from the kidneys down to the urinary bladder.

The urinary (cystic) bladder is a hollow, muscular organ that serves as a temporary reservoir for urine. By contraction of the muscular wall of the bladder, urine is expelled from the body through a tube called the urethra. When the amount of urine in the bladder reaches a certain level, it exerts pressure on certain nerve endings in the bladder wall and causes the urge to empty the bladder. Expelling the urine from the bladder is called urination or voiding.

The urethra is a small tube approximately ¼ inch in diameter, 1½ inches long in the female, and 8 to 9 inches long in the male. The urethra extends from the bottom end of the bladder to the exterior (outside of the body). The external opening of the urethra is concealed between the folds of the labia in the female, and at the distal end of the penis in the male.

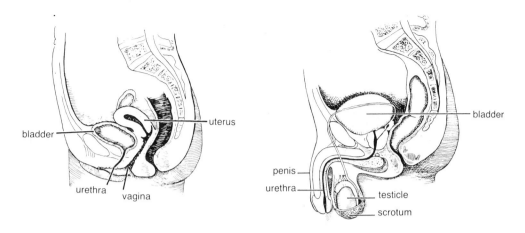

Female urinary system.   Male urinary system.

B. Function of the Urinary Bladder

The mucous membrane is the continuous lining inside the urethra, the ureter, and the kidney pelvis. You will remember that a mucous membrane secretes a lubricating fluid; in other words, it keeps the tissue moist.

The musculature of the bladder wall enables it to expand and hold the accumulating urine. The capacity for urine accumulation varies in relation to the patient's health, disease, fluid intake, the action of food and drugs on the kidneys, and the weather. The normal adult urine secretion is 1000 to 1500 cc (2 to 3 pints) within 24 hours. The desire to empty the bladder occurs when approximately 250 cc of urine has accumulated. Healthy adults do not urinate during their sleeping hours, although some may do so occasionally.

In certain diseased conditions, the bladder may hold as much as 3000 to 4000 cc of urine (3 to 4 quarts). Excessive expansion of the bladder wall causes a condition known as bladder distention. When the bladder is severely distended, extreme caution must be taken to prevent any blow or heavy weight on the bladder region that could rupture (break) the bladder wall. In case of bladder rupture, the patient can die within 8 hours if surgical repair is not done.

C. Common Urinary Infections and Pathogens

Because the urinary tract is dark, moist, and warm, it is an excellent breeding place for germs or pathogenic bacteria.

Cystitis (inflammation of the urinary bladder) is a very common bladder infection caused by any of the following: highly concentrated urine, pathogenic bacteria, injury, irritation, or installation of an irritating substance. Signs of cystitis include frequency, burning, urgency, and often a slight elevation of temperature. Patients with cystitis are very uncomfortable.

D. Characteristics and Components of Urine

The *normal components* are: 95 per cent water, 3.7 per cent organic wastes, and 1.3 per cent combined inorganic wastes, mineral salts, toxins, pigments, and sex hormones.

The *color* of normal urine is described in terms of varying shades of yellow. The color is due to the presence of pigments in the urine. Normal urine is a straw yellow or amber color. The lighter the shade of yellow, the more it is diluted with water.

Abnormal pigments are often found in the urine and they, too, are designated or indicated by color of the urine. Smoky red or dark brown urine denotes presence of hemoglobin or many red blood cells (erythrocytes) from bleeding in some part of the urinary tract. Blue or blue-green urine may be due to a dye or medication the doctor has ordered for his patient.

U
N
I
T
15

The *odor* of freshly voided urine is faintly aromatic but not unpleasant. Variations appear as the result of the ingestion of certain foods, and drugs, or a decomposition of bacteria that changes the urea to ammonium carbonate and then to ammonia. An unpleasant (putrid) odor may indicate pathology.

Since sediments alter the composition of urine when it stands at room temperatures for short periods of time (as brief as 20 to 30 minutes), it is urgent that urine specimens be sent to the laboratory immediately upon collection. Otherwise laboratory personnel may give an erroneous (wrong) urine report and the doctor may in turn prescribe the wrong treatment, based on the laboratory report. Therefore, although this is a small task, it is vitally important to the patient's recovery.

The *specific gravity* is the weight of a given volume of urine as compared with the weight of an equal volume of pure water. In simple terms, it is the thinness or thickness of the liquid urine. The specific gravity is measured by an instrument called the *urinometer*. The normal numerical range is 1.010 to 1.030. Variations of the numerical values are due to the amounts of solids dissolved in the urine. The specific gravity of a healthy individual changes during a 24-hour period within the above normal limits.

The acidity or alkalinity of the urine is measured in units called *pH*. The pH of normal urine is slightly acid, ranging from 5.5 to 7.0.

The abnormal matter in the urine is composed of many pus cells, red blood cells, hemoglobin, occasional kidney stones (calculi), casts (rectangular cells), acetone bodies, albumin, sugar, bacteria, and some parasites. Other chemicals and drugs may be present.

The urine output can be affected by two kinds of drugs: *diuretics*, which increase the flow of urine, and *antidiuretics*, which decrease the flow of urine.

ITEM 1. ASSISTING THE PATIENT TO USE THE BEDPAN

It is necessary for you to know what equipment is needed when the patient has to urinate. The following items are described so that you will be able to assist the patient to use the appropriate equipment.

Bedpan is made of metal or plastic. Each patient has an individual bedpan stored in the bedside stand during his hospital stay.

Bedpan cover is made of cloth or paper, depending upon the agency in which you work. It is used to mask the unpleasant sight and odor of the pan's contents after it has been used.

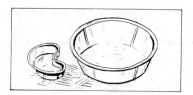 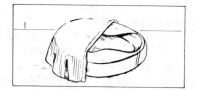

Toilet tissue is used either by you or the patient to clean and wipe the patient's perineal and rectal areas.

The washcloth, towel, soap in its dish, and washbasin with warm water should be available on the patient's bedside stand so that he is able to wash and dry his hands and genital area after using the bedpan.

Now that you know what equipment is required for this lesson, read the following paragraphs carefully. Remember that perfecting your skills enables you to perform a particular task effectively and confidently and gives you an opportunity to listen to the patient's comments.

While you are assisting the patient to use the bedpan, explain the steps that will be taken to make the task safe and easily accomplished. The female patient usually uses the bedpan for both urine and bowel elimination, whereas the male patient uses the bedpan for bowel elimination only.

Given a female patient who wants to void, you are to assist her to use the bedpan.

Important Steps	Key Points

1. Wash your hands.

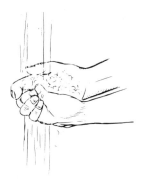

Before starting this task, wash your hands at a nearby sink so that the patient can either see or hear the running water. The sound of running water reinforces the patient's urge to void and makes it easier even though she is in a reclining or flat position in bed.

2. Approach and identify the patient. Explain what you are going to do, and gain her cooperation and confidence.

Adjust the bed to a comfortable working height. This will prevent unnecessary back and leg strain while you are working.

Assess the patient's condition. If she is unable to help, you may need to call for assistance.

3. Obtain the bedpan, its cover, and toilet tissue.

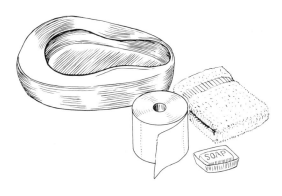

Remove them from storage either in the bedside stand or the patient's bathroom. Since metal bedpans conduct heat and cold, rinsing the pan with warm water will heat the metal so that it will not be uncomfortably cold when the patient sits on it. Place the bedpan cover between the mattress and springs on the side of the bed nearest you so that you can easily obtain it later. Place the toilet tissue conveniently at the patient's side.

4. Provide privacy for the patient.

Keep the patient covered with a bath blanket or a sheet to avoid exposure or embarrassment. If she is in a single room, close the door; if it is a room for two or more, pull the curtains around the bed.

5. Position the patient on the bedpan.

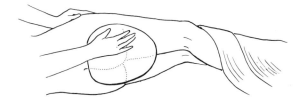

Ask her to roll toward the distal side of the bed, where the siderail is up. While she is lying on her side, place the bedpan under her buttocks with the open, pouring side of the pan toward the foot of the bed. Have the patient return to the supine position and adjust the pan for her comfort and for normal body alignment. Elevate the head of the bed so that the patient is in a sitting position.

U
N
I
T
15

Important Steps	Key Points

6. Take safety precautions.

Put the siderail up, place call signal within easy reach, and leave the bedside to give the patient more privacy.

Some patients attempt to raise their hips rather than turn to get on the bedpan. This method is usually difficult both for the patient and the nursing helper. The patients usually overestimate their strength and are unable to lift themselves high enough off the bed for adequate clearance to slip a bedpan under them easily or without assistance. *Do not attempt to lift the patient by this method.* You will risk hurting yourself and the patient. Encourage her to use the roll method; if she needs assistance in being placed on the bedpan, obtain *additional aid* from your co-workers.

7. Remove the bedpan.

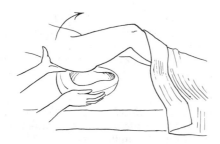

Before removing the bedpan, lower the head of the bed. Ask the patient to turn to the distal side of the bed. Hold the bedpan to avoid spilling its contents while she rolls to her side. Place the bedpan cover on the bedpan, and set it at the foot of the bed or on a chair out of the way.

8. Wipe the perineal area dry with toilet tissue.

Use a continuous stroke from the vulva across the vaginal opening to the rectum (anterior to posterior). This method of cleansing will help prevent rectal bacteria from contaminating or entering the vaginal opening or urinary tract.

9. Empty the bedpan, clean it, and return it to bedside stand.

Observe the following characteristics: color, sediment, amount, and any unusual material in the urine. Pour it into a graduated container to measure the amount voided if patient is on I & O (refer to Unit 17). Empty the urine into the toilet.
    Wash the bedpan thoroughly. Use a brush with a germicidal solution that is usually kept in the bathroom. Remember to return the cleaned equipment to its proper place.

10. Make the patient comfortable.

Give the washcloth, towel, soap, and washbasin containing warm water to her so that she can wash, rinse, and dry her hands. Place the bedside stand and the call signal so that the patient can reach them without strain or discomfort. Adjust the bed to the low position, raise the siderails, and leave the patient in comfort.

11. Obtain the chart.

Record accurately all significant observations made of the urine.

ITEM 2. ASSISTING THE PATIENT TO USE THE FEMALE URINAL

The female urinal is a plastic bottle with a long, wide, spoutlike top; it has a handle, a rectangular base along the side, and a flat, round base at the bottom. It is used by the female patient when she is unable to use the bedpan or commode for voiding. The urinal may be indicated for patients with severe limitations, pain with movement, or extensive sacral ulcers, or for those who prefer it.

Important Steps	Key Points

Follow Item 1, steps 1 through 4.

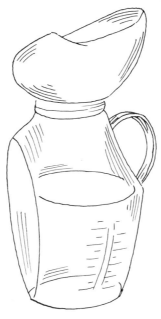

5. Position the patient to use the female urinal.

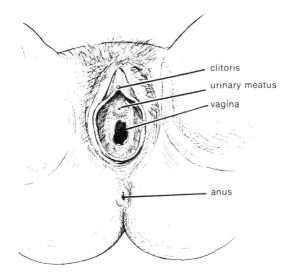

External female genito-urinary organs.

The patient's position will depend on the amount of physical movement and activity that she is permitted.

A. If she is able to stand at the bedside, ask her to stand with her legs apart and bent slightly at the knees. Either you or the patient should hold the urinal in place between her legs. The spout side should be pointing toward the patient's rectum. The handle should be toward the front of the patient. The opening of the urinal should be in direct contact with the perineal area. The extent of body contact with the urinal opening should reach from the rectum to the vagina.

B. If the patient is confined to bed, but is permitted to be in a sitting position, elevate the head of the bed and place two pillows under her buttocks so that she is sitting on the spout of the urinal edge; this will help prevent spilling the contents of the urinal.

If she is permitted to sit on the edge of the bed (dangle position), she will be able to use the urinal without discomfort or difficulty.

C. When the patient must remain flat in bed, yet is permitted to roll from side to side, the urinal can be used. Place it between the

Important Steps	Key Points
	patient's legs using the technique described at the beginning of this lesson. Remember that it is necessary to keep the urinal in direct body contact with the patient (skin to urinal) so that the urine does not leak out.

Follow steps 7 through 11 Item 1.

ITEM 3.   ASSISTING THE PATIENT TO USE THE FRACTURE PAN

The fracture pan is used when patients are unable to sit on a regular-size bedpan. The fracture pan is made of metal or plastic. It is smaller in surface area and height than the regular bedpan. The back part of the pan is approximately 2½ inches high with a wide strip of metal across the top so that the patient is able to sit comfortably. The front, pouring side is high enough to prevent urine from being splashed or spilled in the bed.

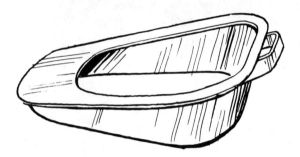

Important Steps	Key Points

Follow steps 1 through 4 of Item 1.

Important Steps	Key Points
5. Position the patient on the fracture pan.	Expose the patient just enough for you to see what you are doing. Have her sit with her knees in a flexed, upright squatting position. Separate her legs so that the pan can be placed between them and slipped under her buttocks. This method is to be used if the patient is able to assist you. If she is unable to do so, use the roll-to-the-side method.
6. Place the call signal within easy reach, raise the siderails, and leave the room to insure privacy.	
7. Remove the fracture pan.	Use the same technique used to put the patient on the fracture pan when she was in the sitting position, with one exception: reverse the initial motion. In other words, pull the pan out from under the buttocks.

Follow Item 1, steps 8 through 11.

ITEM 4. ASSISTING THE PATIENT TO USE THE MALE URINAL

The male urinal is a plastic or metal bottle with a long, round neck, a handle, a rectangular base along one side, and a flat base at the bottom.

The urinal is used by male patients who are limited in physical activity by their illness or injury.

The preliminary and concluding steps used in this task are the same as those in Item 1, "Assisting the Patient to Use the Bedpan." There is one exception to be noted: the use of toilet tissue is omitted. It is not customary for the male patient to use toilet tissue when he urinates since the urine is expelled in a straight single stream and the skin surface of the penis does not get wet.

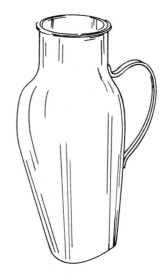

Important Steps

1. Wash your hands.

2. Approach the patient.

3. Obtain the necessary equipment.

4. Position the patient to use the male urinal.

Key Points

The male patient is able to use the urinal when he is in any one of four positions: lying supine (on his back), lying on either the right or left side or in a Fowler's position, or standing at the bedside.

Without Assistance. Give the urinal to the patient so that he can utilize the equipment without assistance. Place the bedpan cover between the mattress and springs of the bed, to be accessible when you carry the bedpan and empty it into the toilet.

With Assistance. If the patient is unable to place the urinal in the proper position to urinate, you will do this for him.

Expose the patient just enough for you to see what you are doing. Separate the patient's legs so there is enough space to permit the urinal to be placed between them without causing pain or discomfort. Hold the urinal with one hand and with your other hand place his penis into the urinal, far enough that it does not slip out when the patient begins to urinate. Hold the urinal in place if the patient is unable to maintain a supporting position with his legs.

The most important aspect of this task is to remember that this is an embarrassing situation for the patient. The task is to be performed in a skillful, matter-of-fact manner, and every effort must be made to keep the patient covered with the bath blanket or sheet.

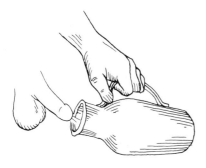

UNIT 15

Important Steps	Key Points

5. If the patient can keep the urinal in place unassisted, put the call signal within easy reach, raise the siderails, and leave the room to insure privacy.

6. Remove the urinal; empty, wash, and store the equipment in its proper place.

Refer to the concluding steps in Item 1.

ITEM 5.   ASSISTING THE PATIENT TO THE BATHROOM

The methods to be used for safety in assisting the patient to the bathroom depend on the degree of physical activity ordered by the physician.

Important Steps	Key Points

1. Wash your hands.

2. Obtain the patient's robe and shoes from the closet or bedside stand.

3. Approach and identify the patient.

4. Adjust the bed to low position and lower the siderail nearest you.

5. Position the patient and assist him to the bathroom.

Ask him to turn so that he is sitting on the side of the bed nearest you. Help him put on his shoes and robe while he is in this position.

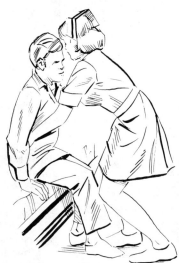

6. Have the patient stand and walk to the bathroom.

If the patient is using a walker or a pair of crutches to aid him in ambulation, refer to the unit on Mechanical Aids for Ambulation and Movement.

7. Help the patient to sit down on the toilet.

When he is seated comfortably, remind him *not to flush the toilet*. Explain that you will do so later after you see the results so that accurate observations can be recorded. Close the bathroom door to insure privacy. If there is a lock

Important Steps	Key Points
	on the door, remind him not to lock it. In the event anything happens to the patient, you will need to help immediately, and of course a locked door would prevent this.
8. Remain within immediate hearing distance of the bathroom.	Never leave the patient unattended.
9. When the patient is finished, have him wash his hands.	Turn the water on and adjust the temperature so that he does not burn himself.
10. Assist the patient to return to bed.	Use the same method to help him return to bed as used in assisting him to the bathroom.
11. Leave the patient safe and comfortable in bed.	
12. Return to the bathroom to clean it up.	

ITEM 6. VOIDED SPECIMEN FOR URINALYSIS

You have learned how to assist the patient in using designated equipment for urination, and now you will learn about tests of urine that physicians need to help in making an accurate diagnosis.

Important Steps	Key Points
1. Wash your hands.	
2. Obtain the equipment: bedpan or urinal, specimen container, specimen label, and laboratory requisition slip.	Specimen containers may vary; some are disposable.

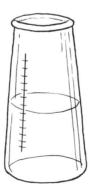

Important Steps	Key Points
3. Approach and identify the patient.	
4. Have the patient void.	Ask the patients on bed rest and those requiring assistance to void into a bedpan or urinal. Refer to the steps in Items 1, 2, 3, and 4. For the ambulatory patient: give the patient the specimen container, and ask him to go to the bathroom, and void either in the container or a collecting basin. The male patient can easily hold the specimen container

UNIT 15

Important Steps

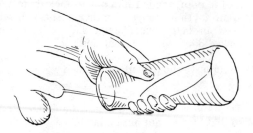

5. Collect the urine specimen.

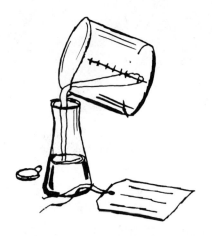

6. Have the patient wash his hands at the sink in the bathroom.

7. Wash the equipment and return it to the proper storage place.

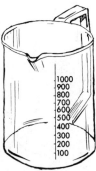

A graduate used to measure fluids.

8. Help the patient back to bed and provide for his safety and comfort.

9. Remove the container of urine from the patient's room.

10. Label the container with the patient's name and room number.

Key Points

in front of him, and as he voids, catch the urine in the container.

The female patient will be able to void directly into the urine specimen container if she is able to stand in a squatting position over the toilet bowl. While she is in the process of voiding, she can hold the urine specimen container underneath the perineal area to catch the urine.

If the patient voids into the bedpan or urinal, pour the urine into a measuring pitcher (commonly called a graduate) and note the amount. Pour at least 4 ounces into the specimen container. Put the lid on the container tightly. Clean and dry the outside of the container.

If any urine has contaminated the outside of the specimen container, take it to the sink in the bathroom and rinse the outside of the container under running water. Dry it with a paper towel and then discard the towel into the wastebasket.

Refer to this step in Item 1.

Use the addressograph (similar to a charge plate in a department store) to print the patient's

Important Steps   Key Points

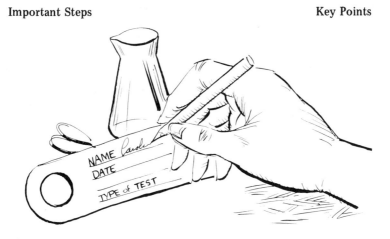

name, and the hospital number of the laboratory requisition and charge voucher. Enter the type of test that is ordered so that the laboratory technician will know what test to perform.

11. Take the specimen to the laboratory immediately.

Urine specimens deteriorate quickly while standing at room temperature. The chemical composition of the urine changes rapidly if it is kept at room temperature for more than 15 minutes. If the urine specimen is left on the nursing unit for a longer period of time, the laboratory will obtain incorrect readings. The laboratory results provide the basis upon which physicians frequently order their treatment and medication. Thus, an incorrect laboratory report due to delay in the delivery of the specimen could cause incorrect diagnosis and medication for your patient.

12. Record on the patient's chart.

Record all pertinent information in the nurses' notes. Record time, amount, color, odor, unusual characteristics, and disposition of the specimen to the laboratory. Charting example:

> 6:15 P.M. Urine specimen with requisition and voucher sent to laboratory. Specimen appeared cloudy and slightly pink. No complaints of pain on voiding. Catamenia present.
> M. Green, SN

U
N
I
T
15

Strain all urine. Occasionally all the urine voided by a patient is strained to catch stones from the kidney or bladder, which may be discharged through the urine. The most common method for straining the urine is to place a fine gauze 4 × 4 dressing over the spout of the graduate (some agencies may use a special sieve). Pour the urine carefully into the graduate; all stones will be caught in the fine mesh gauze. (Discard the gauze after use — take clean gauze for each straining.)

ITEM 7. MID-STREAM OR CLEAN-CATCH URINE SPECIMEN

This procedure is used to obtain a urine specimen for culture and sensitivity. The method provides a specimen that is free from external contamination. Two principles are involved:

one is that the first portion of the urinary stream is discarded and not used for the specimen, and the other is that the external skin surfaces are cleansed to reduce contamination of the urine specimen.

Important Steps	Key Points
1. Assemble the necessary supplies.	You will need a disposable, sterile clean-catch kit or a sterile tray from Central Supply containing cotton balls, a cleansing agent, a specimen bottle, gloves, and a container for sterile water.
2. Wash your hands; approach and explain the procedure to the patient.	Identify the patient by reading the name on the identification band. Ask if he or she can void and provide a urine specimen after the perineal area has been cleansed.
3. Assist the ambulatory patient to the bathroom, OR provide privacy and drape the bed patient.	Have patient wash hands. Place the bath blanket over the abdomen and legs. Fan-fold the top bedding to the foot of the bed. Place the patient on the bedpan (if female) and expose the area.
4. Open the equipment tray and prepare the equipment.	Give direct instructions to ambulatory patients about using the sterile materials. Open the tray and put it within easy reach. Open sterile water flask. Moisten the cotton balls with the liquid cleaning agent.

5. Carry out sterile perineal care.	Refer to the instructions in Unit 33 or follow these steps:
	For female patients:
	  a. Put on gloves.
	  b. Spread the tissue of the vulva apart with the index finger and thumb; do not move them until cleaning is completed.
	  c. Clean the inner surface from the anterior to the anus with one moistened cotton ball; discard the cotton ball.
	  d. Repeat, cleaning the right and left sides of the vulva, using one cotton ball for each wipe from pubic area to anus; discard each used cotton ball.
	  e. Rinse with sterile water.
	  f. Dry area with cotton balls.
	For male patients:
	  a. Put on gloves.
	  b. Hold the penis with one hand, and with the other take a moist cotton ball and begin the cleaning motion at the center and wash outward in a circular manner.
	  c. Repeat the cleansing two times.
	  d. Rinse with sterile water, and dry.

Important Steps	Key Points
6. Ask the patient to void and collect a specimen of the middle portion of the voiding.	As the patient continues voiding in the bedpan or toilet, place the sterile urine bottle in line with the urine stream and collect 30 ml or more for the test. Carefully, place the sterile lid or cap on the specimen bottle. Rinse and dry the outer surface of the bottle.
7. Remove the bedpan or assist the ambulatory patient if needed.	Collect all equipment. Discard as appropriate. Return unused items. Remove the drape and straighten the bedding. Empty the bedpan, rinse it, and return it to the proper storage area.
8. Label the specimen and send to the laboratory with the request slip.	The label should include the patient's name, room number, and other information required by the agency. The requisition slip should note that it is a clean-catch specimen, the date it was obtained, and the tests that are required. Urine specimens should be taken to the laboratory because changes in composition occur when left standing.
9. Record on the patient's chart.	Charting example: 2:30 P.M. Clean-catch urine specimen obtained. Sent to laboratory for culture and sensitivity. M. Green, SN

ITEM 8. 24–HOUR URINE COLLECTION

A number of urine tests require a collection of urine over a period of 24 hours. The most important aspect of this task is that the urine collection must be 100 per cent accurate (every drop of urine must be kept). The laboratory analysis is done to determine the amount of a specified chemical that is excreted through the urine in a 24-hour period. It is the responsibility of all health workers to perform this task skillfully and without error.

Important Steps	Key Points
1. Obtain the equipment. 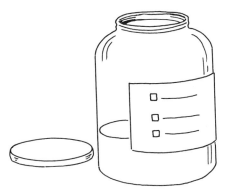	You will need one-gallon jugs, which you can get either from Central Service or the general laboratory (check your agency procedure). The gallon jug is used because it will usually hold the total amount of urine that is voided by the patient over a 24-hour period. If the amount voided over the 24-hour period is more than the gallon jug will hold, add another properly marked jug to the collection. Most special urine specimens will be collected in containers that have at least one strong preservative; therefore, take great care both for yourself and your patient when handling these items.
2. Identify and approach the patient.	Explain this task in detail. Stress the importance of collecting the urine accurately. The 24-hour urine specimen is collected for a variety of reasons: to check total volume of

U
N
I
T
15

Important Steps   **Key Points**

output in a 24-hour period; to detect certain
renal (kidney) diseases; and to detect certain
cardiac (heart) conditions. Check with your
team leader to find out why your patient is to
have a 24-hour urine collection. When you
believe the patient understands, proceed with
the task.

3. Take the equipment to the patient's room.

Label the jug(s) with the patient's name and
room number. Write the time and date that the
collection is to be started, and the time and
date it is to be finished. Put the jug(s) in the
patient's bathroom.

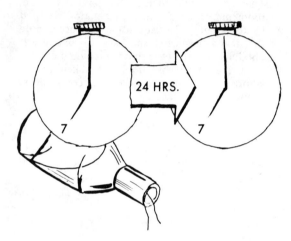

Make a sign (a 6 × 8 card will do) stating that a
24-hour urine collection is in progress, and tape
it at the head of the patient's bed. (Labels may
also be inserted in the Hollister Bed Signs.
Check with your agency for this procedure.)
When the patient voids, ask him to remind the
health worker to save the urine and place it in
the appropriately marked jug.

Some tests require that the urine be kept
cold over the 24-hour collection period. If so,
place the labeled jug(s) in the refrigerator used
for specimen collections. If there is no refrigerator on the unit for this purpose, put the jug(s)
into a pan of ice in the patient's bathroom. You
will have to add ice to the pan as it melts during
the 24-hour period. Remember to empty the
water from the melted ice so there is room in
the pan for ice to be added.

4. Begin the urine collection.

Approximately 5 minutes before the starting
time of the collection, ask the patient to void
into the designated equipment. Discard this
urine specimen into the toilet. Now begin the
collection. Every voided urine specimen should
be measured and poured into the appropriately
marked gallon jug.

5. Have the patient void approximately 5
minutes before the end of the last hour of
the collection.

Add this specimen to the collection.

6. Send the marked gallon jug(s) with the
correctly marked requisition slip and
charge vouchers immediately to the laboratory.

Use the messenger service, dumbwaiter, or a
staff person to deliver it. Remember that
chemical disintegration can quickly take place
when urine specimens are left at room temperature for long periods of time.

7. Tell the patient when the collection is
completed and remove all written notations and equipment from the patient's
room and bathroom.

8. Obtain the patient's chart.

Record the starting time and date, and the
ending time and date of the collection in the
nurses' notes. Include in the record the
measured amount of each voiding with a
notation that it was part of the collection. The

Important Steps	Key Points

last notation in the nurses' notes will be the time at which the collected specimen was sent to the laboratory. *Remember, the test is useless if any of the urine specimens are discarded.* If this should occur, notify the charge nurse and she will notify the physician. The physician will have to decide if the collection is to be restarted. An incomplete collection could add another day to the patient's hospital stay. This is costly to the patient, and therefore it is vital that the task be performed accurately and completely during the first collection period.

Charting example:

3/4/71 7:30 A.M. 24-hour urine specimen collection initiated.   M. Green, SN
3/5/71 7:30 A.M. 24-hour urine specimen collection completed. Sent to lab for VMA.
M. Green, SN

ITEM 9. TIMED URINE COLLECTION

In this lesson you will learn to obtain a timed urine collection. This procedure is determined by the kind of test to be done and the reason the physician is asking that it be done. The physician will determine the fluid intake, the time, and the number of specimens that are required to complete the test. (Some laboratory procedure manuals give the specific procedures for collection of timed urine specimens. Check your agency's Laboratory Procedure Manual.) Timed urine tests are done to determine or confirm glucose tolerance, causes for high blood pressure, and some renal and cardiac diseases.

Important Steps	Key Points

1. Obtain the equipment.

Get the number of urine specimen bottles that will be required from Central Service or the general laboratory. Label each bottle with the patient's name and room number and the date and time of each voiding. Wash your hands.

Note: If some of the specimen collection bottles contain preservatives, remember to use *extreme caution* to avoid spilling any on yourself or on your patients. If the solution does spill, rinse the area vigorously with running water and report at once to your charge nurse.

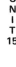

U
N
I
T
15

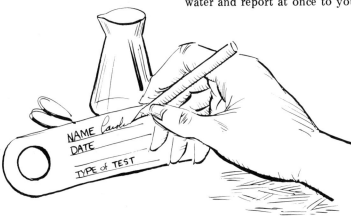

Important Steps	Key Points
2. Identify and approach the patient.	Check the patient's identification. Call him by name. Give him a detailed explanation concerning this task. Stress the importance of collecting the urine accurately. Timed urine specimens may be collected to aid in the diagnoses of a variety of diseases. Although the doctor has probably told his patient the reason for the test, you should ask your team leader why the test is being ordered. When you think the patient understands, proceed with the task.
3. Begin the collection.	Place the labeled bottles in the patient's bathroom and ask him to void. Pour this specimen into the bottle labeled for the appropriate time. The labels may also be numbered in sequence, for example, 1st specimen, 2nd specimen, 3rd specimen.
4. See that the patient takes the required amount of liquid.	Tell him to drink the kind and amount of liquid the physician has requested for the specimen: water must be taken at stated intervals to determine the volume and concentration of the urine; glucose solution must be taken to determine if the patient is a diabetic.
5. Instruct the patient to void at the specified times designated by the physician or laboratory procedures.	
6. Measure every voided specimen and pour each specimen into the properly marked bottle.	
7. Place 6 × 8 cards in easily observed places in the patient's room stating that the collection is in progress.	
8. Tell the patient when the collection is completed, and remove all written notations and equipment from the patient's room and bathroom.	
9. Take the specimens with the requisition and charge vouchers to the laboratory for testing and evaulation.	Refer to step 6, Item 8.
10. Obtain the patient's chart.	Record the time and amount of each voided specimen in the nurses' notes. State that it was a timed urine collection. The last notation should tell where the specimens were sent. *The results of the tests will be useless if the time of each voiding is not accurate.* If an error is made, notify the charge nurse, who will notify the physician, and give you further instructions about whether to start the specimen collection over. This could mean an added day of hospitalization for the patient, which is costly. Specimen collections are extremely important in determining the medical plan of care. *Precise accuracy and attention to detail are mandatory.*

ITEM 10. TESTS FOR SUGAR AND ACETONE IN THE URINE

Patients with diabetes have difficulties using the sugars in food. Sugar is used by the body for energy. Insulin is a normal hormone produced by the endocrine cells called the islets of Langerhans, located in the pancreas. This hormone assists in oxidizing (burning) the sugars in the blood and maintaining the normal limits of blood sugar. However, in the diabetic patient there is less insulin—or none at all—manufactured by the body to aid in the process of burning sugars. A medication (insulin administered by hypodermic or an oral synthetic insulin) is given to the patient to assist him in using the sugars from foods.

To determine how much medication is needed, the doctor measures the amount of sugar that is excreted in the urine. The simple urine test for sugar content is called Clinitest. It is done four times a day (q.i.d.), usually before meals and before bedtime. The testing may be done more frequently if the patient's condition warrants it.

A. Clinitest

A Clinitest kit is ordered from the pharmacy for each diabetic patient. The plastic kit contains a bottle of Clinitest tablets, a test tube, an eyedropper, and a color chart. The kit is usually stored in a safe area in the patient's bathroom. Two strengths of Clinitest tablets are commonly used. One requires 5 drops of urine mixed with 10 drops of water, and the other requires 2 drops of urine mixed with 10 drops of water. Be certain that you have read the instructions on the bottle so that you are following the correct procedure.

Important Steps	Key Points
1. Wash your hands. Approach and identify the patient.	Explain what you are going to do. Part of the diabetic teaching program may be to teach the patient how to perform this simple test. It is important that you fully understand the procedure.

2. Ask the patient to void at the designated time.	A bedpan, or urinal may be used.
	For a double-voided specimen, add these steps:
	  a. Discard the first voiding, which may have been in the bladder for several hours or longer.
	  b. Give the patient a glass of water to drink.
	  c. After an interval of about 30 minutes, ask the patient to void.
	  d. Use the second specimen for the Clinitest.

3. Take the urine specimen to the bathroom or utility room for testing.	Foley catheter specimens: A urine specimen can be obtained for testing diabetic urine from the Foley catheter by cleaning the rubber catheter (near the thick part of the tubing at the drain connection) with an alcohol sponge, then inserting a sterile 25-gauge needle attached to a 2½-cc syringe into the cleaned catheter and removing enough urine for an accurate test.
4. Prepare Clinitest equipment.	Make sure that you have a test tube, eyedropper, Clinitest tablets, color chart, and water available for use.

U
N
I
T
15

Important Steps	Key Points
5. Add 5 drops of urine to the test tube. 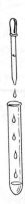	Hold the test tube between the thumb and index finger about ¼ inch from the top rim. Fill the eyedropper with urine. Hold it in a straight position when you place the 5 drops of urine into the center of the test tube. For accurate measurements, do not let the drops run along the sides of the test tube. Rinse the inside and outside of the eyedropper with cold water.
6. Add 10 drops of water to the urine.	The water and urine must be mixed for this test to be accurate.
7. Gently rotate the test tube.	Roll it between your left forefinger and thumb to mix the urine and water. (Reverse hands if you are left-handed.) Place the test tube in the plastic kit for safekeeping until you are ready to add the Clinitest tablet.
8. Remove one Clinitest tablet from the bottle by gently shaking the tablet into the lid of the bottle. Pick up the lid and pour the tablet into the test tube. 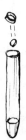	Do not use tablets that are moist or have changed color; these changes cause inaccurate testing. Good tablets are lightly spotted and bluish-white in color. Avoid putting the tablets into the test tube with your fingers because the tablets contain a caustic soda and could irritate or burn your skin. The dissolving tablet causes a boiling reaction and the test tube becomes hot. To avoid burning your fingers, hold the tube near the top. DO NOT ROTATE the test tube during this step. WARNING: If a Clinitest tablet is swallowed, do not have the patient vomit. Give him a glass of water and take him to an emergency hospital immediately. Clinitest tablets can severely burn the esophageal tissues.
9. Compare the color changes of the specimen in the test tube with the color chart.	After 15 seconds (or after the boiling stops), shake the tube gently and compare it with the Clinitest color chart. If the mixture passes through all the colors (blue, green, and orange) during the boiling stage and has a green color for the final stage, the specimen should be retested. Use the same technique, but use only 1 drop of urine to 14 drops of water. Report the results to your team leader.
10. Wash, rinse, and dry the equipment.	Return the bedpan or urinal to its storage space. Close the Clinitest bottle tightly, wipe up spills, and tidy the work area.
11. Record the readings on the patient's chart.	Note the color reaction. Usual color designations are:

Important Steps	Key Points
	Negative—the fluid will be blue, indicating that no sugar is present.
	Positive—the fluid changes in color from dark green to orange; check the color change in the test tube with the block on the color chart indicating the degree of sugar content: trace, 1+, 2+, 3+, and 4+.
	The dosage of insulin is based on the amount of sugar in the urine. The higher the sugar content, the more insulin will be given. Therefore, report the results of the test immediately to your team leader so she can give the insulin. Diabetic patients are usually taught to carry out this procedure themselves.

B. Tes-Tape Test

Another method for testing the content of sugar in the urine is the use of Tes-Tape. As in the preceding item, you will be testing the urine at least q.i.d. (or more often if the condition so indicates).

Important Steps	Key Points
Follow steps 1 through 3 of the procedure used for Clinitest.	
4. Withdraw 1½ inches of Tes-Tape from its dispenser.	This is similar to a Scotch tape dispenser. (Do not use if the tape has turned brown.) On the outside of the dispenser there is printed a color code with percentages indicated for each color.

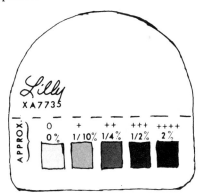

| 5. Tear off the piece of tape. | Holding it between your forefinger and thumb, pull the tape up against the cutting edge on the dispenser and cut it free. |

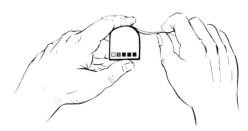

U
N
I
T
15

Important Steps	Key Points
6. Dip the distal end of the tape into the urine specimen.	Remove the tape immediately from the urine. However, be sure it has been moistened uniformly. (Keep your fingers dry.)

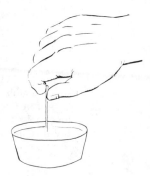

7. Wait one minute.

8. Compare the tape with the color chart on the exterior of the dispenser.	Match the tape with the darkest square of color shown on the dispenser. If the tape indicates ½ per cent or higher, wait one additional minute for final comparison.

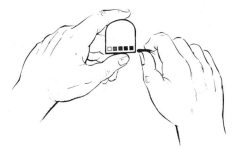

9. Wash, rinse, and dry the equipment.

10. Record the readings on the patient's chart.	Record the color reaction, coded as follows: Yellow — zero per cent (or sugar-free). Varying shades of green from light to dark — 1+ (1/10 per cent); 2+ (1/4 per cent); 3+ (½ per cent); and 4+ (2 per cent or more).
	Again the dosage of insulin given depends on the amount of sugar in the urine.
	Report the results immediately to your team leader so that she can give the prescribed dose of insulin.

C. Test for Ketone Bodies (Acetone) in the Urine

Another commonly performed urine test is the one for ketone bodies (acetone) in the urine. The test can also be used on blood to determine the amount of acetone in the blood. This test is used as an indicator for specific treatment of patients with diabetes, and for unconscious patients to determine whether the coma is due to ketosis, hypoglycemia (low blood sugar), stroke, or other disorders. The Acetest tablet is used for this test.

Important Steps	Key Points

Follow steps 1 through 3 of the Clinitest procedure.

4. Place a clean paper towel on the work surface.

5. Place one Acetest tablet on the paper. — Draw urine up into the eyedropper. Drop one drop of urine on the tablet.

6. Wait 30 seconds. — Compare the color of the tablet with the color chart on the bottle.
Reactions can be negative or positive. If the color of the tablet remains unchanged or becomes a cream color, it is considered to be a negative reaction. If the tablet turns from a lavender to a deep purple, it is considered a positive reaction. It is recorded as slightly, moderately, or strongly positive.

7. Record and report. — Report the results to your team leader and record this information on the patient's chart.

8. Wash, rinse, and dry the equipment. — Return it to the storage area. Check to be sure that the cap is secured tightly on the Acetest bottle. Be sure to wipe up spills. Leave the work area neat and tidy.

D. Ketostix Test

One other frequently used method to determine the amount of acetone (or ketones) in the urine is the Ketostix. It can also be used to determine the amount of ketones in blood. The specially treated strips react when moistened with urine or blood. The variations in color determine the amount of acetone in the urine or blood. (The reaction is similar to that of the Acetest tablets.)

Important Steps	Key Points

Follow steps 1 through 3 of the Clinitest procedure.

4. Remove one Ketostix strip from the bottle. — Close the jar tightly.

5. Dip the designated tip into the urine and then remove it immediately. — The tip is indicated with an arrow-type point. Remember, the urine must be freshly obtained urine so that the result will be accurate.

6. Tap the edge of the strip against the bedpan. — This will remove excess urine.

7. After 15 seconds, compare the Ketostix with the color chart. — The chart is printed on the Ketostix container.

UNIT 15

Important Steps	Key Points

8. Record your readings on the patient's chart.	Indicate the color reaction.
	    Usual color designations are:
	Negative: buff color
	Positive: slightly — lavender
	            moderately — dark lavender
	            strongly — purple
	
	Report the results to your team leader.

E. Keto-Diastix Test

This is a newer method, utilizing a reagent strip that combines the tests for sugar and acetone. The strip changes the urine color by a reaction similar to that in the Ketostix Test. The color variation determines the amount of sugar and acetone in the urine. A bottle of Keto-Diastix is ordered for the patient and kept in his bathroom or bedside stand.

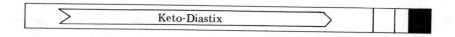

Important Steps	Key Points
Follow steps 1 through 3 of the Clinitest procedure.	
4. Remove one Keto-Diastix from its bottle.	Close the jar tightly.
5. Dip the designated tip into the urine for 2 seconds and then remove it.	Tap the strip gently against the urine container to remove excess urine.
6. Compare the ketone reagent area on the strip to the chart.	Be sure to match it with the Ketone Chart on the Keto-Diastix package.
7. Compare the glucose reagent area on the strip after 30 seconds.	Check the results with the Glucose Chart on the package for the closest matching color.
8. Record your readings on the patient's chart.	Indicate the color reaction; report the results to your team leader immediately.

ITEM 11. FOLEY CATHETHER CARE

In this procedure you will learn how to care for the Foley catheter, or the indwelling catheter, as it is often called. Inserted into the bladder to maintain a continuous free flow of urine, it is used for a variety of purposes: (a) emptying of the bladder to allow an infected area to heal free of contaminated urine; (b) keeping an incontinent patient dry; (c) retraining or restoring normal bladder function; and (d) keeping an accurate intake and output record.

Foley catheters come in various sizes; the size to be used depends on the physical structure of the patient. (The physician may designate the size when he writes the order for the catheter to be inserted.) The Foley catheter has two rubber tubes; the main line is identified by the openings at the tip and at the wide base on the opposite end. The second tube is connected and sealed along the side of the main tube; the end of the tube is fixed in a manner that allows it to be inflated with air or sterile liquid, causing the formation of an inflated balloon around the main tube. The balloon prevents the catheter from slipping out of the urinary tract.

After the catheter has been inserted well into the bladder, the balloon is inflated. You can test to see if the catheter is in place by gently pulling the catheter toward you.

The plastic drain tube with the attached plastic drain bottle or pouch is inserted into the main drain tube of the catheter. The complete catheter drainage setup is known as a closed drainage system.

While the patient is ambulatory, maintain the closed drainage system by pinning the tubing and the plastic bag to the inside of the patient's gown. This will keep the patient from having to hand-carry the equipment.

A number of agencies require that sterile perineal care be given once or twice a day to all patients with an indwelling catheter. Disposable, sterile catheter-care kits are available for this purpose; they contain a drape, gloves, cotton balls, small basin, and pavidone-iodine solution for cleansing.

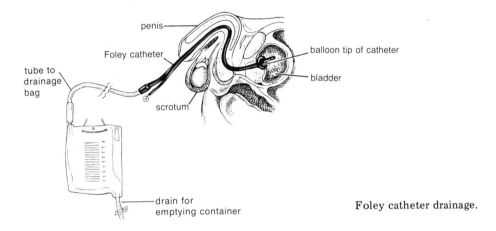

Foley catheter drainage.

Important Steps	Key Points
1. Wash your hands.	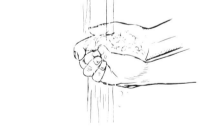
2. Approach and identify the patient.	
3. Position the patient.	
4. Observe his skin at the place of insertion and surrounding area.	Be certain that there is no redness, skin eruption, or swelling at the insertion site or surrounding area. If there are any of these signs, report immediately to your team leader so that she can begin recommended treatment at once.
5. Cleanse the area gently with warm water and soap, rinse, and pat dry.	This is usually done as part of the daily bath. However, if the patient has a Foley catheter in for several days, the proximal end of the catheter should be inspected frequently

U
N
I
T
15

Important Steps	Key Points
	throughout the day and night, and kept free of dried crusts and blood. Sterile perineal care is given according to agency policies. Refer to Item 7, step 5, or Unit 33.
6. Keep the tubing close to the patient's body.	Put tape around the drain tube about 12 to 18 inches from the entry site and secure it to the skin on the patient's thigh. Place the tube so that it is comfortable for the patient and there is no tension or unnecessary pull on the skin. Use nonallergenic tape so that it can be changed when necessary without causing skin irritation. Some agencies recommend placing a piece of tape around the drainage tube about 18 to 24 inches from the entry side into the urethra, and making a side loop through which a safety pin can be placed and pinned to the bottom sheet. Provide enough length on the drainage tube to allow the patient to move freely in bed.
7. Maintain tubing alignment.	The drainage tube should lie on top of the bed in a straight alignment. It must be kept free of kinking, twisting, and added weight pressure. This prevents the tubing from being clamped together and allows urine to flow freely into the bottle at all times.
8. Keep the gravity-flow drainage even.	Pin or tape the longest part of the tube to the bed linen. This prevents the tubing from falling over the side of the bed and keeps it above the drainage bottle to maintain an even, free gravity flow. Attach the drainage container to the side of the bed frame. Change the position of the plastic drainage container as you change the position of the patient.
9. Empty the drainage container. 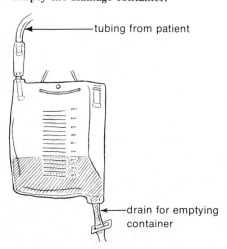 tubing from patient drain for emptying container	Plastic closed drainage containers have a short tube extending from a bottom corner so that the urine can be empted without disconnecting the closed drainage system. Remove the cap from the drain tube and let the urine flow into the graduate pitcher. If urine is spilled on the floor, wipe it up because it causes an offensive odor if left to dry. If the spilled urine was being collected as part of a 24-hour specimen, report the loss immediately to your team leader so that she can take the appropriate action.
10. Measure and discard or save the urine, as indicated by the order.	This method of urine drainage minimizes the risk of reinfecting the urinary tract and of contamination from the environment. Wash your hands.

Important Steps	Key Points
11. Position the siderails.	Leave the patient safe and comfortable. Refer to this step in Item 1.
12. Obtain the chart.	Record all pertinent information in the nurses' notes.

To prevent germs from entering the catheter tubing and causing a urinary tract infection, the Foley catheter should be disconnected only when the physician orders the disconnection.

Important Steps	Key Points
1. Wash your hands.	
2. Approach and identify the patient.	
3. Disinfect the catheter and drain the tube at the connection.	Use a germicidal solution.
4. Place the disconnected tubing ends on a sterile field.	Use two sterile 4 X 4 dressings.
5. Insert a sterile plastic plug into the end of the catheter tubing.	This comes with the catheter set and may be stored at the patient's bedside in a germicidal solution. (Change the solution daily.)
6. Place a sterile cap on the end of the drain tubing.	This comes with the catheter set and may be stored at the patient's bedside in a germicidal solution. (Change the solution daily.) Some agencies keep sterile wrapped plugs and caps in a central storage place, for patient use. If the sterile caps and plugs are not available in your agency, clamp the catheter, and clean the catheter and drain tube with a germicidal solution as you disconnect them. Then place a thick, sterile 4 X 4 dressing around the end of each tube.
7. To connect the drain tube to the catheter, reverse the actions of steps 5 and 6. Remove the cap and plug; insert the drain tube into the catheter tubing.	Store the cap and plug in germicidal solution at the patient's bedside.
8. Follow steps 6 through 12 of Item 11.	

At times the patient will say that he has the urge to urinate. You are to check the catheter and drainage through the tubing. The catheter openings in the bladder may be clogged with solid matter, and the catheter may need to be irrigated with sterile saline to remove it. This, of course, will depend on the doctor's order and your agency procedure. Another source of discomfort may be the position of the catheter in the bladder. The opening may be lying against the bladder wall, or it may be above the urine level so that it is impossible to remove the urine. Gently rotate or move the catheter so the flow will be continuous. The size of the catheter may affect the urine flow, particularly if the catheter tube is too small for adequate drainage. This can cause the bladder to become distended, and internal pressure will be exerted on the sphincter so the patient feels the urge to void.

Remember, the reproductive organs are in the perineal area of the body. Do not be surprised if the male patient expresses concern about a sexual stimulus that may occur while he has the Foley catheter in place. Reassure him that it is a natural phenomenon because these organs are extremely sensitive to external and internal stimulation. Maintain a matter-of-fact, gentle, and comforting manner while you care for the patient.

UNIT 15

PERFORMANCE TEST

In the skill laboratory, you will be asked to perform the following activities for your instructor without reference to any source material. You will need another person to take the part of the patient.

1. Given a patient who is unable to move her legs and assist herself on the bedpan, explain to her how she is to roll and how you are going to place her on the bedpan. In this movement you will assist her to roll safely to the far side of the bed, place the bedpan under her buttocks, position her for comfort, and keep her modestly covered with the bath blanket.

2. Given a patient who is to have a 24-hour urine collection, explain the task to him, stressing the importance of obtaining all the urine voided in the 24-hour period, and telling him that if one specimen is lost, the test is useless. Obtain the equipment from the laboratory, mark the labels correctly on the bottle, and then indicate by signs placed on the bed and in the bathroom that the 24-hour urine collection is in progress.

3. Given a patient who is to have a clean-catch urine specimen collected, explain the task to the patient. Obtain and set up the necessary equipment, position the patient standing over the toilet bowl, and go through the motions of cleaning the patient for the task.

4. Given a diabetic patient who has voided a urine specimen, test the urine for sugar and acetone (using your agency procedure) and practice recording the results on the chart forms.

PERFORMANCE CHECKLIST

URINE ELIMINATION

POSITIONING THE BEDPAN

Demonstrate the procedure for positioning a bedpan.

1. Wash your hands.

2. Identify the patient; explain the procedure to the patient.

3. Obtain the necessary materials.

4. Assist the patient to the lateral position.

5. Place the bedpan appropriately.

6. Return the patient to the supine position.

7. Elevate the patient to the sitting position.

8. Provide the patient with privacy and safety.

9. Lower the head of the bed.

10. Help the patient return to the lateral position.

11. Hold the bedpan during the move to avoid spilling its contents.

12. Remove the bedpan.

13. Assist the patient with personal cleansing if necessary.

14.   Provide for the patient's comfort and safety.

15.   Empty the contents of the bedpan.

16.   Wash the bedpan thoroughly.

17.   Record all significant observations of the urine.

24-HOUR URINE COLLECTION

Demonstrate the procedure for a 24-hour urine collection.

1.   Identify the patient.

2.   Obtain the equipment with the preservative and take it to the patient's room.

3.   Post warning signs.

4.   Store collection jugs in the refrigerator or in buckets, if indicated.

5.   Tell the patient to void approximately 5 minutes before collection begins and discard that urine.

6.   Transfer the urine to an appropriate jug after each voiding; make sure to measure and record the quantity.

7.   Tell the patient to void approximately 5 minutes before the end of the 24-hour collection and add voiding to the specimen.

8.   Mark the jugs correctly.

9.   Mark the laboratory slip appropriately.

10.   Mark the charge vouchers appropriately.

11.   Arrange for immediate transfer of the specimen to the laboratory.

12.   Inform the patient that the collection period is completed.

13.   Remove the written warnings and equipment from the room.

14.   Obtain the patient's chart and record all information pertaining to the collection.

COLLECTION OF A CLEAN-CATCH SPECIMEN

Demonstrate the procedure for collecting a clean-catch specimen.

1.   Identify the patient.

2.   Obtain the supplies and equipment.

3.   Wash your hands.

4.   Explain the procedure to the patient.

5.   Provide for the patient's privacy.

6.   Cleanse the perineal area.

7.   Assist the patient to the bathroom.

8.   Tell the patient to void.

9.   Ask the patient to interrupt voiding.

10.   Collect the specimen after interruption.

11.   Transfer the specimen to the specimen jar.

UNIT 15

12. Assist the patient to bed; provide an opportunity for the patient to cleanse himself.

13. Label the specimen with all appropriate information.

14. Arrange to have the specimen taken to the laboratory with all pertinent information.

15. Return to the patient's room and provide for his comfort and safety.

16. Clean the bathroom.

17. Record the activity on the patient's chart.

DIABETIC TESTING

Demonstrate the procedure for the diabetic testing of a urine specimen.

1. Wash your hands.

2. Identify the patient.

3. Explain the procedure.

4. Obtain the urine specimen.

5. Transport the urine specimen to the work area.

6. Perform the indicated diabetic test.

7. Compare the reading of the test to the color chart.

8. Record the reading on the patient's chart.

POST-TEST

Directions: Choose the answer that will make the statement complete.

1. After the patient is placed on the bedpan, the bedpan cover is conveniently placed:

    a. Between the sheet and spread.

    b. Between the mattress and springs.

    c. At the foot of the bed.

    d. In the bedside stand.

2. After the patient uses the bedpan, the following articles are given to wash her hands and perineal area:

    a. Washcloth, towel, and soap.

    b. Towel and soap.

    c. Towel and washcloth.

    d. Washcloth, soap, towel, and washbasin with warm water.

3. A safe nursing practice after you give a bedpan to the patient is to:

    a. Wash your hands.

    b. Empty the bedpan without using the bedpan cover.

    c. Warm the bedpan.

    d. Leave the bedpan on the floor of the patient's bathroom.

4. The safest method for assisting a patient on the bedpan is to:

    a. Slip the bedpan under her elevated buttock.

    b. Lift the patient onto the pan.

    c. Have the patient roll to the opposite side of the bed, position the pan, and have the patient roll back.

    d. Roll up the head of the bed so the patient can get on the pan.

5. When emptying urine, note and record *unusual* characteristics such as:

    a. Clean, yellow appearance.

    b. pH of 7.

    c. Specific gravity.

    d. Blood-tinged appearance.

6. An important fact to remember when assisting the female patient to use the urinal is to:

    a. Hold the urinal close to her skin.

    b. Use the urinal only when the patient stands.

    c. Have the wheels on the bed unlocked.

    d. Keep the urinal in bed with the patient at all times.

UNIT 15

7. Routine urine specimens are obtained to determine all the following normal characteristics except:

   a. Albumin.

   b. Clear, straw color.

   c. pH of 7.

   d. organic waste products.

8. The fracture pan is described as:

   a. Round with a 2-inch wide opening in front.

   b. Oblong with a curved top and 3-inch opening.

   c. Having a back that is 2½ inches high with a wide strip of metal across the top and a wide, high front.

   d. Kidney-shaped.

9. An important factor to include when giving the urinal to the male patient is to:

   a. Avoid patient embarrassment. Maintain a matter-of-fact manner.

   b. Keep the urinal handy on the bedside stand.

   c. Keep the urinal in the patient's bed.

   d. Give the toilet tissue to the patient.

10. Voided urine decomposes in a short time at room temperature. Therefore, fresh specimens should be sent to the laboratory within:

   a. 60 minutes.

   b. 20 to 30 minutes.

   c. 120 minutes.

   d. 90 minutes.

11. Patients are catheterized for all of the following reasons except:

   a. Keeping incontinent patients dry.

   b. Restoring normal bladder function.

   c. Keeping an accurate intake and output record.

   d. Keeping the urine free of sediment.

12. To obtain a urine specimen from a Foley catheter, use the closed drain system, which means that you must:

   a. Disconnect the drain tube from the catheter.

   b. Remove urine from the collection bag.

   c. Clean the tubing with germicide; use a sterile needle and syringe, and insert it into the tubing and withdraw urine.

   d. None of these.

13. Patients with catheters often feel the urge to void for all the following reasons except:

   a. Catheter may be clogged with solid matter.

   b. There is clear, free-flowing urine.

    c. Catheter may be lying against the sphincter wall.

    d. Catheter may be too small to remove an adequate amount of urine.

14. The most important principle to remember when the clean-catch urine specimen is obtained is to:

    a. Wash your hands.

    b. Use clean equipment.

    c. Use sterile technique in the procedure.

    d. Assist the patient safely to the bathroom.

15. When 24-hour specimens are collected, all of the following are true except:

    a. Have the patient void exactly at the starting time.

    b. Save every voided specimen.

    c. 5 minutes before the starting hour, have the patient void, and discard the urine; and 5 minutes before the finished hour, have the patient void, and save that urine.

    d. The specimen is properly labeled and sent to the laboratory.

16. When a urine specimen in the 24-hour collection procedure has been accidentally discarded, the following must be done:

    a. Tell yourself it doesn't matter, it was only a little bit.

    b. Report to the charge nurse so that she can make the appropriate decision.

    c. Report to the physician and follow his instructions.

    d. Report to the laboratory chief and follow his instructions.

17. When urine is to be collected for a Clinitest procedure, the process of "double voiding" is used; this means that the patient must:

    a. Drink water and void.

    b. Void a specimen to be discarded and drink water; 30 minutes later, void another specimen, which is tested.

    c. Void a specimen to be tested.

    d. Void a specimen to be sent to the laboratory.

18. Clinitest tablets should be placed in the test tube by using:

    a. The bottle lid as the carrying vehicle.

    b. Your thumb and forefinger.

    c. A hemostat

    d. A 2 × 2 gauze pad.

19. Important safety steps to consider when emptying a bedpan or urinal are all of the following except:

    a. Wiping up spilled urine.

    b. Using a germicide to clean equipment after each use.

    c. Lifting the patient from the bed pan.

    d. Keeping the far siderail up as the patient rolls in that direction when the pan is removed.

UNIT 15

20. Important steps used to avoid undue embarrassment to the patient who is using the bedpan are all of the following except:

a. Screening the patient when putting her on the bedpan.

b. Keeping bed covers over her while she is on the bedpan.

c. Keeping your facial and verbal expressions kindly and matter-of-fact.

d. Telling your co-workers that the patient is on the bedpan.

POST-TEST ANNOTATED ANSWER SHEET

1. b. (p. 299)
2. d. (p. 298)
3. a. (Unit 4)
4. c. (p. 299)
5. d. (pp. 297–298)
6. a. (p. 301)
7. a. (pp. 297–298)
8. c. (p. 302)
9. a. (p. 303)
10. b. (pp. 298 and 307)

11. d. (p. 318)
12. c. (p. 313)
13. b. (p. 321)
14. c. (p. 308)
15. a. (pp. 309–311)
16. b. (p. 311)
17. b. (p. 313)
18. a. (p. 314)
19. c. (pp. 299, 300, and 320)
20. d. (pp. 299 and 303)

ASSISTING WITH NUTRITION

I. DIRECTIONS FOR THE STUDENT

Proceed through this lesson. When you have finished, demonstrate to your instructor the methods of feeding an infant and an adult, in the skill laboratory.

For this demonstration, you will need the following:

1. Adult and infant mannequins.

2. Complete meal tray.

3. Baby bottle with formula (or any liquid).

4. I & O (Intake and Output) sheet or form, and pencil.

When you have finished, complete the post-test.

II. GENERAL PERFORMANCE OBJECTIVE

You will demonstrate the knowledge and skills related to basic foods and general nutrition for adults and children, and you will be able to assist the adult and the child with nutrition, after which you will make a record of oral intake and output.

III. SPECIFIC PERFORMANCE OBJECTIVES

When this lesson has been completed, you will be able to:

1. Assist or feed an adult patient and a pediatric patient with solids and liquids.

2. Record oral intake and output accurately.

3. Serve and collect meal trays and nourishments.

IV. VOCABULARY

calorie—the unit of heat required to raise the temperature of one gram of water one degree Centigrade.

carbohydrates—foodstuffs with high starch and sugar content, consisting of carbon, hydrogen, and oxygen molecules. A source of heat and quick energy, they are burned up rapidly by body action.

fats (lipids)—food substances that provide heat and long-lasting energy. Some common fats are lard, olive oil, and butter. They give flavor to foods and act as a regulator for emptying the contents of the stomach. Fats also consist of carbon, hydrogen, and oxygen molecules, but these elements are combined in a different manner from those of the carbohydrate molecule.

kilocalorie—the large calorie of food calories; 1000 times as big as a small calorie; often abbreviated as kcal.

metabolism—chemical transformation (change) of food by which energy is provided for the growth of cells, and substances not needed by the body are decomposed. These substances are excreted by the body as waste products (urine, feces, sweat).

minerals—chemical substances that build and repair tissues; they are important for proper cell function. Some common minerals are calcium, phosphorus, sodium, potassium, iodine, and iron.

nutrition—a branch of science dealing with the scientific laws that govern the food requirements of the human body for growth, reproduction, and energy.

proteins—food substances that build and repair tissues; they are also important in regulating the body processes. Proteins are composed of carbon, hydrogen, oxygen, and nitrogen.

vitamins—chemical substances that aid in body metabolism. When lacking in the diet, they manifest their absence by certain disease conditions. They are used to treat or prevent vitamin deficiency diseases. Some common vitamins are vitamins A, B, C, D, E, and niacin.

V.   KNOWLEDGE BASIC TO THIS LESSON

ITEM 1.   WHAT ARE THE BASIC NUTRITION REQUIREMENTS?

A good diet is important for health. The nutrients in foods are necessary for the growth and repair of tissues, to provide the energy for the body to do work, and to regulate the body processes. If we select and eat a wide variety of wholesome food in the amounts needed to maintain the ideal body weight, we are probably getting an adequate diet. A wholesome diet consists of foods from the basic four food groups, which are described briefly here.

I.   The Milk Group

This group of foods provides a good source for calcium, proteins, and fats. Milk products such as ice cream, cheeses, custards, and milk soups are used to supply some of the milk needs and to add variety. The powdered nonfat and low fat forms of milk contain fewer calories and saturated fat than whole milk, and generally cost less.

The recommended intake of milk is 2 to 3 cups daily for children, depending on their age and size. Teenagers should have 4 cups of milk daily, and adults should have 2 cups, or the equivalent in other milk products. The pregnant woman needs 3 cups a day, and when nursing the baby, the mother needs to increase her milk consumption to a quart a day.

II.   The Meat Group

Proteins in the diet are required for the growth and repair of body tissues, and as the building blocks for enzymes, hormones, and antibodies, which regulate the body processes. The best sources of proteins are red meats, fish, and poultry. Alternative protein sources are eggs, and the legumes, which include beans, peas, and lentils. Whole grains, nuts, and deep green leafy vegetables also supply lesser amounts of protein. Two servings of protein group foods are recommended daily. Although proteins are among the most expensive foods, skill and imagination can help you to prepare nutritious and appetizing dishes economically.

III.   The Cereal and Bread Group

Cereals (the seeds of grasses such as wheat, rye, rice, oats, and so forth) are rich in starch, a carbohydrate used by the body for fuel. The cereal foods are among the most economical of the food groups, and they can be prepared in many ways. The whole grains and enriched grains provide many of the vitamins needed by the body. Four or more servings of bread, dry or cooked cereal, noodles, macaroni products, or rice should be included in the daily diet.

IV. The Vegetable and Fruit Group

The foods in this group are high in vitamins, minerals, and fiber. Vegetables are used in soups, salads, stews, and as separate servings. Fruits contain natural sugars and make wholesome desserts. Both fruits and vegetables are good choices of foods for people who are watching their weight because both are filling and have fewer calories than other compact or concentrated foods like proteins, pastries, and nuts. Four or more servings daily are recommended from this group, including at least one citrus fruit (or other source of vitamin C such as tomatoes), and one of a deep green or deep yellow vegetable that is high in vitamin A.

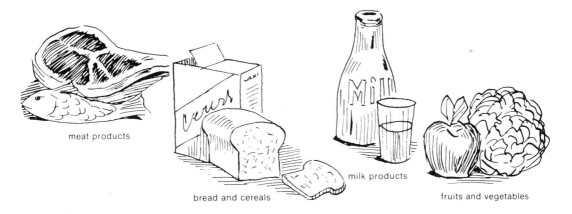

meat products

bread and cereals

milk products

fruits and vegetables

Four basic food groups.

Sick people often are not able to tolerate a normal diet. Illness decreases the appetite and desire for food, and the ability to digest and utilize the food. Often, the diet is withheld for various procedures and tests, or for a period of time as part of the treatment of a disease. Often, the diet is modified to meet the patient's needs; the physician orders a specific type of diet, and the dietician is responsible for seeing that it contains the proper groups and amounts of foods.

During illness, the sick person needs to eat a diet that supplies the nutrients needed to bring his body back to a healthier state. The patient who is ill for only a few days may not suffer much from a decreased intake of food, but the seriously ill patient, or the one who has been ill for a longer period of time is in more danger of not eating enough foods to meet his daily requirements.

Unless enough foods are eaten, body tissues (fat and muscle) are used to supply the energy needed by the body each day. The basic life processes needed to circulate the blood through the body, to move the muscles in order to breathe, and to maintain the body temperature require a certain amount of energy. The sick person with a fever requires 7 per cent more energy for every 1°C elevation in temperature for these basal needs. The average adult patient uses 6 calories an hour resting quietly in bed, about 25 calories when sitting up an hour, and about 30 calories per hour when standing. Additional physical exercise requires greater amounts of energy. Many patients do lose weight during an illness, because of the large amount of energy needed for healing and return to health.

The nurse is responsible for seeing that the patient is served a tray, assisting the patient as needed, or feeding him in order to assure that an adequate diet is consumed. One of your most important duties is to report or record the amount and type of foods the patient has eaten.

U
N
I
T
16

ITEM 2.   WHAT ARE SOME OF THE COMMONLY ORDERED THERAPEUTIC (TREATMENT) DIETS?

Let us examine some of the special diets used in the hospital as part of the treatment of disease conditions.

Full Liquid Diet.   Liquids alone are usually prescribed after surgery, or in cases of acute infections, difficulty in swallowing (dysphagia), or acute inflammation of the gastrointestinal (digestive) tract. As the name implies, this diet consists primarily of liquids or strained, semiliquid foods (such as Jello or custard).

Clear or Surgical Liquid Diet.   The clear liquid diet assures a minimal residue and consists primarily of dissolved sugar and flavored fluids that provide calories but lack other essentials such as fats, proteins, and vitamins. It permits no milk, and is served in the form of ginger ale, sweetened tea or coffee, fat-free broth, and plain gelatin desserts.

Soft Diet.   That is an easily digested intermediate diet that is a compromise between a full liquid and a general diet, consisting of soft foods that are easily chewed and digested, and that contain almost no fiber. These foods represent most of the items on a general diet except that they are chopped or strained for ease in digestion.

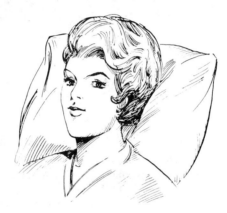

Intestinal disorder — soft diet.

Regular or General Diet.   This is nutritionally prepared to include all items in the four basic food groups. In other words, it represents the normal diet for the healthy person; fried and highly seasoned foods are usually avoided.

Diabetic Diet.   The diabetic diet is prescribed for a specific diabetic patient. This is due to the fact that the dietary requirements differ with each individual, based on the severity of the disease, the type of insulin therapy administered, the amount of exercise performed, and the weight and age of the patient. The diet is usually measured in grams of protein, carbohydrates, and fats (as well as calories) per day.

Bland Diet.   Often used as an adjunct in the treatment of colitis, gallbladder disease, and gastritis, and postoperatively after abdominal surgery, this diet consists of food that is nonirritating. It *excludes* fried foods, onions, radishes, cabbage, coffee, tea, and very hot, very cold, or highly seasoned foods.

Low-Sodium Diet.   The low-sodium diet is prescribed in any illness in which the patient retains fluids in his body tissue. Sodium (salt) is an element that helps retain fluid in the body tissues. It is restricted in such illnesses as cardiovascular and kidney diseases, and complications of pregnancy. The greatest source of sodium is ordinary table salt (sodium chloride). Generally, all processed meats, meat products, and fish, canned vegetables, and many frozen foods contain more salt than is compatible with low-sodium diets. It should be noted that many natural foods also have small amounts of sodium in them; therefore, some of these foodstuffs may be restricted on the low-sodium diet.

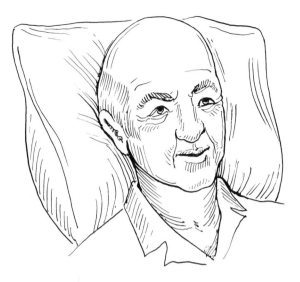

Heart disease — low sodium diet.

ITEM 3. FOOD PREFERENCES

People eat food, not only to satisfy the needs of the body for energy, but also for the feelings of pleasure and satisfaction that accompany eating. Mealtime is a social event for most people, and many joyful occasions in life are celebrated with a feast.

Although food likes and dislikes are an individual matter, many attitudes and habits concerning food are the result of culture and society. National origin influences the types of foods eaten most frequently. Bread is the most important item in the Greek diet, and it is the main course of the meal in many countries. People of German descent like pork, noodles, and sauerkraut. Those of Italian heritage enjoy pastas, greens, and use generous amounts of olive oil in their cooking. People with an Oriental background use rice and fish as staple foods in their diet, and some use strong, spicy herbs for seasoning.

What is considered a food varies from one culture to another. In some places, raw fish, grasshoppers, and fried bat wings are regarded as food delicacies. A French cook prepares gourmet dishes using snails, tripe, and truffles. In the arctic regions, willow greens, salmon, and fish oils are important items in the diet. People in various parts of the United States have strong preferences for some foods. Grits and hominy are popular in many Southern states. Lobster is featured in Maine, baked beans in Boston, and Westerners regard breakfast incomplete unless fried potatoes are served with the ham and eggs.

Food preferences are influenced by religious beliefs. Seventh Day Adventists and the strict Hindus and Buddhists eat no meat. Those of the Jewish faith avoid pork; the orthodox believers do not mix dishes containing meat with those containing milk, and follow other dietary laws.

When people become sick and are hospitalized, they often must make some adjustments in their food preferences and food habits. The patient on a special diet may discover that it doesn't include the foods he usually eats, that spices or seasonings are not permitted, and these changes may be very disturbing to him.

You must understand that the patient's diet is an important part of medical treatment. If the patient is not eating the food in his diet, you should notify your team leader. Other ways may be found to encourage the patient to eat, or the dietician could be called to visit the patient. Often the diet can be adjusted so it is more appealing to the patient without altering the therapeutic effect.

U
N
I
T
16

ITEM 4. WHAT ARE YOUR RESPONSIBILITIES FOR PATIENT NUTRITION?

Nursing personnel cannot separate other elements of patient care from the need to give attention to adequate nutrition. Wash your hands before beginning this procedure. Identify the patient.

A. Before Meals

1. Provide for Elimination. Assist the patient to the bathroom or in using the bedpan/urinal. Offer this assistance before meals without waiting for the patient to ask; interrupting the meal for this activity may cause him physical or psychological distress. Change the infant's diaper, if necessary. Wash your hands.

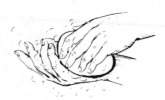

Wash your hands
before serving meals.

2. Give Mouth and Hand Care. Assist the patient to wash his face and hands in preparation for meals. Allow him to brush his teeth (dentures) before his meal. This is important because many sick people have a bad taste in their mouth. If good oral hygiene is not given, their food may taste bad, yet they need nourishment to gain strength.

3. Position the Patient. If he is able, assist him to a chair and place the overbed table in front of him. If he must be in bed, place him in a sitting position, using pillows to support his head if necessary. Ask him if he is comfortable; this is very important if he is to enjoy his meal. Make sure that the overbed table is cleared to receive the food tray.

4. Prepare the Environment. Create an attractive environment for the patient. Be sure that no disturbing articles such as an emesis basin or urinal are in sight during meals. If there are unpleasant odors in the room, spray or place deodorizer in the room. Have the room well-lighted and ventilated, and at a comfortable temperature. Remember, you enjoy your meals more when there is a little "atmosphere"; so will the patient. Wash your hands before serving the tray.

B. During Meals

1. Serve the Diet Trays. Dietary personnel generally prepare the patient's tray either from a central kitchen or from the nursing unit kitchen. Usually, each tray is labeled with the patient's name and room number, and the type of diet. Even though dietary personnel may serve the trays, it is still your responsibility to see that the proper tray is served to your patient. The name on the tray label must match your patient's wristband.

If you are responsible for bringing your patients' trays, first serve those patients who are able to feed themselves. If you bring trays

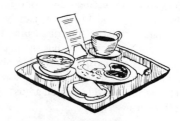

Serve the right tray to
each patient.

first to those who need help, the food for the others will be cold by the time you can return to serve them. Serve one tray at a time to avoid dropping or spilling liquids. When bringing a tray, remember to:

a. Check the name and room number so that you serve the right tray to the right patient.

b. Grasp the tray on the short sides with both hands to avoid spilling.

c. When entering a room with a tray, make sure you have the proper patient by comparing his identification band with the name card on the tray before you place it in front of him.

d. Put the tray on the table with the main dish closest to the patient. Remove the food covers and place them on the bedside table. Assist the patient to butter bread, chop or cut meat and vegetables, and pour his beverage. Place a napkin under his chin. Allow him to do as much as he can. You can proceed easily in most cases and avoid having the patient ask you for assistance.

e. If the patient is in isolation, follow the Isolation Procedure for delivery of food trays. The Isolation Unit comes near the end of the course. You will not be assigned to Isolation patients until you have satisfactorily completed the instructional unit.

C. Feeding Adult Patients

1. Protect the patient's clothing and bed linens with a small towel or extra napkin. Spilling food or fluids is often embarrassing to the patient. It only makes him more aware of his inability to do for himself. Be patient and kind; reassure him that you will help him eat until he is well enough to eat by himself.

2. Position yourself in good body alignment (see lesson, if necessary) at the patient's level. If you are seated (on a high stool or chair), the patient loses his sense of hurry and some of his embarrassment over "causing so much trouble." If you stand beside him, he has the feeling you are hurrying him.

3. There are no set rules as to the amount of each mouthful or the rate at which anyone eats. Estimate the amount of food to be placed on the fork or spoon by the patient's size and age. Older adults, as well as children, take smaller portions at a time and generally require longer periods to chew and swallow. Ask him which food he prefers to start with; some people start with their meat, some with their salad, others with their liquid.

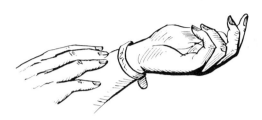

Identify the patient.

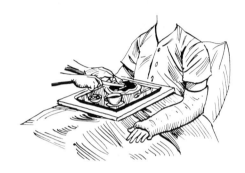

Put main dish closest to patient.

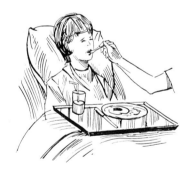

Protect clothing with small towel.

U
N
I
T
16

4. If the patient does not indicate when he wants fluids during his meal, offer fluids after every three to four mouthfuls of solid food. This helps the patient "wash down" food particles. If he wishes, or if it is easier for him, place a straw (preferably flexible) in the cup or glass, grasping the straw at a point near its middle, not at the end which goes in his mouth.

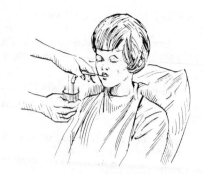

Offer fluids frequently.

5. Allow the patient (or assist him) to wipe his mouth with a napkin at appropriate intervals or as needed. Do not hurry the patient; give small bites, varying the foods. Alternate with liquid. Friendly, interested conversation also helps put the patient at ease and assists his digestion. Test hot food by dropping a small amount on your inner wrist before feeding the patient.

D. Feeding Blind Patients

1. To assist the blind patient who can feed himself place utensils in conventional positions, since that is where he expects to find them.

2. Tell him what foods are being served and give their locations by imagining that the plate is a clock. For example, in the diagram, the bread is at 12:00, the potatoes at 3:00, the beef at 6:00, and the carrots at 9:00.

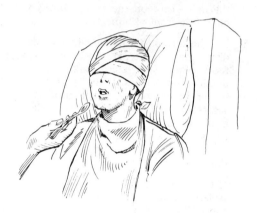

Tell what food is being offered.

3. Try to treat him with every possible respect, giving the help he needs inconspicuously. (Occasionally patients who have had eye injuries or surgery have bandages over both eyes and they require the same procedure as a blind person.)

   When feeding a patient who cannot see, follow the same procedure that is used for all patients who cannot feed themselves.

E. Removing the Tray

Important Steps	Key Points
1. Observe what the patient has eaten.	

Observe what patient has eaten.

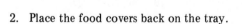

Important Steps	Key Points
2. Place the food covers back on the tray.	Be sure that all items are returned on the soiled tray.
3. Return the tray to the Dietary Department.	Usually trays are taken back to the unit kitchen. From there trays may be returned to the Dietary Department via a dumbwaiter or cart service. Do not leave soiled diet trays on the nursing unit. The dishes and utensils must be washed and ready to serve the next meal. Few agencies have a supply of dishes large

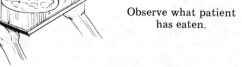

Important Steps	Key Points

Key Points (continued)

enough to permit a set on the nursing unit as well as a clean set in the Dietary Department. Wash your hands.

4. Return to the patient.

Remove the overbed tray. Offer the bedpan/urinal or assist the patient to the bathroom if permitted. Offer a basin and washcloth so that he can wash his hands and face. He may want to brush his teeth after the meal; therefore, you must offer him the opportunity for oral hygiene. Adjust the bed and leave the patient in good body alignment. Tighten the sheets, fluff the pillow and attach the signal cord nearby. Raise the siderails (if indicated). Leave the room neat and tidy.

Reporting and recording your observations about the patient and his diet are very important. The best planned diet is useless unless the patient eats it. These are some of the observations you might make; perhaps you can think of others.

a. How well did the patient eat?

b. What food did he seem to enjoy or dislike?

c. Were the servings of the proper size?

d. What was his attitude toward the diet?

e. Was there any pain or discomfort associated with eating?

f. Did he become fatigued during or after the meal?

g. Were there any conditions that interfered with his ability to eat?

Observation is essential if the patient is to receive maximum benefit from his diet.

5. Ask if there is anything else you can do.

Charting example:

8:00 A.M. Needed much encouragement to eat 1/3 of egg, 1/2 slice toast and 2 tsp of farina.
J. Jones, NA

REMEMBER:

Do not impose your eating habits on the patient.

Occasional friendly comments contribute to a pleasant atmosphere, but lengthy stories are disturbing.

Asking many questions frustrates the patient and interferes with his eating. Perhaps you remember the times when you were in the dentist's chair with various kinds of equipment in your mouth, and the dentist asked questions. How did you feel about it? This is a similar situation.

UNIT 16

ITEM 5.   WHAT YOU MUST KNOW ABOUT FEEDING CHILDREN

A.   Newborn to Two Years of Age

1. Procedure for Feeding Formula. A baby should usually be held while he is being fed. Be sure to cradle his head, neck, and back. (See the accompanying picture.) Holding the infant gives him a sense of security and love, both essential for sound psychological development. Without these, infants can become unresponsive, lose weight, and die.

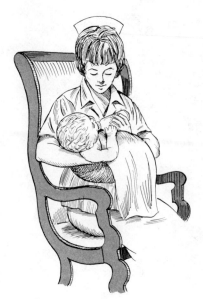

Bottle-feeding.

Never prop the bottle and leave the baby with it. The infant may suck in air or too much fluid too quickly, causing him to vomit. Or he may not be able to vomit the milk, and it could be sucked into his lungs (aspirated), which promptly causes a pneumonia. The result can be dangerous; this type of pneumonia could cause death very quickly.

Infants or toddlers (18 months to 3 years) may require oxygen treatments in an oxygen tent or a Croupette. Because the act of swallowing during eating closes off the airway so that food can pass down the esophagus to the stomach, the infant needs as much oxygen as he can have. Thus, you probably will feed him while he remains in the tent; remember his needs, not yours. Reach through the armlets in the tent or Croupette (or under the edge if your equipment has no arm openings in the side) and support his head and back with your arm as you feed him. Again, this child needs the feeling of love and security that comes from physical contact as you hold him.

Formulas are usually kept refrigerated on the Pediatric and Nursing Units or are ordered from a Central Supply area. The new types of prepared formula need no refrigeration; they are usually stored in an accessible work area near the patients' rooms. The amount, type, and feeding time schedule are ordered by the doctor.

Important Steps	Key Points
1. Approach the infant.	Wash your hands. Identify the child by reading his identification bracelet and compare it with your assignment to be sure that you are feeding the correct formula to the correct child.
2. Obtain the bottle of formula from the storage area.	Verify the label on the bottle to see that it is the correct formula. Check the size of the nipple holes; they should be large enough to permit the baby to get the formula without undue sucking and yet not so large that the milk runs freely. The baby may have difficulty swallowing fast enough, and could choke.
3. Test the size of the nipple holes.	Firmly grasp the bottle in your hand and turn it upside down, with the nipple toward the floor. If a drop of milk gathers on the tip of the nipple, you can be assured that it is the right size. If no milk appears, or the milk flows out

Important Steps	Key Points

Key Points (continued): in a steady stream, discard the nipple and obtain a fresh one.

4. Test the temperature of the formula.

Some formulas must be warmed to take the chill off; for others, this is not necessary. (Check with your agency for its procedure.) If the formula is warmed in a bottle sterilizer, invert the bottle of formula and then let a few drops fall on the inner aspect of your wrist. If it feels hot, it is too warm for the infant. Allow the formula to cool awhile, then test it again before feeding the baby.

5. Pick up the infant.

Carry him like a football — with his head resting in the palm of your hand and his back lying on your arm for support. Hold him close to your body; his feet will fit between your upper arm and your chest. Pick up the bottle of formula.

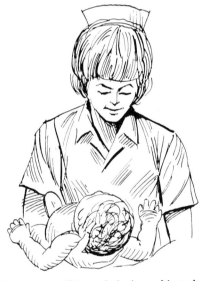

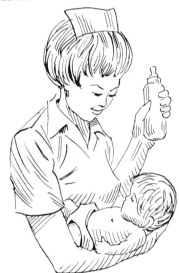

6. Seat yourself in a chair (a rocking chair is preferable).

Place the baby's bottom in your lap and cuddle his neck and head in the bend of your elbow.

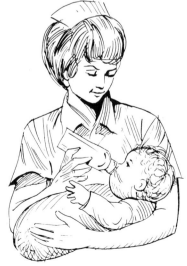

U
N
I
T
16

Important Steps	Key Points

7. Insert the nipple into the baby's mouth.

Rub the nipple gently on the baby's cheek near his mouth. The infant will usually turn his mouth toward the nipple with his mouth open. This is called the rooting reflex and is normal for infants.

8. Hold the bottle to avoid air bubbles.

The bottle should be held at a 45° angle. Be sure that the milk fills the nipple end of the bottle at all times. If you allow the angle to be too great, so that only half of the nipple is covered with milk, the baby will suck air into his stomach, causing it to become distended and painful.

9. Remove the bottle and burp or bubble the baby periodically.

This is usually done after each ounce of formula that is consumed. Raise the baby to a cuddle position with his front side lying on your upper breast. Support his back with one hand while gently patting or rubbing his back with the other hand. This will make it easier to expel any air he might have sucked in.

In some of the newer collapsible feeding bottles, the danger of the baby sucking air into his stomach is almost eliminated. Therefore, you will probably need to burp him only at the end of the feeding.

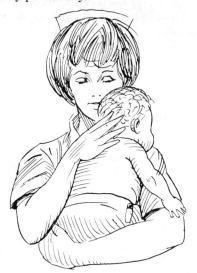

10. Continue feeding.

Continue until the formula is gone, or until the baby seems unwilling to take more. Burp the baby if necessary.

11. Return the infant to his crib.

Be sure that his diaper is dry; if not, change him. Position him comfortably on his side. Be sure that the siderails are up.

12. Rinse and drain the bottle.

Return it to the service area. Tidy the work area.

13. Record the feeding.

Make a notation on the appropriate chart forms. Charting example:

11:00 A.M. 4 oz Similac taken very eagerly. Burped. Diapered. Returned to crib.

J. Jones. LVN

2. **Procedure for Feeding Solid Foods.** Cereals, vegetables, and fruits are usually the first foods introduced to the infant. A small amount of food (usually baby food that comes already prepared in cans or jars) is given with an infant feeding spoon. The spoon should be placed well into the baby's mouth, then pulled outward and upward. If food is not placed well into his mouth, he will push it out again. This is a reflex called the retrusion tongue

reflex; it can be demonstrated by placing a solid or semisolid substance in the front portion of the mouth; the substance will be pushed out almost as quickly as it is placed in the mouth.

When the child is between six and 12 months old, he becomes fascinated with his food. He wants to touch it, play with it, stick it in his hair. *Do not* leave a child for an instant with food in front of him. If you do, guess where you are likely to find it?

B. Feeding the Toddler (18 to 36 Months of Age)

The toddler eats the same food as an older child except that the toddler's meats and vegetables are usually diced or chopped. The early toddler (18 to 24 months) likes to feed himself, and therefore "finger-foods" are introduced. These are items such as diced cooked carrots and chopped beef that the child can feed to himself. During this time, he generally drinks out of a cup. *Do not* serve his liquids in glass containers; at this age he likes to chew and may bite down on a glass. If the child refuses a cup, try offering him a bottle; it may make him feel more secure during his illness.

The older toddler (24 to 36 months) may try to use a utensil to eat with; start with a spoon, not a fork. The fork tines may poke his mouth or gums and prove painful and frustrating for him.

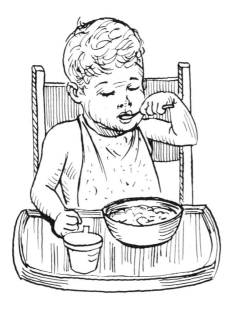

Most three-year-olds self-feed.

C. Feeding the Preschool Child (Three to Six Years)

This age group eats the same foods as the toddler, only in greater quantity. He generally eats with a "junior" fork and spoon, which are smaller than regular utensils. He enjoys eating with other children his age. It is well to have several children eat their meals together at small tables and chairs. Socializing (talking) at mealtimes helps him learn how to act and handle his utensils.

D. After Meals

1. Record the child's intake. Before the tray is removed, write down the amount of fluids taken in on the Intake and Output form. Also check to see if the patient ate well, moderately well, or poorly. Record this on the nurses' notes.

2. Remove the tray to the kitchen or dietary cart. Try not to leave a tray in the patient's room for an extended period of time. Also, the dietary workers have a

UNIT 16

cleaning schedule for trays; they must be washed and ready for serving the next meal.

3. Return to the patient and offer a bedpan/urinal or assist him to the bathroom following a meal.

4. Provide mouth and hand care. Some children brush their teeth and wash their hands following a meal. Give them this opportunity; it is good health practice.

ITEM 6.   HINTS FOR FEEDING CHILDREN

Do Not	Do
Hurry the child.	Praise him at intervals and at the end of the meal.
Punish him for spilling.	Provide opportunities for socializing if possible.
Allow him to drink all his milk first.	Promote and encourage good eating habits.
Leave him unattended by an adult.	
Place dessert on the tray until other foods are eaten.	
Prop the baby's bottle and leave.	

PERFORMANCE TEST

In the skill laboratory, feed your student partner, keeping in mind patient and tray identification procedures. Do not impose your eating habits on the patient, and provide a pleasant environment for him to enjoy his meal.

At the completion of the meal, record pertinent information on the sample nurses' notes.

PERFORMANCE CHECKLIST

ASSIST WITH NUTRITION

1. Provide for elimination before the meal.

2. Give mouth and hand care before the meal.

3. Position the patient and the overbed tray before the meal tray is served.

4. Prepare the environment (tidy the room, remove emesis basins, bedpans, or urinals from the area).

5. Wash your hands before serving the tray.

6. Serve the tray without spilling its contents. Match the tray label with the patient's identification band.

7. Place a napkin under the patient's chin and arrange the food on the tray.

8. Position yourself in good body alignment (standing or sitting) to feed the patient.

9. Test hot foods on the inside of your wrist.

10. Give moderate-sized bites of food. Alternate liquids with solids (1:3 or 1:4). Ask the patient which food he prefers to eat first, i.e., salad, meat, and so forth.

11. Feed slowly, giving him ample time to eat. Carry on a pleasant conversation.

12. Assist with elimination, oral hygiene, and face and hand care on the completion of the meal.

13. Return all dietary items to the appropriate area immediately after the completion of the meal.

14. Leave the patient neat, tidy, and comfortable. Attach the call signal.

15. Tell him the time of your return.

16. Chart your observations on your practice nurses' notes.

POST-TEST

1. Name the four basic food groups:

   a. _____   b. _____

   c. _____   d. _____

2. List at least three nursing measures (responsibilities) to be offered patients before meals:

   a. _____

   b. _____

   c. _____

3. Foods are the sources of three main elements called _____, _____, and

   _____.

4. Complete the following from the Hints for Feeding Children:

   Do not _____

   Do not _____

   Do _____

   Do _____

True or False: Indicate in the column at the left whether the statements are True (mark "T") or False (mark "F").

_____ 5. You must feed all blind patients.

_____ 6. A small packet of salt is acceptable for patients on low-sodium diets.

_____ 7. Milk is not allowed for patients on a clear or surgical diet.

_____ 8. Eating habits are culturally learned.

_____ 9. It is a nursing responsibility to see that patients receive the proper trays.

_____10. Baby bottles may be propped for feeding.

_____11. Toddlers should be left alone to enjoy their meals.

_____12. Warming formulas is only done to take the chill out of them.

_____13. A child's first utensil for feeding himself is a fork.

_____14. Offer the patient fluids only after he has finished all the solid foods.

POST-TEST ANNOTATED ANSWER SHEET

1. a. meat group

   b. milk group

   c. cereals and bread group

   d. vegetables and fruits (pp. 330–331)

2. a. Provide for elimination

   b. Give patient hand and mouth care

   c. Position the patient

   d. Prepare the environment (p. 334)

3. Proteins, carbohydrates, fats (pp. 330–331)

4. *Do not*   Hurry the child.
   Punish him for spilling items.
   Allow him to drink all of his milk first.
   Leave him unattended by an adult.
   Place dessert on tray until other foods are eaten.
   Prop baby's bottle.

   Do   Praise him at intervals and at the end of the meal.
   Provide opportunities for socializing.
   Promote and encourage good eating habits. (p. 342)

5. F   (p. 336)

6. F   (p. 332)

7. T   (p. 332)

8. T   (p. 333)

9. T   (p. 334)

10. F   (p. 338)

11. F   (p. 342)

12. T   (p. 339)

13. F   (p. 341)

14. F   (p. 336)

UNIT 16

Unit 17

FLUID INTAKE
AND OUTPUT

I. DIRECTIONS TO THE STUDENT

Proceed through this lesson. When you have finished, take the post test. See your instructor about an appointment to demonstrate the measuring and recording of fluids.

II. GENERAL PERFORMANCE OBJECTIVE

When you have finished the unit, you will be able to measure accurately oral fluid intake and fluid output, and maintain records as required for determination of fluid balance.

III. SPECIFIC PERFORMANCE OBJECTIVES

Following this lesson, you will be able to:

1. Identify all food items that should be measured as fluid intake.

2. Correctly convert volumetric measurements from English and household units to metric units.

3. Measure fluid volume accurately with a graduated container.

4. Give instructions appropriate to the condition and sex of a patient for voiding of bodily wastes in a manner that will permit their measurement.

5. Keep accurate quantitative records of oral fluid intake and fluid output, and make determinations of total I & O as required by physician's orders.

6. Record appropriate qualitative observations on fluid output.

7. Recognize, note, and report symptoms of edema and dehydration, and conditions of unusual or excessive fluid output.

8. Define frequently used terms that refer to mechanisms and conditions of fluid balance.

IV. VOCABULARY

anuria—failure of the kidneys to secrete urine; total lack of urination.
ascites—collection of fluid in the peritoneal or abdominal cavity.
bladder—a hollow muscular reservoir in the lower abdominal cavity for temporary storage of urine before it is expelled from the body.
dehydration—process that occurs when output of water from the tissues exceeds water intake.
diaphoresis—profuse sweating.
diuretic—an agent or medication that increases the secretion of urine.
edema—a condition in which the body tissues contain an excessive amount of fluid, causing swelling of the tissue; may be localized or generalized in the body.

346

electrolytes—chemicals that in solution separate into charged particles called ions, which can conduct an electrical current; sodium chloride (ordinary table salt) separates into sodium and chloride ions in the body fluids.

fluid balance—a condition of the body that exists when fluid intake approximately equals the amount of fluid lost from the body.

fluid compartments—the main fluid spaces: (1) *intracellular space* (filled with the liquid cytoplasm of cells) contains about two-thirds of the body water; and (2) *extracellular space* (outside cells) includes the space around cells, filled with interstitial fluid, and the space within blood vessels, containing the liquid blood plasma.

force fluids—a special order requiring the patient to take in an additional amount of fluids during short periods of time; often used in cases with fever.

hypodermoclysis—the injection of fluids into the tissues just below the skin (subcutaneous) to supply the body with liquids when fluids cannot be taken by mouth or IV; commonly called clysis.

kidneys—two glandular, bean-shaped bodies situated at the back of the abdominal cavity, one on each side of the spinal column just below the waist, that excrete urine (liquid waste matter).

nourishments—extra foods, usually liquids, given between meals to supplement the diet (e.g., milk, fruit juices, crackers, ice cream, cookies).

oliguria—diminished amount and frequency of urination.

polyuria—excessive secretion and discharge of urine.

urethra—a small tube approximately ¼ inch in diameter, 1½ inches long in the female and 8 to 9 inches long in the male, extending from the bottom end of the bladder to the outside of the body; the urine is expelled through the urethra.

urine—the liquid wastes filtered from the blood by the kidneys, stored in the bladder, and discharged through the urethra.

V. KNOWLEDGE BASIC TO THIS LESSON

ITEM 1. THE IMPORTANCE OF BODY FLUIDS

Water is vital to health and to survival. Body water is essential as the environment for chemical changes occurring in the cells, as the means for keeping the body temperature stable, and to give structure and form to body tissues.

In order for the body to function properly, the water must be in the needed amounts and distributed in the right proportions in the fluid compartments of the body. Body water inside the cells makes up the largest fluid compartment, or about 45 per cent of the total body weight of an adult and even more in a child. Fluid located outside the cells averages 20 per cent of the body weight. It consists of the body water that surrounds the tissues, the blood, the plasma, and the various secretions such as the digestive juices, tears, bile, and spinal fluid, to name a few.

Fluid Balance. The body maintains fluid balance when the amount of water taken in approximately equals the amount of water eliminated. The fluids and foods of the diet provide most of the water needed each day. A small amount of water is produced during cellular metabolism as energy is released. Water is eliminated from the body in the urine, perspiration, feces and exhaled air. Some typical volumes of water intake and output for an adult in a 24-hour period are these:

INTAKE		OUTPUT	
Liquid	1500 ml	Urine	1400 ml
Food	800 ml	Sweat	500 ml
Metabolism	200 ml	Feces	200 ml
		Respiration	400 ml
Totals	2500 ml		2500 ml

UNIT 17

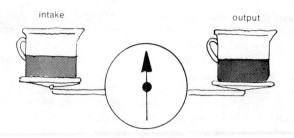

This would indicate fluid balance for this person. The amount of fluid taken in and eliminated varies in health with the temperature, activity, and habits of the person, and other factors. So vital is water to survival that if fluid intake is decreased, the body will conserve fluid by decreasing the amount of urine secreted. This is an important fact for health workers to know.

Fluid and Electrolyte Balance in Illness. Illness can markedly disturb the delicate balance of body fluids and electrolytes. Large amounts of fluids may be lost from the body by diaphoresis (profuse sweating) or in vomitus or diarrhea. Drainage from wounds and nasogastric suction remove body fluids and electrolytes. Of course, hemorrhage or loss of interstitial fluid from a large burned surface disturbs fluid balance. These losses are especially serious for an infant or young child because more of his body tissues are liquid than are those of an adult. Sometimes it is necessary to restrict the oral intake of fluids because of nausea, vomiting, or diseases of the intestinal tract. Most surgical patients are ordered to be NPO (nothing by mouth) for a time both preoperatively and postoperatively. To maintain fluid balance under these conditions, fluids are given parenterally, that is, intravenously (into a vein) or by hypodermoclysis (into the subcutaneous tissue, or under the skin). The latter procedure is often used for infants, young children, and the elderly.

Dehydration. If more fluids are lost from the body than are taken in, dehydration results. The symptoms of dehydration include thirst, dry skin and mucous membranes, constipation, oliguria, and a fall in blood pressure accompanied by a weak, rapid pulse.

Edema and Ascites. Do you recall the fact that body fluids must be distributed properly in the fluid compartments in order to maintain fluid balance? Sometimes, excess fluid accumulates in the spaces around the cells, a condition that is called edema. Symptoms of edema include weight gain, and swelling of the subcutaneous spaces, particularly of the feet and ankles, or of the face and hands.

Fluids can accumulate in the peritoneal (abdominal) cavity, and this condition is called ascites. Symptoms of ascites include weight gain, abdominal distention, and dyspnea (from the abdominal pressure).

Nursing Role in Maintaining Fluid Balance. An important responsibility of the nurse is to assist with the maintenance of body fluid and electrolyte balance. This involves providing and encouraging oral fluids according to individual needs, measuring and accurately reporting fluid intake and fluid loss, and then informing the doctor if the patient is not maintaining an adequate fluid balance so that he can order parenteral fluids if necessary.

The urinary output accounts for the largest volume of water eliminated from the body. In health, the color of urine varies from a light yellow to an amber. The amount of urine produced is influenced by:

1. fluid intake

2. body temperature — fever increases sweating and decreases urine production.

3. blood pressure — a serious drop in blood pressure decreases urine production.

4. age — infants produce three to four times more urine for their weight than do adults.

5. disease conditions — kidney disease may result in either increased or decreased urine production; other disorders also affect kidney function.

Question 1. By now you should know three important uses of body fluids. These are:

a. _____

b. _____

c. _____ .

Question 2. What would a typical daily urinary output be for a healthy adult?

_____ .

Question 3. Match the term with the correct definition.

_____ ascites   a. profuse sweating

_____ dehydration   b. scanty urine output

_____ diaphoresis   c. fluid in peritoneal cavity

_____ edema   d. parenteral fluid

_____ hypodermoclysis   e. swollen ankles

_____ oliguria   f. Na^+ (sodium particles with an
                                       electrical charge)

_____ ion
                                   g. Fluid intake exceeds fluid output

                                   h. Fluid output exceeds fluid intake

ITEM 2. MEASURING

Oral Intake. The average active adult requires from 2000 to 3000 ml (cc) of fluid per day, which is 2 to 3 quarts. Some agencies use cc's or cubic centimeters synonymously with ml (milliliters). See Appendix A for conversion tables.

Generally, the physician orders the recording of I & O for his patient. He sometimes limits the amount of fluid the patient may have in a 24-hour period. If fluids are to be limited check with your team leader or RN for the amount you must give during your 8 hours of duty. *Do not guess.* Many hospitals designate 50 per cent of limited fluids be given on the day shift, 30 per cent for the afternoon shift and 20 per cent during the night hours.

Know how much fluid is contained in a water pitcher and in dietary dishes. This information may be obtained from your team leader or from the dietary personnel. There may be some minor variations from agency to agency.

To check the oral intake at mealtimes, you must look at the tray before it is removed from the patient's room. *Don't* count on the patient or the dietary personnel to tell you. This is *your* responsibility. The fluids you must measure on the tray include: water, coffee, tea, Jello (gelatin), ice cream and sherbet, carbonated drinks, wine, consommé, juices, milk, cream, milk shakes, infant cereals, and broth or soup.

Because dietary items are served in household measures (cups, bowls and glasses), you will have to convert these into ml measurements. List them in numbers of ml (or cc), and record

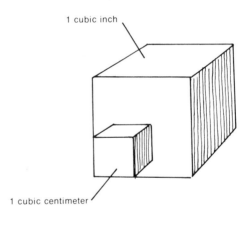

1 cubic inch

1 cubic centimeter

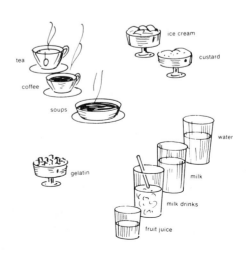

tea

coffee

soups

ice cream

custard

water

milk

milk drinks

gelatin

fruit juice

the time they were taken. Some agencies also want you to list the type of fluid, e.g., orange juice 180 ml. Write this in the column headed *Intake* on the I & O record.

The method of measuring the amount the patient drinks from the water pitcher may be one of the following:

Record each amount of liquid the patient drinks.

Measure the amount left in the water pitcher and subtract it from the amount in a full pitcher.

If the patient can take only ice chips by mouth, ask your team leader or dietitian to determine the number of ml per ice chip. However, you may estimate that there are approximately 5 ice chips to an average ice cube (see Appendix A for ml in average ice cube).

At the end of your 8-hour tour of duty, you will add the total intake and write the amount on the I & O record. Some patients are on I & O at more frequent intervals, and if so, you would add intake when specified and enter it on the record. I & O may be recorded every hour for some seriously ill patients.

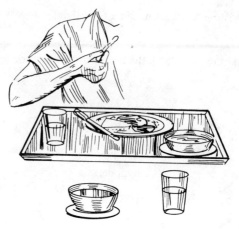

Fractions: 1/2 bowl of soup; 2/3 glass of milk
Metric: 180 cc. ÷ 2 = 90 cc.
            240 cc. ÷ 3 = 80 cc.

ITEM 3. URINE OUTPUT

Generally, urinary output ranges between 30 ml (cc) to as much as several hundred ml per hour depending on the amount of intake. The average urinary output in a 24-hour period is 1400 to 1600 ml; you should report an output of less than 500 ml in a 24-hour period. In health, urinary output is approximately equal to the volume of liquids taken in.

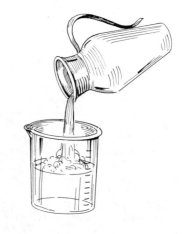

To measure urinary output, pour the urine from the bedpan or urinal into a measuring cup, commonly called a "graduate." Place the cup on a flat surface for accurate measurement. Note the level reached by the top of the fluid. Record under the column marked *Output*. Designate the time and the amount in ml. If you notice when pouring the urine in the toilet that it is a different color from the usual yellow or amber, or smells sweet or sour, note this on the patient's chart. Describe the color, amount, and odor, and report them to your team leader immediately.

If the patient is ambulatory, be sure to tell him that you are measuring his urine output. Ask him either to urinate into a urinal or bedpan (placed under the toilet seat), or to use a measuring cup and save the urine for you to dispose of later. If the patient has diarrhea, you may follow the same procedure as with urine, for it too is excreted fluid. If he has vomited into a container, measure the contents as output. If not, estimate the amount of vomitus as small, moderate, or large. Describe the color and odor on the nurses' notes. If a patient has diarrhea, or is vomiting or sweating profusely (diaphoresis), indicate this in the nurses' notes and report to your charge nurse. Also, if these conditions are present, the patient may have less urinary output because he is losing fluid through these other routes. You will practice recording these remarks on a sample of the nurses' notes and I & O sheet at the completion of this lesson.

Given a patient who has been placed on I & O, instruct him in the agency procedure, and practice measuring and recording his intake and output.

Preliminary to the Steps

Find out if the patient is on I & O.

Determine from your team leader or Kardex if the patient is on I & O, and at which time interval: every 2, 4, or 8 hours? Determine the specific amount to be given within your 8-hour tour of duty (sample of the Kardex is included with this unit).

Ask if a conversion table is available.

Ask your team leader if there is a list that converts household measures to ml. If not, you might ask the team leader to obtain one from Dietary.

Important Steps	Key Points
1. Tell the patient that you are recording his fluid intake and output.	Explain that all the fluids taken in (by mouth, IV, clysis) and all fluid output are to be measured. Ask him to urinate or void in a graduate, bedpan, or urinal, and *not to flush it down the toilet*. Some patients will record their own intake. If so, provide a pencil and the record for the patient. This may be done *if* it is an acceptable agency policy. Place an I & O Record in the patient's room. This is determined by the agency policy. Write the patient's name and room number and the date on the form. (Sample forms are included at the end of this unit.) Remember — items considered as intake are: water (H_2O), Jello (gelatin), ice cream, carbonated drinks, consommé, milk, milk shakes, broth or soup, coffee, tea, sherbet, wine, juices, cream, and infant cereals.
2. Check the water pitcher when beginning your tour of duty.	Some agencies have the off-going personnel fill water pitchers — if so, check to see if it is full and how many ml (cc) it holds; each agency has its own measurement-equivalent charts. If it was not filled, and the patient is not on restricted fluids, fill the pitcher with fresh water. *Remember* to check to see if the patient is NPO (nothing by mouth) for surgery or tests.
3. Check fluids at meals and nourishment times.	Check the patient's tray *before* removing it from the room. Check the amount of fluids taken in, convert household measures to ml (cc)

UNIT 17

Important Steps	Key Points
	and record on the Intake Record. If your agency prefers, record the amount, type of fluid, and time taken.
4. Record intake.	Intake may be totaled and recorded every 1, 2, 4, or 8 hours on the patient's chart, and either on the special I & O sheet or the nurses' notes (check your agency procedure). The fluid in the water pitcher may be recorded by the number of glasses of water taken *or* by subtracting the amount left in the pitcher from the total amount it holds. Follow your agency policy.
5. Measure output. 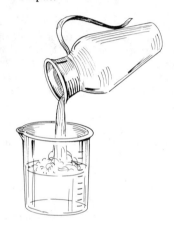	If the patient is ambulatory, remind him that you are measuring his output, and he must save all output for you to measure and record. Ask a male patient to void (urinate) in a urinal, which you can leave in the bathroom, or in the graduate. For female patients, either place the bedpan under the toilet seat or ask the patient to void into the measuring cup (graduate). Pour the urine into the graduate. Place the graduate on a flat surface. Read the number at the top of the fluid level.
6. Record the output.	Make a note on the I & O Record each time the patient urinates so you don't forget. Remember, if he vomits into a basin, or has diarrhea in a bedpan, you should measure these the same as urine. Be sure to indicate if the output is urine, diarrhea, or vomitus. In the nurses' notes, make a comment if the patient sweats profusely (diaphoresis), for this too is output.
7. Dispose of output.	If a specimen is not needed for analysis, pour the output into the toilet. Pour cold water into the graduate, rinse it, and empty it into the toilet — not the sink. Flush the toilet. Return the container to the storage area — usually in the bedside stand.

VII. ADDITIONAL INFORMATION FOR ENRICHMENT

Your instructor will give additional reading assignments if you are interested in learning more about fluid balance for your patient.

Accurate measurements and recordings of Intake and Output amounts are critical for some patients and are vital for patients for whom these procedures are ordered. Your strict attention to the accurate measurement and recording of the information is a clear indication to the patient of your concern and interest in his welfare. The information is also extremely valuable and necessary to the physician so that he can prescribe further therapies for his patient. Be alert and accurate.

WORKBOOK ANSWER SHEET

Question 1. a. to regulate body temperature and make body fluids, such as blood and digestive juices.

b. to help eliminate waste products; as a major constituent of cells.

c. for the movement of solutes between cells and blood.

2. 1400 – 1600 ml

3. c.

h.

a.

e.

d.

b.

f.

PERFORMANCE TEST

I. For this performance test you will need the Oral Intake and Output Unit, an Intake/Output Bedside Record (see pages 356–357), a pen, water, and the equipment set up in the skill laboratory for these experiments.

A. Identify the *paper cup*. Fill it to the top. Using a graduate pitcher to measure, answer the following:

    1. How many ml does it hold? _____

    2. How many ml would be needed to fill the paper cup half-full? _____

    3. Fill it half-full and note the level. Repeat the procedure for one-third full _____

       and two-thirds full. _____

B. Identify the *water glass*. Fill it to the top. Answer the following:

    1. How many ml does it hold? _____

    2. Number of ml when one-third full? _____

    3. Number of ml when half-full? _____

    4. Number of ml when two-thirds full? _____

Fill the glass to each of the above levels and note the water level.

C. List four items that you would be recording on the *I & O* sheet.

    1. _____ .

    2. _____ .

    3. _____ .

    4. _____ .

D. 1. Refer to the Bedside Intake/Output sheet and record how many ml the soup bowl will hold. _____

    2. Fill the soup bowl with this amount to check your answer. If the patient drank all but *four* tablespoons of his soup, how many ml would he have consumed? (1 tbs = 15 ml) _____

    3. How many ml would be left in the soup bowl? _____

E. Refer to the Bedside Intake/Output sheet and fill the water pitcher *half-full*.

    1. How many ml would this take? _____

    2. How many ml would be needed to fill the water pitcher two-thirds full? _____

    3. How many ml would be needed to fill the water pitcher one-third full? _____

    4. How many ml would be needed to fill the water pitcher one-fourth full? _____

F. Refer to the Bedside Intake/Output sheet and note the ml contained in a small (sm) emesis basin and in the standard (std) emesis basin.

    1. Record in ml the difference in amounts between a small emesis basin and a standard emesis basin. _____

    2. If a patient vomited 250 ml, how full would a standard emesis basin be? _____ Fill the basin with this amount of water to check your answer.

II. For this test you will need the following equipment:

1. I & O record form.

2. Graduated container.

3. A set of bottles or any containers, arranged in random order, each containing some quantity of water previously measured and recorded by the instructor, and labeled as follows:

    a. Urine specimen 2:30 P.M.

    b. Urine specimen 3:45 P.M.

    c. Urine specimen 4:30 P.M.

    d. Vomitus 3:00 P.M.

    e. Water pitcher: Contents as of 4:00 P.M.
                  Filled to 2000 ml capacity at 2:00 P.M.

    f. One pint of orange juice

4. Toilet and sink available for use in test.

Instructions to the student: You have a patient on 2-hour I & O. His record is complete through 2:00 P.M., which is the end of the last I & O period. The sample form as filled out represents his I & O since 2:00 P.M. You are to measure and record his I & O in the order in which they normally would have been recorded according to the times shown on the labels on the bottles. Carry out all operations just as you would if these were actual specimens. You have 20 minutes to complete this assignment.

INTAKE – OUTPUT RECORD

BEDSIDE RECORD

Mrs. Jane Rowe   *333*

PATIENT'S NAME   ROOM NO.

INTAKE		INTRAVENOUS SOLUTIONS	OUTPUT		
7-3:30 LIQUIDS	C. C.	C. C.	VOIDED	EMESIS	DRAINAGE ETC.
8^{00} fruit juice	100 cc.	1000 CC.	7^{30} 300 cc.		
9^{30} water	210 cc.	5% D/W			
11^{15} water	210				
11^{30}		500 cc. 5% med.	11^{00} 500 cc.		
12^{15} coffee	180 cc.		2^{00} 400 cc.		
3-11	100	1500	1200		
11-7					

EQUIVALENTS

CUP	180 CC	SOUP BOWL CHILDS	110 CC
PAPER CUP LG	210 CC	SOUP BOWL ADULTS	190 CC
PAPER CUP MED	150 CC	SOUP BOWL LARGE	210 CC
WATER GLASS	210 CC	WATER PITCHER	950 CC
FR JU GLASS	150 CC		
TEA POT	250 CC		
JELLO	100 CC	EMESIS BASIN STD	500 CC
ICE CREAM	120 CC	EMESIS BASIN SM	300 CC

154-1 Saint Johns's Hospital — Santa Monica, California

1050SR

SAINT JOHN'S HOSPITAL
SANTA MONICA, CALIFORNIA

Mrs Jane Rowe RM. 333

#1279356   Dr. Doe

INTAKE AND OUTPUT SUMMARY

	Oral Fluids c.c.	Parenteral Fluids c.c.	Weight of Patient	Urine c.c.	Emesis c.c.	Drainage (Wangenstein) etc. c.c.	Excess persp., diarrhea or hemorrhage	Total Intake c.c.	Total Output c.c.
Date: 3/15/72									
7-3	700 cc.	1500 cc.		1200 cc.	0	0	0	220 cc.	1200 cc.
3-11									
11-7									
TOTAL — 24 Hour Period									
Date: 3/16/72									
7-3									
3-11									
11-7									
TOTAL — 24 Hour Period									
Date: 3/17/72									
7-3									
3-11									
11-7									
TOTAL — 24 Hour Period									
Date: 3/18/72									
7-3									
3-11									
11-7									
TOTAL — 24 Hour Period									
Date: 3/19/72									
7-3									
3-11									
11-7									
TOTAL — 24 Hour Period									

Form No: 150-I
5/63

UNIT 17

PERFORMANCE CHECKLIST

Measurements will vary according to the size of the cups, glasses, soup bowls, water pitchers, and emesis basins used.

ORAL INTAKE AND OUTPUT

1. Measure and record intake and output in correct sequence (as indicated by time tables).

2. Measure each output specimen correctly and enter results in ml or cc in correct column. Clean and store equipment appropriately.

3. Convert pint measurement correctly to ml or cc.

4. Measure contents of water pitcher correctly and calculate water intake correctly; refill as required.

5. Calculate and enter correct totals for 2:00 to 4:00 P.M. intake (e and f) and output (a, b, and c).

6. Measure and record 4:30 P.M. urine specimen after calculation and entry of 2:00 and 4:00 P.M. totals.

7. Make complete record on I & O form for 2:00 to 4:00 P.M.

8. Complete assignment within a time limit of 20 minutes.

APPENDIX A

CONVERSION TABLE

Metric Measurement	Apothecary Measurement	Avoirdupois Measurement
1 ml or 1 cc	15 minims	
4 ml or 4 cc	60 minims	1 teaspoon
30 ml or 30 cc	1 fluid ounce	1 ounce
500 ml or 500 cc	1 pint	
1000 ml or 1000 cc	1 quart	
240 ml or 240 cc	1 cup (8 ounces)	
15 ml or 15 cc	1 tablespoon	
4 ml or 4 cc	1 teaspoon	
40 ml or 40 cc	1 average size ice cube (equal to 10 teaspoons)	
	5 ice chips to 1 ice cube	

Note: Because different agencies use dishes of varying sizes, *be sure* to ask for a table converting household measures to metric (cc or ml) measures used in your agency.

POST-TEST

Situation: Your patient is an adult male. His intake and output are to be recorded every four hours. Total intake and output were last recorded at 12 noon. At 12:30 P.M. the patient had lunch. He was served a bowl of soup (10 ounces), a cup of Jello (gelatin) (8 ounces), and one-half pint of milk. When you removed the tray, the milk and Jello (gelatin) had been consumed. Six tablespoons of soup remained in the bowl. His water pitcher at noon contained 900 ml. At 2:00 P.M. he urinated; you measured his output as 25 ml. At 3:00 P.M. he urinated again; you measured his output as 35 ml. At 3:15 P.M. he vomited (into a container; you measured the amount as 80 ml. At 4:00 P.M. you checked his water pitcher; it contained 600 ml of water.

1. The patient's fluid intake at lunch should be recorded as:

    a. _____ ml of soup

    b. _____ ml of milk

    c. _____ ml of Jello (gelatin)

2. You should record his total intake and output for the period from _____ to _____ at _____ .

3. His total fluid intake for this period is _____ ml.

4. His total fluid output for this period is _____ ml.

5. His urinary output indicates that he might have _____ .

6. If you have an ambulatory patient on Intake and Output, you should: (check the correct items only)

    a. _____ remove his water pitcher so that his fluid intake can be controlled.

    b. _____ tell him not to drink any fluids during the night.

    c. _____ make sure he has a container in which to urinate.

    d. _____ tell him to inform you whenever he needs to urinate.

    e. _____ tell him not to flush his urine down the toilet.

    f. _____ provide the patient with materials for recording his own urinary output if this is agency policy.

    g. _____ if the patient is NPO, allow him to drink only water.

    h. _____ if the patient vomits, note the color and odor of his vomitus.

    i. _____ if the patient sweats profusely, note the color and odor of his sweat.

    j. _____ measure and record all fluid intake except what the patient drinks at regular meals.

    k. _____ if a urine specimen is not needed for analysis, pour the urine into the toilet and rinse out the graduate into the sink.

7. When you measure or observe the amount of urine or vomitus, you should also observe its _____ and its _____ and describe these observations in your _____ .

U
N
I
T
17

8. Indicate by check marks which of the following items should be included among a patient's fluid intake:

a. water _____   e. custard _____   i. spinach _____

b. tea _____   f. gelatin _____   j. noodles _____

c. milk _____   g. fruit juice _____   k. cheese _____

d. apples _____   h. ice cream _____   l. potatoes _____

9. Indicate by check marks which of the following are factors that affect the amount and rate of urine production:

a. fluid intake _____   d. pain _____

b. dehydration _____   e. body temperature _____

c. body weight _____   f. kidney disorders _____

POST-TEST ANNOTATED ANSWER SHEET

1. a. 210 (p. 356)

    b. 250

    c. 240

2. 12 noon to 4:00 P.M.; 4:00 P.M. (p. 350)

3. 1000 (p. 349)

4. 140 (p. 350)

5. edema (p. 348)

6. c, d, and e (p. 350)

7. odor, color, nurses' notes (p. 351)

8. a, b, c, e, f, g, and h (p. 349)

9. all (p. 348)

CHARTING

I. DIRECTIONS TO THE STUDENT

Study this lesson thoroughly. Note the word that applies to the part of the body or behavior, then note the terms defining the idea that describes a body part or action. Following this section, you will find standardized, acceptable, technical terms that may be used in charting. Although the terms suggested for use in charting do not make complete sentences, they are clear, concise, and accurate.

Visualize a situation to be charted, for example, the morning bath given and an enema given. Check the sample charting provided, then use the listed terms to write a sample charting assignment. Be prepared to describe in acceptable technical terms an observation, treatment, or situation suggested by the instructor.

Refer to this lesson frequently for ideas on how to describe patient care, treatment, observation, or reaction to therapy. Refer to the sample charting provided as a guide.

II. GENERAL PERFORMANCE OBJECTIVE

You will be able to enter a written account on a patient's chart of the patient's health history, the therapy given, the patient's reaction to therapy, and your observation of a patient situation. Use of suggested charting terms will provide a safe, legally acceptable account of a patient's situation.

III. SPECIFIC PERFORMANCE OBJECTIVES

Upon completion of this module, you will be able to:

1. Record information legibly.

2. Properly record information pertaining to the patient that will assure safety for him, the hospital, and the health worker.

3. Describe the exact time, effect, and reaction of the patient to therapy or treatment rendered.

4. Describe the character and amount of drainage, vomitus, stools, urine, or hemorrhage (bleeding) from the body.

5. Describe the type, onset, location, and duration of pain.

6. Note the time, type of visit, examination, and reaction of the patient when the physician or other health worker attends to him.

7. Describe the patient's condition — usual, unusual, or changed.

8. Adapt to the requirements of different health facilities.

9. Use clear, concise terms that plainly describe a situation pertaining to the patient and that will be quickly understood.

10. Use problem-oriented record (POR) charting.

IV. INTRODUCTION

Charting: The Written Picture. Charting presents a written picture of occurrences and situations pertaining to a patient. All records are strictly confidential and are not to be read or discussed by anyone except the physician or persons directly caring for the patient in a hospital or medical care facility.

Charting is required for each medication, treatment, or nursing procedure. Accounts of the patient's condition and activities must be charted accurately and in clear terms. Terse statements are essential. The chart is a legal document and is the property of the hospital or health facility. The law requires that a record be kept of the patient care. Charting must be done so that it is meaningful days, months, or years later in case it must be used in court. This is why standardized charting terms are used. Each medical worker knows and recognizes the meaning of these terms and they are not likely to be misconstrued in court. Practice charting your activities as you complete the specific instructional unit.

Accounts of the patient's condition are hand-printed or written, and signed with a handwritten signature of the person doing the charting. Only standard medical abbreviations and terms are used. If you are in doubt about abbreviations, consult a medical dictionary or books of terms and abbreviations.

Viewed from a legal standpoint, charting is one of the most significant duties that the health worker performs. Charting the admission of a patient is especially important because it provides a written picture of the patient when he is admitted. By using the form, one may call attention to many things that otherwise might be forgotten. These things are described in correct charting terms in the nurses' notes, as indicated in the following samples. It is especially important to note all the subjective symptoms and even more important to note all the objective symptoms, such as abrasions, burns, pressure sores, or any abnormal appearance of a body part. A notation is also made of the patient's mental condition.

It is essential to record on the chart that the physician was notified of the patient's condition. The time when he was called should be noted as well as the symptoms or change in a patient's condition that required the call.

Problem-Oriented Record (POR). The hospital care of patients has traditionally been divided into medical care and nursing care, each recorded in separate parts of the patient's chart. Since the late 1960's, a new system of recording has gained acceptance as a method of focusing on patient care, not medical or nursing care. This is the problem-oriented record, or POR, first introduced by Dr. Lawrence Weed. POR provides a method of communicating *what*, *when*, and *how* things are to be done in order to meet the needs of the patient.

The problem-oriented record contains four basic parts: the data base, the problem list, the plan, and the progress notes. The precise form these records take will vary greatly between agencies. The data base contains information of a routine nature about the patient, including a general health history, the findings of the physical examination, and the results of physiological and laboratory tests. It also contains information about the patient's lifestyle, family, and social relations, as well as his response to illness as determined in the nurse's assessment. The data base is a collection of information that can follow the patient from the hospital to an outpatient basis and back again. It isn't necessary to repeat the process of making out a new data base every time someone else takes care of the patient, although new information can be added to the record to provide an up-to-date description of the patient.

In the POR, a problem is some situation or aspect of the patient's health that interferes with his physical or psychological comfort, or his ability to function, or that threatens his survival. From the information provided by the data base, the patient's problems are identified and listed on a form that is usually the first document in the patient's chart. The list of problems is dynamic; new problems are added as they develop and others become inactive as they are resolved. If POR is used in your agency, the problem list provides you with immediate information about the patient's needs for care. The plan for actions related to managing the problem is included as part of the progress notes.

The POR progress notes are a section of the chart that contains the findings, assessment, plans, and orders of the doctors, nurses, and other therapists involved in the care of the patient. All chart on the same form, and the progress notes are charted using the SOAP format.

S = Subjective information obtained from the patient, his relatives, or a similar source.

O = Objective information based on the health team's observations of the patient, the physical examination, or diagnostic or laboratory tests.

A = Assessment, which refers to the analysis of the patient's problem.

P = Plan of action to be taken to resolve the problem.

Progress notes contain the date and the title of the problem with the information recorded in the SOAP format. It is not necessary to chart all problems each day, nor will it be possible to include each SOAP element in each note. After the initial plan, additional plans are the changes and revisions made as a result of the evaluation of the previous action.

An essential element of the POR system of charting is the flow sheet. Flow sheets are used to record routine information, recurring observations, and data that are repeatedly recorded. Flow sheets are designed by the agency to include the information needed to show routine nursing care and specific treatments. Vital signs, baths, bowel movements, diet, pain, medications, and other activities are included on these forms. Flow sheets may be used for specific assessment data, such as in the CCU for cardiac function and blood gases, for diabetes, for head injuries, and so forth.

In summary, POR charting accomplishes the following:

1. Focuses on the patient and his problems.

2. Improves communications among all those caring for the patient.

3. Reduces the cost of health care by deleting needless duplication of information and recording.

4. Provides for confidentiality by allowing release of information on specific problems, and separation of sensitive data without the need to release the whole chart.

5. Provides control of the quality of care by making the patient data, assessments, and plans available to those giving care so there is less chance that some problem will be overlooked.

6. Provides a method for evaluating the importance and meaning of the patient's concerns.

Charting Error Correction. It is possible to make an error when charting. Since the chart is a legal document, an erasure is not permitted. If a word is wrong or misspelled, or is written on a wrong chart, it may be corrected in the following manner:

Note that an error was made by writing "sitz bath" instead of "shower." It is legally correct to draw one line through the incorrect word or error and write the word "error" above it, and then proceed with the charting. It is suggested that sample charting be done on scrap paper before writing on the chart until you are sure of how you want to describe an action. Words that you are unsure of should be looked up in the dictionary.

If you charted an entry on the wrong chart, you may need to recopy an entire page of notes. Cross out the error as stated above. Place the incorrect page at the back of the chart.

Remember, *all* charting becomes a permanent part of the patient's legal record. *Never* destroy incorrect charting; it must be kept with the patient's chart. Remember that the original cannot be copied by you unless you sign your name after the original signature, i.e., Jane Doe, RN/Mary White, NA. The preferred method is to have the person who charted the original note rewrite his own signature.

V. CHARTING PROCEDURE

Problem-Oriented Charting. When using the POR system of charting, the first record on the chart is usually the Master Problem List with all the problems listed using Arabic numbers. The data base information is included in the chart along with the Progress Notes, forms for reports of laboratory and diagnostic procedures, consents, and various flow sheets used by the particular agency. Observations, orders, and data regarding the patient's problems are charted on the Progress Notes by the doctors, nurses, and therapists, using the SOAP format. All write on the same form, so you may find entries made by the nurse following those made by the respiratory therapist, and the doctor's notes entered after those of the nurse.

Flow sheets supplement the Progress Notes charting. Routine types of care and information are recorded on the flow sheets, while the unusual or exceptional data are charted on the Progress Notes. Some examples of charting on the Progress Notes are included below:

Example 1. SOAP format (initial admission)

Date	Time	Problem	Progress Notes
6/11	7 P.M.	1	Admitted at 6:30 P.M.

      S Complains of feeling warm and restless.

      O Face appears flushed, skin warm to touch.
           T 101°F.   P 120.   R 24.   B/P 160/90.

      A Fever of unknown origin.

      P Call physician for treatment orders; provide tepid water sponge bath.

          Retake temperature 10–15 minutes after sponge bath.

| 6/11 | 8 P.M. | 2 | |

      S Complains of being hot. States neck is stiff and hurts. Headache and feeling of nausea.

      O Appears flushed; skin unusually warm.
           T 104°F.   P 132 Thready.   R 28.   B/P 166/90.
           Projectile-type emesis.
           Body position — opisthotonos.

      A Fever with meningeal irritation.

      P Notify physician of elevated temperature and opisthotonos position in bed. Give ordered aspirin gr. X and an alcohol sponge bath. Place on NPO and await further orders.

Retake temperature q. 15 minutes and continue close observation.

Example 2. SOAP format (problem from Master Problem List)

Date	Time	Problem	Progress Notes
1/5/75	8 A.M.	2	Abdominal Pain

    S   Complains of pain in upper right quadrant. States pain radiates to right shoulder and is precipitated by meals. States he feels nauseated but unable to vomit.

    O   Patient is pale and appears acutely ill.
Diaphoretic and splints abdomen.
Patient is taking $FeSO_4$ at present.
T 100°F.   P 112.   R 22.

    A   Recurring abdominal pain.

    P   Put on NPO and notify physician.

    4   Obesity

    S   (no subjective data)

    O   Wt. 240; Ht. 5'6".

    A   Obese.

    P   Consult with dietitian and physician re diet.

General Charting. Each individual health facility has chart forms designed to meet the needs of that institution, and you must use your own institution's chart forms. The collection of chart forms for an individual patient becomes the patient's chart. Health workers may have different responsibilities for completing chart forms in a specific agency.

Charts vary among health facilities but generally include the following forms:

General Forms

1. Physician orders — for the physician to write his guiding orders.

2. Graphic sheet — for recording the temperature, pulse respiration, blood pressure, and possibly the weight of the patient.

3. Medication sheet — for noting the medications and intravenous fluids that are given to the patient.

4. Nurses' notes — for listing the patient's complaints (subjective symptoms), what you observe (objective symptoms), the patient's morale and reaction to therapy, and the nursing care given to the patient.

5. History and physical — for the physician to enter the findings of his examination.

6. Progress sheet — for the physician to keep a continuing account of the patient's progress.

7. Laboratory sheet — for entering the returns of the laboratory findings.

UNIT
18

Special Forms

1. Social history — for listing patient's name, address, religion, nearest of kin, and other information of this type.

2. Inhalation sheet — for recording the administration of oxygen and forced inhalations.

3. Physical therapy sheet — for records of treatments.

4. Consultation sheet — for the use of physicians who are called in to examine a patient in order to make a possible diagnosis.

5. Surgical or treatment consent — for the patient to authorize surgery or treatment.

6. Other — for recording blood pressure, intake–output, diabetic information, and other individual reports.

VI. GENERAL RULES FOR CHARTING

1. Entries on the patient's chart should be printed or handwritten. After completing the account, sign the chart with one initial and your last name, and your title (NA, LVN, RN), e.g., J. Jones, RN; S. Smith, LVN; M. White, NA.

2. Ditto marks may *not* be used.

3. Do not erase. Erasures provide reason for question if the chart is used later in a court of law. If a mistake is made, a single line should be drawn through the mistake and the word "error" printed above it. Then continue your charting in a normal manner, for example:

error
10 A.M. ~~S.S. enema given. Solution returned clear.~~ S. Smith, LVN
10.A.M. Fleet's enema given. Solution returned clear. S. Smith, LVN

4. Record *after* completing each task for the patient, and sign your name correctly after each entry.

5. Be exact in noting the *time*, *effect*, and *results* of all treatments and procedures.

6. Describe clearly and concisely the character and amount of drainage, vomitus, stools, and urine. Record patient complaints and general behavior. Describe the type, location, onset, and duration of pain.

7. Note the time of the physician's visit, examination, and treatments.

8. Leave no blank lines in the charting. Draw a line through the center of an empty line or part of a line. This prevents charting by someone else in an area signed by you.

9. Check with the hospital or health facility to learn the color of ink used there for charting. Usually blue or black ink is specified because it can be microfilmed. Red ink does not microfilm.

10. Chart the time that the patient leaves the unit for treatment, surgery, or diagnostic procedure, and the time of return.

11. Use standard abbreviations.

12. Postoperatively, chart the patient's pulse, respiration, blood pressure, general condition, time of reaction from anesthesia, condition of wound dressing, and other pertinent factors about the patient placed in your care.

13. Chart the time of death, the name of the doctor certifying the expiration, the date when the deceased patient was transferred to the mortuary, the disposition of the patient's belongings, and the name of the mortuary.

14. Print the proper headings on all new pages added to the chart. Addressograph each page.

15. Use the present tense. Never use the future tense, as in "patient to be ambulated." Also, it is not necessary to use the term "patient" on the chart; the chart belongs to the patient, and all notations are about him.

16. Spell correctly. If you are not sure about the spelling of a word, use the dictionary at the desk to look it up.

VII. SPECIFIC CHARTING SUGGESTIONS

Record vital information regarding the patient in the space designated for it. In POR charting, much of the daily care of the patient and routine treatment is charted or checked off on the flow sheets. For more traditional charting, you may be expected to record patient care in more detail. These entries include:

1. General baths and packs — record an accurate description of each treatment.

2. Dressings — chart the appearance of the wound, any drainage, and the type of dressing applied.

3. Diet — chart the type and amount of food taken, as well as the amount of fluids.

4. Output — chart emeses, BM (bowel movement), wound drainage, urine, perspiration, and the amount obtained from suction.

5. Hot and cold treatments — chart the temperature of applied heat, the type, how long applied, and where applied; chart any cold measures applied, the type, and how long and where it was applied.

6. Infant feedings — chart the amount, the time given, whether there was regurgitation, how the food was taken.

7. Menstruation — note the number of pads used, the kind of discharge, and the odor.

8. Body care — chart the hour; whether it was back care, care of decubitus (if needed), mouth care, and so forth; the type of bath; and the positioning. Indicate special procedures or appliances used. State the patient's body positioning and describe any required supports.

9. Ambulation — chart the time, distance, and how the patient tolerated walking.

10. Diagnostic tests — note the time, the type, any unusual occurrences, the patient's reaction, and the outcome.

11. Specimens — identify and label each one. Chart the time and kind sent to the laboratory.

12. Patient progress — note the time of any change and describe his condition (usually done by the physician on this form).

13. Admission — record the patient's full name, hospital number, room number, age, B/P, T, P, R, height, weight, and allergies, the last date he took cortisone, and whether he wears dentures or contact lenses. Note any prostheses and independent valuables, identification band number, the chief complaint, known diagnostic tests, and whether he was admitted ambulating, by wheelchair, or by gurney.

14. Oxygen — chart the time oxygen was begun and when discontinued, and the method used (mask, catheter, or tent).

15. Medication — note the time, amount, and method of medication given.

16. Sleep — the time slept during the day as well as at night.

17. IV — chart the time that IV was begun, the kind, where given, and the number of drops per minute. Also record the time that the IV was completed, the amount, the condition of the tissue, and the patient's reaction. (Usually the entry-level nurse would not chart items mentioned in the first statement; in some instances, however, she may chart items noted in the second statement.)

18. All procedures that were accomplished — the type, time, and outcome, and the patient's reaction.

19. Mental state — chart any mental symptoms, his state of consciousness, convulsions, or untoward behavior. State the patient's general attitude, and the time, place, and outcome of such symptoms.

20. Bleeding or unusual discharge.

21. Surgical preparation.

22. Discharge or death of the patient — follow the procedure of the health facility and chart all information pertaining to the patient.

VIII. COMMONLY USED ABBREVIATIONS

Others may be found in a dictionary or in books on medical terminology.

Abbreviation	Meaning
āā	of each
abd.	abdomen
a.c.	before meals
ad lib.	as needed
A.M.	morning
amb.	ambulatory, walking
amt.	amount
approx.	approximately (about)
ax.	axillary (armpit)
b.i.d.	twice per day
BMR	basal metabolic rate

Abbreviation	Meaning
BM	bowel movement
BP	blood pressure
BRP	bathroom privileges
C	centigrade
c̄	with
ca	cancer
cc (c.c.)	cubic centimeters
CD	communicable disease
cmpd.	compound
clysis	hypodermoclysis (fluid given under skin)
c/o	complains of
DC	discontinue
dist.	distilled
dr	dram (measurement)
ECG (EKG)	electrocardiogram (tracing of heart function)
EEG	electroencephalogram (brain wave tracing)
ER	emergency room
elix.	elixir
exam	examination
ext.	extract
F	Fahrenheit
Fe	iron
fld.	fluid
GI	gastrointestinal (stomach and intestinal)
gm	gram (measurement)
gr	grain (measurement)
gtt (sing.—gt)	drops (measurement)
GU	genitourinary (pertaining to organs of reproduction and urinary excretion)
h	hour
hi-cal	high calorie
hi-vit	high vitamin
Hgb	hemoglobin
H_2O	water
h.s.	bedtime
invol.	involuntary (without knowledge of)
irrig.	irrigate
I & O	intake and output
IV	intravenous (within vein)
kg	kilogram (weight)
lab.	laboratory
lb	pound
liq.	liquid
LLQ	left lower quadrant (left lower section of abdomen)
LUQ	left upper quadrant
M	minim (measurement)
med.	medical (or medication)
mid.	middle
min.	minute
mg	milligram (measurement)
no.	number
noc.	night

Abbreviation	Meaning
NPN	nonprotein nitrogen (content of blood)
NPO	nothing by mouth (nulli per os)
O_2	oxygen
OB	obstetrics
OR	operating room
O.D.	right eye
O.U.	each eye
O.S.	left eye
oz	ounce
P	pulse
Ped. or Peds, or Pedi	pediatrics
per	by or through
p.o.	per os, or by mouth
post-op	postoperative (after surgery)
p.r.n.	when necessary
pre-op	preoperative (before surgery)
psych.	psychology
pt.	patient
PT	physical therapist
q.d.	every day
q.h.	every hour
q.i.d.	four times per day
q.o.d.	every other day
q.s.	quantity sufficient
R or resp.	respirations
RBC	red blood cell
RLQ	right lower quadrant (right lower quarter of abdomen)
RUQ	right upper quadrant of abdomen
sol.	solution
SOS	one time only if needed
sp. gr.	specific gravity (measure)
SS	soapsuds
ss	one-half
stat.	at once
staph	staphylococcus (germ)
tab	tablet
TL	team leader
TPR	temperature, pulse, respiration
VD	venereal disease
via	by way of
WBC	white blood cell
wt.	weight

IX. NUMBERS AND SYMBOLS COMMONLY USED IN CHARTING

These are standard and are used most frequently. Others may be found in a dictionary, books of medical terminology, or pharmacology books.

One	$\dot{\mathrm{i}}$	Five	$\bar{\mathrm{v}}$
Two	$\ddot{\mathrm{ii}}$	Six	$\bar{\mathrm{vi}}$
Three	$\dddot{\mathrm{iii}}$	Seven	$\bar{\ddot{\mathrm{vii}}}$
Four	$\bar{\mathrm{iv}}$	Eight	$\bar{\dddot{\mathrm{viii}}}$

Nine $\overline{\text{ix}}$ grain gr

Ten $\overline{\text{x}}$ one-half $\overline{\text{ss}}$

Eleven $\overline{\text{xi}}$ one and one-half $\overline{\text{iss}}$

Twelve, etc. $\overline{\text{xii}}$ three ounces ℥ iii

and et, +, &   two drams ʒ ii

greater than >   number #, no.

less than <   with $\overline{\text{c}}$

dram ʒ   without $\overline{\text{s}}$

ounce ℥

X. ANATOMICAL REGIONS OF THE ABDOMEN

1. right hypochondriac area
2. epigastric area
3. left hypochondriac area
4. right lumbar region (in back and side)
5. umbilical (navel) area
6. left lumbar area (side and back)
7. right iliac
8. hypogastric area
9. left iliac
10. genitourinary area

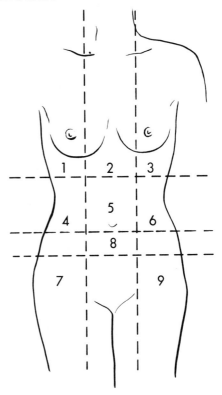

Regions of abdomen.

XI. COMMON DESCRIPTIVE TERMS

Word	Idea to be Charted	Terms Suggested
abdomen	appears black and blue in color	bruised (appears); ecchymotic
	bloated; filled with gas	tympanitic; distended
	hurts when touched	sensitive to touch; tender
	hard; boardlike	rigid
	large; extends out	protruding
	soft; flabby; flat	soft; flaccid; flat

Word	Idea to be Charted	Terms Suggested
amounts	large amount	copious; excessive; profuse
	moderate amount	moderate; usual
	small amount	scanty; slight; small
appearance	thin and undernourished	emaciated
	fat, overweight	obese
	seems very sick	acutely ill
	fails to notice things	apathetic, indifferent
	extremely worried; nervous	anxious; shows anxiety
	appears to have blue color	cyanotic
	extremely happy; fails to accept reality as it is	euphoric
	skin appears yellowish	jaundiced
appetite	craves certain foods	parorexia
	desire to eat material not accepted as food	perverted appetite
	eats everything served and asks for more food	hearty appetite
	appears never to get enough food	insatiable appetite
	eats all food served	good appetite
	eats little of food served	poor appetite
	loss of appetite	anorexia
arm (extremity)	shoulder to elbow	upper arm
	elbow to wrist	lower arm
	with much extra tissue	plump to obese
	appears puffy or swollen	edematous; edema
attitude	afraid; worried	anxious; fearful
	does not believe what is said	distrustful; suspicious
	fixed idea (right or wrong)	obsession
	behavior that forces self or ideas on others	aggressive
	insists upon false belief	delusion
	centers attention upon self	introvert
	"don't care" attitude	apathetic
	not interested in surroundings	indifferent
	happy, carefree	cheerful; optimistic
	seems to feel guilty and worries about unreal things	appears depressed
back	upper back	shoulder area; thoracic area; interscapular
	small of back	lumbar area
	end of spine	sacral area
	buttocks	gluteal area
	humped back	kyphosis
	sway back	lordosis
	curved back	scoliosis
bath	given when patient arrives	admission bath
	entire body	complete bath

Word	Idea to be Charted	Terms Suggested
	face, neck, arms, back, and genitals	partial bath
	special bath	state method and materials used
	taken in bed	bed bath
	taken in tub or special tub	tub bath or sitz bath
belch	noise made in mouth area	eructation; burping
bleeding	in large amount and in spurts	spurting blood; profuse
	very little	oozing; minimum amount
	nosebleed	epistaxis
	blood in vomitus	hematemesis
	blood in urine	hematuria
	blood in sputum	hemoptysis
blister	raised area on skin filled with water	vesicle
blood pressure	the reading on a measuring instrument	B/P 120/80 (example), strong, weak
breast	each appears the same size	of equal size
	inflammation	mastitis
	large; hard	engorged
	appears average for that person	developed normally
	nipple always depressed	inverted nipple
	period of milk formation	lactation
breath	taking in air	respiration; inspiration
	breathing air out	respiration; expiration
	difficult breathing	dyspnea
	short time without breathing	apnea
	rapid breathing	hyperpnea
	cannot breathe lying down	orthopnea
	snoring sounds of breathing	stertorous respiration
	unpleasant odor	halitosis
	increasing dyspnea with periods of nonbreathing	Cheyne-Stokes respiration (a terminal breathing condition)
	no breath from suffocation	asphyxia
	large amount of air taken	deep breathing
	small amount of air taken	shallow breathing
	abnormal variation of breath	irregular respiration
	sweet, fruitlike odor	fruity, sweet
care	wash face and hands, perform toilette	A.M. care
	wash face, hands, and back, give backrub, perform toilette	P.M. care
	special attention to mouth	special mouth care
	special attention to back	special back care
chest	abnormally shaped	deformed
	looks rounded front and back	barrel-chest
	looks abnormally small	shrunken

UNIT 18

Word	Idea to be Charted	Terms Suggested
chill	came on quickly	sudden onset
	how long it lasts	duration of (state time); prolonged, short, persistent, or intermittent
	extent of chill	moderate, severe, or slight
color of excretion: urine	without color	clear; colorless
	normal urine	straw colored to amber
color of excretion: feces	resembling clay	clay-colored BM
	looks black as tar	tarry BM
	tinged with blood	blood-tinged
coma	does not respond to stimuli	coma (partially comatose or profound coma)
consciousness	aware of surroundings	alert — conversant; fully conscious
	partly conscious	lethargic; semiconscious
	not conscious, but can be aroused	stuporous
	unconscious, cannot be aroused	comatose
consistency	remains together, retains shape	formed
	running like water	liquid
	thick and sticky	concentrated; viscous
	looks like mucus	mucoid
convulsion	muscles contract and relax	clonic tremor or convulsion
	muscle contraction maintained for a time	tonic tremor or convulsion
	localized muscle contraction	spasm
	began without warning	sudden onset
	abrupt start and end of spasm or convulsive seizure	paroxysm
cough	coughs all the time	continuous
	coughs up material	productive
	coughs over long period of time	persistent
	coughs without producing material	nonproductive
	coughs with a "whoop"	a whooping cough
	coughs with certain attacks	paroxysmal
	various types	loose; deep; dry; painful; exhaustive; tight; hacking; hollow
decay	teeth	caries
	tissue	necrosis, necrotic
defecation or bowel movement	bowel movement	feces; stool; defecation
	excessive	diarrhea
	gray color	clay-colored
	dark, liquid	brownish-black, loose
	soft material	soft; formless; or soft-formed stool

Word	Idea to be Charted	Terms Suggested
	constipated	hard-formed stool expelled with difficulty; pelletlike
dizziness	feeling of being unstable, unsteady	vertigo
drainage	watery, from the nose	coryza
	sticky	viscous
	contains pus	purulent
	watery; bloody	sanguineous or serosanguineous
	fecal (contains bowel material)	fecal
	contains mucus and pus	mucopurulent
	from vagina after delivery	lochia
dressings	dressing over original one	dressing reinforced
	dressing removed; reapplied	dressing changed
	sterile dressings	sterile dressing applied
ears	wax in ears	cerumen
	ringing sensation	tinnitus
	dizziness	vertigo
	abnormal shaped	deformed
emesis	material coming from mouth	emesis
	produced by effort of patient	self-induced
	ejected forcefully without warning	projectile
	blood particles in content	blood-tinged
	material given to produce vomiting	emetic
enemas	liquid given to induce expulsion of feces	cleansing enema
	for nourishment	nutritive
	to rid gas	carminative
	to expel worms	anthelmintic
	to remain for some time	retention
	to soothe and protect	emollient
	for diagnostic exam	barium
expectoration	spitting up saliva	expectorate
	much or little amount	profuse, or small or scant
	spitting up blood	hemoptysis
	mucus with blood particles	blood-tinged
eyes	ability to see well	visual acuity
	nearsightedness	myopia
	farsightedness	hyperopia
	inability to see clearly	blurred vision
	dilation of pupil	enlarged pupil
	small, pin-point pupil	pupil contracted; "pin-point"
	sees double (two of things)	diplopia
	squinting	strabismus
	puffy; appears swollen	edematous
	drooping eyelids	ptosis
	whites of eyes appear yellow	jaundiced
	appear staring; will not move	fixed

UNIT 18

Word	Idea to be Charted	Terms Suggested
	eyeball appears to stick out of socket	exophthalmia (as in hyperthyroidism or goiter)
	inflammation of socket and lid lining	conjunctivitis
	stye on eyelid	hordeolum
	other terms to describe	burning, smarting, clear, dull, inflamed, sunken, bloodshot, crossed
face	without normal color	pale
	unusually pink	flushed
	broken areas of skin	acne or rash
	black and blue colored	appears bruised
	expressions	defiant, angry, sad, fearful, worried, happy, anxious, dissatisfied, stressful, pained
	scars and pits	pockmarked
faint	losing consciousness	syncope
feet	reddened; blistered	pressure area present
	puffy, appears swollen	edematous
	other terms to describe	warm, cold, hot, painful, gangrenous
fever	no evidence of fever	afebrile
	temperature above normal	pyrexia
	greatly above normal	hyperpyrexia
	elevated temperature suddenly returns to normal	crisis (peak of anything)
	elevated temperature gradually returning to normal	lysis (falling)
fingers	appear square across and curved at the end	clubbed (as in some cardiac conditions)
	coming to fine point at end	tapering
gas	digestive tract appears full (with or without sounds)	flatus
	distention caused by gas	flatulence
gums	tender, inflamed	gingivitis
	pulling away from teeth	receding; shrunken
	other terms to describe	bleeding, spongy, firm, pink
hair	clean, good appearance	clean; glossy
	unclean, coarse	dirty; greasy; coarse
	absence of hair	alopecia
	other terms to describe	tangled, neglected, bleached, dyed, uncombed
hallucination	abnormal senses not observed by others	hallucination
	hearing	auditory hallucination (voices or sounds)
	sight	visual hallucination (visual images not observed by others)

Word	Idea to be Charted	Terms Suggested
	smell	olfactory hallucination (abnormal odors)
	taste	gustatory hallucination
hands	abnormally large	massive
	fingers square and curved	clubbed fingers
	shaking continuously	trembling
	other terms to describe	dirty, rough, wet, dry, hot, cold, broken nails
head	forehead	frontal
	near ear	temporal
	side of head at top part	parietal (right or left)
	back of head	occipital
	unusually large head	macrocephalous
	unusually small head	microcephalous
heartbeat	irregular rate	arrhythmia
	slow rate, under 60	bradycardia
	fast rate, over 100	tachycardia
hives	hives (raised areas on skin)	urticaria
	itching	pruritus
joints	bent	flexion
	straightened	extension
	turned downward	pronation
	turned upward	supination
	revolve around	rotation
	move away from center line	abduction
	move toward center line	adduction
	stiff joint	ankylosis
	inflammation	arthritis
	stretching or wrenching	sprain
legs	between knee and hip	thigh
	thigh to knee	upper leg
	knee to ankle	lower leg
lice	animal parasites on body	pediculi
	of head area	pediculosis capitis
	of body area	pediculosis corporis
	of pubic area	pediculosis pubis
lips	pale, lacking normal color	pale
	blue in color	cyanotic
	with tiny cracks	fissured; cracked
	blistered appearance	herpes simplex (cold sore)
lungs	abnormal sounds	rales
memory	loss of memory	amnesia
mucous	relates to a sensitive membrane or lining	e.g., mucous lining of the intestinal tract
	relates to drainage from a mucous membrane	clear; yellow; sanguineous (bloody); purulent (pus)
muscle	loss of normal tone or size	atrophy

Word	Idea to be Charted	Terms Suggested
	inflammation	myositis
	stretching	strain
nails	blue in color	cyanotic
	other terms to describe	clean, dirty, broken, manicured, brittle
nose	nosebleed	epistaxis
odor	not pleasant; pungent; spicy	aromatic
	like fruit	fruity
	unpleasant	offensive; foul
	belonging to a particular thing	characteristic
pain	much pain	severe
	little amount	slight
	comes in seizures	spasmodic
	spreads to certain areas	radiating
	begins suddenly	sudden onset
	hurts when moving	increased by movement
	other terms to describe	dull, aching, faint, burning, throbbing, gnawing, acute, chronic, generalized, super-ficial, excruciating, un-yielding, cramping, shooting, darting, colicky, continuous, shifting, agonizing, piercing, intense, cutting, transient, localized, remittent, persistent
paralysis	face muscles unable to move	facial paralysis
	leg muscles unable to move	paraplegia, right or left
	one side of the body	hemiplegia, right or left
	four extremities unable to move	quadriplegia
	single limb unable to move	monoplegia
perspiration	large amount	profuse, excessive
	small amount	scanty or slight
positions of the body	flat on back	dorsal
	on left side (right leg flexed)	Sims'
	dorsal, head elevated, knees extended	Fowler's
	on back with heels brought close to buttocks, knees bent	lithotomy
	on back, knees flexed	dorsal-recumbent
	resting on knees and chest	knee-chest
	on back, pelvis higher than head	Trendelenburg's
	on abdomen, head turned to one side	prone
pulse	force of blood exerted against artery wall	(taken at) radial; temporal; femoral; pedal; carotid; apical
	number of beats per minute	rate
	rhythm	regular or irregular

Word	Idea to be Charted	Terms Suggested
	beat missed	intermittent
	over 100 per minute	rapid
	slow in rate	slow
	beats indistinct (rapid)	running
	beats hardly perceptible	thready
	rapid, distinct beats	bounding
	cannot be felt	imperceptible
sensation	feeling experienced	tingling; burning; stinging; prickling; hot; cold
skin	terms to describe	pale, red, moist, dry, clear, coarse, tanned, scaly, thick, loose, rough, tight, infected, discolored, jaundiced, mottled, calloused, edematous, excoriated, abraded, bruised, oily, painful, scarred, black, brown, white, pink, clammy, rash, wrinkled, smooth
sleep	unable to sleep	insomnia
	tired when awakens	awakes fatigued
speech	unable to be understood	incoherent
	meaningless	rambling, irrelevant
	runs words together	slurs
	difficulty in speaking	dysphasia
	unable to speak	aphasia
	other terms to describe	stammering, stuttering, hoarse, feeble, fluent
symptoms	observed by the patient	subjective
	observed by others	objective
teeth	false teeth	dentures
	decay	caries
	collection of material on	sordes
	other terms to describe	decayed, notched, crooked, protruding, broken, loose, irregular, dirty
tongue	terms to describe	dry, furrowed, cracked, raw, coated, swollen, ulcerated, pink, inflamed
throat	difficulty in swallowing	dysphagia
	inability to swallow	aphagia
treatment	preventative	prophylactic
	gives temporary relief	palliative
urination	pass fluid from bladder	void; micturate; urinate
	unable to control	incontinent; involuntary
	large amount	diuresis
	no urine passes	anuria
	frequent night urination	nocturia
	frequent and much urination	polyuria
	pus in urine	pyuria
	blood in urine	hematuria

Word	Idea to be Charted	Terms Suggested
	sugar in urine	glycosuria
	albumin in urine	albuminuria
	scantiness of urine	oliguria
	wetting bed	enuresis
	stones in urine	calculi
	other terms to describe	cloudy, with sediment, straw-colored, coffee-colored, excessive amount
wounds	surface	superficial
	without infection	clean wound
	pus discharges from	suppurating
	infected	infected
	torn	lacerated
weight	overweight	obese
	thin, underweight	emaciated

In most hospitals, charting of the time on a patient's records is done according to military practice. The following illustrations indicate how to calculate military time, beginning after midnight. The third and fourth numbers indicate minutes after the hour, for example 1025.

Twenty-four-hour clock charting compared to regular time charting.

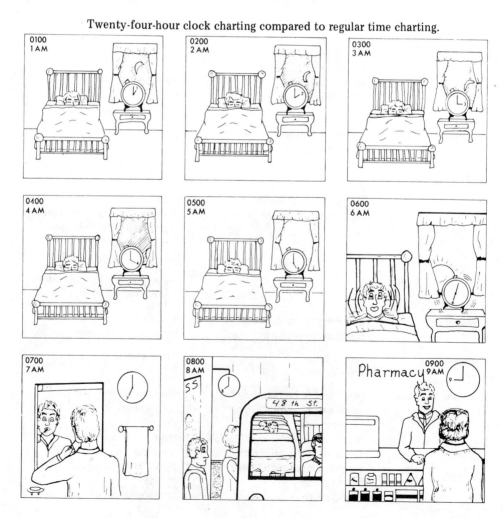

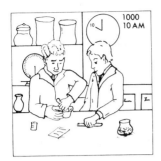

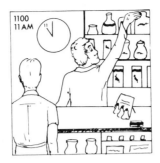

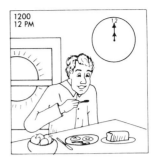

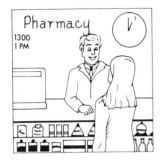

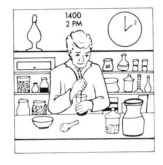

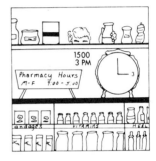

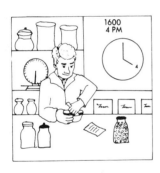

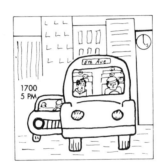

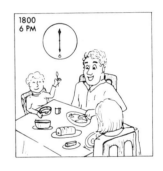

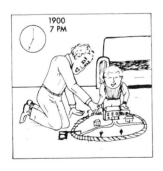

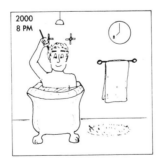

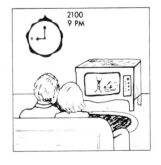

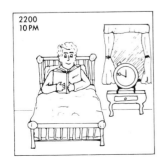

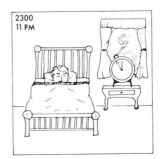

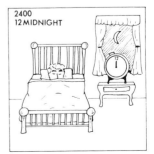

UNIT 18

XII.   ADDITIONAL INFORMATION FOR ENRICHMENT

Legal action may be taken against a person who falsifies a patient's chart. Legal action may also be taken against a person who helps falsify a chart. Information of this sort includes:

1. Concealing real nature of an operation.

2. Deceiving insurance companies.

3. Concealing information to protect a doctor or hospital from consequences of a mistake.

Charts may or may not be requested as a part of a court proceeding. To be legal and accepted as evidence, charting must be signed. This chart is a part of the hospital or health facility, and families should not read it.

A patient may decide to leave the hospital without stated permission from the attending physician. It is the duty of the health worker to ask the patient to sign a "release" paper supplied by the health facility and to enter such action in the chart.

A signed consent form for an operation is a legal requirement, and the health worker is responsible for getting such a form signed by the patient and entering it in the patient's chart.

Accurate charting of medicine and treatment is as important as their correct administration. The nature of these measures may lead to litigation if correct administration and charting are not carried out.

Charting is currently done in most hospitals, but in the near future large hospitals will probably convert to the "computer" system; entering information in a patient's chart will therefore be the duty of one person assigned to that task. However, information will still be required from the health worker and must be supplied in the terms indicated in this module.

POST-TEST

Item A: Explain what the following forms are used for (refer to page 365):

1. Physician order sheet _____

    _____

    _____

2. Graphic sheet _____

    _____

    _____

3. Medication sheet _____

    _____

4. Nurses' notes _____

    _____

5. History and physical _____

    _____

    _____

6. Progress sheet _____

    _____

    _____

7. Laboratory sheet _____

    _____

    _____

Item B: Read the sample charting given to you on page 385. Identify the charting errors and then chart the information correctly on your nurses' notes on page 386. Refer to pages 366–367 for the "General Rules for Charting."

Item C: Define the following abbreviations. Refer to pages 368–370, "Commonly Used Abbreviations."

1. p.r.n. _____

2. h.s. _____

3. NPO _____

4. stat. _____

5. ax. _____

6. q.d. _____

7. b.i.d. _____

8. cc _____

9. ECG _____

10. noc. _____

Item D: Define the following terms. Refer to pages 371–380, "Common Descriptive Terms."

1. admission bath _____

2. hearty appetite _____

3. lumbar area of back _____

4. "don't care" attitude _____

5. thigh _____

6. upper leg _____

7. lower leg _____

Item E: Read the following Case History and prepare problem-oriented charting using the SOAP format discussed on pages 364–365.

Mr. A. was the victim of a car accident. There was cessation of motion and loss of sensation in his lower extremities. He has no control over his bowels or bladder content.

He is known diabetic maintained on 30 units of protamine zinc insulin daily. Regular insulin is used to supplement the 30 units of protamine zinc insulin when urine sample test shows 4 + sugar.

The physical examination revealed no muscle strength or sensation in the body below the umbilicus. There was spasticity of his lower extremities. No abrasions appeared on the body.

Laboratory Findings:

Serum cholesterol 300 mg%

Fasting blood sugar 250 mg%

Urine sugar 4+ Acetone: moderate

Note: Identify and list problems according to No. 1, No. 2, and so forth; then prepare problem-oriented charting and ask your instructor to evaluate your work.

Item F: Read the additional information about Mr. A and prepare a POR progress note using the SOAP format. Check with your instructor for additional help.

Mr. A. refused his lunch and supplemental orange juice. He took 30 units or protamine zinc insulin in the A.M. He refused to talk to his wife when she visited. He turned his face to the wall and said, "Let me alone!" He appeared pleasant before the visit from his wife.

NURSES' RECORD

DATE 4/17/72	HOSPITAL DAY 2	POST-OP. DAY 1	DATE	HOSPITAL DAY	POST-OP. DAY

	NIGHT	DAY	EVENING		NIGHT	DAY	EVENING
CHARGE NURSE				CHARGE NURSE			
MEDICINE NURSE				MEDICINE NURSE			

VISITS DOCTOR		TIME			VISITS DOCTOR		TIME		
DOCTOR					DOCTOR				

WEIGHT	TIME				WEIGHT	TIME			
	BLOOD PRESSURE					BLOOD PRESSURE			

DIET Regular	APPETITE AM	NOON	PM	DIET	APPETITE AM	NOON	PM

O₂ LITERS ☐ NASAL ☐ TENT ☐ CONTINUOUS ☐ MASK ☐ PRN

☐ BED REST ☐ BED BATH ☐ ORAL CARE
☐ CHAIR ☐ TUB BATH ☐ EVENING CARE
☐ BRP ☐ SHOWER ☐ SIDE RAILS UP ☐ AM ☐ HS
☐ UP AD LIB

☐ VOIDING ☐ ENEMA ☐ HARRIS FLUSH
☐ STOOL ☐ SITZ BATH

O₂ LITERS ☐ NASAL ☐ TENT ☐ CONTINUOUS ☐ MASK ☐ PRN

☐ BED REST ☐ BED BATH ☐ ORAL CARE
☐ CHAIR ☐ TUB BATH ☐ EVENING CARE
☐ BRP ☐ SHOWER ☐ SIDE RAILS UP ☐ AM ☐ HS
☐ UP AD LIB

☐ VOIDING ☐ ENEMA ☐ HARRIS FLUSH
☐ STOOL ☐ SITZ BATH

TIME		TIME	
	From O.R. Moaning — says she has pain in leave leg. M. Walker	10p	Patient checked
		12p	" "
		6A	Patient not complaining of dis-comfort
		6³⁰	" " "
			M. W. LVN
850	Patient turned to side. Dr. Reed here. Jones L.V.N.	0100	Patient up about / error Back to bed
		0200	Pt. crying c̄ pain.
11AM	Patient to be dangled at side of bed. Pulse apparently strong and regular. Henrietta F. RN		Morphine gr ¼ given for pain. Joan Jones R.N.

E-09-0288

NURSES' RECORD

DATE		HOSPITAL DAY		POST-OP. DAY		DATE		HOSPITAL DAY		POST-OP. DAY	
	NIGHT	DAY		EVENING			NIGHT	DAY		EVENING	
CHARGE NURSE						CHARGE NURSE					
MEDICINE NURSE						MEDICINE NURSE					
VISITS DOCTOR			TIME			VISITS DOCTOR			TIME		
DOCTOR						DOCTOR					
WEIGHT	TIME					WEIGHT	TIME				
	BLOOD PRESSURE						BLOOD PRESSURE				
DIET			APPETITE AM	NOON	PM	DIET			APPETITE AM	NOON	PM

O_2 LITERS ☐ NASAL   ☐ TENT   ☐ CONTINUOUS
_____   ☐ MASK   ☐ PRN

☐ BED REST   ☐ BED BATH   ☐ ORAL CARE
☐ CHAIR   ☐ TUB BATH   ☐ EVENING CARE
☐ BRP   ☐ SHOWER   ☐ SIDE RAILS UP   ☐ AM   ☐ HS
☐ UP AD LIB

☐ VOIDING   ☐ ENEMA   ☐ HARRIS FLUSH
☐ STOOL   ☐ SITZ BATH   _____   _____   _____

O_2 LITERS ☐ NASAL   ☐ TENT   ☐ CONTINUOUS
_____   ☐ MASK   ☐ PRN

☐ BED REST   ☐ BED BATH   ☐ ORAL CARE
☐ CHAIR   ☐ TUB BATH   ☐ EVENING CARE
☐ BRP   ☐ SHOWER   ☐ SIDE RAILS UP   ☐ AM   ☐ HS
☐ UP AD LIB

☐ VOIDING   ☐ ENEMA   ☐ HARRIS FLUSH
☐ STOOL   ☐ SITZ BATH   _____   _____   _____

TIME		TIME	

E-09-0288

BOWEL ELIMINATION

I. DIRECTIONS TO THE STUDENT

Proceed through this lesson using the workbook as your guide. In the skill laboratory you will need to practice the enema and irrigation procedures on the Chase doll. After you practice the procedures and complete the lesson, arrange with your instructor to take the post-test for this lesson.

You will need the following items for your study and practice:

1. Disposable or reusable enema unit.

2. Lubricant.

3. Solution as ordered by doctor.

4. Bedpan and cover.

5. Irrigating graduated pitcher, 1000 ml.

6. Roll of toilet tissue.

7. Chux or pad for buttocks.

8. Irrigating bag, plastic apron, and tubing.

9. Stool specimen container.

10. Rectal tube.

11. Unsterile examining (rectal) gloves.

Please read the following paragraphs carefully. They will tell you exactly what you will be expected to know and how to assist the patient to establish and maintain regularity in the elimination of waste products from the large intestine. If you feel that you have sufficient knowledge and skills to do the performance test accurately without further study of the lesson, please discuss this with your instructor. All students are expected to perform accurately the skills required in the test without use of reference materials.

II. GENERAL PERFORMANCE OBJECTIVE

You will be able to demonstrate your ability to assist the patient to establish and maintain regular elimination of waste products from the large intestine, using methods appropriate to the patient's age, physical condition, and disease.

III. SPECIFIC PERFORMANCE OBJECTIVES

Upon completion of this lesson, you will be able to:

1. Identify some of the abnormal conditions manifested in the appearance of the patient's stool, such as the presence of blood, mucus, iron, and worms or other parasites.

2. Collect a stool specimen and prepare it correctly for examination in the laboratory.

3. Promote the patient's regular elimination of waste products from the large bowel through nursing measures related to the patient's prescribed diet, fluid intake, exercise, and rest.

4. Reduce incontinence of feces in patients of any age through methods of habit training and retraining.

5. Assist evacuation of feces and flatus in the hypoactive bowel through the use of the enema, rectal tube, or Harris flush.

6. Examine for the presence of constipated stool in the rectum and promote its evacuation by the use of suppositories, and cleansing or retention enemas.

7. Assist and teach the patient with a colostomy or ileostomy to irrigate his bowel in order to cleanse it of fecal material, to prevent obstruction, and to establish a habit of regular evacuation.

IV. VOCABULARY

Many new words are introduced in this lesson. These words are frequently used by doctors and nurses, and you will need to learn their meanings. Because there are so many new words, those that are related are grouped together.

1. **The Small Bowel (total length 22 to 23 feet in the adult)**
   duodenum—an 8- to 10-inch portion of the small intestine connected to the lower end of the stomach and to the jejunum.
   ileum—the twisting intestine between the jejunum and the large intestine, about 13 feet long in the adult.
   ilium—part of the pelvic bone.
   jejunum—the section of the intestine between the duodenum and the ileum, about 9 feet long in the adult.
2. **The Large Bowel (total length 4 to 6 feet in the adult)**
   anus (anal)—the outer opening of the rectum between the buttocks and beyond the lower tip of the sacrum.
   appendix—a small wormlike pouch about 7.5 cm long at the end of the cecum.
   cecum—the pouch at the junction of the small intestine and the ascending colon with the appendix at the lower end.
   colon—the large intestine from the cecum to the rectum, which is divided into the ascending colon, the transverse colon, the descending colon, and the sigmoid.
   rectum—the lower part of the large intestine between the sigmoid and the anus, about 5 inches long.
   sigmoid—the lower part of the descending colon, which is shaped like the letter "S."
3. **Some Diseases and Surgical Conditions**
   appendicitis—inflammation of the appendix.
   colitis—inflammation of the colon.
   colostomy—an incision into the colon to form an artificial opening (stoma).
   diverticulitis—inflammation and distention of little pouches throughout the colon.
   hemorrhoids—dilated blood vessels in the anal area.
   ileostomy—an incision into the ileum of the small intestine to form an artificial opening (stoma).
   polyps—growths attached to mucous membranes of the nose, bladder, colon, or uterus.
   ulcerative colitis—a severe inflammation of the colon with open sores of the membrane lining.
4. **Contents of the Bowels**
   bile—an important digestive juice secreted by the liver, stored in the gallbladder; substances in bile give the brown color to feces.
   chyme—the partially digested food and digestive juices; the liquid mass found in the intestines.

electrolytes—substances of a solution capable of conducting an electrical impulse or charge; important electrolytes in the body are sodium, chloride, calcium, potassium, iron, and others.

feces—the waste material following digestion; the stool.

flatus—gas in the digestive tract (flatulence is the distention of the abdomen due to gas in the intestines).

mucus—a slippery, slimy fluid secreted by mucous membranes and glands.

parasites—organisms that live upon or in another organism or body called the host; common parasites in the intestinal tract are amoebas, flukes, pinworms, round-worms, hookworms, and tapeworms.

stool—feces; the waste matter discharged from the bowel.

5. Words Pertaining to Movement of the Intestines

constipation—sluggish action of the bowels; compacting of the feces into a hard, dense mass.

defecation—the evacuation of the bowel.

diarrhea—frequent movement of the bowels, increased number of stools per day, often liquid or semiliquid.

hyperactive—excessive movement; irritable.

hypoactive—decreased movement; less than normal.

incontinence—inability to retain feces or urine; lack of voluntary control over sphincters.

peristalsis—contraction of successive portions of the intestines followed by relaxation, which propels food content, fluids, and flatus onward.

sphincter—a circular muscle that opens and closes an opening, such as the sphincter of the anus.

6. Other Words Used in the Lesson

hemorrhage—excessive flow of blood out of the blood vessels; an abnormal amount of bleeding.

proctoscopy—examination of the rectum by instrument.

sigmoidoscopy—examination of the sigmoid colon by instrument.

stoma—mouth or opening, or an artificially created opening.

suppository—a cone-shaped, medicated substance that is inserted in the rectum, vagina, or urethra where it dissolves and is absorbed.

Question 1.   That makes quite a vocabulary list. Now let's see what progress you have made in learning what the words mean. In the following list, all but one of the words on each line are related to the others. Place a check mark before the word that does not belong.

a. ____sigmoid   ____ rectum   ____mucus   ____ anus

b. ____cecum   ____ ileum   ____duodenum   ____jejunum

c. ____intestine   ____ tract   ____bowel   ____ colon

d. ____appendicitis ____ diverticulitis ____colitis ____ flatus

e. ____chyme   ____electrolytes ____suppository ____ bile

f. ____polyp   ____feces   ____waste products ____stool

Question 2.   Three of the words in your vocabulary are spelled in an unusual way, with the letters "r-r-h" in sequence. Match the word with its meaning and spell the word correctly.

a. _____ an excessive amount of bleeding.

b. _____ increased number of bowel movements.

c. _____ dilated blood vessels around the anus.

ITEM 1. THE IMPORTANCE OF BOWEL ELIMINATION

Why do you need to learn about the elimination of wastes from the bowel? Emptying a bedpan filled with stool, or feces, seems to be one of the more unpleasant tasks that nursing workers do. The sight and odor are often very unpleasant. To some of you, it might seem that we should rush through this part and get on to some more important lesson. Nevertheless, bowel elimination happens to be one of the most important subjects we study.

What are the functions of the bowel that make it so important to health? They can be stated simply as those related to the absorption of nutrients and those related to the elimination of waste products.

Absorption of vital nutrients, electrolytes, and water takes place in the small intestine and in a portion of the large intestine as the liquefied food mass moves out of the stomach and down the bowel. Elimination of the waste products at regular intervals indicates free passage of the food mass through the bowel in the time allowed for the absorption process. Absorption is reduced when the bowel moves the food mass along too quickly, or when the bowel moves so slowly that waste products collect in the absorbing parts, or when the bowel becomes obstructed or blocked. The causes of these conditions in the bowel *may* be serious enough to endanger the life of the patient.

The body must get rid of the waste materials that are produced in the process of converting food into usable substances, which are delivered to the cells with oxygen. These waste products of the body are eliminated through the skin, lungs, kidneys, and bowel. The bowel is the most important excretor of the more solid wastes of the body. The solid wastes consist of by-products of the digestive process, indigestible stuffs, water, and matter from the intestinal tract itself, such as secretions, dead bacteria, and sloughed cells.

The appearance and the composition of the stool are important indicators of conditions in other parts of the digestive system. Obstruction or disease of the bowel may be detected by observing the stool for changes in color, the absence of color, and the presence of unusual matter such as blood. Changes in bowel habits may indicate a growth, obstruction, or disease.

In this lesson, you will learn more about the functions of the intestinal tract; conditions that change the normal composition and appearance of the stool; such problems related to elimination as distention, constipation, diarrhea, and incontinence; and ways to assist the patient to achieve and maintain regular elimination of waste matter from his bowel.

Question 3. The two main functions of the intestines are:

a. _____ and b. _____.

Question 4. Select the best answer(s) to complete the following statement. The patient's life may be endangered when absorption in the bowel is reduced by:

a. blockage of the bowel by twisting itself closed.

b. change in the color of the stool.

c. slow movement with no stool passed in five days.

d. quick movement with ten stools in one day.

e. all of the above.

Question 5. State four of the problems related to the function of elimination.

a. _____ , b. _____ ,

c. _____ , d. _____.

ITEM 2. BRIEF DESCRIPTION OF THE INTESTINAL TRACT

The intestinal tract is a muscular tube that extends from the stomach to the anal opening at the skin surface. The intestines are approximately six times the length of the body. In the adult, this would average about 8.5 meters, or 33½ feet.

The inner surface of the intestine has innumerable circular folds that greatly increase the area for absorption. Through this surface, nutrients, water, vitamins, and electrolytes are absorbed into the blood stream. A rich supply of blood vessels around the intestines transports the absorbed materials to the cells of the entire body.

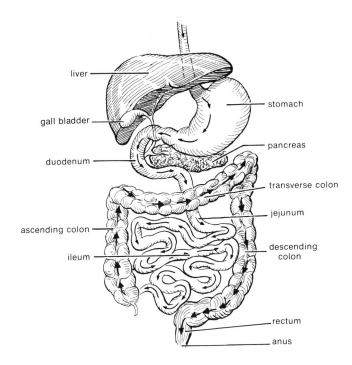

The intestinal tract and related digestive organs—liver, stomach, pancreas, and gallbladder.

The walls of the intestines also have circular muscle fibers that contract or enlarge the size of the tube, as well as longitudinal and oblique muscle fibers that allow stretching and turning of the tube.

The *small intestine* comprises the *duodenum*, the *jejunum*, and the *ileum*. The duodenum is connected to the lower end of the stomach. The jejunum forms the middle section of the small intestine, and the ileum, or twisted intestine, is the lower section that is joined to the cecum of the large bowel.

As the liquefied food mass (*chyme*) enters and passes through the small intestine, it is mixed with intestinal digestive juices. Absorption of nutrients takes place mainly in the small intestine. Electrolytes are also absorbed in the upper portion of the small intestine, and some water is absorbed in the ileum, but greater amounts are absorbed in the large intestine.

The *large intestine* provides a frame for the small intestines in the abdominal cavity. The *cecum with the appendix* is at the lower right corner of the frame and is attached to the *ascending colon*. The *transverse colon* crosses the abdomen at about the level of the navel, and the *descending colon* goes down the left side where it joins the *sigmoid*. The sigmoid

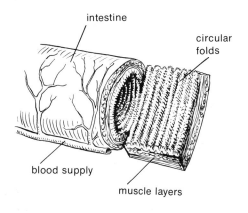

Cut-away section of intestines, showing circular folds.

colon, which gets its name from its "S" shape, crosses the abdominal cavity toward the back.

The lower segment of the large intestine is the *rectum*, and the *anus* is the outer opening of the bowel to the skin.

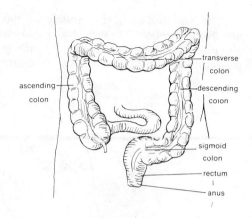

The main functions of the large intestines are (1) to absorb water and electrolytes, and (2) to temporarily store the residual waste products as feces. As an example of the water-absorbing capacity of the large intestine, about 500 ml of chyme enters the bowel daily and all but 50 to 100 ml of water is absorbed.

Numerous bacteria are present in the normal bowel. They are found in the absorbing portion of the large intestines where they digest small amounts of food roughage, form some of the vitamins (namely vitamins K, B_{12}, and thiamine), and produce gas, or *flatus*, as a result of this bacterial activity.

The large intestine forms a frame of the abdomen.

Question 6. A child's intestinal tract is approximately _____ times as long as his body.

Question 7. The long length of the intestinal tract and the circular folds provide greater surface for _____ to take place.

Question 8. The various parts of the intestinal tract have been described. In the following list, indicate the parts of the small intestine with an "S" and those of the large intestine with an "L."

a. ____ ileum   b. ____ rectum   c. ____ colon

d. ____ jejunum   e. ____ cecum   f. ____ duodenum

g. ____ anus

Question 9. The two functions of the large intestines are a. _____

and b. _____ .

ITEM 3. CHARACTERISTICS OF FECES

The digestion of food is similar to the refining of oil. Food enters the body as raw fuel and is changed by the digestive juices. The usable parts are converted to nutrients, and these are absorbed into the small and large intestines. The unusable part, or the waste product, is passed into the colon where most of the water and electrolytes are absorbed. It is then passed into the sigmoid and rectum for storage as feces until it is evacuated from the body.

Normally, the feces are composed of three-quarters water by weight, and one-quarter solid material. The solid material consists of about 30 per cent dead bacteria and 70 per cent undigested roughage from food, fat, protein, and inorganic material. The brown color of the normal stool is caused by bile (one of the digestive juices), and the odor is the result of bacterial action on the foods that have been eaten.

In the newborn infant, the stool is characteristically dark greenish-black (meconium) for the first two to three days of life. The stool of a breast-fed baby has an orange-yellow color and a strong smell; the stool of a bottle-fed baby has a brownish-yellow color if the formula given him contains malt sugars.

The color of the feces may be changed by certain drugs that the person may be taking. Vitamins and other drug perparations containing iron give the stool a black color throughout. Chlorophyll may impart a green color to the stool.

Question 10.   Feces consist of one-fourth _____ and three-fourths _____ .

Question 11.   The color of the normal stool in an adult is _____ and in

the bottle-fed baby it is _____ .

ITEM 4. BLOOD IN THE STOOL

Before you empty feces from any patient's bedpan or flush the toilet, you should find out whether a specimen of the stool is required for laboratory examination, *and* you should observe the stool for any noticeable changes from the normal-appearing stool. The most serious change is the presence of blood in the stool.

Blood in the stool should always be regarded as a serious matter until it has been determined otherwise. A small amount of bleeding from hemorrhoids or an irritation caused by straining at stool may clear up without any treatment. The serious causes of blood in the stool include hemorrhage from ulcer in the stomach or duodenum, severe inflammation or irritation as in ulcerative colitis or diverticulitis, cancer, or diseases that cause hemorrhage. When you *observe blood in the stool*, you should *report it promptly*, *record* it on the patient's chart, and *save* the stool so it can be inspected by the doctor for amount of blood and clues as to when the bleeding occurred.

Bleeding that occurs in the upper gastrointestinal tract (stomach or small intestine) shows up in the feces as dark, almost black, in color, and tarlike in consistency. During the hours that it takes the blood to move through the intestines, it undergoes partial digestion, which changes blood to the dark tarry substance. A dark tarry stool indicates that the hemorrhage occurred hours earlier, probably from the area of the stomach or the small intestine. The partially digested blood is found thoroughly mixed in the entire contents of the stool.

Bright red blood in the stool, a sign of a recent hemorrhage or one that occurred in the large bowel, will be found on the surfaces of the stool and in pools, but not mixed throughout the stool. The color indicates that the blood has not undergone digestion in the upper part of the bowel, nor has it been in the intestinal tract for hours.

Question 12.   One of your patients, Mr. Long, has just had a bowel movement that is black in appearance and tarry in consistency. This means that the stool contains

_____ , which probably came from the (duodenum) (cecum) (sigmoid colon). (Circle one.)

Question 13.   Mr. Long's hemorrhage probably occurred (10 minutes) (10 hours) (10 days) ago.

Question 14.   Hemorrhage in the large intestine produces a _____ appearance of the stool.

ITEM 5. OTHER ABNORMALITIES OF THE FECES

One of the most easily observed changes in the stool is a difference in color. Color varies according to the foods eaten, but the normal stool is brown, except in infants or patients receiving formula in tube feedings, whose stools are a dark yellow. The color of the stool is important in the care of patients with disease of the digestive system because it may indicate a need to change the diet. This is especially important for the patient with an ileostomy since his stool is evacuated through an opening in the ileum of the small bowel before maximum absorption of nutrients, electrolytes, and water has occurred.

Some of the abnormalities that can occur in the color of stools are listed along with the condition that this color indicates. Clay color, or pale white, indicates the absence of bile or an obstruction that prevents its passage into the intestines. Chalky white color is due to chalky substance swallowed by the patient or instilled into the lower intestinal tract for X-ray purposes. Light tan color indicates undigested fat in the stool. Green, watery stools, mainly seen in infants, indicate too much sugar.

Other abnormal characteristics of feces are the presence of large amounts of mucus, pus, or parasites, such as worms. Unusual amounts of mucus in the stool indicate an irritation or inflammation of the inner surface of the intestines. The mucus coats the stool and gives it a slimy appearance. The presence of pus indicates drainage of an ulcer that is inflamed or infected. The most *common parasitic worms* found in the intestines are the *tapeworm*, the *pinworm*, and the *roundworm*.

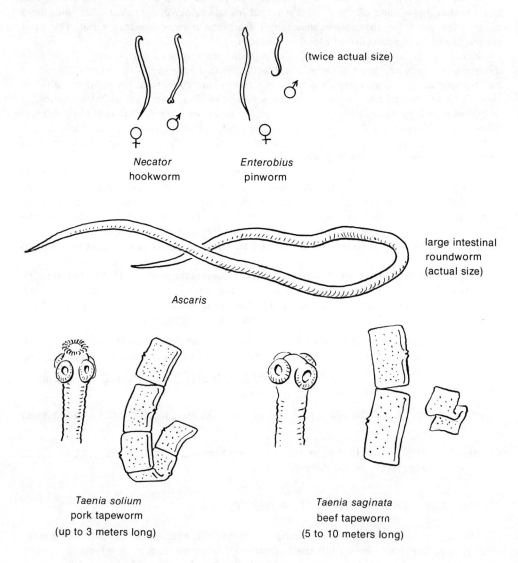

Types of parasites.

Question 15. Too much sugar in a baby's diet irritates the bowel and produces stools that are a. _____ and b. _____.

Question 16. Pale, clay-colored stools are due to the absence of _____.

Question 17. A slick, slimy appearance of the stool is caused by _____.

ITEM 6. MOVEMENT IN THE INTESTINES

The *chyme* (liquefied food mass) is passed along the intestines by means of movement of the muscular tube. This movement is called *peristalsis*. In peristalsis, the circular muscle layer of the intestine contracts to squeeze and propel the portion of chyme and gas ahead of it. The circular, longitudinal, and oblique muscle layers in the segment ahead of the contracted part will expand and lengthen to accommodate the entering mass. The rumbling noise that can occasionally be heard coming from the abdomen is caused by the peristaltic movement of liquid mass and gas along the intestinal tract.

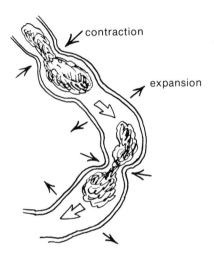

Peristalsis.

The feces are propelled along the lower intestines by peristalsis until they reach the storage portion in the lower sigmoid colon and the rectum. As more feces collect here, the rectum is filled, and the pressure on the sphincter of the anus causes the urge to open and defecate. The abdominal muscles contract to help force the evacuation of the rectum, and pass the feces through the anus.

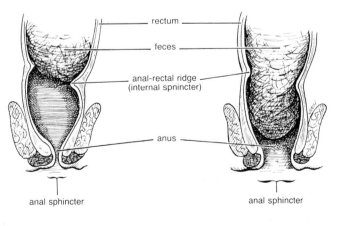

Anus closed.   Anus open.

Question 18.   Movement in the intestines is caused by contraction and expansion of the

a. _____ , b. _____ , and c. _____ muscle layers.

Question 19.   The movement is called _____ .

Question 20.   When feces fill the rectum, what causes the urge to defecate?

_____ .

ITEM 7. BOWEL CONTROL TRAINING

In almost every culture, the child is expected to learn early in life to control the elimination of stool from his bowels. Control is usually accomplished between the ages of two and three; the child can then curb the urge to defecate for a period of time to allow him to get to the bathroom or toilet. The child's success in controlling his bowels becomes a sign of progress toward personal independence, a step toward growing up. It also gives him the feeling of being more socially acceptable to his family and others.

To establish bowel control in the child, it is essential to observe the child's diet, fluid intake, exercise, and rest inasmuch as these factors influence his ability to regulate his bowels.

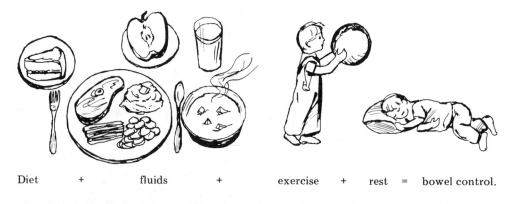

Diet   +   fluids   +   exercise   +   rest =   bowel control.

The diet should contain roughage adequate to give bulk to the stool. The young child should take 800 to 1000 ml of fluids per day, which include water, milk, juices, soups, Jello, and others. Adequate sleep and exercise are necessary for good health and the proper functioning of the intestinal tract.

The frequency of bowel movements depends on many factors and varies among individuals. It is normal for some people to have a movement every day, for others to have one every other day, and for a few to have a movement every three days. The important thing is that the bowel movements occur on a regular basis. The time of the bowel movement also differs. Many adults have elimination following breakfast, but it can occur at other times of the day. Infants usually have two or three movements per day following feeding, and the young child often has his bowel movement shortly after breakfast or lunch.

Habit training for bowel control depends on recognizing the urge to defecate, establishing a regular time for elimination, providing a comfortable position, and allowing sufficient time.

Signs of the urge to defecate are a rumbling noise in the abdomen, expelling of flatus, and restlessness caused by the feeling of fullness in the rectum. The child should be toiletted at a regular time each day, usually after breakfast or after lunch. He should be placed in a comfortable position on a potty chair, a small commode, or toilet with a child-sized seat on it. No more than 20 minutes should be allowed. The child should be reminded frequently and encouraged to move his bowels. Playing with toys distracts the child from the task to be done.

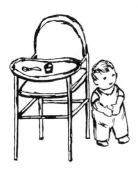
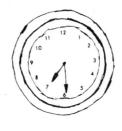
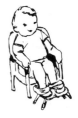

Bowel training.

Question 21.   Bowel control in children is usually accomplished by age _____ .

Question 22.   To help establish bowel control, attention should be given to the child's

a. _____ , b. _____ , c. _____ and

d. _____ .

Question 23.   It is essential for your good health to have a bowel movement every day.

True _____   False _____

ITEM 8.   THE HYPOACTIVE BOWEL AND CONSTIPATION

A reduction or absence of peristaltic movement of the bowel results in the hypoactive bowel. Conditions that cause the hypoactive bowel are surgery, injury, disease, and bed rest. In the normal person, lack of sufficient roughage in the diet and decreased exercise may produce a sluggish or hypoactive bowel. Certain drugs such as narcotics and tranquilizers also reduce the activity of the bowel.

Constipation, one of the most common problems of the hypoactive bowel, is the irregular evacuation of feces from the bowel, causing them to become more compacted and hard while in the rectum. As additional feces are formed, they fill greater portions of the colon as well as the rectum. Constipation tends to occur when muscle tone is lacking because of inadequate exercise, irregularity of bowel movements, a sedentary life, or when there is worry, anxiety, or fear.

The treatment includes plenty of exercise, lots of liquids, a good diet with sufficient roughage, setting a regular time for defecation, and avoiding emotional stress. When ordered by the doctor, enemas are used to empty the rectum, laxatives to stimulate bowel activity, and suppositories to stimulate the urge to defecate.

ITEM 9.   THE ENEMA

An enema is the introduction of fluid into the rectum and colon by means of a tube. Rectal enemas are usually given to stimulate peristalsis and the urge to defecate. The cleansing enema is used to wash out the waste products or feces from the bowel when they have not been properly eliminated, when the bowel is to be examined by X-ray or proctoscopy, or when the bowel is distended by flatus.

The *kind* and the *amount of fluid* used in the enema will often be prescribed by the doctor, and will vary depending on the age and condition of the patient, the preference of the doctor, and the purpose of the enema. The most common solutions are the tap water enema (TWE) using water obtained from the faucet, the saline enema using a saline (salt) solution, and the soapsuds enema (or SSE) using a small amount of liquefied soap in water.

When other types of enemas are ordered, you may need to consult the nursing procedure book of the hospital for the ingredients and the proportions to use in the enema.

The amount of solution to be used is usually between 500 ml (cc) to 1000 ml (cc) for adults; a smaller quantity is required for children. The solution should run in slowly to avoid discomfort and pain as the rectum is distended by the fluid. Hold the container approximately 12 to 18 inches above the patient's anus; a greater height creates too much pressure so that the fluid runs in too rapidly and causes painful distention of the rectum and colon. It also stimulates the urge to defecate immediately so that the patient cannot retain the fluid.

The temperature of the solution should be about 40.5°C (105°F). If a bath thermometer is not available, you can test the temperature of the fluid by pouring a small amount over your inner wrist. It should be warm to touch, but not hot. Solution that is too cool usually can't be retained; hot solutions may damage the tissues of the rectum.

The position of choice when giving an enema to a bed patient is the left lateral position with the hips slightly elevated. This allows the fluid, aided by the force of gravity, to flow downward along the natural curve of the rectum and descending colon. Although the right lateral position can be used if necessary, the patient may only be able to absorb a smaller quantity since that solution has to overcome gravity to enter the sigmoid colon. If the patient is unable to turn to the other side, the supine position can be used. Enemas should not be given to a patient seated on the toilet unless it is intended only to stimulate the urge to defecate. In a sitting position, the fluid cannot flow to other parts of the colon; it merely dilates the rectum and is rapidly expelled.

Question 24. For a cleansing enema given to an adult, indicate the specific information in connection with the following:

a. Kind of solution used _____.

b. Amount of solution _____.

c. Temperature of the solution _____.

d. Height of the solution container above the anus _____.

Question 25. State at least two possible reasons for the patient to have difficulty retaining the solution.

a. _____.

b. _____.

ITEM 10. PROCEDURE FOR GIVING A CLEANSING ENEMA

In the skill laboratory, practice assembling the supplies needed for giving an enema, and carry out the procedure using the Chase doll or other model with an anal opening. Review the steps of the procedure until you are familiar with them before you give an enema to a patient in the clinical setting.

Given a patient in bed who can turn to his side, assemble the supplies, prepare the enema, and give it to the patient so that it will effect an emptying of the rectum without undue discomfort.

Important Steps	Key Points
1. Collect the materials needed: an enema tray or disposable enema unit with a cover, lubricant, solution, paper towel, and Chux or pad for placing under the buttocks.	The enema tray or the disposable unit should have the same items: a container to hold the solution, tubing with a clamp to regulate the flow, and a rectal tube with a rounded tip to insert into the rectum. In the commercial enema, such as FLEET, these are in one unit. Other disposable enema kits contain a plastic bag, tubing, and a tip. The kit is charged to the

Important Steps   **Key Points**

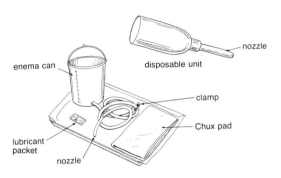

Enema tray.

patient and is discarded after use. In some
agencies, the kit is cleaned and reused by the
same patient as needed.

2. Prepare the solution as ordered by the
    doctor.

For tap water enema (abbreviated to TWE), fill
the container with warm water from the faucet
(approximately 1000 ml). For a soap solution
enema (abbreviated to SSE), add 1 ounce of
liquefied mild soap, like Ivory, to 1000 ml of
warm water.

For a saline enema, use a prepared solution
that has been warmed to 105° by setting the
flask in a pan of hot water. The temperature of
all solutions should be about 105°F (40.5°C).
Carry the enema unit to the patient's room.

Omit this step when using the commercially
prepared enemas, which are ready for use.

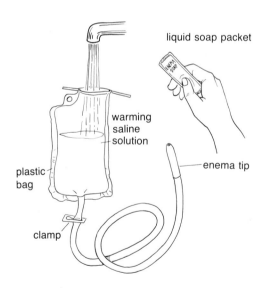

Preparing soapsuds enema.

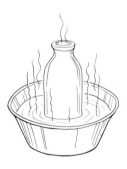

Warming saline solution.

3. Approach and identify the patient, explain
    what is to be done and why, and enlist his
    cooperation.

Wash your hands. Check the patient's wristband
to assure that the name is the same as the one
for whom the enema is ordered. While few
patients like the idea of an enema, most are
cooperative.

Important Steps	Key Points

4. Prepare the patient.

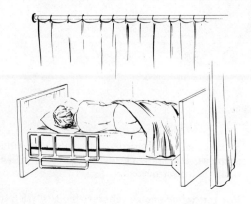

Provide privacy by closing the door, screening the bed, or pulling the cubicle curtains.

Avoid giving enemas at mealtimes, when other patients are eating in the same room, or during visiting hours unless visitors are asked to leave the room. It is embarrassing both to the patient and to others.

If at all possible, work from the right side of the bed so that the patient can turn on his left side. (The enema solution flows through the rectum and sigmoid colon to the descending colon more easily in this position.) Raise the bed to a comfortable working height. Lower the siderail if one is used, and adjust the bed to a flat position. Place the Chux or pad under the buttocks. Fold back the upper bedding and replace it with a bath blanket. Avoid exposing the patient's body. Turn him on his left side.

5. Prepare to give the enema.

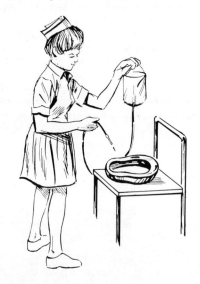

Place the enema unit on a chair near the area where you are working and place a bedpan near it. Open the packet of lubricant and lubricate the end of the rectal tube (about 1 inch). Open the clamp and allow the solution to run through the tubing to expel the air. Use the bedpan to collect this solution. Close the clamp on the tubing.

6. Insert the rectal tube.

Tell the patient about each step as you go along. Ask him to take deep breaths through his mouth to relax the anus and rectum. Insert the lubricated rectal tube *slowly* and *gently* about *4 inches.*

7. Instill the solution into the bowel.

Open the clamp on the tube and *allow the solution to flow slowly into the bowel.* Hold the solution *container 12 to 18 inches above the anus.* Regulate the flow according to the patient's ability to retain it. When the patient has discomfort, stop the flow by kinking the tubing or clamping it and instruct the patient to take deep breaths through his mouth until the cramping and urge pass. Then continue until the patient can retain no more, or the can is empty except for the fluid in the tubing.

8. Remove the rectal tube.

Do not allow all of the fluid in the tube to flow in, but clamp the tubing. If all the solution runs

Important Steps	Key Points

	in, air may get into the rectum and cause more discomfort to the patient. Withdraw the rectal tube gently and quickly. Place the soiled end in the paper towel.
9. Assist the patient to the bathroom or onto the bedpan.	If the patient goes to the bathroom, ask to see the results before the toilet is flushed.
	Roll up the bed so that the patient is in a sitting position unless contraindicated by his condition. Place the toilet tissue and his call light within reach.
10. Observe the results of the enema.	When the enema and stool have been expelled, remove the bedpan if used and assist the patient to clean the anal area if needed. Note the color, amount, and consistency of the stool. Take the bedpan, empty the contents, and clean and return it to the patient's unit.
11. Provide for the patient's comfort.	Remove the Chux or pad from under the patient. Replace the top covers. Provide water and a towel so that patient can wash his hands. Place him in the desired position, adjust the bed for comfort, and raise the siderail. Ventilate the room when possible to get rid of the odor, or use a room spray deodorizer if needed.
12. Remove all enema equipment.	Wash the enema container, tubing, and rectal tube in soapy water; rinse and dry them. If it is a disposable unit, discard it. Return reusable equipment to the proper place for sterilizing, and put soiled linen in the laundry hamper. Wash your hands.
13. Report and record as appropriate.	Report to the team leader or the nurse in charge that the enema has been given, and describe the results. Record this information on the patient's chart, and the time the enema was given. Charting example:
	2030. FLEET enema given. Large amount of dark brown stool expelled. J. Jones, NA

ITEM 11. THE RETENTION ENEMA

Often an oil-retention enema is ordered for a patient who is constipated. The oil must be retained in the rectum to soften and coat the hardened feces. Between 120 ml and 180 ml of warm oil is instilled rectally in the same manner as the cleansing enema, except that the oil should be retained at least 30 minutes. An Asepto syringe, rectal tube or small catheter, and a small pitcher or funnel to hold the oil may be used instead of the usual equipment. Mineral oil or olive oil is most commonly used. There are several prepackaged retention enemas on the market. Follow the same procedure as when giving a cleansing enema.

ITEM 12. THE USE OF RECTAL SUPPOSITORIES

In some settings, the beginning worker in nursing may not be allowed to insert rectal suppositories. *Check with your instructor; she may omit the next two items.*

UNIT 19

Rectal suppositories consist of a semisolid material that melts readily; they are somewhat cone-shaped and approximately 1½ inches long. They are made for many different purposes: some relieve pain or irritation, some contain drugs that the patient cannot take by mouth, and others promote bowel movements. The latter may do so (1) by stimulating the inner surface of the rectum and increasing the urge to defecate, (2) by forming gas that expands the rectum, or (3) by melting into a lubricating material to coat the stool for easier passage through the anal sphincter.

Rubber or plastic gloves should be worn when inserting the suppository into the rectum. After it has been inserted through the anal sphincter, the suppository should be guided by the index finger along the wall of the rectum to a point beyond the anal rectal ridge that is about 2 to 3 inches from the outer sphincter. The suppository will be ineffective if it is pushed into the fecal mass. Correct and incorrect placement of the suppository is shown in the following sketches. Correct placement is essential to assure that the suppository melts and serves its purpose.

Question 26.   Purposes for using rectal suppositories are a. _____ ,

                 b. _____ , or c. _____ .

Question 27.   When placed correctly, the rectal suppository

         ____a.   stimulates the outer surface of the rectum.

         ____b.   is in contact with the inner surface of the rectum.

         ____c.   melts inside the fecal mass in the rectum.

         ____d.   lies between the anal sphincter and the anal rectal ridge.

ITEM 13.   PROCEDURE FOR INSERTING RECTAL SUPPOSITORIES

You should go through the steps of this procedure several times in the skill laboratory in order to become familiar with it. Most schools do not have lifelike models of the anus and rectum, and you will not be able to insert the suppository and get the "feel" of it in the rectum until you reach the clinical area.

For your practice situation, you are to insert a rectal suppository to stimulate a bowel movement in a bed patient who can be turned on his side.

Important Steps	Key Points
1. Collect the items needed: the correct suppository, a rubber or plastic examining glove, lubricant, and a paper towel.	Check the doctor's orders for the type of suppository to be used and obtain it from the team leader or nurse in charge. The glove used to protect your hand need not be sterile unless specified because of surgery or chance of infection in the anal region.
2. Approach the patient, check his identity, explain what you plan to do, and enlist his cooperation.	The crucial point is to identify the patient correctly. The name on the patient's wristband should be identical to the name on the doctor's order. Unless it matches, do not proceed further. Most adult patients will be cooperative and eager for relief from their constipation. Children cooperate better if they have become used to having rectal temperatures taken, and if it is explained that the suppository will not hurt.
3. Prepare the patient.	Provide for privacy by closing the door, screening the patient, or pulling the cubicle curtain. Wash your hands. Place the suppository, glove, and towel on the bedside table.

Important Steps	Key Points

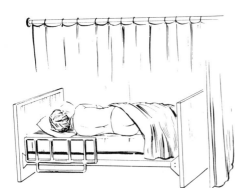

Adjust the bed to a nearly flat position, and lower the side if it is used. Place the patient in a Sims' position with his uppermost leg flexed and his back to the proximal side of the bed. Fold the top bedding obliquely back over the hips to expose the buttocks. Lower the pajama pants or fold the hospital gown out of the way.

4. Insert the suppository rectally.

Unwrap the foil or plastic covering of the suppository, leaving it on the wrapper. Put the glove on your dominant, or working hand, and take the suppository between thumb and index finger, and lubricate it. With your other hand, draw the top gluteal fold upward and toward the head to expose the anus. Ask the patient to take a deep breath at the time you insert the suppository; this helps to relax the anal sphincter. Slip the suppository into the anus, and with your gloved index finger guide it along the wall of the anus and rectum for 3 inches or the length of your finger. Withdraw you finger, and hold both buttocks tightly together for a few seconds while the patient breathes deeply until the urge to expel it has passed.

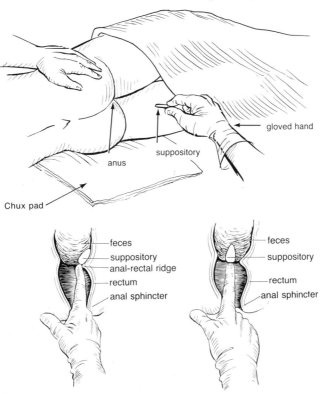

Correct placement.   Incorrect placement.

Important Steps	Key Points
5. Remove the glove.	Take the cuff of the glove, and pull it down over the hand so that the glove turns inside out. Place the soiled glove on the paper towel, and fold it closed.
6. Provide for the patient's comfort.	Turn the patient to his back. Inform him that he should retain the suppository for 15 to 20 minutes if possible. Leave his call light so that he can signal you to assist him to the toilet, onto a commode, or onto the bedpan. Adjust the top bedding and the bed for the patient's comfort, and raise the siderail. If he can get onto the bedpan himself, he may feel more secure if the bedpan is placed under the covers at his side, with a roll of toilet paper within his reach.
7. Remove the used items.	Take the suppository wrapper and the towel containing the soiled glove from the room. Discard the wrapper and towel; rinse the glove in soap and water and return it to the central processing department, or discard it if it is a disposable one.
8. Report and record as appropriate.	Record the type of suppository given, the time given, the time it acted, and the results. Note the color, amount, and other characteristics of the feces. Charting example: 0930. Glycerin suppository inserted. J. Jones, NA 1005. Large amount of soft brown formed stool expelled with large amount of flatus. Patient states he is much relieved. J. Jones, NA

ITEM 14.   DISTENTION OF THE HYPOACTIVE BOWEL

A second problem related to the hypoactive bowel is that of distention. Abdominal distention is caused by flatus (gas) when peristalsis is reduced or absent. Distention and "gas pains" occur frequently following abdominal surgery. The discomfort and pain are due to the stretching of the intestines, and to the spasms of the muscle layers. The goal of treatment is to reduce the amount of flatus into the bowel.

Procedures that you will use include the enema, irrigations such as the Harris flush, and use of the rectal tube.

Question 28.   In the hypoactive bowel, peristaltic action is (increased) (decreased).

Question 29.   Two common conditions that result from a hypoactive bowel are

a. _____ and b. _____ .

ITEM 15.   THE HARRIS FLUSH

One of the most effective methods of stimulating the hypoactive bowel to reduce the abdominal distention caused by flatus is the Harris flush. (In some parts of the country, it is called a colonic irrigation.) This is a means of irrigating the rectum and colon with fluid, then, with the rectal tube still in place, lowering the solution container (or irrigating can) 12 to 18 inches below the anus so that the fluid flows back into the container. The *alternate filling and draining of the colon* continues at least 4 or 5 times, or until there is no further release of gas. Since the fecal material, as well as flatus and the solution, may drain into the container, the contents may become thick and offensive. It can be emptied into the bedpan, and clear solution added to the irrigating container.

In the skill laboratory, you will need to practice collecting the equipment and carrying out the steps of the procedure for giving a Harris flush. The Harris flush follows the same procedure as the one used for giving a cleansing enema, except for the alternate instilling of fluid into the colon, and draining of it out. Unless ordered otherwise, 1000 ml of tap water is used at 40.5°C (105°F).

Given a patient with moderate abdominal distention following surgery of the abdomen three days ago, you are to give a Harris flush to reduce the flatus.

Important Steps	Key Points
Follow steps 1 through 6 for the cleansing enema, Item 10.	
7. Instill 200 to 300 ml of the solution into the patient's bowel.	Hold the irrigating can 12 to 18 inches above his anus. Regulate the flow according to the patient's ability to retain it. When the patient has discomfort, stop the flow by kinking the tubing or clamping it, and instruct him to take deep breaths through his mouth until the cramping and urge pass.
8. Drain the solution from the bowel.	Lower the irrigating can to a point 12 to 18 inches below the anus and allow the solution and flatus to flow back into the can. Fecal material may also flow back into the can. If the solution becomes thick with fecal particles, it may be emptied into the bedpan, and more clear solution poured from the pitcher into the can.
9. Repeat steps 7 and 8 until there is no further evidence of flatus.	You should continue the flushing of the bowel at least four to five times to ensure the release of flatus.
Steps 10 through 13 are the same as for the cleansing enema, Item 10.	Charting example: 2045. Harris flush given. Solution returned clear with a large amount of flatus expelled. Abdomen soft. States feeling very relieved. J. Jones, NA

ITEM 16. USE OF RECTAL TUBE FOR RELEASE OF FLATUS

When a patient is uncomfortable because of flatus in the lower bowel, a rectal tube can be inserted in the anus. This allows the gas to be expelled without the patient's straining to open the anal sphincter. The procedure is simple and effective. Obtain a rectal tube, lubricate the end, and take it to the patient's bedside in a hand towel or paper towel. Turn the patient to his side and gently insert the rectal tube about 4 inches. The free end of the rectal tube should be placed in the folded hand towel in case there is some expulsion of fecal liquid. The *rectal tube should not remain in the anus more than one-half hour*. It should be removed and reinserted after several hours if the patient again has discomfort. Severe irritation of the lining of the rectum can occur from prolonged insertion. When treatment is completed, rinse the rectal tube and return it to the central processing department. If disposable rectal tubes are used by your agency, discard the tube into the designated waste container. Charting example:

1115. Rectal tube inserted. Much flatus expelled.   J. Jones, NA
1145. Rectal tube removed. Patient states he is greatly relieved.   J. Jones, NA

ITEM 17. THE IRRITABLE OR HYPERACTIVE BOWEL

Hyperactivity of the bowel means that there is excessive movement in that area. Any condition that causes irritation of the intestines can cause hyperactivity of the bowel. The hyperactive, irritable bowel is seen in cases of diarrhea of all kinds, ulcerative colitis, diverticulitis, and certain other diseases.

Excessively strong and frequent peristaltic action moves the chyme rapidly through the intestines because the food mass may also serve as an irritant to an already irritated bowel. This rapid movement of the chyme in the bowel reduces the amount of time available for the intestines to *absorb* the nutrients, electrolytes, and water. It causes numerous bowel movements per day that generally are liquid or semiliquid in consistency.

The problems related to the hyperactive bowel are lack of enough food to nourish and repair the cells of the body; loss of electrolytes, which disturbs the chemical composition of the body fluids; and dehydration, which reduces the amount of water available for the body fluids. These conditions pose a serious threat to the patient's life. For example, infants and small children may die in a matter of 24 hours or less as a result of severe diarrhea.

The objectives of treating the hyperactive bowel are to reduce the irritability *and* to maintain adequate levels of nutrition, electrolytes, and water in the body. This requires vigorous treatment by the doctors and nurses. It is very important for the nurse worker to record the number and character of the stools per day, and the amount of food and fluid taken by the patient. It is also essential to provide an emotionally calm atmosphere for the patient.

Question 30. The rapid movement of chyme in the hyperactive bowel interferes with

_____ .

Question 31. An increase in the number of bowel movements per day is called

_____ .

Question 32. Disturbance of the chemical composition of body fluids is caused by loss of

_____ .

ITEM 18. COLLECTION OF A STOOL SPECIMEN

Review the following procedure several times to become familiar with it before you collect a stool specimen from a patient in the clinical area.

Given a doctor's order to obtain a stool specimen for specific laboratory tests, inform the patient about the procedure and after he has had a bowel movement, collect a portion of the stool, place it in a specimen container, complete the laboratory request for examination, and then promptly send the specimen and request slip to the laboratory.

Important Steps	Key Points
1. Gather the items needed: two tongue blades, a plastic or cardboard container with lid, and a paper towel.	Take them to the patient's unit and store them near the bedpan or the bathroom. This will serve to alert whoever cares for the patient that a stool specimen is needed. When the nurse answers the patient's light to remove the bedpan, supplies will be convenient for use in collecting the specimen.
2. Approach the patient, check his identification band, explain that a stool specimen is needed, and enlist his cooperation.	It is necessary to inform and get the cooperation of all patients, but especially the patient who has bathroom privileges so that he won't flush the stool away and delay the collection of the specimen for a day or more.

Important Steps	Key Points

3. Tell the patient how to assist in the collection of the specimen.

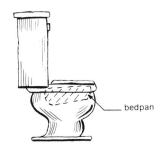

bedpan

He should be asked to:

    a. use the bedpan or bedside commode when he has the next bowel movement,

    b. save the stool, and

    c. notify the nurse that he has had a stool for the specimen.

The bedpan may be placed on a chair for use by the patient who has bathroom privileges, or the bedside commode may be used. In some cases, a bedpan will fit in the toilet bowl under the toilet seat as shown.

4. Collect a specimen of the stool after the patient has defecated.

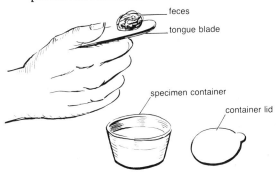

feces

tongue blade

specimen container

container lid

Take the bedpan and your supplies to the bathroom where you will empty the pan after obtaining the specimen. Write the *patient's name, his room number* or *ward*, and the *date* on the lid of the container. Often the label is on the container. You may need to put the information in both places. Use one or both of the tongue blades to transfer approximately one tablespoon of stool to the container. Put the lid on the container, wrap the soiled tongue blades in the paper towel, and drop them into the wastebasket. Empty and clean the bedpan or commode pan, and return it to its proper place.

5. Complete the laboratory request (requisition) slip.

Check the name of the patient and the name on the lab slip to see that they are identical. This is *vitally important.* An incorrect label will cause the laboratory to give the wrong information on a patient. The doctor could therefore order incorrect medicines or treatments for his patient because of an error in labeling a specimen.

6. Assure the prompt delivery of the specimen and the request slip to the laboratory.

Stool specimens should be examined while still warm (at or near body temperature) and while still fresh. Time and changes in temperature alter the stool. As an example, bright red blood begins to clot, dry out, and turn dark, and certain disease-causing organisms may die and thus fail to be detected. Make sure the specimen is taken to the lab immediately. (Some laboratories accept stool specimens only during specified hours. Check your agency procedure.)

7. Record and report as appropriate.

Report to the team leader or nurse in charge that the specimen has been obtained and sent to the laboratory. Record on the patient's chart that the specimen has been sent to the lab; note the date and time, and anything unusual about the stool. Charting example:

1110. Moderate amount of brown soft-formed stool. Specimen with requisition to lab.
                        J. Jones, NA

ITEM 19. INCONTINENCE OF FECES

Some patients lose the ability to control their bowels during a serious illness or hospitalization. This condition is called *incontinence*. The patient may become incontinent of feces whether his bowel is hypoactive, hyperactive, or normal. Incontinence generally occurs in patients who are not fully aware of where they are or what is going on. This lack of awareness may be due to the patient's physical disease or illness, or to his mental condition. However, whenever possible you should attempt to retrain and assist the incontinent patient to control the regularity of his bowel movements.

Even patients who are not fully aware of what is going on about them often realize that they have had a bowel movement and have soiled themselves or the bedding. Such a patient often has feelings of being less of a person, loses some of his self-respect, becomes embarrassed, or suffers from anxiety and fears that he has lost all control over what is happening to him. When you take care of an incontinent patient, it is important not to judge, scold, or fuss at him.

The treatment for incontinence is *retraining* in *bowel control habits*. In the beginning, it will take more time to try to establish bowel control habits than to clean up the soiled patient and change his bed. In the long run, however, you will help the patient to regain his self-respect as well as control of his bowels. Special effort should be made to help the very elderly patient overcome incontinence. It should be pointed out that incontinence of urine or feces is one of the major reasons for admitting the elderly patient to the extended-care facility or nursing home.

The method of retraining the incontinent patient is the same as that used for training a child to control his bowels. You must see that the patient eats an adequate diet, that his daily fluid intake is at least 2500 ml, that he gets the proper amount of sleep and rest, and that he gets exercise within the limits imposed by his illness. Set a regular time for evacuation based on his prior bowel habits and your observation of when the incontinent movements tend to occur. The patient should use the bedpan or commode, or be taken to the toilet. He should be given privacy and allowed at least 20 minutes for his bowels to move. Many doctors order rectal suppositories to stimulate defecation on a regular schedule in the retraining period. One way of using suppositories in habit training is to give one every day for the first week, then every other day for the second and third weeks, and thereafter only as needed to maintain a regular movement every two to three days.

Question 33. Incontinence of feces means _____ .

Question 34. The treatment for incontinence is _____ .

Question 35. Two benefits to the patient that result from retraining bowel control habits

are a. _____ and b._____ .

ITEM 20. FECAL IMPACTION

Fecal impaction means that the rectum and sigmoid colon become filled with fecal material. As the fecal material remains in the bowel for several days, it becomes more compacted, contains less water, and consequently becomes quite hard, and difficult or painful to pass through the anus.

The most obvious sign of fecal impaction is the absence of (or only a small amount of) bowel movement for more than three days. Another important sign of a possible fecal impaction is the passage of small amounts of semi-soft or liquid stool so that there is staining and soiling of the bed linens. This occurs as bacterial action of the fecal material continues to work on the outer surfaces of the hardened impacted mass, liquefying small portions of it. It is the result of the body's effort to remove the obstructing mass.

Fecal impaction should be suspected when a patient has a hypoactive bowel with constipation, or lack of bowel movement for three days or more. As in the case of bowel incontinence, this condition usually occurs in patients who may not be fully aware of their surroundings owing to their physical condition, illness, or mental state of confusion. The very young and the very old patients are especially prone to develop fecal impaction.

The nursing treatment of a fecal impaction is to *examine* for the presence of an impaction, *manually break it up*, and *remove* portions of the fecal mass. This should be followed by the use of suppositories, enemas, or laxatives as ordered by the physician. Again, emphasis should be on the *prevention of fecal impactions* by taking measures to ensure regular evacuation of the waste products from the bowel of each patient.

ITEM 21. PROCEDURE FOR REMOVAL OF FECAL IMPACTION

In the skill laboratory, go through the steps of the procedure several times until you are familiar with it. If a lifelike model of the anus and rectum is available, it can be used to help you get the feel of examining the rectum for impacted stool before you perform the procedure in the clinical area.

In this procedure, you are to examine the rectum for the presence of hardened stool, manually break it up, and remove such portions as you can in an older patient who is able to turn on his side.

Important Steps	Key Points
1. Collect the items you will need: a pair of rubber or plastic gloves, toilet paper, bedpan with cover, paper towel, lubricant, and Chux pad.	Check with the team leader or the nurse in charge to find out if there are any reasons for not carrying out the procedure. Gloves need not be sterile unless specified by the RN. The Chux is used to protect the sheets from possible soiling during the procedure.
2. Approach the patient, check his identification band, explain what you plan to do, and enlist his cooperation.	This procedure is often *uncomfortable for the patient*, so when possible you should have someone assist you who can reassure and comfort the child, aged patient, or patient who may be mentally disturbed. Wash your hands.
3. Prepare the patient.	Provide privacy by closing the door, screening, or pulling the cubicle curtain. Raise the bed to working height. Place the patient in Sims' position, and slip the Chux under his hips. Fold the top bedding back obliquely over his hips to expose his buttocks. Fold the hospital gown out of the way or lower the pajama pants. Place the bedpan and toilet tissue on a chair that is close to the bed and within your convenient reach in order to avoid strain or injury to yourself.
4. Examine the patient rectally for fecal impaction.	The person assisting you should reassure him, hold his hand or support his shoulder in Sims' position, and help explain what is being done. Put on the gloves, use lubricant on your index finger, and *gently* insert it into the anus. The index finger should follow the wall of the rectum in a slightly curving motion. As the finger comes in contact with feces in the rectum, note the consistency; then move the finger into the lower portion of the fecal mass, again noting the consistency.
5. Break up and remove the fecal impaction.	With the examining index finger, dislodge or break off a small amount of fecal material and gently remove it, placing it in the bedpan. Continue removing as much fecal material as you can reach with your finger, or until the patient's discomfort warrants discontinuing the procedure. Remove the soiled gloves and place them in a paper towel.

Important Steps	Key Points
6. Remove the remaining fecal material.	Often, the stimulation of removing the impaction manually will create the urge in the patient to defecate. Help the patient to the bathroom, or place the patient on a clean bedpan and provide toilet paper. If he is unable to defecate, follow up by carrying out the doctor's order for a suppository, enema, or laxative.
7. Provide for the patient's comfort.	Wash and dry the patient's anal area. Remove the Chux from under his hips. Position him comfortably in good alignment and adjust his bed to the desired position. Leave his call light within reach, raise the siderail if used, and ventilate the room or use a deodorizer if necessary to get rid of the odors.
8. Remove the used items.	Observe the characteristics of the fecal material in the bedpan; then remove it from the room, empty the pan, clean it, and return it to its proper place along with the roll of toilet paper. Remove the soiled Chux and the gloves in the paper towel. Discard gloves of the disposable type.
9. Report and record as appropriate.	Record the presence of the fecal impaction, the time, and the characteristics of the feces, such as color and consistency. Record any additional procedures, such as giving an enema or a suppository. Report the results of these procedures to the team leader or the nurse in charge. Charting example:
	1045. Rectal examination for fecal impaction. Moderate amount of brown hard feces removed manually. B. Rose, SN

ITEM 22. COLOSTOMIES AND ILEOSTOMIES

The first successful colostomy was performed in 1793. Today, thousands of people have colostomies, and a smaller number have ileostomies. Most of them have learned to manage their ostomy and to lead a normal life again. Part of the patient's adjustment and rehabilitation depends on how well the nurse and others help him adjust to having a stoma.

Colostomy refers to an opening, or *stoma*, made through the abdominal wall into the colon. Waste materials drain through the stoma and bypass the lower portion of the diseased or injured colon. Colostomies are performed to allow an injured or inflamed bowel time to heal, or they are performed after removal of a tumor, such as cancer.

The management of the ostomy depends on the location of the stoma and the portion of colon that remains. Since the main functions of the large intestine are to absorb water, solidify waste material, and store feces until it is eliminated, the further down the colon the colostomy is located, the more the discharge will resemble a normal bowel movement. In fact, one can live with the entire colon removed or inactive, as in the case of an ileostomy. Various types of ostomy are shown in the following illustrations.

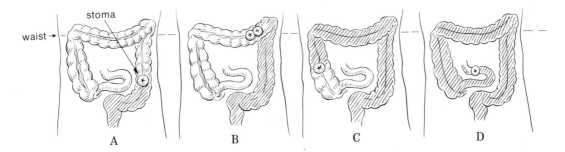

a. Descending colon: Solid stools; controlled by irrigations.

b. Transverse colon: May be single opening or double-barrel — one barrel active with drainage, the other inactive. Stool is toothpaste consistency or semiliquid. May be controlled by irrigation.

c. Ascending colon: Frequent, liquid, semiliquid; difficult to control.

d. Ileostomy sites: Liquid, runny stool; no control.

Colostomies of the sigmoid, or descending, colon are the easiest to manage and to control because they are closer to the end of the large intestines. People who have colostomies in this area are able to regulate themselves so well by using irrigations that they generally can get along without a colostomy bag much of the time and need not worry about an accidental discharge. A colostomy of the ascending, or transverse, colon is sometimes referred to as a "wet" colostomy because the discharge is semiliquid and tends to flow at intervals during the day and night. The discharge of a "wet" colostomy may contain digestive enzymes that are irritating to unprotected skin surfaces. Refer to the unit on special skin care for information on how to protect the skin around the colostomy.

Care of the Patient with a Colostomy

A patient who has a new colostomy must make many adjustments following surgery. It is understandable that such a patient is worried and fearful about being different now from other people, about their friends acceptance of them, and about their own feelings regarding the colostomy and loss of control over bowel actions. Perhaps most of all, he is concerned about the possibility of recovering from a disease that has required this extreme type of surgery.

As a skillful and understanding health worker, you can do a great deal to help the patient through this difficult time. First, you need to develop skills in using the colostomy appliances, in giving skin and stoma care, and in assisting the patient to gain control, if possible, through irrigations. Give frequent reassurances to the patient and his family that many people in all walks of life live with an ostomy and conduct normal daily activities. If there is an ostomy club in your community, the patient can derive considerable benefit from sharing experiences with others who also have colostomies or ileostomies. You may be able to assist further by advising him about the proper diet for helping to control the type of drainage and odors. Some foods, such as those of the cabbage family, beans, onions, and often, asparagus, cause increased flatus and odors. Finally, you can provide a calm, matter-of-fact atmosphere, and encourage him to resume normal patterns of living. We know that emotions affect the bowel, and patients who are tense or upset will reflect this physically by developing an upset colon and increased drainage.

Ostomy Appliances

Generally, surgeons now attach an appliance on the patient's colostomy at the time of the operation, or soon thereafter. This appliance is a device for collecting the drainage from the stoma. A patient with a colostomy usually wears a lightweight plastic bag over the stoma that can be discarded after each use. The plastic is made to resist odors, but occasionally the bag may inflate with gas and look like a balloon if the patient has a lot of flatus. You can make a small hole in the top of the bag and allow the gas to escape.

Although there are many kinds of appliances on the market, most are variations of these three basic types:

1. Cloth belt supporting a two-piece combination of a disposable bag and reusable mounting ring, which may have an inner sealing ring of karaya gum, a substance that protects the skin from irritation.

2. One-piece bag with an attached square of adhesive around the stoma opening that can be worn without a belt.

3. One-piece bag with a gasket that uses no adhesive, but is worn with a belt.

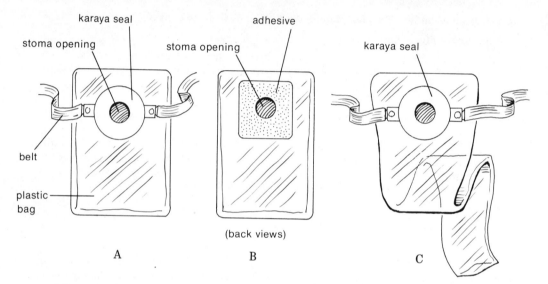

a. A karaya seal stoma bag helps promote postoperative healing. It is secured with belt.

b. Simple "stick-on" type of stoma bag, using adhesive on skin.

c. Ileostomy stoma bag, 12 to 16 inches long. Can be drained through end, then reclosed or clamped.

A person who has an ileostomy usually wears a two-piece appliance. Because he has continuous drainage from the stoma, he must keep that drainage from flowing directly onto the skin, and he therefore needs a bag that can be emptied without removing the appliance, and then be reclosed.

Stoma bags come in a variety of sizes and it is important to have one that fits closely around the stoma. Because stomas tend to shrink as healing occurs, it may be necessary to remeasure the stoma to ensure the correct size opening. Manufacturers also produce irrigations sets which contain all the equipment the patient needs for self-care. Refer to Unit 21, pages 457 to 460 for instructions on stoma care and changing bags.

Preparing the Patient for Self-care

As soon as the patient's postoperative condition improves, he should become involved in the care of the stoma and skin, and also learn how to control the drainage from the stoma. First have him watch while you change the bag and clean the skin around the stoma several times. Next, ask him to change the bag on the appliance and clean the area around the stoma. When he has become accustomed to doing this, encourage him to learn to do his own irrigations. Reassure him that he can resume normal activities much sooner if he does not have to depend on someone else for this care.

ITEM 23. COLOSTOMY IRRIGATIONS

A colostomy irrigation is simply an enema given through the stoma. Irrigations are done to (1) cleanse the intestinal tract of wastes, (2) establish control or regular evacuation of the colostomy, and (3) prevent obstruction of the bowel. For patients with a new colostomy, irrigations are carried out only with a doctor's order.

Irrigations may begin as soon as two to four days after surgery, when fecal drainage begins to come through the stoma. Remember the following rules when using colostomy irrigations to establish control of the drainage.

1. Irrigations should be done at the same time each day. Plan with the patient and select a time that will be convenient after he arrives home as well. The time should permit undisturbed use of the bathroom for about one hour.

2. One hour should be allowed for the irrigation. The patient may be able to clamp the end of an irrigator drain and carry out other activities, but he should not feel rushed or pressured for time.

3. Irrigations should continue daily until control is established. Control means that there is no spillage of fecal material from the colostomy during a 24-hour period. Control can be established within a three- to ten-day period, and then maintained by irrigations every other day, or as needed.

Procedure for Irrigating a Colostomy

Given a patient who underwent a colostomy of the descending colon five days ago and is making a good recovery, you are to irrigate the colostomy with the patient sitting on the toilet or commode. You must be skillful and your manner should be accepting of the patient as a person.

In the skill laboratory, assemble the equipment required to give a colostomy irrigation and practice each step by using a Chase doll or a similar model.

Important Steps	Key Points
1. Obtain an irrigator set containing an an irrigator, irrigator drain, ostomy belt, and lubricant.	The irrigator set can be used by the patient after he leaves the hospital. If a set is not available, assemble the equipment — an enema can, a number 16 or 18 French catheter, a lubricant, a pitcher, and an irrigating drain or a plastic apron.

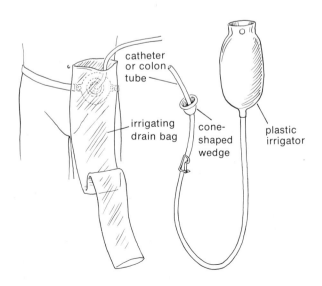

catheter or colon tube

irrigating drain bag

cone-shaped wedge

plastic irrigator

Important Steps	Key Points
2. Approach the patient, explain what is to be done and why, and enlist his cooperation.	Be sure that you are doing the irrigation at the same time as on the previous day in order to establish regularity and control.
3. Prepare the patient.	Assist him to the bathroom and provide privacy so that others cannot intrude during the procedure. Have him sit on the toilet and help him remove and dispose of the soiled colostomy bag. Wash your hands. Have a disposable irrigating drain ready to attach to the belt, or place it over the stoma if the drain has a valve to insert the catheter through. Pull his gown or pajamas out of the way to keep them from soiling.
4. Prepare the solution.	Regular tap water is used, unless saline or some other solution has been ordered by the doctor. Water should be warm — about body temperature. Clamp the tubing of the irrigator, add 1000 ml of lukewarm tap water, and expel the air from the tubing.
5. Insert the catheter into the colostomy stoma.	Lubricate about 2 inches of the catheter. Insert it into the stoma about 4 inches. A cone-shaped plug placed at that distance prevents the catheter from being inserted too far and keeps the water from leaking out. If the catheter is hard to insert, *do not force it*. Open the clamp on the tubing and allow the water to flow gently, or rotate the catheter as you insert it. You could injure the colon by forcing the catheter.

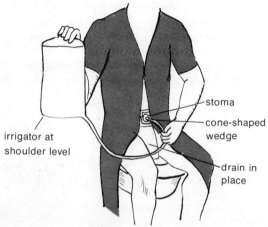

irrigator at
shoulder level

stoma

cone-shaped
wedge

drain in
place

Colostomy irrigation sitting on toilet.

6. Instill the solution into the colon.	Hold the irrigator no higher than the patient's shoulder level. Holding it higher would cause too much pressure, and water would come out as fast as it goes in. Cramps are caused by water that is too cold or being run in too fast. Run the solution in. Do not use more than 1000 ml.
7. Have the patient expel the fluid.	Make sure that the irrigator drain bag is in place over the stoma opening. The first gushing return of water and fecal drainage goes directly down into the toilet. It may take up to one hour for all the fluid to return. Later, with more experience in irrigating, the patient may fold up the end of the drain, clamp it, and engage in other activities while waiting for the rest of the water and stool. If no water returns, it may be due to the fact that the catheter is

Important Steps	Key Points

inserted too far, or that insufficient water was used, or that not enough time has been allowed to expel it.

8. See that the patient is comfortable.

When all the water and stool have been expelled, remove the irrigating drain. Assist the patient as needed to clean the skin around the stoma and dry it. Attach a clean bag over the stoma. Help him back to bed after he has washed his hands. Adjust the bed to a comfortable position. Leave the signal light and bedside stand within reach.

9. Clean the equipment and return it to the proper place.

Rinse any stool from the irrigating drain and dispose of the soiled drain. Clean and dry the irrigator and tubing. If it is the private property of the patient, store it in the bathroom or unit for future reuse.

10. Report and record as appropriate.

Report to the team leader or the nurse in charge that the colostomy irrigation has been given; report the time and the results. Also report the patient's reaction to the procedure, any unusual appearance of the stoma, or any change in the patient's condition. Charting example:

1400. Tap water, 800 ml as colostomy irrigation. Solution and moderate amount of soft brown stool expelled. Did own stoma care and applied new colostomy bag.   J. Jones, LPN

Irrigation Procedure for a Bed Patient

An alternative method involves giving a colostomy irrigation to the bed patient. Use the same equipment and procedure as you would with the patient who can get up to go to the bathroom. However, after instilling the water into the stoma, place the irrigating drain securely around the opening to make sure that it doesn't leak. Either clamp the end of the drain or let the contents of the drain flow into a bedpan at the side of the bed.

ITEM 24.   CONCLUSION OF THE LESSON

You have now completed the lesson on bowel elimination. When you feel sure that you know the vocabulary, the abnormal characteristics of the feces, the problems related to the hypoactive and hyperactive bowel, and the methods of control of the bowel, and when you have practiced the procedures used, arrange with your instructor to take the post-test.

V.   ADDITIONAL INFORMATION FOR ENRICHMENT

The bowel is part of one of the major systems of the body. In this lesson on bowel elimination it has been possible to include only a small part of what is known about the bowel and its function. Those of you who have a special interest in learning more about nursing problems related to the bowel may wish to study further.

Some areas that might be of interest to you are listed:

1. Information related to the anatomy and physiology of the intestinal tract.

   a. Absorption of nutrients through the mechanisms of active transport and diffusion.

    b. Electrolytes, and their function in body fluids and in the regulation of the body's acid-base balance.

    c. Types of bacteria present in the bowel, the function of the "good guys," and the identity of the "bad guys."

    d. The role of the liver and bile in the digestive process.

2. Causes of diseases related to the bowel; treatment and nursing care of patients with these diseases.

    a. Diarrheas and dysentery.

    b. Ulcers of the stomach or duodenum.

    c. Ulcerative colitis.

    d. Diverticulitis.

    e. Cancers of the bowel.

    f. Sprue and other nutritional diseases.

    g. Obstructions and intussusception of the bowel.

    h. Parasite and worm infestations of the bowel (common in children living in underdeveloped countries). Some cases are so severe that worms are regurgitated from the stomach and infest the lungs as well.

3. Other areas of study suggested by material in the lesson.

    a. Effects of various drugs on the bowel, especially the hypoactive and the hyperactive bowel.

    b. Incontinence problems of elderly patients.

    c. Indications, preparation, and procedure for proctoscopy and sigmoidoscopy.

    d. Preoperative and postoperative care of the colostomy patient.

    e. Altered body image and psychological impact created by the artificial anus.

    f. Special challenges to nursing care presented by the patient with an ileostomy.

    g. Procedure for irrigating a double-barrel, or two-loop, colostomy.

4. It is highly recommended that you contact the local chapter of the Colostomy Club, which is part of a national organization, United Ostomy Association, Incorporated (there are chapters in many cities). A member of the club could be invited to speak to a group about his operation, his feeling about it, the problems he has encountered, and the way he controls his colostomy.

When you have found a topic of interest to you, look up reading material on the subject in your library. If you have some difficulty finding appropriate literature, contact your instructor, who may be able to help you find it.

WORKBOOK ANSWER SHEET

Question 1. a. mucus

           b. cecum

           c. tract

           d. flatus

e. suppository

f. polyp

Question 2. a. hemorrhage

b. diarrhea

c. hemorrhoids

3. a. absorption

b. elimination of waste products

4. a., c., and d.

5. a. distention

b. diarrhea

c. constipation

d. incontinence

6. six

7. absorption

8. a. S, b. L, c. L, d. S, e. L, f. S, g. L

9. a. absorption of water and electrolytes

b. storage of waste products

10. solid material; water

11. brown; brownish-yellow

12. blood; duodenum

13. 10 hours

14. bright red blood

15. a. green

b. watery

16. bile

17. mucus

18. a. circular

b. longitudinal

c. oblique

19. peristalsis

20. pressure or weight on the sphincter

21. three

22. a. diet

b. fluids

c. exercise

d. rest

23. false

Question 24.   a.   tap water, saline, or soap solution, or as ordered by physician

b.   1000 ml

c. $105°F$ or $40.5°C$

d.   12 to 18 inches

25.   Any two of the following:

a.   rectum overdistended with fluid

b.   solution is too cool

c.   solution is too hot

d.   solution is running in too fast

e.   solution container is held too high

26.   a.   to relieve pain

b.   to give medications

c.   to promote bowel movement

27.   b.

28.   decreased

29.   a.   distention

b.   constipation

30.   absorption of water, nutrients, and electrolytes

31.   diarrhea

32.   electrolytes

33.   inability to control elimination of feces

34.   retraining for bowel control

35.   a.   control or continence of bowels

b.   regain self-respect

PERFORMANCE TEST

In the skill laboratory, your instructor will ask you to demonstrate your knowledge and skill in performing four of the following six activities without use of reference material:

1. Describe five unusual or abnormal conditions of the stool that you could observe visually.

2. Given a recent postoperative patient with constipation due to a hypoactive bowel, you are to demonstrate the preparation and the procedure for giving a cleansing enema.

3. Given a recent postoperative patient with abdominal distention, you are to demonstrate the preparation and the procedure for giving a Harris flush.

4. Given a patient who has called you to empty feces from his bedpan, describe the steps you would take to collect a specimen of the stool and prepare it for the laboratory.

5. Given a patient who is incontinent of feces, you are to describe the measures that you would use in retraining the patient to control his bowels.

6. Given a patient with a recent colostomy of the sigmoid colon, you are to demonstrate the preparation and the procedure for irrigating the colostomy as the patient sits on the toilet. (This is an optional performance test, used at the discretion of your instructor.)

PERFORMANCE CHECKLIST

BOWEL ELIMINATION

IDENTIFICATION OF ABNORMAL FECES

1. Observe the color of the feces to detect abnormalities

    a. Brown — normal.

    b. Green — too much sugar in the infant's diet.

    c. Greenish-black (meconium) — newborn infant.

    d. Orange-yellow — breast-fed infant.

    e. Green — from chlorophyll.

    f. Color of the stool is affected by some drugs.

    g. Clay — lack of bile secretion.

    h. Chalky white — ingestion of X-ray preparation solutions.

    i. Light tan — undigested fat.

2. Observe the stool for the presence of blood.

    a. Bright red blood — hemorrhage in lower bowel, or hemorrhoids.

    b. Dark brown to black blood — bleeding high in the GI tract.

3. Check the stool for mucus; mucus indicates irritation or inflammation of the intestinal lining.

4. Look for parasitic worms: tapeworms, roundworms, and pinworms.

5. Observe for pus, which indicates an infection in a portion of the intestinal tract.

6. Check for constipation.

7. Check for diarrhea.

ENEMA

1. Collect the materials needed and wash your hands.

2. Prepare a solution as ordered (temperature at 105°F).

3. Take the solution to the patient's room and put it on a chair near the bed.

4. Identify the patient.

5. Explain the procedure and enlist the patient's cooperation.

6. Wash your hands.

7. Prepare the patient correctly: screen him for privacy, drape and position him, adjust the bed height, and lower the siderails.

8. Prepare to give the enema

   a. Lubricate the tube about 1 inch.

   b. Expel the air from the tube.

   c. Allow the solution to run into the bedpan.

   d. Clamp the tube.

9. Gently insert the rectal tube 4 inches into the patient's rectum.

10. Clamp the tube.

   a. Run the solution slowly.

   b. Hold the can 12 to 18 inches above the anus.

   c. Clamp the tubing and wait if the patient complains of cramps; instruct him to breathe deeply through his mouth.

11. Remove the rectal tube and place it in a paper towel.

12. Remove the bedpan.

   a. Empty it and observe the contents.

   b. Clean the bedpan.

   c. Store the bedpan.

13. Leave the patient comfortable.

   a. Permit him to wash and dry his hands.

   b. Use a deodorizer if available and needed.

14. Record the activity on the chart.

HARRIS FLUSH

1. Collect the equipment.

2. Identify the patient and inform him about the procedure.

3. Prepare the patient.

4. Wash your hands.

5. Prepare a rectal tube:

   a. Lubricate the tube.

   b. Expel the air from the tube.

6. Insert the tube 4 inches into the patient's rectum.

7. Raise the can 12 to 18 inches above the patient's anus.

8. Unclamp the tube and insert 250 to 300 cc of solution.

9. Regulate the flow with the patient's ability to retain the solution.

10. Drain the solution from the colon by lowering the can to 12 to 18 inches below the anus.

11. Repeat steps 4, 5, and 6 until there is no more flatus.

12. Remove the rectal tube and place it in a paper towel.

13. Provide for the patient's comfort.

14. Remove the equipment; clean it and return it to storage.

15. Record the treatment on the patient's chart.

COLLECTION OF STOOL SPECIMENS

1. Gather the necessary equipment: two tongue blades, a specimen container and lid, and a paper towel.

2. Wash your hands.

3. Collect the specimen.

4. Remove the bedpan and take it to the appropriate work area.

5. Write the patient's name and room number, and the date in the proper place on the container.

6. With a tongue blade, transfer at least 1 tablespoon of stool from the bedpan to the specimen container.

7. Put the lid on the container; wrap and discard the tongue blade.

8. Empty, clean and return the bedpan to storage.

9. Complete the laboratory requisition. Check the patient's name on the requisition and on the specimen container to be sure they are the same. Be sure to use the correct lab slip, indicating the type of test ordered, the date, and the time the stool was passed.

10. Take to the lab at once (stat). Explain why a delay in taking the specimen to the lab would alter the stool and give a false reading.

11. Record on the patient's chart.

BOWEL TRAINING

1. Describe measures used in retraining the incontinent patient.

   a. Adequate diet.

   b. Adequate liquids, at least 2500 cc of liquid daily.

   c. Sleep and exercise within the patient's physical limits.

   d. Regular time for bowel evacuation based on his prior habits.

   e. Allowance of at least 20 minutes for bowels to move.

   f. Suppository, used on the doctor's order. Given daily at the same time for the first week, then every other day the second and third weeks, and then p.r.n.

COLOSTOMY IRRIGATION

1. Assemble the equipment.

2. Wash your hands.

3. Identify the patient and explain the procedure.

4. Provide privacy, and prepare the patient for the procedure.

   a. Assist him to the toilet.

   b. Remove his soiled colostomy bag.

   c. Prepare the irrigating drain and attach it to the belt.

5. Prepare the solution — 1000 ml water at body temperature.

   a. Pour 1000 ml of solution into the irrigator bag.

   b. Expel the air from the tubing, then clamp it shut.

6. Lubricate the tip of the catheter.

   a. Insert it into the stoma about 3 to 4 inches.

   b. Unclamp the tubing and allow the solution to run for easier insertion of the catheter.

7. Instill the solution, holding it no higher than the level of the patient's shoulder.

8. After instilling 500 to 1000 ml of solution, remove the catheter.

9. Place an irrigating drain over the stoma.

10. When all the solution and stool have been expelled, remove the irrigating drain.

11. Cleanse and dry the skin.

12. Attach a clean colostomy bag; allow the patient to do this as soon as he is able.

13. Have the patient wash his hands, and provide for his comfort.

14. Clean and return the equipment to storage.

15. Record the treatment on the patient's chart.

POST-TEST

Matching: Match each of the items in Column I with the item in Column II that best describes it. Items in Column II may be used more than once.

Column I

_____ 1. colitis

_____ 2. rectum

_____ 3. duodenum

_____ 4. chyme

_____ 5. ileum

_____ 6. appendicitis

_____ 7. sigmoid

_____ 8. flatus

_____ 9. hemorrhoids

_____10. bile

Column II

a. part of the small intestine

b. part of the large intestine

c. part of the contents of the intestines

d. disease of the intestines

e. none of the above

Multiple Choice: Select the correct or best answer for the following questions. There is only one best answer for each one.

11. In the adult, the length of the intestinal tract is approximately:

    a. 20 feet long

    b. three times the body length

    c. 16 feet long

    d. six times the body length

12. The important function of the small intestine is to:

    a. connect the stomach to the colon

    b. absorb nutrients and electrolytes

    c. provide storage for waste products

    d. absorb water and gases

13. One important function of the large intestine is to:

    a. absorb nutrients

    b. aid in the digestion of foods

    c. absorb water

    d. aid in transporting chyme

14. Movement in the intestines by alternate contractions that squeeze the contents forward is called

    a. constipation

    b. peristalsis

    c. distention

    d. incontinence

15. Frequent, rapid movement of intestinal contents that results in many watery stools per day is called

   a. diarrhea

   b. diverticulitis

   c. peristalsis

   d. hemorrhoids

16. If an obstruction or twisting of the small intestine prevents the chyme from moving past the obstacle, the result is

   (1) some discomfort, but not serious

   (2) loss of nutrients and electrolytes

   (3) a serious threat to person's life

   (4) decreased bowel movements

   a. All of above, b. (2), (3), and (4), c. (1), (2), and (4), d. (3)

17. Mrs. Shortly was admitted to the hospital two days ago after vomiting some blood. She passed a small stool that was black and tarry in appearance. The reason for the color of the stool is:

   a. mucus

   b. parasites

   c. blood

   d. medications

18. Today Mrs. Shortly had barium while in X-ray for a GI series. The barium causes the color of the stool to appear:

   a. white

   b. green

   c. brown

   d. red

19. In most cultures of the world, children are taught to control their bowel movements by the age of:

   a. one year

   b. 18 months

   c. three years

   d. three and one-half years

20. When training the young child to gain voluntary control of his bowel movements, the mother or nurse should do all of the following *except*:

   a. give frequent encouragement while the child is sitting on the toilet.

   b. provide roughage in the diet to give bulk to the stool.

   c. establish a regular time for bowel elimination.

   d. take the child off the "potty" after 5 minutes even if there has been no movement.

21. An older person in the hospital has not had a bowel movement for several days. In the last few hours, the patient has passed two very small, semiliquid bowel movements. The nurse suspects that the patient has:

a. an inadequate diet

b. an impaction

c. diarrhea

d. a hyperactive bowel

22. The most common problem that people with a hypoactive bowel have is:

a. constipation

b. impaction

c. obstructions

d. infections

23. The treatment of constipation includes all of the following *except*:

a. avoidance of emotional stress

b. medication for pain or discomfort

c. laxatives and enemas

d. a moderate amount of exercise

24. When giving an enema to a patient in bed, the best position for instilling the solution is:

a. a prone position

b. a right lateral Sims' position

c. a supine position

d. a left lateral position

25. The lubricated rectal tube is inserted into the anus a distance of about

a. 2 inches

b. 4 inches

c. 6 inches

d. 8 inches

26. How high above the patient's buttocks does the nurse hold the solution container when giving an enema?

a. 4 to 6 inches

b. 6 to 10 inches

c. 10 to 12 inches

d. 12 to 18 inches

27. The reason for holding the container at the correct height is to:

a. make the solution run in more quickly

b. have the water go up higher in the colon

c. avoid increasing the pressure of the water

d. keep the nurse's arm from getting too tired

UNIT
19

28. All of the following may be reasons for a patient to have difficulty taking and retaining the enema solution *except*:

    a. he takes panting breaths through the mouth

    b. the solution is too cool

    c. the solution is too hot

    d. the solution is running in too fast

29. The correct position of the rectal suppository is:

    a. lying in the sphincter of the anus

    b. pushed into the fecal mass

    c. at the flexure of the sigmoid

    d. in contact with the lining of the rectum

30. The most common purpose for giving a Harris flush or colonic irrigation is to:

    a. relieve distention caused by flatus

    b. cleanse the bowel of fecal material

    c. promote the absorption of fluids

    d. remove bacteria from the intestinal tract

31. A rectal tube that is left in the patient's rectum for more than 30 minutes can cause:

    a. total removal of all gases from the abdomen

    b. irritation of the rectum and anus

    c. increased absorption of water from the bowel

    d. hyperactivity of the large intestines

32. Patients who have a colostomy can more easily control the drainage from a stoma located in the:

    a. ileum

    b. ascending colon

    c. sigmoid colon

    d. transverse colon

33. Important things the nurse can do for the patient with a new colostomy would include all of the following *except*:

    a. Be skillful in using the colostomy appliance

    b. Provide an accepting and matter-of-fact atmosphere for care

    c. Tell the patient not to worry and that he'll be okay

    d. Inform him about some of the gas-forming foods

34. The colostomy appliance often used for the patient following surgery contains a karaya seal because the karaya:

    a. controls the amount of drainage from the stoma

    b. cushions and reduces the pressure of the drainage bag

    c. keeps the odors from escaping into the drainage bag

    d. protects the skin against the irritation of the drainage

35. When the patient takes (or is given) a colostomy irrigation, care should be taken to:

    a. hold the solution no higher than the patient's shoulders.

    b. alternate irrigation time from morning to evening

    c. make sure the procedure is completed within 30 minutes.

    d. keep the irrigating water hot, or over $140°F$

POST-TEST ANNOTATED ANSWER SHEET

1. d. (p. 388)	19. c. (p. 396)
2. b. (p. 388)	20. d. (p. 396)
3. a. (p. 388)	21. b. (p. 408)
4. c. (p. 388)	22. a. (p. 397)
5. a. (p. 388)	23. b. (p. 397)
6. d. (p. 388)	24. d. (p. 398)
7. b. (p. 388)	25. b. (p. 400)
8. c. (p. 389)	26. d. (p. 400)
9. d. (p. 388)	27. c. (p. 398)
10. c. (p. 388)	28. a. (p. 398)
11. d. (p. 390)	29. d. (p. 402)
12. b. (pp. 390–391)	30. a. (p. 404)
13. c. (p. 392)	31. b. (p. 405)
14. b. (p. 395)	32. c. (p. 411)
15. a. (p. 389 and 406)	33. c. (p. 411)
16. b. (p. 390)	34. d. (p. 412)
17. c. (p. 393)	35. a. (pp. 413–414)
18. a. (pp. 393–394)	

VOLUME 2

Unit 20

ADMISSION, TRANSFER, AND DISCHARGE

I. DIRECTIONS TO THE STUDENT

You are to proceed through the lesson with this workbook as your guide. Practice the tasks using the different types of equipment with the mannequin or a student partner in the skill laboratory. After you have completed the lesson and the practice, arrange with your instructor for the post-tests.

II. GENERAL PERFORMANCE OBJECTIVE

You will be able to admit, transfer, or discharge a patient correctly while demonstrating concern for his physical and emotional well-being as well as for his personal belongings.

III. SPECIFIC PERFORMANCE OBJECTIVES

After finishing this lesson, you will be able to:

1. Make observations of the patient's physical and emotional condition at the time of admission and record them.

2. Explain the hospital environment and routine to the patient, including the operation of the electric bed controls, the TV controls, and the nurse-call communication system.

3. Take care of the patient's personal belongings during his stay in the hospital or during his transfer to another location.

4. Prepare the patient and his belongings for discharge.

5. Complete the necessary admission, transfer, and discharge forms.

IV. VOCABULARY

Words commonly used in charting the procedures for this unit can be found in the unit on Charting. Practice charting these procedures, using the terms listed. When you are able to use these words effectively and correctly, you will have increased your vocabulary greatly.

V. INTRODUCTION

The admission of a patient to a health care facility is understandably a difficult time for him and his family. The patient is frightened and may be having pain or discomfort. Your kindness, courtesy, concern, patience, and confidence in what you are doing are vitally important. You must also convey the assurance that everything in his records will be kept strictly confidential by you and other health personnel.

The preliminary routine admission procedures (obtaining personal facts for the admission record, getting a signed general consent for care, assigning the patient to a bed, applying the patient's identification bracelet) are usually handled by the Admitting Office staff. They may be a part of the Business Office section or the Nursing Service, depending on the agency. (Emergency admission procedures may vary from the routine admission procedure.) Although each agency has its own policies, the general procedure is similar.

After completing the first admitting procedures, the admitting office will notify the nursing unit by telephone that the patient will be arriving shortly to occupy a specific bed. Other information is also given in this call: the patient's full name, the physician's name, the diagnosis, and other details affecting his admission to the unit.

The patient will be sent to the unit on foot, in a wheelchair, or on a stretcher, depending on his condition. He will be accompanied to the nursing unit by a volunteer, a member of the escort service, or someone from the admitting office or the nursing unit to which he is going, depending on agency procedure.

The patient's admission chart will go with him; usually it is carried by the health worker. The chart will include the admission record, the consent for care, and sometimes, the doctor's order. Occasionally, preadmission laboratory work has been completed, and such reports will be included with the chart.

The first contact that the patient and his family have with the health personnel is crucial. You should therefore take this opportunity to greet the patient warmly by name, and introduce yourself. Be helpful in any way you can—answer questions that the patient or his family may ask. This should be done by every health worker who meets the newcomer and his family, regardless of responsibility to the particular patient.

ITEM 1. PREPARATION OF ROOM FOR NEW PATIENT

Upon notification that a patient will be admitted, prepare the patient's room for his arrival.

Important Steps	Key Points
1. Open the bed.	Turn back the covers, fluff the pillow, and adjust lights, temperature, and ventilation.
2. Lower the bed.	This makes it easier and safer for the patient to get in. (Place the bed in high position if the patient comes to the room by stretcher.)
3. Place a gown on the bed.	The patient usually changes into the hospital gown as soon as he is settled in his room. If he is not too ill, he may prefer to wear his own sleeping garments.
4. Assemble admitting equipment.	Obtain a urine specimen container, sphygmomanometer and stethoscope, thermometer, admission checklist (if used), and any other special equipment your team leader suggests, such as oxygen equipment or an IV standard. Await the arrival of the patient.

ITEM 2. PATIENT'S ARRIVAL AT HIS ROOM

Upon arrival of the patient to the unit:

Important Steps	Key Points
1. Greet the patient.	Call him by name and check his identification band. Give his chart to the ward clerk or nurse.
2. Introduce yourself.	Tell the patient and his family, "I'm Miss Olsen, the nurse's aide (or nursing student) assigned to

Important Steps	Key Points

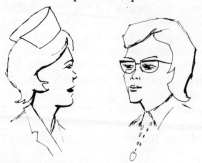

take care of you." Be warm, friendly, and courteous. First impressions should make the patient feel that he has been expected. Sometimes patients arrive on the unit before the admission notice has been relayed to the unit, or before the patient formerly occupying the bed has left the room. If this happens, explain the delay and maintain a warm, courteous manner. Escort him to an area that will be comfortable until the situation is resolved.

3. Take the patient to his room.

Wash your hands. Gain his cooperation by giving him an explanation of the environment. Introduce him to his roomates if he has been admitted to a multiple bed unit.

4. Provide privacy for the patient.

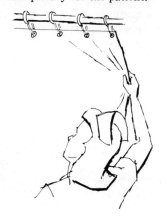

Pull the curtains to give him privacy as he changes either into the hospital gown or his own sleeping garments. Provide assistance if the patient needs it to change and prepare for tests or treatment to begin. Be sure the room is warm and free of drafts. When a screen or curtain is not available (and for a private room) be sure that the corridor door is closed.

5. Obtain a urine specimen.

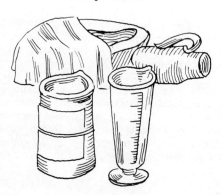

Ask the ambulatory patient to go to the bathroom, taking the container so he can void into it. Have the bed rest patient use the bedpan or urinal. (Refer to Unit 15, Urine Elimination.)

Excitement or apprehension often acts as a stimulating force in elimination, making this a good time to obtain the urine specimen. If the patient is unable to void, however, leave the container at the bedside for later use.

6. Help the patient put his belongings in the appropriate storage place.

Hang his clothes neatly in the closet. Place personal hygiene articles in the bedside stand (toothbrush, comb, brush, and deodorant). Put the empty suitcase in the closet or ask the family to take it with them.

When you handle the patient's clothing, be alert for pediculi (lice) or bedbugs. If you find

Important Steps	Key Points

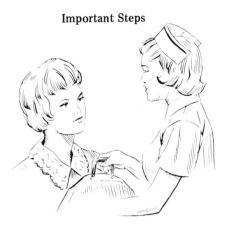

any, notify the nurse so that appropriate measures can be taken immediately and treatment begun for the patient.

a. Handle valuables properly.

Tell the patient that valuables and money worth more than $2 should be taken home by his family or put in a special valuables envelope and placed in the business office safe until his discharge. Record the envelope number and storage area in the nurses' notes or on the admitting interview note.

b. Handle medication appropriately.

Explain to the patient that medications brought to the hospital should be taken home by his family or taken to the pharmacy for safe-keeping. They will be returned when he is discharged (record this information in the nurses' notes.) If he refuses to give his valuables or medications to you, refer the matter to the charge nurse. She will assume the responsibility for the appropriate action, following the agency regulations.

7. Assess the patient's physical and emotional well-being.

Record the information on the admitting record as you proceed. Later, transfer it to the patient's chart. (When Problem Oriented Charting is utilized, an admitting sheet designed for the nursing assessment interview is used.) Look at Unit 18, Charting, for a list of descriptive terms.

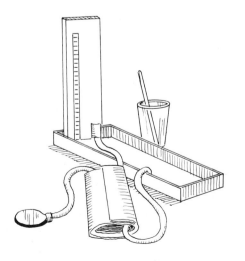

a. Take the T, P, R, and BP.

b. Weigh the patient (use either the portable scales or the health scales in the treatment unit).

c. Observe the patient carefully during the entire procedure for:

(1) general condition (good, alert, drowsy, emaciated or thin, and so forth).

(2) condition of his skin (clean, dirty, dry, bruised, cut, birthmarks, and so forth).

(3) difficulty in breathing (dyspnea).

(4) coughing: kind (dry, wet, hacking) and product (amount, color, odor, and so forth).

Important Steps	Key Points

(5) breath (odor).

(6) level of consciousness (alert, partly conscious, comatose).

(7) pain (location and type).

(8) speech (fluent, articulate, inco-
herent), and language (English,
Spanish, French, and so forth).

(9) complaints, e.g., "I have a headache."

(10) ability to move easily.

(11) ability to hear (deafness).

(12) ability to see (blindness).

(13) protheses (wigs, dentures, bridges,
glass eye, contact lenses or eyeglasses, artificial leg, and so
forth).

All of these must be recorded on the patient's
chart.

8. Explain the use of hospital equipment.

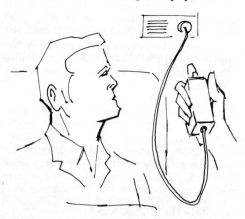

Demonstrate how to use the *call button* and
intercom (communication system) for calling
the nurse. Attach the call light conveniently
within the patient's reach; demonstrate the use
of the bathroom emergency call button. Explain how to operate the bed controls for the
bed; demonstrate the operation of the TV
controls; and explain how to use the telephone
for outside calls. Be sure that the telephone is
easy to reach.

Because each of these items may vary from
agency to agency, follow your agency procedure.

9. Explain the hospital routine.

Tell the patient when meals will be served, for
example, 8 A.M., 12 noon, and 4:30 P.M.
Explain the visiting hour regulations: afternoon
2 to 4 P.M., evening 7 to 8:30 P.M. These vary
among agencies, so tell him your agency's
visiting hours.

There are Public Health Regulations that
prohibit children under 14 years of age from
visiting (exceptions can be made in critical
cases, however, so check your your team
leader). This is done to minimize the possibility
of children bringing infectious diseases to already sick patients and to keep the children
from contact with patients who have infectious
disease.

Special Care units (obstetrics, pediatrics,
Coronary Care Unit (CCU), Intensive Care Unit
(ICU, etc.) have special visiting hours. Check

Important Steps	Key Points

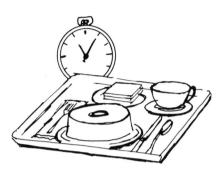

your agency regulations. Exceptions are also made for critically ill or preoperative patients.

Visitors are usually limited to two at a time per patient. This is done for several reasons:

a. To avoid overtiring the patient, who usually makes an effort to entertain visitors.

b. Because of limited space and chairs available for visitors in the patient's room.

c. To keep the noise level at a minimum. Many people crowded into a small area tend to talk loudly.

Explain that laboratory and X-ray procedures may be done on admission, or they may be taken care of later, after the patient arrives on the floor. If the patient is scheduled for surgery, explain that surgical preps (shaves) are usually done on the evening of admission by someone from the operating room. Inform him about the volunteer service to obtain newspapers, toilet articles, reading materials, and so forth.

Describe the uniforms and duties of various personnel the patient will have contact with, such as nurse's aide, orderly, LVN (LPN), RN, student nurses of several types from various programs, and personnel from other departments, such as housekeeping, dietary, and maintenance.

10. Provide for the patient's safety.

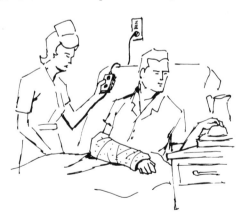

Lower the bed to its lowest position. Raise the siderails if indicated (observe your agency rules). Place the call light within easy reach, also the TV and bed controls. Have the bedside stand near the bed so that the patient will not have to reach (and possibly fall out of bed). Arrange the bedding and the patient for comfort and proper body alignment.

11. Report and record.

Transfer information from your admission form to the nurses' notes. Report any unusual findings to your team leader. Take the urine specimen (properly labeled) immediately to the laboratory. Charting example:

1740. White male admitted ambulatory. To bed in 602, appears alert and in good condition. States he is in for general cardiac workup.

Important Steps	Key Points
	Valuables sent home with wife. Urine specimen obtained, sent with requisition and charge voucher to the laboratory. Oriented to equipment in room and to general hospital routine.

B. Olsen, SN

TPR/BP/weight are recorded on the graphic sheet and may also be recorded in the nurses' notes, depending on agency procedures.

ITEM 3.   TRANSFER PROCEDURE

Transfers, moving a patient from one bed to another, or to another room or unit, are common occurrences in health agencies. They are necessary for a variety of reasons:

1. The patient requests a private or semiprivate room on admission. If none is available, he must wait and stay in a multi-bed room until a private one is vacated.

2. The patient's condition changes and he must be moved to a special care unit, such as ICU, CCU, or isolation room. Certain persons in a room may not get along; therefore, one must be moved so that both can rest.

3. The patient may request a bed by the window when it becomes available.

A patient may be apprehensive about a transfer requested by the doctor. You must reassure him and explain why he is being transferred. Be sure that the room to which he is going is ready for his occupancy.

Important Steps	Key Points
1. Wash your hands, identify the patient, and collect his personal items.	Explain that he is being transferred. It helps to use a utility cart or a wheelchair in transporting his personal items and supplies. Check the bedside stand, clothes closets, dressers, and bathroom. Be sure to take all of his clothes, luggage, personal items, and dentures. If these items are lost during the transfer, you may be held responsible. Collect all his equipment, such as the bedpan, washbasin, and emesis basin, and take them with the patient to the newly assigned room.

2. Transfer the patient.	Move the patient by wheelchair or stretcher, depending on his condition, to his new room. Remember to use good body movement both for yourself and your patient during this procedure. Take the necessary safety precautions (use safety belts if available; use equipment that is in good working order). Push

Important Steps	Key Points

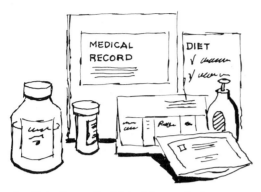

the wheelchair or stretcher in the correct manner. The patient may be moved in his own bed if his condition warrants it. You will need assistance in moving the bed.

Take the patient's chart and medications with you when you are transferring him to another unit.

3. Help the patient into his new bed.

Position him for comfort and safety. Adjust the siderails if indicated. Place the call button, bed and TV controls conveniently. Put the bedside stand near the head of the bed in easy reach. Store his supplies and equipment in the bedside table. Get fresh water and a pitcher of ice for him (if permitted).

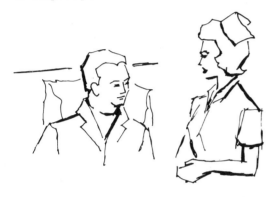

4. Introduce the patient to his new room-mate.

It is also helpful to introduce him to his new ward personnel. Leave the patient neat and comfortable.

5. Return the weheelchair or stretcher to the storage area.

Remove soiled linen from the stretcher and replace it with clean linen, ready for the next usage.

6. Go back to the patient's former unit.

Strip the room of used linens and supplies. Make it ready for terminal cleaning by housekeeping personnel or nursing personnel, according to your agency procedure. After cleaning, a closed bed is made for new admission. Be sure that the room is neat and restocked with admission equipment (bedpan/urinal, emesis basin, washbasin, gown, and so forth).

7. Report and record.

Note the transfer on the patient's chart, including the time, old room number and bed, new room number and bed, and means of transfer (wheelchair or stretcher). Chart any unusual occurrences. Give the chart and medications to the charge nurse. Give an oral report on patient's condition. Charting example:

1045. Transferred to room 407 via wheelchair. All personal items including dentures with patient.   B. Olsen, SN

Important Steps	Key Points
8. Receiving the transfer patient.	The assigned personnel will assist in getting the patient to bed and settled. The charge nurse will take the patient's chart, his medications, and a verbal report from nursing personnel bringing the patient to the unit (specimens required, special care needed, procedures to be completed). Be sure to introduce the patient to the new staff. Make him feel welcome. Be courteous and friendly.
9. Explain routines.	If routines in new area are different (meals, visiting, and so forth, they should be thoroughly explained to the patient and his family.
10. Record on patient's chart.	Make a note of the time, method of transportation, and general condition of the patient at time of the transfer. Charting example: 1055. Received on unit via wheelchair from room 602, in good condition. To bed after orientation to unit routines and introductions. P. Shaw, SN

ITEM 4.   PLANNED DISCHARGE PROCEDURE

The vast majority of patients leave the hospital after talking it over with their doctor, who then writes an order authorizing the discharge. Often the patient discharge involves planning by the doctor, nurses, family, and social workers. Patients are normally happy to go home, but they are often weak and need your careful, considerate assistance. Before the patient can be released from a nursing unit, certain financial arrangements must be made with the business office. These arrangements can be handled by the patient or his relatives. The business office will notify the nursing unit when these arrangements have been made.

If the doctor wrote orders for medications to be sent home with the patient, be sure that they are available on the nursing unit. Occasionally, the patient will have a special diet to follow. Be sure that the dietitian has conferred with the patient or his relatives before he is discharged.

Patients may be discharged by ambulance service, and a time is usually scheduled for the departure. Make sure that the patient is completely ready for discharge when the ambulance personnel arrive. Again, be courteous and helpful as you assist the patient in packing his personal belongings and leaving the hospital.

Important Steps	Key Points
1. Obtain the discharge order.	The order will be written by the physician, and you will be given the assignment by your team leader.
2. Wash your hands, identify and patient, and explain the procedure to him and his family.	Ask for their cooperation. Determine the expected time of discharge and the time when family, friends, or ambulance will arrive to take him home.
3. Obtain the patient's valuables from the safe.	In order to release them to the patient, he must first sign the release tab on the valuables envelope indicating that he has received the items. The signed receipt will either be attached to the patient's chart or returned to the business office for filing.

Important Steps	Key Points
4. Check any home care instructions for the patient.	Make certain that the patient or his family has received home care instructions concerning: a. Medications that are sent with him. b. Special diet (from the dietition). c. Future appointments with the doctor (send the appropriate forms and directions). d. Information about which activities are permitted and which are restricted after the patient returns home.
5. Check any dressings or bandages.	The team leader will determine if they should be changed; see that it is done if indicated. Usually the entry-level nurse does not do the actual dressing change; the LVN or RN will complete the procedure.
6. Assist the patient to dress and pack. 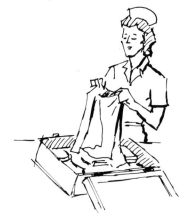	Help him pack his belonging; check the bedside stand and clothes closets for all his belongings. Assist him to dress as needed. If the patient asks questions you cannot answer about his condition or what he is to do at home, immediately ask the team leader to clarify them.
7. Verify that the business office procedure has been completed.	Most agencies require a special release form that must be completed for the business office before the patient can leave. The patient or a member of the family will have to go to the business office to take care of the financial arrangements. (Follow your agency procedure.)
8. Obtain a wheelchair and utility chart to transport the patient's belongings.	Assist the patient into the wheelchair, and secure the safety belts. The excitement of "going home" often causes the patient to overestimate his physical strength, making him feel that using the wheelchair is not necessary. Do not be influenced by these feelings; keep the patient safe by using the wheelchair. Transport his luggage on the utility cart. Most institutions require the use of wheelchairs for patients being discharged.
9. Transport the patient and his belongings to the waiting vehicle.	Most agencies have a discharge area where the patient is protected from the weather when getting into the car. Assist the patient with his belongings into the car.

Important Steps	Key Points
	Remember: the patient is eager to get home. Therefore, as you approach the car, remind him to remain safely in the wheelchair until you have come to a stop, put on the brakes, released the safety belt, and opened the car door.
10. Return the wheelchair and utility cart to the storage area.	Some agencies have a special area for returning supplies so they can be cleaned before reuse. In any event, when you return the equipment, be sure it is clean (you may need to wipe it with a cleaning solution) and in good working order. If it needs repair, attach a repair notice on it and notify the maintenance department either by phone or requisition.
11. Go back to the patient's room, strip the bed, and prepare for terminal cleaning.	In most agencies, nursing personnel are responsible for this activity, but the actual cleaning is done by the housekeeping department.
12. Report and record.	Report to your team leader and ward clerk that the patient is gone. Chart the discharge on the nurses' notes. Information should include the time, the means of transport (stretcher or wheelchair), a statement about the patient's general condition, his destination (home or another health facility), and any other appropriate comments. It is helpful to note the name and location of the other health agency for future reference. Sign your name and title. Remove the chart from the chart holder and put it in the area designated for discharge charts. If Problem Oriented Charting is utilized, follow the discharge summary procedures designated by the agency. Charting example:
	1430. Discharged via wheelchair to home in good condition. Dietary instructions and medication were explained. Patient stated all personnel were most kind, thorough, and conscientious. B. Olsen, SN

PERFORMANCE TEST

1. Read through the following situation. Record the appropriate information on the nurses' notes.

   On December 22, 1970 at 2:15 P.M., a Caucasian male, age 63, was admitted via wheelchair to room 466. He undressed and was assisted to bed. Vital signs 98.2—82—22, BP 122/82, Wt. 152 lbs., Ht. 6 ft. He was alert but appeared to have difficulty moving his right arm and leg. He complained of nausea and vomiting, and stated his stomach hurt. While assisting him to bed, you noticed a small bruise on his right ankle and a large reddened area on his sacrum. A urine specimen was obtained and sent to the lab. His doctor was notified.

2. Given a partner in the skill laboratory, you will prepare the "patient" and carry out the procedure for admission, transfer, or discharge. You will assemble the necessary equipment, supplies, and records, explain to the patient what you are going to do, follow the procedure established in the lesson, and practice the charting of your activity on the nurses' notes. Explain *what* you are doing and *why* so that both the "patient" and your instructor will be able to follow your line of reasoning.

PERFORMANCE CHECKLIST

ADMISSION, TRANSFER, AND DISCHARGE

ADMISSION

1. Adjust the height of the bad on notification that a patient is to be admitted (low if the patient is ambulatory; high if he is on a stretcher).

2. Prepare the environment: open a bed, adjust the lights, temperature, and ventilation.

3. Provide a hospital gown and towels.

4. Assemble the admitting equipment: urine specimen container, sphygmomanometer, stethoscope, thermometer, and admission checklist.

5. Await the patient's arrival.

6. Greet the patient and check his identification band.

7. Give the chart to the nurse.

8. Introduce yourself.

9. Take the patient to his room.

10. Wash your hands.

11. Pull the screen.

12. Assist the patient into a gown (his own or the hospital's).

13. Obtain a urine specimen.

14. Hang his clothes neatly in the closet.

15. Inspect the clothes for pediculi.

16. Inquire about his valuables and medications, take the necessary steps.

17. Do the patient physical inventory: temperature, blood pressure, weight; observe objective symptoms and elicit subjective symptoms from the patient.

18. Explain hospital procedures: the call signal and emergency call system, and the television and bed controls.

19. Explain the agency schedules and procedures: meals, visiting, laboratory and X-ray exams, prep, volunteer service, uniforms, and types of personnel.

20. Provide for his safety: lower the bed; position the siderails; check the controls; and make sure there is a bedside stand nearby.

21. Leave the patient comfortable and in good body alignment.

TRANSFER

1. Wash your hands, identify the patient, and explain the procedure.

2. Collect the patient's personal items.

3. Obtain a stretcher or wheelchair to transport patient.

   a. Obtain a utility cart if needed to transfer the patient's personal items.

   b. Check the equipment for safety.

4. Transfer the patient to the new location.

   a. Use good body movement for yourself and the patient.

   b. Use a safety precaution with the mechanical aid, i.e., a safety belt.

5. Take the chart and medications and deliver to charge nurse.

6. Install the patient in the new unit and leave him neat and comfortable.

7. Introduce his new roommate and staff.

8. Return the stretcher or wheelchair to the storage area.

9. Return to the patient's former unit and strip the room for a terminal cleaning.

10. After the room is cleaned, restock the supplies, and make it ready for a new admission.

11. Chart the procedure on nurses' notes.

DISCHARGE

1. Obtain the discharge order.

2. Wash your hand, identify the patient, and explain the procedure to the patient.

3. Obtain his valuables.

4. Check to see if special instructions have been carried out, e.g., take-home medications provided, special diet instructions given.

5. Check dressings or bandages, and change them if necessary.

6. Assist the patient to pack and dress (make sure all personal items are packed).

7. Verify the final business office clearance.

8. Obtain a wheelchair and utility cart for transportation, and check their safety features, i.e., safety belts.

9. Transport the patient and his belongings to the discharge area.

10. Assist patient into his car.

    a. Use good body movement for the patient and yourself.

    b. Use safety principles, i.e., lock the wheels of the chair.

11. Return the wheelchair to the storage area.

    a. Clean and check the wheelchair for needed repairs.

    b. Prepare a work requisition if repairs are needed.

12. Return to the patient's room, strip it and make it ready for a terminal cleaning.

13. Make the room ready for a new patient after the cleaning is completed.

14. Record the activity on nurses' notes.

POST-TEST

Directions: Choose the answer that makes the statement complete.

1. When the patient's room is prepared for admission, all of the following instructions are true except:

   a. lower the bed

   b. turn back the covers, fluff the pillow

   c. adjust the lights, temperature, and ventilation

   d. a hospital gown is mandatory for all patients

2. The items used for the admission assessment include all of the following except:

   a. urine specimen container

   b. scantron paper

   c. sphygmomanometer, stethoscope, and thermometer

   d. admission checklist

3. When the patient arrives on the nursing unit, the nursing personnel's tone of voice in the introduction should be:

   a. distant, cool

   b. warm and courteous

   c. matter-of fact

   d. annoyed, irritated

4. When the patient has been taken to his room, you do all of the following except:

   a. wash your hands, give a detailed explanation of the environment

   b. introduce him to his roommate

   c. obtain a urine specimen at exactly 4 P.M.

   d. be alert for pediculi or bedbugs when handling his clothes

5. Explain to the patient that valuables worth $2 or more, and medications brought with him are handled in all the following ways except:

   a. left in the patient's bedside stand

   b. put in a properly marked, sealed envelope and placed in the business office safe until the time of his discharge

   c. properly marked and put in the drug room for safekeeping until his discharge

   d. sent home with the family

6. Assessing and recording the physical well-being of the patient includes the following except:

   a. taking the TPR, BP, weight, and height

   b. noting the color of his suit and shoes

   c. observing the patient's general condition, skin condition, difficulty in breathing, level of consciousness

   d. noting coughing, pain, speech, hearing, seeing, and prostheses

7. Explaining the use of hospital equipment and hospital routine is vital to the patient's well-being. These include all of the following except:

   a. call button and intercom system

   b. bathroom emergency call button

   c. meal times and visiting hour regulations

   d. children under 14 years of age are permitted to visit at any time and in any area of the hospital

8. When patients are transferred from one area to another, all of the following instructions are true except:

   a. take all of his personal items and supplies

   b. transfer the patient by wheelchair or stretcher

   c. oral reports are an unimportant part of the transfer procedure

   d. transfer the chart and medications

9. When the patient is discharged, you do all of the following except:

   a. obtain the discharge order and business office clearance slip

   b. help the patient obtain his valuables from the business office safe

   c. check that the patient has his home care instructions, medicine, diet, activities

   d. notify the security office that the patient is discharged

10. When you take the patient to the discharge area in the wheelchair, all of the following are true except:

   a. all patients are to walk to their waiting vehicle

   b. safety belts are secure

   c. remind the patient to remain in the wheelchair until you stop, apply the brakes, release the safety belt, and open the car door

   d. assist the patient and his belongings to the car

POST-TEST ANNOTATED ANSWER SHEET

1. d. (p. 429)

2. b. (p. 429)

3. b. (p. 429)

4. c. (p. 430)

5. a. (p. 431)

6. b. (pp. 431–432)

7. d. (p. 432)

8. c. (pp. 434–435)

9. d. (pp. 436–437)

10. a. (p. 437)

Unit 21

I. DIRECTIONS TO THE STUDENT

Read this lesson carefully. It will provide some of the basic knowledge and techniques for giving special skin care to patients such as those who are incontinent, who are in a cast or traction, or who have a colostomy or ileostomy.

II. GENERAL PERFORMANCE OBJECTIVE

When you have finished this unit, you will be able to give special care to the geriatric and incontinent patient, to the patient in a cast or in traction, and to one with an ileostomy or colostomy, while maintaining good body alignment both for the patient and yourself, and providing a safe, comfortable environment.

III. SPECIFIC PERFORMANCE OBJECTIVES

On completion of this unit, you will be able to:

1. Identify specific skin indications, such as cyanosis, increased redness, or broken skin, that could lead to a decubitus, and begin appropriate preventive measures.

2. Prevent decubitus ulcers by examining the patient's skin and removing pressure from bony prominences (such as the sacrum or heels) by correctly changing the patient's position and using appropriate supportive aids.

3. Detect signs of impaired circulation in an extremity in a patient who has a cast, and start appropriate nursing measures to prevent further impairment.

4. Change an ileostomy or colostomy appliance, using clean technique, observing the skin condition, and applying the appropriate ointment, while reassuring the patient.

5. Clean and cut the patient's toenails or fingernails according to your agency procedure.

IV. VOCABULARY

abrasion—a scraping of the skin, a minor injury.
compound fracture—a broken bone that has an accompanying skin wound, i.e., the bone protrudes through the skin.
cyanosis—bluish color caused by decreased oxygen content in the blood.
decompose—to decay; to break down chemicals to a simpler form.
decubitus ulcer—a bedsore or pressure sore occurring over any bony prominence, caused by prolonged pressure on the skin covering that area, which decreases the circulation.
dermis—the second layer of the skin (commonly called the true skin).
epidermis—the outer layer of skin.
evaporation—the changing from liquid form to vapor (steam).
excoriation—damage or abrasion to skin caused by chemicals or burns, for example, diaper burn on an infant.

444

gangrene—death of tissues due to lack of circulation.

incontinence—inability to retain feces or urine; lack of voluntary control over anal or urinary sphincter.

involuntary—lack of voluntary control over anal sphincter, inability to retain feces.

necrosis—death of tissue from any cause.

orthopedics—treatment of abnormalities and diseases of the musculoskeletal system.

scapula—a large, flat, triangular bone of the shoulder.

sebaceous glands—oil-secreting glands of the skin.

simple fracture—a broken bone that does not have an accompanying skin wound.

sweat (perspiration) glands—glands in the skin that secrete a salty, colorless liquid; they keep the body cool by the process of evaporation.

traction—an arrangement of ropes, pulleys, and weights that exerts a pulling force on a part of the body that requires this type of treatment.

wound—a break in the continuity of soft tissues due to trauma (injury).

V. INTRODUCTION

Care of the skin is basic to all nursing care. It is not only a part of your daily routine, but also a special procedure in certain cases such as newborn infants, geriatric patients, incontinent patients, and patients who are immobilized over a long period of time because of a cast, traction, or paralysis. Frequent bathing of all or parts of the body prevents skin irritation from perspiration, urine, feces, or drainage. Bathing should depend on the regular habits of the individual as well as the condition of the skin. Some people take daily baths; others bathe only once or twice a week because of excessive dryness of the skin. Of course, certain areas must be washed daily: groin, underarms, face, hands, perineum and body creases.

Structure of the Skin. Skin is a remarkable part of the body. Its condition provides us with one indicator of the general health of the patient. The outer layer of the skin, called the epidermis (often referred to as "false skin"), constantly sheds dead cells. It also acts as a barrier between the individual and his environment by protecting him against physical attack on the underlying tissues, and preventing microorganisms and other foreign substances from entering the body.

The dermis is the layer directly below the epidermis and is called the true skin. This layer is made up of tissue that contains hair follicles imbedded in bundles of smooth muscle, sweat glands, sebaceous glands, blood vessels, and nerve endings. Thus the skin also has a sensory role, i.e., the skin is sensitive to touch and temperature. The skin also acts as a regulator of body fluids and temperature. The sweat glands excrete waste products from the body, and the evaporation of these waste products has a cooling effect, thereby helping to regulate the body temperature.

The skin varies in thickness in different parts of the body; for example, the eyelid is paper thin, while the sole of the foot and the palm of the hand are very thick because they must withstand much abuse, wear, and tear.

Functions of the Skin. To recapitulate, the skin serves several functions:

1. It acts as a protective barrier against microorganisms.

2. It is a sensory organ that enables the body to feel pain, pressure, and temperature.

3. It shields body tissue from injury.

4. It insulates against heat and cold.

5. It aids in elimination of waste products.

6. It helps produce vitamin D for body use.

In caring for your own skin as well as your patient's, you must be aware of several significant facts:

One route for eliminating waste products from the body is provided by the sweat glands of the skin. Other routes are the urinary tract and the alimentary tract. The accumulation of these products on the skin must be gently washed away to rinse off dead skin cells, and to prevent burning, or excoriation, of the skin caused by the chemical reaction of decomposed urine, feces, sweat, or drainage.

Oil is secreted by the sebaceous glands in the skin and helps to prevent dryness. If the skin becomes excessively dry through the aging process, damage to the sebaceous glands, or excessive washing away of protective skin oils, it may break open. Pathogenic organisms can gain entry to the underlying body tissues and set up an infection.

Sometimes rubbing alcohol is used to toughen the skin. Alcohol coagulates the protein in the cells of the skin much as heating will coagulate the white of an egg. Alcohol also provides a cooling effect because it rapidly evaporates from the skin. Therefore, an alcohol sponge bath is often used to assist in bringing a patient's elevated temperature to normal limits. However, some authorities believe that alcohol causes excessive dryness of the skin. For this reason, it may be better to use an oil or lotion to keep the skin well lubricated.

ITEM 1. SKIN CARE FOR INCONTINENT PATIENTS

One of the early lessons we learn in childhood is to become "toilet-trained." When adults, for any reason, cannot maintain their excretory control of urine or feces, they become demoralized and embarrassed. Loss of control occurs more often in patients who are elderly, paralyzed, or lacking full mental awareness. Chemicals in the urine and feces soon become irritating if left on the skin and lead to burned areas, or excoriation. It is essential that these patients be kept clean and dry at all times. This means that you will be checking them frequently for soiled skin and linen.

Patients who are incontinent must be treated with kindness and understanding. Assure the patients that you will help them regain as much control as possible. Use retaining methods, and toilet them at regular intervals before the incontinence occurs. Your goal should be to supply the patient with a bedpan before he soils himself. Don't scold, threaten, or abuse the patient in any way. Never put a diaper on these patients: it is a degrading practice and demoralizing to the patient. In addition, a wet diaper causes further skin irritation from the acid content of the waste products, and this leads very quickly to rashes, open sores, and decubiti.

Remember to treat the incontinent patient with dignity and respect. Many of these patients fear being dependent on others to take care of their elementary body functions, so they need your reassurance, patience, and understanding. You should accept their right to feel fearful, sad, or even belligerent at finding themselves in the situation of being unable to control their bowels or urination.

In the clinical setting, after practice in the skills laboratory, cleanse the soiled skin, change linens, and provide for the comfort of an incontinent patient. You will assist the patient to take care of his excretory functions:

Important Steps	Key Points
1. Wash your hands. Approach and identify the patient, and enlist his cooperation.	He may be very uncomfortable from lying in a wet or soiled bed. He may also be very embarrassed that he needs your assistance for this very routine activity. Further, he may be angry because he had to wait for you. Meet him with kindness, courtesy, understanding and acceptance. Fold the top linens back to inspect the situation so that you can determine what supplies you will need. Re-cover the patient.
2. Assemble the necessary supplies.	Obtain clean linens (drawsheet, bottom sheet, gown). If the patient is soiled, bring a basin with warm water, mild soap, a washcloth, a towel, and toilet tissue to the bedside stand.

Important Steps | **Key Points**

You may need a bedpan to put soiled toilet tissue in if you have to remove excess fecal material before beginning the cleansing process.

3. Provide for privacy.
Close the door of the room and pull the cubicle curtain if you are not in a private room. Drape the patient for modesty, using the top covers.

4. Position the bed.
Place the bed in the working level position to avoid undue backstrain. Have the patient roll on his side away from you in the Sims' position (obtain assistance if the patient can't move for you).

5. Remove the soiled linen and wash the soiled skin.
Loosen the soiled linens as needed or remove the soiled Chux. Wash the patient's skin gently with warm water and mild soap; rinse the soap off the skin thoroughly. Pat the skin dry carefully with the bath towel. Be sure that it is thoroughly dry. Inspect the skin carefully for evidence of beginning skin breakdown such as the development of an excoriated or reddened area.

6. Apply ointment, lotion, or powder to the patient's buttocks.
Each agency has routine measures for applying these substances for the prevention of decubitus ulcers.

7. Give back care.
Give a backrub and massage for possible pressure areas over the sacrum, shoulders, and hips. Use lotion or powder as recommended by your agency. Gently massage *around* any reddened areas noted on the patient's back.

8. Put a clean gown on the patient and remake the bed.
Adjust the gown to keep wrinkles from gathering under the patient, and to provide for free movement. Proceed to make an occupied bed.

9. Provide for the patient's comfort.
Remember: it is important to change the patient's position *at least* every *two* hours to avoid undue pressure over bony prominences. You should rotate positions systematically, from right side to back, to left side, to stomach (if permitted), and so forth. Thus during an 8-hour shift, these positions should be changed at least four times. Make sure that he is positioned in good body alignment. Proceed with bowel training (if indicated) as discussed in the unit on Bowel Elimination.

10. Remove the soiled materials.
Place the call signal within easy reach. Be sure the patient knows where it is located and how to operate it.

Leave the room neat and tidy. Return soiled supplies to designated places. Clean and store the bedpan (if used) and the washbasin.

11. Report and record.
Report any unusual skin condition to your team leader. Record the time of the change and the procedures performed: backrub, partial

Important Steps   Key Points

bath, ointment application, and so forth. Charting example:

1110. Incontinent. Back washed and rubbed.
Skin color is pink, no broken areas noted.
Turned to left Sims' position.   J. Jones, LVN

ITEM 2. PRESSURE SORE: THE DECUBITUS ULCER

You will recall from the earlier unit on Positioning the Bed Patient that changing the
patient's position will be one of your most frequent activities. Three purposes of this
responsibility are (1) to relieve pressure, (2) to provide comfort, and (3) to prevent
contractures. In this section we are particularly concerned with the effects of pressure on
certain bony prominences due to the patient remaining in the same position for a prolonged
period of time, either lying down or sitting up.

You will recall that every part of the body has weight. This weight exerts pressure when
it comes in contact with another object, such as the bed. Remaining in one position over a
prolonged period of time causes the body weight to exert pressure on the skin, blood vessels,
and muscles at the areas where the body is in contact with the bed or chair. The evidences of
pressure can easily be observed by closely inspecting the skin over the bony prominences of
the scapulas, trochanters, knees, elbows, heels, and sacrum.

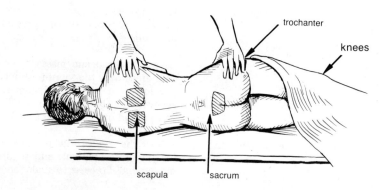

You will observe that the skin very quickly becomes reddened, often within 30 to 60
minutes. Because the blood vessels are compacted by the weight of the body pressing against
the bed surface, the circulation is usually slowed down and a resulting mottled look appears
on the skin. The skin may have a dusky, cyanotic, or bluish, color. Continued compression
of the blood vessels decreases the supply of oxygen and nutrients to the surrounding tissues,
resulting in *necrosis*, or death of the tissue which leads to the formation of a decubitus ulcer
or pressure sore.

Although a decubitus ulcer may develop after only a few short hours, particularly in the
aged or poorly nourished patient, the process of curing one often takes many weeks and
sometimes years of very devoted nursing care. Therefore, it is imperative that you remember
the old adage, "an ounce of prevention is worth a pound of cure."

The impaired circulation, with the resulting redness or mottled appearance of the skin,
can be further aggravated by heat, soiled or wet bedclothes, and irritation of the skin from
decomposing substances such as perspiration, urine, feces, or vaginal discharges. You will
recall from the unit on handwashing that these are environmental factors that also provide
breeding places for germs. Wrinkles in the bedding, crumbs and foreign substances in the
bed, and friction from restless moving about in the bed, along with any or all of the above,
can be forerunners to the development of pressure sores.

The prevention of pressure sores is the responsibility of the nursing staff. When a patient develops a decubitus, it is often considered a sign of neglect and poor nursing care. It is much easier to prevent a bedsore than to cure one. You must therefore observe your patient's skin frequently and change his position at least every 2 hours to keep decubitus ulcers from developing.

You can prevent pressure sores by:

1. Careful, frequent observation of the color of the skin. Skin that is red, blue, or mottled signifies impaired circulation.

2. Changing the patient's position at least every 2 hours.

3. Restoring circulation to a deprived area by rubbing *around* a reddened area. Do not massage the reddened skin itself because it has already suffered temporary damage. Use a circular motion, starting at the reddened area and moving outward in an ever-widening circle. This will rush the stagnant venous blood away from the affected area and replace it with fresh arterial blood. The friction causes the blood vessels to dilate and bring more blood to the area, and more nutrients and oxygen are delivered to the affected area.

4. Keeping the patient dry and clean at all times. The application of small amounts of fragrant powder helps to keep the skin dry. However, large amounts of powder can accumulate and cause pressure to the skin when the patient lies on the powder accumulation for long periods of time.

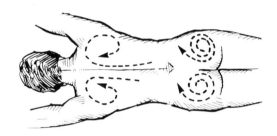

5. Avoiding any mechanical or physical injury to the skin from improper fitting of splints, braces, casts, and prostheses, or from burns caused by excessively hot or cold applications such as hot water bottles, ice bags, heating pads, heating lamps, and so forth.

Specific treatments for the care of a decubitus ulcer are usually ordered by the physician, although some nursing departments have recently developed nursing procedures that they may institute when a decubitus is first discovered. When the decubitus is large and far-advanced, surgical intervention with a possible skin graft may be indicated. Thus it is imperative that nursing personnel work diligently to prevent decubitus ulcers from developing.

Given an elderly male patient, severely undernourished and emaciated (extremely thin), who has been lying on his back for two hours, change his position to the left Sims' position, using good body alignment principles both for yourself and your patient, observing his skin condition and taking appropriate steps as indicated.

Important Steps	Key Points
1. Wash your hands. Approach and identify the patient. Explain what you are going to do.	Identify your patient by name. Speak to him warmly and reassuringly. Ask him to assist you if possible. Since he is elderly, he may feel that he is too weak to be bothered. Explain the need to change his position in order to keep a sore from developing on his back.

Important Steps	Key Points
2. Adjust the bed to a working height.	This will keep you from straining your back muscles as you handle your patient. The bed should be flat; this will prevent undue friction when moving your patient across the bed. Lower the bedrail on the proximal (near) side if indicated.
3. Provide privacy.	Shut the door of the room or pull the cubicle curtains. Fold the top linen back, but avoid unnecessary exposure of the patient.
4. Place the patient in the left Sims' position.	Turn him to his left side and flex the right leg (top) so that it does not rest on the left leg (bottom). The right arm can be flexed on the bed in front of him so that his hand is near the pillow, palm down.
5. Align and support the patient in good position.	Make sure that he is not lying on his left arm. Place his head, neck, and back in a straight line. Place his legs in a parallel position with knees slightly flexed (bent). His right arm may be flexed across his abdomen or supported on his body at the hip or on a pillow. Place a pillow under the head and neck to prevent muscle strain. Put a pillow under the right leg for support from knee to foot. Take this opportunity to closely inspect the bony prominences over the scapula, sacrum, elbows, and heels for redness.
6. Massage the back and bony prominences.	Frequent brief massages or backrubs with lotion or alcohol when changing your patient's position not only improve the circulation but help to relax the patient. Use firm rotary-friction strokes learned in your lesson on backrubs. If you should find evidence of beginning pressure areas, start prompt action. Massage the area carefully to increase the circulation. Make a special note to change the patient's position every two hours. Remember, *you* are the one who can prevent pressure sores from developing.
7. Use protective aids to reduce pressure on the skin.	You will want to use all the protective aids possible to reduce pressure in the patient who already has signs of impaired circulation. Plan to turn him frequently, give back care, and use antidecubitus pads, heel protectors, alternating air-pressure pads, and other protective devices.

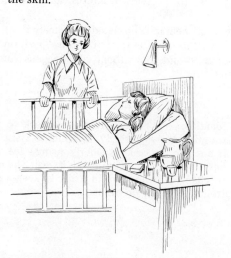

Important Steps	Key Points
8. Provide for the patient's comfort.	Put the call light within easy reach. Elevate the head of the bed slightly if the patient prefers. Spread an extra blanket over him if he is cool. Place the bedside stand with his personal items within easy reach. Raise the siderail if indicated.
9. Report and record as appropriate.	Report to team members any reddened area or evidence of pressure, and the methods used to reduce pressure or increase circulation. Explain your time schedule for changing his position and have it entered on the patient's nursing care plan by the charge nurse. This will alert all who are concerned with the patient around the clock to provide special back care. Charting example: 0310. Position changed to left Sims'. Reddened area on sacrum massaged. Placed on antidecubitus pad. J. Jones, NA 0345. Sleeping quietly. J. Jones, NA

This can be one of your most important and satisfying procedures. You can be particularly pleased with your performance if you prevent bedsores from beginning, or from advancing after they are discovered.

ITEM 3. CAST AND SKIN CARE

People with diseases or injuries involving the bones and joints generally require immobilization for long periods of time so that healing can take place. Fractures of bones must be immobilized in the correct position until they have healed. Casts, splints, surgical pinning or repair, and various types of traction are used to prevent movement in the bones or joints.

Those who have a simple fracture of a bone in an extremity may be able to resume many of their normal activities after a cast has been applied to the part. Healing can be expected to occur within four to six weeks. Serious or multiple fractures, however, may require lengthy hospitalization (possibly months) and different combinations of casts or traction. Because of such prolonged inactivity, it is vital that general hygienic care be carried out daily. This includes attention to diet, rest, cleanliness, elimination, alignment, care of the skin, and prevention of pressure.

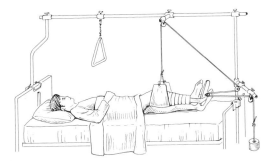

Leg traction.

Care of Patients with Newly Applied Casts

As a nurse, you need to become familiar with the general procedures of providing skin care and checking circulation while working with patients in casts and traction. After a brief explanation about casts we'll consider the patient who has just returned to the unit with a new cast.

There are a number of preparations used in making casts, but plaster of Paris has been the most widely used material. It is available in powder form or in specially prepared strips. When moistened with water, plaster can be shaped or molded into casts for any portion of the body. Various types of plastic or acrylic materials are also used in making casts. Purported advantages of these over the plaster cast include more rapid drying, better resistance to breaking or cracking, lighter weight, and greater porousness, which allows air to circulate more readily. Various types of casts are shown here.

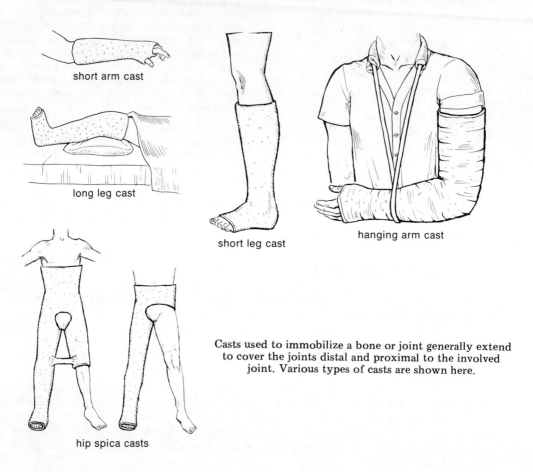

short arm cast

long leg cast

short leg cast

hanging arm cast

hip spica casts

Casts used to immobilize a bone or joint generally extend to cover the joints distal and proximal to the involved joint. Various types of casts are shown here.

Casts are applied, adjusted, split, or removed only by the doctor or a cast room technician working under the doctor's direction. When a cast is to be used, a length of stockinette material is put over the body part, which is then wrapped with soft wadding material; then the plaster or plastic cast is applied. After that procedure the nursing care of the patient begins as follows:

1. Check the circulation in the part every hour for 24 to 48 hours, and then at least every 4 hours thereafter, unless specified otherwise by the doctor's orders or agency policies.

2. Allow time for drying; plaster takes between 24 and 48 hours to dry, although the plastic casts may dry in a few hours. Some agencies permit the use of fans or hair dryers to hasten the drying of the cast, but you must avoid chilling the patient.

3. Support the casted portion of the body at all times until the cast is dry. If the cast is on an extremity, elevate the part above the level of the heart to reduce possible swelling.

4. Keep the cast whole and intact. Do not twist or apply pressure on the wet cast. Even finger print indentations on a cast may cause pressure on underlying tissues.

Circulation Check

Nurses must frequently check the circulation of any body part that has had a cast applied. You must do this deliberately and thoroughly, and then record the information. Check the circulation every hour for the first 24 to 48 hours, and then at least once every four hours. Look for signs of impaired circulation and listen carefully to possible complaints of discomfort by the patient. Complaints of pain involving any area under the cast should never be taken lightly because the pain may be the only sign of pressure on a bony prominence, or it may indicate impaired circulation. Unless you act promptly, the tissues will die, causing a condition called gangrene; this means that cellular death has occurred because of poor or inadequate blood circulation to the body part in the cast.

Five specific areas must be checked for one or more of the cardinal signs of impaired circulation:

1. Temperature — coldness.

2. Color — paleness or cyanosis.

3. Movement — numbness or inability to move.

4. Pain — burning or tingling.

5. Edema or swelling.

First, feel the part to check its temperature, and then ask the patient to move or wiggle the part. At the same time note the color of the skin and whether there is swelling. Even when the patient is asleep, check the circulation by observing the temperature, color, swelling, and movement of the part. If you find any of the signs of impaired circulation, notify the nurse at once. Delays in restoring adequate circulation to an extremity have led to nerve and tissue damage, and even to amputation. Remember that not all of the signs of impaired circulation need be present for severe damage to occur.

Skin Care and Cast Care

Immobilizing a body part with a cast often causes tightness or pressure after even the *slightest* change in position from the time the cast was first applied. The most common pressure areas are located around the top and bottom edges of the cast, and over any bony prominences. At the top or bottom edges, you may be able to rearrange some of the wadding to provide more room and relieve the pressure. If this doesn't work, notify the nurse who may be able to try other methods before notifying the doctor. Pressure over bony prominences, such as the ankle, knee, or wrist, should be reported to the doctor; he will cut a window in the cast over the area, or bivalve the entire cast and secure the two halves in position with Ace bandages or tape.

When the plaster cast dries, small bits of plaster break off the cast or drop off the skin. If these crumbs fall inside the cast, they cause discomfort and irritate the patient's skin. Some of this can be prevented by washing the dried plaster off the skin, and by covering the raw edges of the cast. You can fold the stockinette material down over the edges of the cast and secure it with adhesive tape. Small strips of adhesive tape can also be used to "petal" or enclose the raw, uneven edges. However, long pieces of tape applied in a running manner usually do not cover tightly enough or remain in place for long.

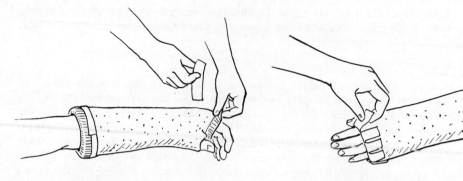

Pull stockinette over edge
and secure with tape.

Use short strips of adhesive tape
to "petal" edges.

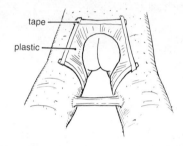

tape

plastic

Methods of smoothing
rough edges of cast.

Line opening of spica and body casts with
plastic material to keep cast dry and clean.

Patients frequently complain about the skin itching under a cast after a week or so. A soothing lotion may help relieve itching near the edge of the cast where you can reach it. You must discourage the patient from using long objects to reach under the cast and scratch the itching area. This can easily break the skin, after which it can become infected. Moreover, the warm, dark, and moist atmosphere under the cast can cause bacteria to flourish if once introduced.

When healing has occurred and the cast is removed, the underlying skin is dry, crusty, and flaking. Although the outer layer of skin is constantly being shed by the body, the dead skin cells accumulate on the skin when it is covered by a cast. You will have to soak off this layer of old, dead skin by using oil or lotion; do not just pull it off. Also, be sure to caution the patient not to scrub the area too vigorously because this may damage the tender skin.

Traction

Traction, a device utilizing a pulling force by means of weights, is employed to maintain parts of the body in extension and in alignment. At the same time, the patient may be partially immobilized, but the primary purpose of traction is alignment. There are two major types of traction: skin and skeletal. In skin traction, an adhesive bandage such as moleskin is applied directly to the skin and then attached to weights by means of ropes and pulleys. Skeletal traction requires the use of steel wires, pins, or tongs surgically put into the bone and then attached to the weights. Slings, girdles, and elastic bandages work on the same principle as skin traction. Various types of traction are shown in the illustrations on the opposite page.

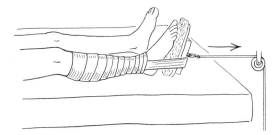

Skin traction of a lower extremity. This is Buck's traction with no elevation of leg from bed. Russell's traction is similar, but requires overbed frame and elevation of lower leg.

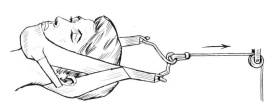

One type of skin traction using head halter.

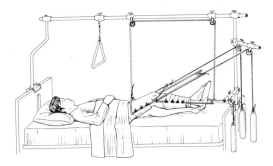

Balanced traction to align broken bone in thigh. Pin is inserted in bone below knee for skeletal traction. Note overbed frame and trapeze bar.

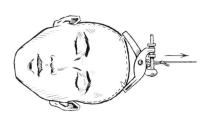

Skeletal traction with use of Crutchfield tongs inserted in skull bone.

Traction may appear to be a complex device, but it simply consists of a system of ropes, pulleys, and weights attached to part of the body. The weights are counteracted by the patient's own weight, and this provides the pulling force. The weights of the traction must be freehanging in order to exert the required force; check frequently to make sure that these weights are not resting on the floor, or hooked under the bed frame. The patient's body should be lying free in bed, so that his feet do not rest against the foot of the bed if the force is in that direction.

The patient who has traction on a portion of his body, like the patient in a cast, needs to have his position changed frequently. You must also give him skin care to prevent pressure areas from developing, and use aseptic technique to prevent infection at the sites where pins, wires, or tongs are inserted.

Given a patient with a long leg cast who is perspiring and in poor alignment, you are to provide care, position him, and check the circulation in the casted leg.

Important Steps	Key Points
1. Approach your patient, explain what you are going to do, and gain his cooperation.	Wash your hands. Check the patient's identification band. Explain why his body must be kept in proper alignment during the healing process, and the importance of keeping the bed dry to prevent discomfort as well as pressure sores. Also, explain the need for him to continue moving about and exercising his muscles to keep them healthy.
2. Adjust the bed to a working height.	Lock the wheels to keep the bed from moving away from you during the procedure. Waist-high beds make it easier for you to work without putting strain on your back muscles.

Important Steps	Key Points
3. Collect clean linen as needed.	Inspect the bed for dryness and cleanliness. Change linen as necessary. Since the patient is perspiring freely, you will need a basin of warm water, soap, and a bath towel to bathe and dry the skin. Immaculate personal cleanliness is a significant part of the fracture patient's care.
4. Check the circulation of the part.	Feel the toes or fingers of a leg or arm in a cast. Note the temperature, color, and movement of the part. Instead of asking the patient if he has pain, try having him describe how the cast or the extremity feels. Look also for *swelling* of an extremity. To prevent swelling, the extremity can be supported or raised on a pillow.
5. Check the edges of the cast.	Inspect for rough or frayed areas around the edges of cast. When the cast is dry enough for tape to stick to it, smooth off its edges. Rough edges can cause pressure on the skin. Redness and discomfort are the first signs. Swelling often occurs in the limb after a cast has been applied; this causes tightness at the edges of the cast.

6. Check for dryness of the cast.

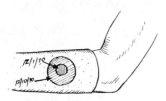

Short arm cast
with bloody seepage.

When a new cast is put on, the plaster of Paris takes time to set (there are fast, medium, and slow-setting types). When the cast is wet, it is shiny and white. When it dries, the cast becomes dull and gray. During the drying process, leave the cast uncovered so that the air can circulate fully to help it dry. It takes more than 24 hours for a cast to dry thoroughly.

Because a new cast is wet, elevate or support it with pillows covered with plastic. The cast shrinks slightly while drying; therefore, check the patient's circulation every hour during the drying period. If the fracture was repaired by a surgical operation (an open reduction), there may be some seepage of blood through the cast. Mark the extent of the seepage in pencil around the seepage area on the outside of the cast along with the date and time. If the area enlarges, report this at once to the doctor.

7. Check pressure areas.

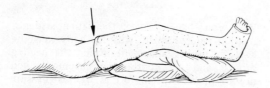

Long leg cast.

Depending on where the cast has been applied, you will need to observe carefully to prevent pressure areas from developing. If the patient has a long leg cast, the cast should be supported so that the anterior (front) of the top of the cast does not cause pressure at the groin. (See the sketch of the long leg cast.) You can do this by placing a pillow under the calf of the leg.

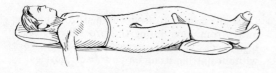

Body cast.

If the patient is in a body cast, you must make sure that his respirations are not obstructed. You will need additional pillows, which provide support to permit maximum breathing and to minimize pressure on the skin at the edges of the cast.

Important Steps	Key Points
8. Have the patient assist you in shifting his position. 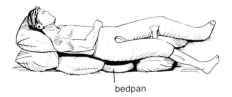 bedpan	It is good for him to be involved in this activity because it helps to exercise his muscles. Also, he can tell you if he is comfortable while moving and being repositioned. The trapeze is especially useful to help the patient raise his hips when you are placing a bedpan under him.

Pillow supports are helpful if properly placed when the patient is on a bedpan. (See accompanying sketch.) If the cast becomes soiled with urine or feces, it soon gives off a very offensive odor, which not only is embarrassing to the patient, but is disagreeable to everyone. You will need to keep all casts clean and dry. From time to time they may have to be covered with plastic, stockinette, or fresh pieces of plaster of Paris bandage. You can lightly sponge the cast with soap and water after it has become completely dry.

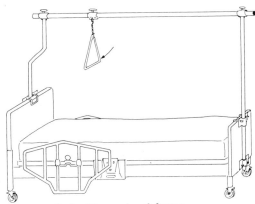

Bed with overhead frame
and trapeze bar.

9. Leave the patient comfortable.	After changing the linen, aligning the patient's position, utilizing various supportive aids (pillows, sandbags, and trochanter rolls), and inspecting his skin and cast for trouble spots, position the patient in correct body alignment. Put the call button within reach. Offer him a drink of fresh water and tell him when you will return.
10. Chart.	Record your observations and pertinent patient comments. Charting example:

1045. Position and linen changed. Toes move and are warm to touch, and pink in color. No swelling and no complaints of pain.
                                                        J. Jones, L.V.N.

ITEM 4.   SKIN CARE FOR THE PATIENT WITH A COLOSTOMY

As was explained in the unit on Bowel Elimination, a colostomy is formed by bringing a segment of the colon through the abdominal wall and making a stoma through which fecal material is eliminated. The colostomy is often a life-saving procedure, but many patients have difficulties in coping with their feelings about this drastic change in the functioning of their bodies. When caring for such patients, you will have to be warm but matter-of-fact; you must listen when they express their feelings. As soon as they are psychologically ready, you should teach them how to take care of the skin and the drainage.

Beginning practitioners in nursing are not expected to change the colostomy dressings in the early postoperative care of patients who have colostomies or ileostomies. However, once their bowel movements have become somewhat regulated, you may be expected to dispose of the collected drainage and to cleanse the skin around the stoma.

The purpose of skin care is to avoid any excoriation of the skin by the digestive juices that are often present in the fecal drainage. The acid and enzymes in the digestive juices literally eat away the outer layer of the skin. An area denuded in this way is painful and may easily become infected. The lower the location of the colostomy in the intestinal tract, the less the amount of irritating substances in the drainage. The skin must be carefully protected in patients who have had ileostomies or colostomies of the ascending colon because the drainage in these parts of the intestines still contains digestive juices.

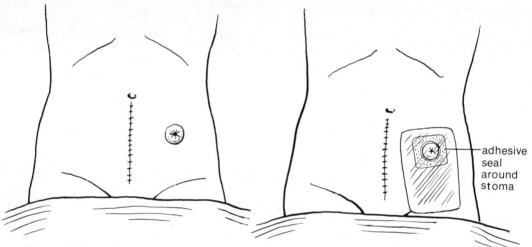

Stoma of descending colon with healed midline suture lines.

Disposable plastic bag in place over stoma.

In the skill laboratory, become acquainted with the colostomy materials. Examine different types of collecting bags used on ileostomies, and the disposable stoma bags used for colostomies. Then practice the procedure of changing a colostomy bag, paying particular attention to the patient's skin around the stoma.

Important Steps	Key Points
1. Approach and identify the patient. Explain what you plan to do and gain his cooperation.	Wash your hands. Check the patient's identification band. Describe the clean dressing procedure. The patient is usually anxious to have the drainage bag removed. Adopt a calm, matter-of-fact manner and handle the procedure as you do when giving a bedpan or changing a child's diaper.
2. Assemble the equipment needed.	Most ostomy appliances and materials are ordered for the patient and should be in the room. You will need disposable stoma bags, medication if ordered, water and soap, and clean linen if his gown or bedding has been soiled.
3. Provide for the patient's privacy.	Close the door of the room, or pull the cubicle curtains. Avoid chilling the patient.

Important Steps	Key Points
4. Place the patient in a supine position and put the bed at a comfortable working height.	Having the patient in Fowler's position is best because it allows him to see easier and become more involved. Fold the top bedding across his lower abdomen and expose only the portion where you will be working.
5. Remove the bag filled with drainage.	Most disposable plastic stoma bags are stuck to the skin with a hypoallergenic adhesive. The adhesive may be part of the bag itself, or a gasket attached to the bag that can be hooked to a belt for added security. Use toilet paper to remove excess drainage from the stoma and skin surfaces. Put the soiled tissue on an old newspaper for later disposal. Empty the contents of the bag into the toilet and dispose of the bag.
6. Cleanse the skin and stoma.	Wash them gently with soap and water, and pat them dry. Avoid using friction on the stoma. Inspect the skin areas; redness is the first sign of irritation.
7. Apply special powder or ointment around the stoma, if ordered.	Following surgery, many doctors order karaya gum powder, or other medications such as Amphojel, zinc oxide, lanolin, or Vaseline to protect the skin from the drainage.
8. Apply a clean stoma bag.	The opening in the bag should be the correct size. If too large, it leaves skin surfaces exposed, and if too small, it puts pressure on the stoma. The stoma does shrink during the first few weeks and months, so it should be measured again for correct fit. The adhesive backing on the disposable bag sticks directly onto the skin. Fasten the belt to the gasket of the bag if a belt is used.
9. Provide for the patient's comfort.	Change any linen if necessary. Remove soiled items and tidy the room. Offer a fresh drink of water and ask if there is anything else the patient needs. Leave the call light within reach.
10. Report and record on the patient's chart as appropriate.	Record the time, amount, color, and consistency of the drainage in the bag as well as your observations about the condition of the skin. Charting example: 1410. Colostomy drainage bag changed. Moderate amount of soft brown stool. Skin around stoma shows no sign of irritation. J. Jones, LPN

ITEM 5. USE OF PERMANENT STOMA BAGS

Patients who have ileostomies or colostomies of the ascending or transverse colon commonly use the permanent stoma bag to collect the drainage that flows day and night. The continual flow requires frequent removal of the drainage to keep it from irritating the stoma and skin. Pulling off the disposable stoma bags with the adhesive backing irritates the skin and leads to severe excoriation by the drainage. This damage to the skin must be prevented if at all possible. The permanent, nondisposable stoma bag is one method used to reduce skin irritation.

The permanent drainage collecting bag is firmly attached to the skin with a cement. It is removed only when the drainage seeps under the seal, or if there is a need to deodorize or to replace the bag. An opening at the bottom of the bag can be unplugged or unclamped to allow the removal of the collected drainage. You can use an Asepto syringe and tap water to flush out the inside of the bag before reclosing it.

To care for the patient who has a permanent stoma appliance, follow the procedure in Item 4 except for the following variations in the steps:

Important Steps	Key Points
Remove the Drainage from the Bag	
Follow steps 1 through 4, Item 4.	
5. Unplug or unclamp the bottom of the bag and remove the drainage.	The bag can be drained into a plastic or stainless steel basin. Measure the amount, record it on the output record, and flush it down the toilet.
6. Rinse the inside of the bag.	Use tap water and an Asepto syringe. Instill the water into the bag. Then hold the end of the bag shut and swish the water around without pulling on the seal. Drain and use more clear water to rinse. Close the bottom of the bag.
Omit steps 7 and 8 of Item 4.	You will not be able to reach inside the bag to apply medication to the skin or stoma, nor will you replace the bag since it remains in place for days and even weeks.

Complete and chart the procedure.

Apply the Permanent Stoma Bag

If possible, arrange to observe when the ostomy nurse specialist changes the permanent stoma bag for the patient. After the used bag is removed, the skin is thoroughly cleansed to remove the old cement and other material. Medication is used to protect any exposed portion of the skin and the stoma before a new bag is reapplied.

Important Steps	Key Points
Follow steps 1 through 7, Item 4.	
8. Apply the first coat of cement around the stoma and the ring or gasket of the bag.	Follow the directions on the appliance package for measuring the opening for the stoma. Use an applicator to apply the cement. Cover an area at least 1 inch larger than the ring or gasket will cover. Let the skin area and the gasket dry completely; allow 30 to 60 seconds.
9. Apply a second coat of cement.	Again cover both the skin area and the gasket or ring of the bag.
10. Place the ring or gasket on the skin covering the stoma.	Press it firmly to the cemented area of the skin. Hold it in place until the two are tightly stuck together.
11. Attach it to the belt.	

Complete and chart the procedure.

ITEM 6. CARE OF FINGERNAILS AND TOENAILS

This is one aspect of personal care that most patients can handle for themselves. However, you may need to do it for the patient who cannot because he is unconscious, blind, confused, unsteady, or in a cast or traction.

Usually nail care is accomplished at the time of the regular bath. The nails should be kept clean, and trimmed according to your agency regulations. Do not cut the toenails or fingernails of a diabetic patient or one who has circulatory disease of the lower extremities until you have checked your agency's regulations.

Since nails frequently can become tough and thick, soak the hands and feet for 15 minutes in warm, soapy water before attempting to cut the nails. The soaking will soften the nail and the cuticle (the outer portion of the skin surrounding the nail) sufficiently so that you can easily cut or file the nails and gently push back the cuticle with an orange stick.

Nails are cut straight across to prevent them from growing into the skin along the sides, which causes pain or infection, and a condition called ingrown nails. Ingrown toenails may require a surgical procedure to correct. Manicured cuticles prevent hangnails (a partly detached piece of skin at the base of a fingernail), which are painful and unsightly, and the source of possible infections.

If it is necessary for you to observe the color of a patient's nailbeds, for example, after surgery or cast application, it may be necessary to avoid the use of colored nail polish on the patient. Well-cared for toenails and fingernails are an essential part of good grooming for your patient as well as for yourself.

ITEM 7. CONCLUSION OF THE LESSON

You have now concluded the unit on special skin care. When you have practiced the procedures so that you know how to do them, arrange with your instructor to take the post-tests. You will be expected to demonstrate your skills in giving skin care and to tell your instructor what you are doing in each step, and why.

PERFORMANCE TEST

In the skill laboratory or the classroom, your instructor will ask you to perform the following procedures without reference to any source material.

1. Given an elderly patient who has had surgical repair of a fractured hip, provide special skin care after the patient has been incontinent of urine.

2. Given a patient with a head injury who has been lying in one position for about two hours, provide care to prevent the formation of decubitus ulcers.

3. Given a young boy with a long leg cast applied three hours ago, check for signs of pressure or impaired circulation to the limb, and describe how you would care for the drying cast.

4. Given an older woman who had a colostomy of the descending colon six days ago, remove the partially filled stoma bag and replace it with another.

PERFORMANCE CHECKLIST

SPECIAL SKIN CARE

SKIN CARE FOR THE INCONTINENT PATIENT

1. Wash your hands.

2. Approach the patient, identify him, and explain what you are going to do.

3. Pick up the required supplies: clean linen, soap, and water.

4. Provide privacy.

5. Adjust the bed to working height.

6. Assist the patient to turn onto his side.

7. Remove the soiled linen.

8. Wash the urine from his skin, then dry it thoroughly.

9. Give him a backrub and massage possible pressure areas.

10. Put a clean gown on the patient; remake his bed.

11. Provide for the patient's comfort; attach the signal light; raise the siderails.

12. Remove the soiled materials.

13. Report and record.

SKIN CARE TO PREVENT DECUBITUS ULCERS

1. Wash your hands.

2. Approach and identify the patient; explain the procedure.

3. Provide privacy.

4. Adjust the bed to working height.

5. Turn the patient to a left Sims' position.

6. Align and support the patient in good position.

7. Inspect the skin of his back; give him a backrub and massage over the bony prominences.

8. Use protective aids to reduce pressure.

9. Provide for the patient's comfort. Rearrange the bedding neatly, raise the siderails, and secure the call light within reach.

10. Report and record as appropriate.

CIRCULATION AND CAST CARE

1. Wash your hands.

2. Approach and identify the patient; explain the procedure to him.

3. Adjust the bed to working level.

4. Check the circulation in his toes.

    a. Note their temperature, color, and movement.

    b. Check for complaints of pain.

    c. Observe for signs of swelling.

5. Check the dryness of the cast.

6. Look for signs of pressure around the edges of the cast.

7. When the cast is drier, finish the rough edges with tape or stockinette.

8. Reposition the patient; support the cast when he is being moved.

9. Provide for the patient's comfort.

10. Report and record as appropriate.

CHANGING A COLOSTOMY STOMA BAG

1. Wash your hands.

2. Approach and identify the patient; explain the procedure.

3. Assemble the equipment needed.

4. Provide privacy.

5. Place the bed at a comfortable working height.

6. Have the patient in supine or semi-Fowler's position.

7. Remove the bag filled with drainage, and discard it.

8. Cleanse the skin and stoma.

9. Apply medication or ointment if ordered.

10. Apply a clean bag to the stoma and attach it to the belt if one is used.

11. Provide for the patient's comfort.

12. Report and record as appropriate.

POST-TEST

Matching: Select the phrase from Column 2 that best describes the words in Column 1. Write the letter designating that phrase in the blank space in Column 1.

Column 1	*Column 2*
_____ 1. necrosis	a. damage to skin from chemicals
_____ 2. dermis	b. excretion of perspiration
_____ 3. decubitus	c. the first, or outer, layer of skin
_____ 4. abrasion	d. inability to control feces and urine
_____ 5. cyanosis	e. circulation of blood in arteries and veins
_____ 6. sebaceous gland	f. a pulling force on the body
_____ 7. incontinence	g. the second, or true, layer of skin
_____ 8. excoriation	h. excretes an oily substance
_____ 9. epidermis	i. damage to the skin by scraping
_____10. traction	j. death of tissues
	k. skin color change caused by insufficient oxygen
	l. damage to skin due to pressure

Multiple Choice: Circle the letter of the best answer for each of the following questions.

1. When you give a bath or special skin care to a patient, the layer or structure of the skin that you touch is:

   a. muscle

   b. epidermis

   c. dermis

   d. follicles

2. The nerve ending and the blood vessels of the skin are located in which layer or structure?

   a. muscle

   b. epidermis

   c. dermis

   d. follicles

3. When the continuous surface of the skin has been damaged or broken as in an abrasion or decubitus ulcer, the body has lost some of its ability to:

   a. resist infections

   b. take in oxygen supply

   c. eliminate waste products

   d. maintain body alignment

4. A possible disadvantage to the use of alcohol when giving a backrub is that:

   a. it evaporates and cools the body

   b. it removes oils and waste products from the skin

c. it toughens and dries out the skin

d. it coagulates oxygen in the tissues

5. In some patients, pressure can cause the beginning of a decubitus within a matter of hours. When you observe the *first* sign of pressure, you should immediately do which of the following?

a. make sure that the skin 's clean and dry

b. turn the patient at least every two hours

c. use padding or protective aids to reduce pressure

d. massage around the reddened skin area to stimulate circulation

6. In caring for the patient who is incontinent, you should keep his skin clean and dry, and:

a. use padding or disposable diapers to catch the urine or feces

b. offer the bedpan or urinal frequently for retraining

c. check the bed linens frequently to see if they are soiled

d. remind the patient that he made extra work for you by soiling the bed

7. For the bed patient, pressure over a bony prominence such as the sacrum can result in:

a. necrosis, and formation of a sore or ulcer

b. reddening of the skin due to impaired circulation

c. decreased supply of nutrients and oxygen to the tissues

d. a, b, and c

e. a and b

8. A patient has had a cast applied for a fracture of his leg and now complains of pain in the ankle area. His toes are warm to touch and of normal skin color, and he can move them. You would conclude that:

a. the patient is a complainer

b. the pain is normal because of the fracture

c. the cast may be causing pressure

d. the signs do not indicate impaired circulation

9. A sharp object should not be used by the patient to scratch the itching areas under his cast because:

a. he may poke holes in the cast, or damage it

b. infection may occur if the skin is broken

c. the itching is just caused by accumulated dead skin

d. he would not be able to feel it if he injured himself

10. Excoriation often occurs in the skin around the stoma of an ileostomy or a colostomy as a result of:

a. excessive flatus, and the odor of the drainage

b. decreased circulation of blood to the area

c. poor absorption of fluids in the colon

d. action of digestive juices in the drainage or feces

11.   The ointment used around the stoma of a colostomy:

      a.   cements the colostomy bag in place

      b.   lubricates the stoma for passage of the feces

      c.   provides a protective covering for the skin

      d.   allows easier cleansing of the skin

12.   Before trimming the nails of a patient who has diabetes or circulatory disease of the legs, you should:

      a.   check with your team leader for instructions

      b.   soak the patient's hands or feet in warm, soapy water

      c.   plan to do this task as part of the bath procedure

      d.   check for hangnails around the cuticles

POST-TEST ANNOTATED ANSWER SHEET

1. j. (p. 445)	1. b. (p. 445)
2. g. (p. 444)	2. c. (p. 445)
3. l. (p. 444)	3. a. (p. 445)
4. i. (p. 444)	4. c. (p. 446)
5. k. (p. 444)	5. d. (p. 449)
6. h. (p. 445)	6. b. (p. 446)
7. d. (p. 445)	7. d. (p. 448)
8. a. (p. 444)	8. c. (p. 453)
9. c. (p. 444)	9. b. (p. 454)
10. f. (p. 445)	10. d. (p. 458)
	11. c. (p. 459)
	12. a. (p. 461)

PREOPERATIVE CARE

I. DIRECTIONS TO THE STUDENT

This lesson includes the psychological and physiological preparation of the patient for surgery. Proceed through all the steps. When you finish, practice both the psychological and physiological preparation with another student or an instructor.

II. GENERAL PERFORMANCE OBJECTIVE

Upon completion of this unit, you will be able to prepare a patient for a surgical operation.

III. SPECIFIC PERFORMANCE OBJECTIVES

When you have finished this unit, you will be able to:

1. Provide the patient with privacy and safety during the preoperative preparations.

2. Procure a surgical consent from the patient if agency policy permits.

3. Explain to the patient the reasons for preoperative laboratory procedures.

4. Safeguard the patient from any food or fluids in the specified period before surgery.

5. Provide personal hygiene as required during the preoperative preparation.

6. Eliminate safety hazards to the patient after he receives the preoperative medications.

7. Instruct the patient and his family regarding his return to the recovery room and the location of the waiting rooms for relatives.

8. Complete a preoperative checklist accurately.

IV. VOCABULARY

anesthesia—a partial or complete loss of sensation, with or without loss of consciousness, as a result of disease, injury, or administration of a drug.
  general—complete, affecting the entire body, with loss of consciousness.
  local—affects a local or specific area only.
  spinal—causes loss of sensation from the hips down, induced by injecting a drug into the lower end of the spinal column.
asphyxia (asphyxiation)—a lack of oxygen in the blood and the increase of carbon dioxide in the tissues and blood.
aspirate—to breathe in; to get foreign material in the lungs.
barbiturates—a group of drugs used as sedatives or relaxants.
bladder sphincter—the plain muscle around the opening of the bladder.
catheter—a tube for evacuating or injecting fluids through a natural passage, e.g., a urinary catheter.

cyanosis—a Greek word for the slightly bluish-gray or purple discoloration of the skin due to a deficiency of oxygen and an excess of carbon dioxide in the blood. (Oxygen in the blood makes it look red and gives the skin a pink tone.)

hematocrit (Hct)—a test that measures the volume percentage of red blood cells in whole blood.

hemoglobin (Hgb)—the essential oxygen carrier of the blood, found within the red blood cells, and responsible for the red color of blood.

hemorrhage—abnormal discharge of blood, either external or internal.

laparotomy—the surgical opening of the abdomen; an abdominal incision.

mastectomy—excision, or surgical removal, of a breast.

narcotics—a group of drugs producing stupor, sleep, or complete unconsciousness; used to allay pain. (Regulated by federal laws.)

nasogastric tube—a small tube that is passed through the nose (naso) down to the stomach (gastric) for the purpose of taking materials out of or putting materials into the stomach.

NPO—nothing by mouth (Latin, nulli per os).

prosthesis—an artificial organ or part, such as an artificial limb, eyeglasses, and dentures.

red blood cell (RBC)—the laboratory count of the number of red cells (erythrocytes) in the blood.

thoracotomy—surgical incision of the chest wall.

venipuncture—withdrawal of blood from a vein by using a needle and syringe.

white blood cell (WBC)—the laboratory count of the numbers of white cells in the blood, which are also called leukocytes.

Prefixes and Suffixes for Surgical Procedures

cardio-:   heart (as in cardiac).

cyst-:   bladder (as in cystoscopy)

gastro-:   stomach (as in gastrotomy).

hemato-, hem-: relating to the blood (as in hemoglobin).

nephro-:   kidney (as in nephrectomy).

oophoro-:   ovary (as in oophorectomy).

pneumo-:   air, lung (as in pneumonectomy).

vaso-:   vessel, vein (as in vasoconstrictor).

-cele: tumor, cyst; hernia (as in cystocele).

-ectomy: cutting out, cutting off (as in appendectomy).

-oma: tumor (as in fibroma).

-ostomosis, -ostomy: to furnish with a mouth or an outlet (as in colostomy).

-otomy: cutting into (as in thoracotomy).

-plasty: revision, molding, or repair of tissue.

-pexy: fixation; anchoring in place.

V. INTRODUCTION

The physical and psychological preparation for surgery begins in the physician's office when he examines the patient and decides that surgery is necessary. It is then that the physician explains the surgical procedure to the patient, helping him to understand the effect that it will have on his life; at this time, the patient has an opportunity to express his concern and feelings about the procedure. After they have completed their discussion, the physician's office nurse schedules the surgery at the appropriate hospital and reviews the specific requirements for admission with the patient.

The psychological impact of this impending operation on the emotional well-being of the patient can be categorized in various ways: fear, shock, anger, denial, acceptance, resignation, or relief. Fear of the diagnosis is probably the greatest concern. The patient may also fear mutilation (e.g., the amputation of a leg), unconsciousness and the inability to know or control what is happening, pain or death, separation from his family, and the effects of surgery on his home and employment. The nurse should provide an opportunity for the patient to describe his reactions and feelings to this stressful situation.

For some patients, religious faith is a source of strength. Contact with a clergyman of the patient's faith and the sacraments of his church are especially important before impending surgery.

The physician writes orders for the preoperative preparation, and the anesthesiologist orders the preoperative medication. In many hospitals, the writing of these orders cancels all previous orders. Be sure to check the specific details of the orders with the registered nurse.

Consents

The patient is asked to sign a statement showing that he consents to have the surgery performed. If the patient is a minor or is confused or comatose, the next of kin with legal responsibility will be asked to sign the consent for the patient. This consent implies understanding of the nature of the surgery to be undertaken. A signed consent is required for each surgical procedure regardless of the length of time the patient stays in the hospital. In this way, the patient is protected from having surgery to which he has not consented, and the hospital and the doctor are protected against claims that unauthorized surgery has been performed. The department responsible for signing and witnessing consents is determined by individual hospitals. Know the policy of your institution before securing a consent.

Vital Signs

The patient's temperature, pulse, respiration, and blood pressure are taken at designated intervals throughout the preoperative days and nights. Any deviation noted in these readings helps the physician to determine existing abnormalities that would indicate the need for a delay in surgery.

Laboratory Procedures

It is customary to collect urine and blood specimens from the patient for routine testing the day before the scheduled surgery. (Emergency surgery requires collection of specimens immediately in the emergency room, or as soon as the patient arrives on the nursing unit and is put into his bed.) A designated amount of blood is removed by venipuncture in order to determine the patient's complete blood count (CBC), hemoglobin (Hgb), and hematocrit (Hct). The results of these studies help to detect the presence of infection, and the general ability of the body to provide oxygen to tissue, and to withstand blood loss and the added stress of surgical injury to tissues. The physician may order a blood typing and crossmatch for a specific number of pints of blood if he knows or suspects that the blood lost during surgery will need to be replaced.

A clean specimen of urine is obtained and tested. The results of the test determine the presence of infection or abnormalities in the patient's urinary system that may alter the schedule of the surgery.

X-ray (Radiology) Procedures

A chest X-ray is taken preoperatively to determine the condition of the patient's lungs. The result may influence the type of preoperative medication ordered as well as the kind of anesthesia used during surgery.

Food and Fluid

The patient is usually given a regular meal the evening before surgery unless he is on a special diet or NPO. The patient scheduled for early morning surgery is NPO from 12 midnight of the previous evening until the surgeon permits fluids to be taken orally during the postoperative recuperative period. Food and fluid restrictions are necessary because an empty stomach will prevent the danger of food aspiration if the patient's reaction to the anesthesia should cause vomiting. The patient scheduled for afternoon surgery or for a local or spinal anesthesia may be allowed a light breakfast or fluids until about six hours before surgery. It is a serious error if the patient is accidentally fed before surgery because it means surgery will be delayed. Rescheduling the surgery and prolonging the hospitalization would cause greater anxiety and expense for the patient. You must remove all food and liquids from the patient's bedside and put an "NPO for Surgery" sign on or over the patient's bed as a constant reminder to all persons who are in contact with the patient. Stress the importance of this restriction to the patient's family and friends in case the patient requests fluids. The temptation to quench his dry mouth with "just a few sips" of liquid is often difficult to resist.

Elimination

It is most important that the patient empty his bladder just before surgery. Offer a bedpan or urinal to the patient or have him go to the bathroom if he has not had any preoperative medication. Do not try to hurry the patient; often the anxiety about surgery makes the bladder sphincter contract, so that elimination requires more time than usual.

Turn on the bathroom cold water tap (hot water may cause the bathroom to steam and become too warm); the sound of the water (suggestion) may effect some relaxation of the bladder sphincter.

If the patient has an indwelling catheter, empty the catheter drainage bag immediately before he goes to surgery. Record the amount of urine removed on the proper record (nurses' notes, Intake & Output record).

Enemas are ordered and usually given the evening before surgery, although in some cases they are given the morning of surgery. An enema is given preoperatively so that the patient will be spared the strain and exertion of moving his bowels during the immediate postoperative period, which could cause hemorrhage in the operative area. General anesthesia and other drugs produce relaxation and hypoactivity of the intestines. Finally, some types of abdominal surgery require cleansing of the colon to remove all fecal material in order to lessen possible contamination of the wound during or following the operation.

Skin Preparation of the Operative Site

The purpose of skin preparation (commonly called a prep) is to make the skin as free of microorganisms as possible, thus decreasing the possibility during surgery of bacteria entering the wound from the skin surface. Skin preparation is usually performed the afternoon or evening before surgery. A wide area of the skin is prepared because this further reduces the possibility of infection. Cleanliness of the skin and removal of hair from its surface (without injury or irritation of the skin in the process) are fundamental. Hair is shaved because microorganisms cling to it and may be a source of infection to the operative site.

Plain soap and warm water are often used for cleansing the skin. However, antiseptic solutions are sometimes preferred because they are particularly effective in reducing the number of microorganisms on the skin and thereby decreasing the possibility of infection in the operative site. Each agency establishes its own "prep" procedure.

Personal Hygiene

Shampoo. Most patients will shampoo their hair before admission for surgery. If the patient has been hospitalized for some time preoperatively, he may (if he is able and the doctor gives permission) have a shampoo at the hospital.

Bath. The patient should bathe thoroughly the evening before or the morning of surgery. If surgery is scheduled for very early in the morning, it is best to have the patient bathe the evening before.

Nails and Hair. Details of personal grooming such as trimming the nails and shaving should be completed before surgery. All metal objects such as bobby pins should be removed from the hair; during surgery they may be lost or could injure the patient's scalp. Long hair may be braided to keep it neat and out of the way. Most hospitals provide turbans or some similar head covering for patients to wear to the operating room. These serve the double purpose of preventing the straying of loose hair in the operating room and keeping the patient's hair clean and in place during the operation and the recovery from anesthesia.

Attire. The patient is given a clean hospital gown. If a female patient asks permission to wear her own gown or pajamas, explain that sometimes patients perspire a good deal and need to have their gowns changed while still in the recovery room. Also, her gown may be soiled or lost in the hospital laundry. Neither the operating room nor the recovery room has facilities to take care of a patient's clothing if it has to be changed while in one of these units. For added warmth, some hospitals provide patients with long, white cotton stockings or boots to wear to the operating room.

Prostheses. In most hospitals, the patient is asked to remove dentures so that they will not become broken or dislodged and cause respiratory obstruction during the administration of anesthesia. This includes all bridges, partial plates, and full dentures. Other prostheses such as glasses, contact lenses, or limbs must be removed before surgery. Be sure that the small items are placed in a container labeled with the patient's name and room number. Dentures should be kept moist with water or a denture cleansing solution. All prostheses are costly and easily broken or lost; *take extra care to keep them safe.* You may find yourself paying for the patient's broken or lost dentures or glasses.

Mouth Care. All patients should have thorough mouth care before surgery; a clean mouth makes them more comfortable and prevents the aspiration of particles of food that may be left in the mouth. Chewing gum is not permitted since it too may be aspirated.

Makeup. Because the color of the face, lips, and nailbeds is watched carefully for cyanosis during surgery by the anesthesiologist, patients are asked to remove their makeup and nail polish. Cyanosis may be caused by certain gases and drugs, asphyxiation, or any condition interfering with the entrance of air into the respiratory tract or lungs.

Jewelry. Jewelry should be removed for safekeeping. A valuable ring might slip off the finger of an unconscious patient and be lost, or stones may be loose and fall out. If the patient prefers to leave his wedding band on, it may be taped to the finger, or a piece of gauze may be threaded under it and tied to the wrist. Be careful not to tie it too tightly so as to impair circulation. Although taping the ring is the most common safeguard used, some patients are allergic to tape of any kind, and gauze would then be preferred.

The policies for preoperative preparation are designed for the safety of the patient and his property. Try not to lose sight of this, or to enforce meaningless rules as an assertion of authority or discipline. Sometimes exceptions can be made by the physician if in doing so the patient will be spared acute embarrassment.

Preoperative Medication

Usually medications are given to help the patient relax before surgery. Sedatives are often given the evening before surgery to help the patient sleep. About an hour before surgery a narcotic such as morphine or Demerol is administered to relieve apprehension. Although he may awaken or be awake when he is taken to the operating room, the medication dulls the patient's awareness of the experience and makes it easier for him to relax and take the anesthetic.

Atropine may be administered with the narcotic to dry up (lessen) respiratory secretions if a general anesthetic is to be given. This decreases the likelihood of respiratory complications resulting from aspiration of secretions. Atropine will make the patient's mouth feel very dry. Explain this to the patient so that he will not become concerned about this discomfort.

Postoperative Instructions for the Patient and Family

Instruct both the patient and his family that the patient will go to the recovery room following surgery. He will remain in the recovery room until he is awake and responding, and the nurses will be checking his dressings and taking his blood pressure frequently.

The family should be directed to the area designated for those awaiting a patient in surgery. This ensures that the surgeon will see them as soon as he is able after surgery. If the surgical waiting room has no facilities, you may show the family where the cafeteria and restrooms are located.

Checklist for Preoperative Care

Some hospitals put a checklist or reminder sheet on the front of the chart of each preoperative patient. You are required to initial and note the date and time of the activities you are responsible for performing in the preoperative period.

The items in this checklist may include:

1. Operative consent signed and on the chart.

2. Blood report on the chart.

3. Urine report on the chart.

4. X-ray report on the chart.

5. Identification wristband on the patient.

6. Operating area prepared.

7. Enema(s) given.

8. Douche given.

9. NPO at _____.

10. Tube inserted: Nasogastric _____ Catheter _____ Other _____

11. Jewelry removed: _____

12. Prosthesis: What removed _____

         What remained on _____ _____

13. Hair prepared or covered.

14. Bathed and gowned for surgery.

15. Voided or catheterized.

16. Morning TPR, BP charted.

17. Preoperative medication given.

18. Bed lowered and siderails up.

19. To surgery: Time _____ Date _____

         Wristband checked by   _____

                              (O. R. Personnel)

                       _____

                            (Floor Personnel)

ITEM 1. PREPARATION PROCEDURE FOR THE DAY BEFORE SURGERY

Explain the preoperative routine to the patient. Wash your hands and identify the patient.

Important Steps	Key Points
1. Take and record the patient's vital signs.	Record them on the graphic sheet and on the preoperative list.
2. Collect a urine specimen.	Explain to the patient that a urine test is routinely done before all surgical procedures

Important Steps

Key Points

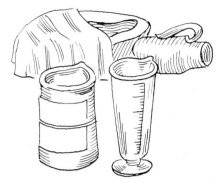

are accomplished. (Refer to Unit 15, Urine Elimination, Item 6.)

3. Explain the laboratory and X-ray procedures.

Tell the patient that a lab technician will be taking some of his blood for tests. These tests are done to ensure that he can safely tolerate the surgery. At this time, tell him that he will be going for a routine chest X-ray. (Do not give specific times for these procedures because a change may cause him greater anxiety.)

In some agencies, the pre-op laboratory and X-ray work is done at the time of admission to the hospital *before* the patient is sent to his room. In this case, step 3 would be omitted.

4. Prepare a consent form (usually done by the RN or ward clerk).

Consent forms are generally kept at the nursing station. In the area designated (usually upper left- or right-hand corner of the form), write or stamp the patient's name, age, sex, and room number, the hospital number, the doctor's name, and the date. Ask the RN to check for accuracy when you are completing the surgeon's name and kind of surgery.

5. Follow your agency's policy to obtain the patient's signature on the consent form.

Take the consent form, a pen, and a clipboard or some stable backing for the form to the patient's bedside. It is easier for him to sign if the consent is placed on a stable surface. Ask him to read the consent carefully. Do not try to answer questions that you are unsure of; refer these to the RN who will notify the doctor if necessary. Ask the patient to sign his full name. You may sign as witness with your full name *if agency policy permits.* (Refer to Unit 31, Consents, Releases, and Incident Reports.)

6. Explain food and fluid restrictions.

If the patient is on an unrestricted diet, he will receive a regular dinner the evening before surgery. If not, he will receive his special diet. Tell him that after midnight, his water pitcher will be removed and he may not have anything to eat or drink, not even a sip of water. This is to ensure an empty stomach at the time of surgery. If surgery is scheduled late or if a local anesthesia is to be administered, and if the doctor ordered it, explain that he may have a light breakfast or liquids until a specific time, and then will be NPO.

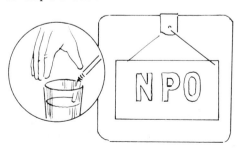

Important Steps	Key Points
7. Give an enema if ordered	Explain that an enema is given to remove the contents of the lower bowel for the purpose of preventing incontinence during surgery and straining during the postoperative period.
8. Explain the need for skin preparation. 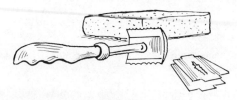	Tell the patient that some time during the evening before surgery, an OR technician or other designated person will come in to clean and shave the area surrounding the site of the incision. The purpose of this is to remove as many bacteria as possible in order to prevent infection of the operative site. Remember that bacteria cling to the shafts of hair.
9. Provide personal hygiene.	If the patient wishes a shampoo, and an order is obtained, give the shampoo. Remove nail polish if worn. Use acetone or nail polish remover. Explain that the anesthesiologist checks the color of the nails as an indication of the amount of oxygen the patient is getting. If surgery is scheduled for very early in the morning, the patient may wish to take a bath the night before; see that this is made possible.

ITEM 2. PREPARATION PROCEDURE FOR THE DAY OF SURGERY

Important Steps	Key Points
1. Wash your hands, approach the patient, identify him, and explain what you are going to do.	
2. Take the patient's vital signs and record them.	Take his temperature, pulse, blood pressure, and respirations, and record them on the nurses' notes on the patient's chart.
3. Give A.M. care. 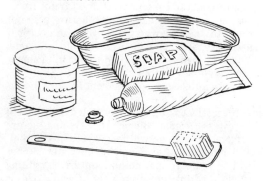	Assist the patient to wash his face and hands, and to clean his teeth. If dentures are worn, ask him to remove them and place them in a labeled denture cup. (Use the same procedure for a partial plate or bridges.) Make sure that the denture cup is clearly labeled with the patient's name and room number on it.
4. Give hair care.	Brush the patient's hair neatly. If it is long, you may braid it for neatness. (Refer to Unit 32, Special Care of the Hair, Item 2.) If the hospital requires a turban or head covering, place it around the hairline, and secure it by taping it.
5. Dress the patient in a hospital gown.	Assist him to remove his own pajamas and put on a hospital gown. Explain that the hospital gown is used in case it is soiled by perspiration

Important Steps	Key Points

or drainage, and also to ensure that the patient's belongings will not be lost.

6. Remove the patient's makeup and jewelry.

Explain that makeup becomes smeared by perspiration during surgery. Also, the anesthesiologist is better able to check the skin color if it is not covered with makeup. Ask the patient to remove her jewelry so that it is not lost during surgery. Put the jewelry in the place provided for safekeeping. If the patient wants to keep a wedding band on, either tape it to the finger or thread a gauze strip under the ring and tie the gauze around the wrist securely, but not so tight as to stop circulation.

7. Encourage voiding (just before preoperative medication).

If the patient is able, assist him to the bathroom, or assist him with the bedpan or urinal immediately before he takes his preoperative medication. A full bladder in surgery can easily be cut; thus it is extremely important that *the bladder be empty*. Explain that the medication will make him sleepy and he will not be allowed out of bed after his injection because he may fall and hurt himself.

8. Apply safety measures after preoperative medication.

Place the bed in the low position with siderails up. Caution the patient to remain in bed and not to smoke.

9. Tell the patient about the recovery room.

The patient and his family should be told that he will be in the recovery room until he is awake. *Do not* give any definite period of time because if the time is extended, it will increase everyone's anxiety. Explain that in the recovery room the patient's dressings, blood pressure, and general condition will be checked frequently.

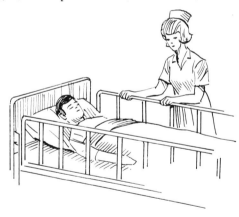

10. Direct the family to the waiting room facilities.

Show them where the waiting area for surgery and the restrooms are located. Also, tell them where coffee, tea, or food may be purchased.

11. Complete your checklist.

Check each item for which you are responsible; write your initials and the time. Notify the RN when the list is completed. Record in the appropriate place on the nurses' notes or the surgical checklist.

12. Assist with the transfer of the patient to the OR cart.

When the OR orderly comes to take the patient to surgery, check the name of the person he is to pick up; check the chart for the correct

Important Steps   **Key Points**

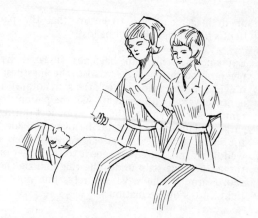

person, and then check the patient's wristband. The patient's hospital number is included in the name check. *All of these must match.* Assist in moving the patient from bed to cart, using proper body alignment, balance, and movement. When he is on the cart, secure the straps for safety. Sign off the chart in the nurses' notes by writing "Patient to surgery," the time, the date, your first initial and last name, and the category. *Both* you and OR personnel must sign the checklist at the bottom, indicating that both of you have identified the patient's wristband.

You may go with the orderly to the OR area with a female patient if this is the agency policy.

VI. ADDITIONAL INFORMATION FOR ENRICHMENT

Preoperative care is essential to the patient. It can be used as an opportunity for teaching good health practices that he should observe after surgery. It also provides an opportunity to answer some of his questions and lessen his fears.

You may wish to know more about preoperative care for a specific patient. Your instructor will give you additional reading assignments. In some agencies you may observe surgery when it is performed on your patient. This, of course, requires permission from your instructor, charge nurse, and operating room supervisor. (Check your agency regulations on this matter.)

PERFORMANCE TEST

1. Complete the nurses' notes and preoperative checklist for the following situation. Read through the case and record the appropriate information on the nurses' notes and on the preoperative checklist.

   A young woman, 26 years of age, was admitted by stretcher to room 223 at 0745. She was complaining of severe pain over the entire abdomen. The intern ordered an ice bag to be applied to the abdomen. The TPR were: (rectal) 101.4°F − 92 − 22. At the time of admission, the patient was unable to void; however, two hours later she voided 400 cc. A urine specimen was sent to the laboratory. The lab technician drew blood for a CBC. When Dr. Sommers called at 0930, the patient was still complaining of pain and was extremely nauseated although she had not vomited. Dr. Sommers visited shortly thereafter to examine the patient and to write the history and physical reports. He then scheduled the patient for an appendectomy for 6:30 that evening. The consent for surgery was signed by the patient.

   The OR technician performed the surgical skin prep, and a cleansing enema was given by the nurse's aide. Since her pre-op medication was ordered to be given by the RN at 5:00 P.M., the patient was prepared for surgery at 4:30 P.M. The TPR remained the same as it was on admission with a BP of 124/72. The patient voided at this time. She had no dentures but she did remove her contact lenses, hair pins, and nail polish. A solid gold watch and $20.00 in four bills were placed in a valuables envelope and locked in the nurses' station.

   The pre-op medication was given at 5:00 P.M., and the bed was placed in the low position with the siderails up. The patient slept until 6:25 P.M., at which time she was taken to surgery via stretcher.

2. With a partner in the skill laboratory, prepare the patient for a cholecystectomy that is scheduled for tomorrow at 0900. Follow the steps outlined in your procedure. Record your activities on practice nurses' notes.

PERFORMANCE CHECKLIST

PREOPERATIVE CARE OF A PATIENT

1. Complete the preoperative entry in the nurses' notes, observing the following rules:

   a. Print or write legibly.

   b. Print or write with blue ink; sign each entry with your handwritten signature and title.

   c. Write the date and time of the entry, and the effect; record the results for each activity.

   d. Do not skip lines.

   e. Correct an error by drawing one line through the error, with an error notation written above. If a whole page needs retyping, the old and new pages are included as a permanent part of the chart.

   f. Describe clearly and concisely the appearance, behavior, character, and drainage of excreta, and the type, location, and duration of pain.

   g. Use standard abbreviations.

    h. Enter each preop activity with a complete description, the time, the date, and your signature.

    i. Sign specimens out to the laboratory in the stated manner (from the unit on Urine Elimination) and follow other laboratory and X-ray procedures.

    j. Chart the prep, noting the time, type, and person performing the prep.

    k. Chart the disposal of valuables.

2. Complete the preoperative checklist with the required information on the form (observing the above rules).

PREPARATION PROCEDURE FOR THE DAY BEFORE SURGERY

1. Wash your hands; identify the patient, and explain the procedure.

2. Take the vital signs.

3. Collect the urine specimen.

    a. Correctly label the specimen and attach a label to the prepared requisition.

    b. Provide for the transmittal of the specimen to the lab.

4. Explain the laboratory and X-ray procedures that will occur.

5. Prepare a surgical consent form and obtain the patient's signature.

6. Explain the food and fluid restrictions.

7. Give an enema.

8. Explain the "prep."

9. Provide personal hygiene, for example, shampoo, shower, oral hygiene, and removal of nail polish.

10. Chart the activities on the patient's chart.

PREPARATION PROCEDURE FOR THE DAY OF SURGERY

1. Wash your hands, identify the patient, and explain the procedure.

2. Take the vital signs.

3. Give A.M. care, care for the hair, and dress the patient in a hospital gown.

4. Remove any makeup and jewelry.

    a. Put valuables in a secure place (with the family or in the agency's safe).

5. Have the patient void (be able to explain why this is necessary).

6. Apply safety measures (bedrails up, bed in the low position, and smoking articles removed).

7. Explain the recovery room procedure to the patient and his family.

8. Direct the family to the waiting room.

9. Complete the preoperative checklist.

10. Assist in transferring the patient to the OR stretcher.

POST-TEST

Directions: Choose the answer that will make the statement complete.

1. Preparation for surgery usually starts:

   a. when the physician examines the
       patient and makes his diagnosis.

   b. when the patient has signed the
       consent for surgery

   c. when the office nurse schedules
       the surgery

   d. when the patient is admitted to
       the hospital

2. The greatest concern the patient has is:

   a. fear of mutilation

   b. fear of death

   c. fear of the diagnosis

   d. fear related to family separation

3. All the following aspects of the admission preoperative procedures are pertinent except
   for:

   a. signed consents

   b. vital signs

   c. appropriate laboratory tests

   d. skull X-rays

4. Food and fluids are usually withheld the night before surgery from:

   a. 4 A.M. to 7 A.M.

   b. 6 A.M. to 9 A.M.

   c. 12 MN until early morning surgery
       has been accomplished

   d. 2 A.M. to 6 A.M.

5. The patient should empty his bladder before surgery:

   a. at 7 A.M. the morning of surgery

   b. immediately before the patient
       goes to the OR

   c. at 9 A.M.

   d. at 4 A.M.

6. The reasons that enemas are usually given the evening before surgery are listed below;
   all are true except:

   a. to avoid the strain and exertion of
       moving the bowels during immediate
       post-op period

   b. to avoid an involuntary bowel
       movement during surgery

   c. to obtain a stool culture

   d. to avoid an involuntary bowel
       movement in the recovery room

7. All of the following are true except:

   a. skin prep is done to make the skin
       as free of microorganisms as
       possible

   b. skin prep is performed the afternoon
       or evening before surgery

   c. the area of skin to be prepped is
       usually 1 inch in diameter

   d. hair is shaved because microorgan-
       isms cling to it

8. All of the following aspects are true except:

   a. the physician may order hair
       shampooed if necessary

   b. the bath can be given the evening
       before or in the early A.M.

   c. the patient may wear his own
       clothes to surgery

   d. all prostheses are costly and should
       be stored in a safe place during
       surgery.

9. All of the following aspects are true except:

     a. mouth care should be given

     b. makeup and jewelry should be removed and put in a safe place

     c. makeup and nail polish should be left on

     d. Demerol and atropine are often used for preop medications

10. While the patient is in the recovery room the patient's family should be directed to all except:

     a. the waiting room

     b. the cafeteria

     c. the rest room

     d. the recovery room

POST-TEST ANNOTATED ANSWER SHEET

1. a. (p. 468)
2. c. (p. 468)
3. d. (p. 469)
4. c. (p. 469)
5. b. (p. 470)
6. c. (p. 470)
7. c. (p. 470)
8. c. (p. 471)
9. c. (p. 471)
10. d. (p. 471)

POSTOPERATIVE CARE

I. DIRECTIONS TO THE STUDENT

You are to proceed through this lesson using the workbook as your guide. In the skill laboratory, you will need to practice gathering the necessary equipment and preparing the bedside unit to receive the patient from the recovery room or from surgery. Following your practice sessions and the completion of the lesson, you should arrange with your instructor to take the post-test for this lesson.

You will need the following items for your study and practice:

1. Thermometer.

2. Sphygmomanometer.

3. Stethoscope.

4. Paper tissues or wipes.

5. Emesis basin.

6. IV standard.

7. Suction machine.

8. Intake & Output record.

9. Drainage bottle and tubing, or disposable GU set.

10. Extra linen as needed — gown, sheets, towel, washcloth, and so forth.

11. Nurses' record.

Please read the following paragraphs carefully. They will tell you exactly what you will be expected to know and how to provide safe postoperative care during the period immediately after surgery, and in the later period after recovery from anesthesia. If you feel that you have sufficient knowledge and skills to complete the performance test accurately and to take the written test with at least 80 per cent accuracy, discuss with your instructor the possibility of proceeding directly to the post-tests.

II. GENERAL PERFORMANCE OBJECTIVE

You will be able to assemble the required equipment and provide postoperative care to the unconscious or helpless patient recovering from anesthesia, or the patient who has fully recovered from anesthesia. You will do this to protect the patient's safety by the early detection and prevention (when possible) of postoperative discomforts and complications. Proper care at this time will promote his recovery and rehabilitation.

III. SPECIFIC PERFORMANCE OBJECTIVES

Upon completing this lesson you will be able to:

1. Maintain open breathing for the unconscious or helpless patient through the use of an artificial airway, the proper positioning of the patient, and the suctioning of secretions from the mouth and throat.

481

2. Observe for signs of shock or hemorrhage by taking and recording the vital signs every 15 minutes during the period immediately after surgery, by frequently inspecting the dressings for signs of unusual bleeding, and by checking any drainage or vomitus for the presence of blood.

3. Ensure the safety of the patient by using siderails on the bed to prevent falling, by not leaving the unconscious or anesthetized patient alone, and by setting up the post-op unit completely and correctly.

4. Accurately record the Intake and Output from all sources as indicators of the patient's fluid and electrolyte balance, connect all tubes to suction or drainage as appropriate, and keep the IV running in the vein.

5. Provide comfort for the patient, and relief from pain by handling him carefully, frequently turning him or changing his position, avoiding unnecessary noise or confusion, and anchoring the drainage tubes. If pain persists, notify the team leader or the nurse in charge without delay.

6. Prevent respiratory complications by changing the patient's position at least every two hours, instructing him to breathe deeply and to cough, and supporting the operative site during coughing.

7. Maintain an adequate urinary output from the patient by offering him sufficient fluids, checking for signs of urinary retention, and promoting the elimination of urine by voluntary voiding or the use of a catheter when ordered by the physician.

8. Reduce or relieve the discomforts related to the patient's gastrointestinal tract (i.e., nausea, vomiting, gas pains, and constipation) through appropriate medical and nursing measures.

9. Provide for the patient's personal needs during the anesthesia recovery period by changing his gown and bed linen as needed, washing perspiration or secretions from his body, and assisting with his personal hygiene, usually for several days, giving particular attention to oral hygiene.

10. Provide passive exercise of the unconscious or helpless patient's arms and legs at least twice a day, encourage active exercise by the alert patient, and promote the goal of early ambulation.

IV. VOCABULARY

By this time you have learned the meaning of most of the words used in the lesson, inasmuch as they were in the vocabularies of other lessons that you have studied. However, there are some that may be new to you. Study the words and their meanings carefully before proceeding further into the lesson.

1. **Words related to postoperative complications**

apnea—stopped breathing; lack of respiration.
atelectasis—a diffuse blockage of tiny air sacs in the lungs caused by bits or plugs of mucus, or by a surgical opening into the chest cavity.
embolism—obstruction of a blood vessel by a foreign substance, i.e., air bubble, fat globule, purulent matter, or blood clot.
embolus (plural is emboli)—an embolism floating in the blood stream.
evisceration—the separation of layers of an incisional wound with the exposure or protuberance of an organ of the body through the separation or opening.
hemorrhage—excessive flow of blood out of the blood vessels; an abnormal amount of bleeding.
hypoxia—decrease in the supply of oxygen.
hypoventilation—decreased or reduced column of air taken into the lungs.

shock—a clinical syndrome resulting from inadequate circulation, or impending circulatory collapse, due to various causes.

thrombus—a blood clot that develops within a blood vessel, either attached to the vessel wall or lodged within the vessel; called a thrombotic embolus when it becomes dislodged and circulates in the blood system.

thrombophlebitis—a condition in which inflammation of the vein wall has preceded the formation of the thrombus.

2. Words related to the level of consciousness

coma, comatose—state of being unconscious; unresponsive to stimuli.

conscious—state of being awake; responsive, alert.

disoriented—state of being confused; lack of response or inappropriate response to stimuli.

semi-conscious (semi-comatose)—state of being able to respond to physiological stimuli, but capable only of reduced response to mental stimuli.

unconscious—state of being unaware; unresponsive to all stimuli.

3. Other words used in the lesson

airway—the air passages of the body: the mouth, nose, larynx, pharynx, trachea, bronchi, and lungs; also, a plastic or metal tube inserted in the mouth and pharynx to insure clear air passage.

aseptic—a condition free of contamination or germs; sterile.

anesthesia—the absence of pain; drugs that block perception of pain; general anesthesia, such as is induced by ether, produces unconsciousness; local anesthesia, such as is induced by Novocain, blocks sensation of pain with no loss of consciousness.

cannula—a short hollow tube or pipe, usually made of plastic; often used instead of a metal needle on an IV.

cyanosis—bluish color of tissue resulting from lack of oxygen.

electrolyte balance—dissolved chemicals in such body fluids as blood and serum, capable of conducting an electrical charge; ionized particles in balance.

larynx—the voice box.

pharynx—the back of the throat (part of the air passages).

pulmonary—refers to the lungs and the function of breathing.

V. INTRODUCTION

The Importance of Postoperative Nursing Care

The operation is over. The surgeon has used his knowledge, skills, and talent to perform an operation designed to prolong the patient's life or to improve the quality of some aspect of that life. However, the very nature of the operation produces injury and stress to the patient's body. The anesthesia administered during the surgery reduces the patient's ability to respond to the stimuli from within himself and from the surrounding environment. This, then, is the state of the patient as he enters the postoperative period: his body has undergone a deliberate injury, and his response to stimuli has been reduced.

The patient has literally entrusted his life and welfare to the doctors and nurses during surgery and the postoperative phase of his illness. If something were to go wrong, the patient often could not even signal for help, much less take steps to correct the problem himself. The surgical injury combined with the reduced ability to respond to stimuli make the patient dependent upon the help and assistance of the nurse. The less the patient is able to respond, the more the nurse must be his eyes, ears, touch, judgment, and muscles, as well as his physiological watchdog.

In postoperative nursing, the *helping* and *caring* aspects of nursing become dramatically clear. The patient recovering from a spinal anesthesia is unable to turn himself, so the nurse turns him frequently. The unconscious patient is unable to control the secretions trickling down his throat, so the nurse controls them by positioning and by suctioning. In helping the patient, the nurse is guided by the doctor's orders for postoperative treatment and therapy, but the helping aspect of nursing is evident even as the nurse bathes perspiration from the patient's forehead, or adjusts the light so that it doesn't shine directly in his eyes.

The caring aspect of nursing is the feeling that is extended to the patient and experienced by him. It is the part of nursing that requires being with the patient, tending to his needs, heeding his responses, protecting him from dangers, and providing him with compassion, tenderness, concern, consideration, and respect. Through this caring aspect of nursing, we are able to nurse the patient, not just the disease.

The helplessness of the postoperative patient makes it essential that the nurse worker have the skills and knowledge to help maintain the life processes, provide safety and comfort, and prevent complications. This lesson is designed to give you the *beginning skills* that you will need in order to provide postoperative care to patients under the direction of the doctor and the nurse.

Question 1.   In the postoperative period, the state of the patient is characterized by

a. _____ , and   b. _____ .

Question 2.   The functions of nursing consist of the   a. _____ ,

and   b. _____ aspects.

Question 3.   Orders for the postoperative care of the patient are written by:

a.   the charge nurse

b.   the doctor

c.   the ward clerk

d.   the anesthesiologist

ITEM 1.   WHERE POSTOPERATIVE CARE IS GIVEN

Regardless of the location in which postoperative care is given, the same meticulous and skillful nursing care is required. The surgical patient receives postoperative care in (1) a recovery room, sometimes called the PAR (Post-anesthesia Room), (2) an intensive care unit (ICU), or (3) his own room.

Following surgery, most patients are taken to the recovery room, which is generally located near the operating rooms. It is staffed with skilled nurses, and equipped with all the things needed to handle most postoperative emergencies. There, doctors and anesthetists from the operating room check on the condition of the patients frequently and can be reached quickly when needed.

Postoperative patients remain in the recovery room until they have reacted from the anesthesia, or are able to respond to the stimuli around them; this generally takes from two to six hours. During this period the nurses give constant and complete care to the patients, with particular attention to the vital signs, which are taken every 15 minutes. When the patient has reacted and the vital signs are stable, the doctor writes an order to transfer the patient to his own room on the nursing unit. Recovery rooms in many smaller hospitals are not open during the night hours when only emergency surgery is performed.

Intensive care units have been established in many hospitals to provide highly specialized and complex nursing care in one central area. Some surgical patients are taken directly to the ICU following a complex and serious operation. The patient may remain there for several days if his condition continues to be unstable. As a beginning worker in nursing, you *should not* be assigned to work in the recovery room or an ICU until you have gained clinical experience.

Postoperative care of the patient mainly takes place in his own room. Before the availability of recovery rooms became widespread, all patients were returned from the operating room directly to their rooms. The nursing staff on the unit stayed with the patient until he reacted from anesthesia, and continued his care through the recovery period until he was discharged from the hospital. In hospitals that have recovery rooms, the patient will already have reacted from the anesthesia before he is returned to his room. However, you will need to check the patient frequently during the first 72 hours or so, and provide greater assistance for his personal needs during this early postoperative period.

Question 4.   As a beginning worker in nursing, where would you most likely give postoperative care to the patient? _____.

Question 5.   When is the patient transferred from the recovery room to his own room?

_____.

ITEM 2.   PREPARING THE POSTOPERATIVE UNIT

In order to provide postoperative care to the patient, whether in his room or in the recovery room, certain equipment is essential. You should prepare the unit and collect the equipment before the patient arrives, so that observation and care of the patient can begin immediately. The patient's bed should be made up as a postoperative bed, as described in your lesson on bedmaking. Even if the patient has reacted from the anesthesia, it is easier to transfer him onto the bed if the top bedding has been folded back. Many patients will experience some nausea and vomiting, or have some drainage, so the bed should be protected with a pad or towel at the head, and a plastic sheet, drawsheet, pad, or Chux on the middle portion of the bed. These pads can easily be changed if they become soiled.

On the bedside stand, supply the following items: tissues, an emesis basin, a thermometer, a sphygmomanometer, a stethoscope, nursing records, paper, and a pencil. Even the reacted patient should have his vital signs checked every 15 minutes at least four times after arriving in his room. When the vital signs have been stable for some time, the doctor or the nurse may instruct that they be taken less frequently or discontinued. Most patients who have had major surgery will also have an IV running during the early postoperative period in order to supply the fluids that they are unable to take orally. An IV stand should be at the bedside to hold the bottle of fluids.

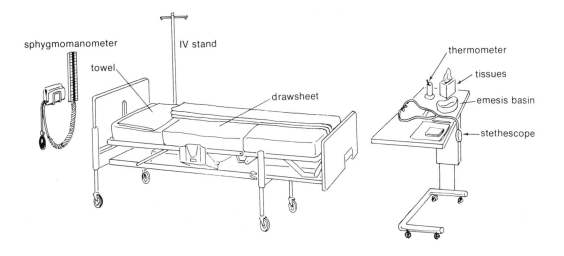

Other equipment may be needed at the bedside, depending upon the type of operation performed, or the patient's condition. The team leader or the nurse in charge will be able to tell you what may be needed. For instance, some patients will have Levin tubes that will be connected to suction machines or wall suction outlets, some may have urinary catheters that will need to be connected to drainage sets; some may need special traction or weights after orthopedic surgery; or, others, who have had tonsils removed, may require ice packs to soothe their throats.

Question 6. List seven items that should be placed in the patient's unit in order to provide postoperative care.

a. _____ b. _____ c. _____ d. _____

e. _____ f. _____ g. _____ .

Question 7. The fully reacted patient who has just arrived in his room from the recovery room should have his vital signs checked:

a. once each day until he is discharged

b. twice a day routinely

c. every four hours during the day

d. every 15 minutes, at least four times

ITEM 3.   PROCEDURE FOR PREPARING THE POSTOPERATIVE UNIT

In the skill laboratory, you should practice the procedure of collecting the required equipment and preparing the patient's bed so that postoperative care can be given to provide for his safety, to reduce or prevent complications, and to promote his recovery.

Important Steps	Key Points
1. Confer with your team leader or the nurse in charge for special instructions.	Based on her knowledge about the patient's condition and the type of surgical procedure being performed, the nurse may ask you to have special equipment or supplies at the bedside, e.g., a urine drainage set, a throat or gastric suction machine, oxygen equipment, or orthopedic appliances.
2. Collect the equipment and supplies needed and take them to the patient unit.	Use a utility cart to collect items and transport them to the unit. In preparing most postoperative units, you will need: linen for the bed, including a rubber or plastic sheet and drawsheet; a box of tissues; a sphygmomanometer; a stethoscope; nursing records; an IV standard; and paper and a pencil. A thermometer is usually in the patient unit; if not, be sure to take one with you.
3. Make a postoperative bed.	Follow the instructions given in the lesson on bedmaking. The top bedding should be folded to the side or to the bottom of the bed, the rubber sheet and drawsheet used to protect the middle portion of the bed, and the pillow placed on the overbed table or on a chair. The bed should be equipped with siderails for safety.
4. Arrange the other items at the bedside.	Place the IV standard at the side or the foot of the bed. On the bedside stand, place the tissues, emesis basin, thermometer, sphygmomanometer, stethoscope, and Intake & Output record. Arrange other special equipment if needed.
5. Prepare for stretcher access to the bed.	Move furniture, such as chairs, out of the way so that there is a clear path at least 4 feet wide from the entrance of the room to the side of the bed for the stretcher transporting the

Important Steps | Key Points

patient. It is often easier to transfer the patient from the stretcher to the bed if the bed is pulled out so that the head of the bed clears the front of the bedside stand.

ITEM 4. CARDINAL RULES FOR POSTOPERATIVE CARE

1. *Maintain an open airway and adequate respiratory function.*
2. *Take vital signs until the patient's condition is stable.*
3. *Maintain fluid balance, and record fluids taken.*
4. *Check the operative site for excessive drainage.*
5. *Provide for the patient's safety.*
6. *Provide for the patient's needs.*

Each of these cardinal rules will be explained in greater detail as we progress. The physiological needs of the surgical patient are of paramount importance. Once these needs are met, his psychological and social needs can be met. First things first; it does little good to help reduce the patient's anxiety about his job when he is hemorrhaging. Attend to the hemorrhage first, then his anxiety.

ITEM 5. MAINTAIN ADEQUATE RESPIRATORY FUNCTION

Every person must breathe and take in sufficient oxygen in order to live. Respiratory function, or breathing, is often compromised in the surgical patient. The combination of drugs given to produce anesthesia or to reduce pain, as well as the body response to the trauma of surgery itself, affects respiratory function. The respirations become shallow, and the rate of breathing is usually slow. This reduces the amount of air moving in and out of the lungs, a condition called hypoventilation. Hypoventilation results in a corresponding decrease in the amount of oxygen available to the body. Decreased oxygen produces a condition called hypoxia, although decreased oxygen supply can be due to other causes besides hypoventilation, such as the breathing of air at high altitudes, or an obstruction or infection in the lungs that interferes with the absorption of oxygen into the bloodstream.

Common early signs of decreased respiratory function are (1) shallow breathing, and (2) a slow respiratory rate. Late signs of respiratory distress are rapid, gasping types of respirations, and cyanosis (dusky, bluish color of the skin and the nailbeds).

Immediate Postoperative Care. In the recovery room, one of the main concerns of the nurse is to maintain an open airway and adequate respirations in the surgical patient. The nose, pharynx, larynx, trachea, bronchi, and lungs are the parts that make up the airway. The airway can become obstructed when the patient's jaw and tongue relax so that the tongue falls back into the pharynx, or when secretions collect and block the passage of air.

The unconscious patient will usually arrive in the recovery room with an airway that was inserted by the anesthetist to keep the tongue in place and the air passages open. (An airway is shown in the sketch.) By turning the unconscious patient's head to one side, you can help to keep his tongue from obstructing the airway.

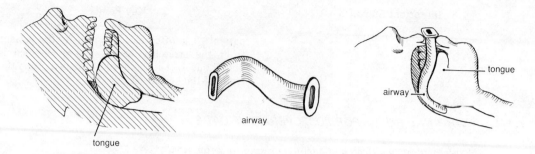

Tongue blocking pharynx.

Airway in place.

Saliva, mucus, and other secretions often collect in the back of the unconscious patient's throat and interfere with breathing. Such secretions may be drawn into the lungs, where they cause irritation to the lung tissue and further interfere with breathing. You can tell by the moist, rattling sounds of his breathing whether secretions are obstructing his passageway. These should be suctioned from the mouth and throat as soon as possible. Again, the patient's head should be turned to one side, so that some of the secretions can drain from the corner of the mouth.

To prevent other respiratory complications, the patient must be turned every two hours to relieve the pressure on the lungs so that all parts of the lung can expand with air. When the patient has reacted from the anesthesia, he should be encouraged to take at least five deep breaths, cough, and move his arms and legs every one to two hours. If he is unable to move himself, the nurse must give passive exercise.

Convalescent Postoperative Care. Health workers continue to monitor the respiratory function of postoperative patients long after they leave the recovery room and return to their own rooms. During the days and sometimes weeks that follow in the convalescent phase, the patients need to be reminded to turn, cough, and take at least five deep breaths every hour while awake. These actions often cause considerable discomfort to patients following certain types of surgery, so they often need encouragement to cough and deep breathe, as well as assistance to turn from side to side.

Many postoperative patients will have doctor's orders for special treatments by the respiratory therapist to improve their breathing and ventilation. The principle involved in most postoperative treatment is to have patients breathe deeply and expand all areas of their lungs more fully. A number of simple types of breathing devices may be ordered for use with your patients, such as blow gloves, blow bottles, inspirators, rebreathers, and others. Some specialists have reservations about their use, since patients may merely expire or use air from the oral passages to blow, and show little or no evidence that they are taking a deeper breath with the use of the device. However, you will need to follow your agency's policies and orders as written, and give instructions to the patient that emphasize taking in deep breaths and inflating the lungs adequately.

Question 8. Hypoventilation should be suspected when the respirations are

a. _____ , and b. _____ .

Question 9. The unconscious patient should be turned every _____ hours.

Question 10. The common obstructions of the airway are a. _____ and

b. _____ .

Question 11. Why is it advisable to turn the unconscious patient's head to one side?

_____ .

ITEM 6. TAKE VITAL SIGNS UNTIL THE PATIENT'S CONDITION IS STABLE

The vital signs comprise measurement of the temperature, pulse, respiration, blood pressure, and level of consciousness. These can be abbreviated and called T, P, R, and BP. The vital signs are indicators of the physiological condition of the patient. Specifically, the blood pressure and the pulse rate reveal the state of the circulatory system; the respiratory rate is concerned with the breathing function. The temperature and the level of consciousness indicate the functioning of the central nervous system and the brain.

The normal ranges for the T, P, R, and BP are given in Unit 14, The Vital Signs. For a particular individual, the vital signs may fall anywhere within the normal range, or they may be above or below the normal range, yet be usual for that person. Thus, the normal range for the specific patient should be determined by comparing his present vital signs to those taken when he was well, or in a stable condition. Stable vital signs refer to T, P, R, and BP readings that do not vary from the patient's other *recent* measurements, but may or may not fall within the patient's usual, or normal, range. For example, a patient normally has a pulse rate between 72 and 80 beats per minute. However, for several days after surgery, his pulse rate ranged between 88 and 100; this pulse rate would be described as stable, even though it is higher than his normal rate.

The level of consciousness should be recorded as part of the vital signs. Various levels of consciousness are described as:

1. Unconscious — The patient does not respond to stimuli and the reflexes are absent; he is unable to swallow or to blink his eyes. General anesthesia produces unconsciousness.

2. Semiconscious — The patient can respond to painful stimuli and move about restlessly, and he has reflexes (e.g., he can swallow), but he has difficulty understanding or responding to verbal directions.

3. Disoriented — The patient may be able to respond to all stimuli, but is confused about reality with respect to persons, time, place, or events. His speech is often irrelevant and his behavior may be inappropriate.

4. Conscious — The patient is able to respond to all stimuli, is alert, and is in command of his intellectual skills.

Immediate Postoperative Care. During the time the patient is in the recovery room, the vital signs must be taken every 15 minutes and recorded. The doctor may order that vital signs be taken less frequently after the patient has responded from the anesthesia and the vital signs have remained stable for one hour or more.

Convalescent Postoperative Care. Vital signs must be taken and recorded for postoperative patients at least once a day during the usual hospital stay. However, they are taken more frequently in most hospitals. Vital signs should be taken whenever the nurse or health worker wants to check on the patient's physiological condition. Even slight changes in these signs may be the first clue that the patient is developing a postoperative complication. A rise in temperature may indicate an infection; a fall in the blood pressure with an increase in the pulse rate may be an early sign of shock or hemorrhage. A slow respiratory rate should alert the nurse to problems associated with hypoventilation. These changes should be reported to your team leader without delay. Vital signs are an important part of postoperative care.

Question 12. Mrs. Lily returned from the recovery room a short time ago. You have taken the vital signs and have noted the following:

	BP	P	R
1115	128/78	88	20
1130	112/70	100	20
1145	108/60	112	20

     a.   What might this indicate to you? _____ .

     b.   What should you do now? _____ .

Question 13. How would you describe the respiratory rate above? _____ .

Question 14. Mr. Willis had surgery last week and his vital signs have been within the normal ranges for several days. However, this morning his temperature was 37.6 C (approximately 99.8 F) at 0600. How often should you take his vital

signs today? _____ .

ITEM 7. MAINTAIN FLUID BALANCE AND RECORD FLUIDS

During surgery, the patient has lost blood and tissue fluid as a result of the surgical procedure. Moreover, fluids have undoubtedly been restricted for several hours before surgery. These lost fluids need to be replaced either during surgery or in the early postoperative period. Fluid balance is essential for the efficient functioning of all body systems, especially the heart and circulatory systems, and for the promotion of the healing process.

Maintain the Fluid Balance. How much fluid is needed to keep the patient in fluid balance? The fluid intake should generally equal the output, or loss, of fluids. During a 24-hour period, the average adult eliminates 1200 to 1500 ml of urine, and loses another 800 to 1000 ml through the lungs, skin, and feces for a total of 2000 to 2500 ml of fluids. Therefore, in order to maintain balance, the adult should take in 2000 to 2500 ml of liquids daily.

The trauma of surgery interferes with the fluid balance of the body. Body metabolism alters the need for fluids, bleeding and oozing occur from the incision, and body fluids are often drained off through tubes (e.g., Levin tubes) used to remove gastric juices. Many patients suffer from a lack of appetite and may also be nauseated after surgery. These conditions affect the amount of fluids the postoperative patient needs and affect the way they are to be given. The doctor orders the kinds of fluids, the amount, and the route. Typical orders for fluids postoperatively are:

1. NPO (nothing by mouth), followed by an order for IV fluids.

2. Clear liquids as tolerated.

3. Full liquid diet.

4. Force fluids to 2000 ml daily.

5. Limit fluids to 1200 ml daily.

In order to keep track of the postoperative patient's fluid balance, a careful Intake & Output record is kept. All fluids given to the patient are recorded and all output is measured from all sources if possible.

Immediate Postoperative Period. The doctor's post-op orders will state the kinds and amounts of fluids the patient is to have. Patients are often NPO for one or more days following major surgery under a general anesthetic. Intravenous fluids are given during this time to replace fluids lost in surgery and to maintain the fluid balance. Blood transfusions are given to replace large blood losses. IV fluids are ordered so that a certain amount runs into the vein in a specified period of time; a sample order follows: 1000 ml of 5% D/W, IV in 12 hours. This means that 1/12 of the 1000 ml in the bottle should be absorbed every hour and that at the end of 12 hours all of the fluid will have run in. The nurse adjusts the rate of flow so that the proper amount runs in, observes the needle site frequently to assure that it is in the vein, and supports the IV site when moving the patient.

In the recovery room, oral fluids are never given to unconscious or semiconscious patients because the swallowing reflex is diminished or absent. Surgical patients who have had a spinal or local type of anesthesia are usually allowed "fluids as tolerated" by the doctor in the post-op orders. The conscious patient is given small sips of water at a time; more can be given later if he is able to keep it down.

It is important that the kidneys continue to function and produce urine after surgery. The patient should void (pass urine) within the 8- to 12-hour period following an operation. Be sure to report to the charge nurse if any surgical patient is unable to void within 8 hours. Some postoperative patients will have a catheter in place so that the urine in the bladder drains continually and the amount of urine produced within a specified time can be quickly measured in the drainage bag. Note the amount of urine in the bag and check the drainage system at least every hour when your patient has an indwelling catheter. Hourly measurement of urine output is easier when you use a urometer instead of a soft pliable collection bag.

Convalescent Period. When the postoperative patient returns to his room on the nursing unit, his fluid balance must be maintained and the recording of his intake and output continued. All fluids taken in by the patient, whether orally or by IV, are recorded on the Intake and Output sheet. All output, including urine, vomitus, and drainage from all tubes, should be measured and recorded. The Intake and Output record provides the doctor and nurse with valuable information about the patient's fluid balance. However, you should know about each patient's fluid intake and output without a written order from the doctor to record intake and output.

Many doctors order a specific amount of fluids for the postoperative patient. For example, some orders read "Force fluids to 2000 ml daily" and others state "Limit fluids to 1000 ml q.d." The rule of thumb is to give 50 per cent of the fluids during the day shift, 30 per cent on the evening shift, and 20 per cent during the night. The amount for each shift should allow some fluids for each meal period, and some to take with medicines or between meals. Keeping a plastic medicine cup at the bedside is convenient for measuring liquids taken in smaller amounts.

Question 15.   What is meant by fluid balance? _____ .

Question 16.   An adult, convalescing well after surgery, has a total output of 2150 ml for

the 24-hour period. What should his intake have been? _____ .

Question 17.   When is the patient expected to void following surgery? _____

_____ .

ITEM 8.   CHECK THE OPERATIVE SITE

Dressings. When the patient has come from surgery or the recovery room, you should check the operative site as soon as possible. Look to see if the dressing over the wound is dry and in place so that it protects the wound. Some dressings may have a small amount of slightly bloody drainage on them, and it is important to check them frequently to see whether the bleeding continues or increases. Be sure also to check the bed linen for signs of bleeding. Cases have occurred in which the dressing appeared dry, but blood seeped under it and formed a pool beneath the dressing.

One word of caution: Do not change or reinforce a surgical dressing unless you are specifically instructed to do so by the doctor or the nurse in charge. Report to them about any bleeding or drainage that has soiled the dressing, because this may be a sign of complications.

Drainage Tubes. You should find out if the patient has tubes in place, and whether these are to remain clamped or connected to suction. The tubes should be secured to the bed in such a way that they do not pull on the patient. Moreover, they should not be kinked or lying under the patient's body. The usual tubes are a urinary catheter, which is attached to the urinary drainage tubing and bag; a Levin or other type of gastrointestinal tube attached to suction; a nasal tube, which carries oxygen; and various tubes or drains left in an incision to assist in the flow of drainage. Commonly used drains would be catheters, Penrose (cigarette) drains, chest tubes, and others.

Question 18.   The most common types of tubes the patient may have following surgery are

a. _____ , b. _____ , and c. _____ .

ITEM 9.   PROVIDE FOR THE PATIENT'S SAFETY

The preoperative medication, the anesthesia, and the injury produced by the surgery all combine to reduce the patient's response to the stimuli in his environment. He is less aware of what is happening to him and what is occurring around him. He is dependent upon others to protect him from dangers at this time. The hospital and the nurse workers are legally responsible for protecting the patient and preventing harm to him. Assemble all needed equipment at the patient's bedside before he arrives from the operating room.

The patient who is not fully conscious, as well as the one who is under the influence of medication, needs protection from harm; he can respond to some stimuli, yet is not fully awake or aware of dangers. Like the unconscious patient, he should have a nurse worker in constant attendance during the early postoperative period. This means that you must be in the room where you can readily see him and be at his side to help him within a second or so.

Siderails.   Make it a habit to use siderails on the bed for the postoperative patient. Siderails help to keep him from falling out of bed, especially when he is not fully aware of his surroundings. If the patient is extremely restless, it may be helpful to attach a safety belt around his waist and to the mattress support of the bed. (The safety belt, or similar restraining device, should not be attached to the immoveable frame because raising the head or foot of the bed will squeeze the patient unduly.) In some recovery rooms, postoperative patients are kept on stretchers instead of being transferred into beds. These stretchers should be equipped with siderails and safety belts for the patient's security. Siderails also can be used to assist the patient in turning; he can hold one siderail while turning himself toward it.

Positioning.   Changing the patient's position is another way of providing for his safety. You should know and use the procedures to immobilize or support parts of the body, and to reduce pressure areas in the postoperative positioning in which (1) no head pillow is used for the unconscious patient or for 8 hours following a spinal anesthesia, and (2) the patient's head is turned to one side when in the supine position so that secretions can drain from his mouth, and his tongue cannot fall back into the throat to block the air passages.

Prevent Infection.   One of the most important ways to provide for the patient's safety is to prevent the possiblity of infection. The patient's resistance to infection is decreased by the surgery. You can reduce the chance of infection by washing your hands before and after working with each patient, by maintaining sterility around the incisional wound, by turning the patient frequently to prevent respiratory infections, and by avoiding contact with patients when you yourself have a cold, sore throat, boils, or other type of infectious disease.

Question 19.   To reduce the possiblity of danger or harm to the postoperative patient, you would take the following steps:

a._____ , b._____ , c._____ , d._____ .

Question 20.   Which of the following statements refers to a measure that provides for the patient's safety?

a.   The nurse closely observes the patient to help maintain his respiratory and circulatory functions.

b.   When turning a patient who is receiving an IV, care is taken to prevent dislodging the IV needle from the vein.

c.   After assisting the patient to use the bedpan for voiding, the nurse washes her hands before taking the patient's vital signs.

d.   Every two hours, the nurse assists and encourages the reacted patient to breathe deeply, to cough, and to turn.

ITEM 10.   PROVIDE FOR THE PATIENT'S NEEDS

Orientation.   As the patient begins to respond from the anesthesia, he needs reassurance from the nurse and he must be oriented as to time, person, and place. You may need to repeat the reassurances several times, for although the patient reacts and seems to talk rationally, the medications and anesthesia diminish his ability to remember. He needs to be reassured that the operation is over, that he is doing well, that you are there to watch over him closely, and that he is in the recovery room (or his own room), and he may even need to be told the date and time.

When caring for the patient still under the effects of anesthesia, *do not* slap the patient's face, yell at him, or shake him in an effort to make him react or rouse more quickly. The response you would get from the patient would not be a true awakening from anesthesia, but a defensive response to avoid pain or hurt. The patient's body needs time to break down the chemicals in the medications and anesthesia, and to begin excreting, or getting rid of, them before he can emerge from their effects.

Personal Hygiene. During the postoperative period, the patient will need your assistance for his personal hygiene. He should be encouraged to take care of many of his hygienic and personal needs as he gains strength in the days following surgery. On the first day after surgery, the patient may be able to brush his teeth and wash his face and arms without becoming overfatigued or uncomfortable. You will need to provide the supplies and to finish bathing him. During the patient's bath period, you should see that his joints are put through the range-of-motion exercises. When the patient is resting in bed, his body should be in good alignment, with supportive aids to maintain good position, and with protective aids to reduce and prevent formation of pressure areas.

Early Ambulation. It is common practice to get the patient out of bed hours after surgery, instead of keeping him in bed for prolonged periods, which adds to his discomfort and delays his recovery. These harmful effects of bed rest were discussed in the lesson on Patient Movement and Ambulation. You should remain with the patient the first few times that he is out of bed. Assist him to dangle his feet at the side of the bed for a few minutes so that his circulatory system can adjust to his change of position. When he no longer feels dizzy or light-headed, assist him to stand, take a few steps, and sit in a chair. In the postoperative orders, the patient's doctor will specify when the patient is to be ambulated, how often, for how long a period of time, and with what, if any, limitations.

Discomfort. The patient will suffer from various discomforts following surgery, the most common of which are pain, abdominal distention and "gas pains," nausea, vomiting, and constipation. He may also develop complications and must be observed closely for signs of these. The postoperative discomforts and complications are discussed in greater detail in the following items.

ITEM 11. DISCOMFORTS FOLLOWING SURGERY

Although the discomforts are less serious than the complications of surgery, the patient may feel miserable unless they are promptly and effectively relieved.

Pain. A certain amount of pain is expected after surgery, the most severe occurring during the first 48 hours. It will normally decrease with each passing day. The doctor's orders for postoperative care prescribe the medication to be given for pain. However, there are things you can do to help relieve the pain. You should make the patient comfortable by helping him turn or change his position, by giving him a backrub, and by other measures. When a patient complains of pain, try to find out what kind of pain and the probable cause. If it is pain in the operative site, he should have his medication promptly because minutes seem like hours if he has to wait. Often a lesser amount of medication will be needed if given promptly. If pain persists over a period of time, a larger dose usually will be needed. Often you will find that the patient has less pain if he can talk about his worries and anxieties. The patient may resist turning, doing his exercises, or getting up during the first few days when pain is severe. You should discuss with the team leader the best time for assisting the patient with these activities in relation to his medication for pain.

Nausea and Vomiting. Vomiting is less a postoperative problem today than it was some years ago when ether was the main agent used in general anesthesia. Ether is still used but not to the extent it was in the past. Although vomiting is less likely, most patients will have some nausea and lack of appetite after surgery.

One of the goals for the postoperative patient is to regain the normal function of his gastrointestinal tract as soon as possible. Generally, patients will begin to take food and fluids within a short time after recovering from the anesthesia. You can help to overcome nausea and vomiting by the following actions: begin by giving small sips of liquid. Tap water (not ice water), tea, and ginger ale are tolerated best, although small children may want only milk. If the patient seems nauseated, suggest that he take several deep breaths through his mouth until the feeling passes. Abrupt movements should be avoided. If the fluids are retained, the patient may take more. When his meal tray arrives, he should be encouraged to taste the food even if he does not have an appetite. If he is nauseated, the sight of a tray of food may lead to vomiting. It would be better to ask him in advance if he would like to try one or two items from the tray, and then take only those in to him.

Care of the Vomiting Patient. You can provide emotional support and physical cleanliness for the patient who is or has been vomiting. The patient is naturally distressed by his discomfort, his illness, and the fact that he is dependent upon someone else to clean up the vomitus. It is important that you perform this task skillfully and effectively in a matter-of-fact, pleasant, and gentle manner.

Important Steps	Key Points
1. Closely observe a patient who complains of nausea or who may vomit (for example, a patient who is recovering from anesthesia, one who is on certain medications or therapy, or one who is acutely ill).	Put the emesis basin and tissues within the patient's reach. Ask him to use the call signal if he vomits, or if you can be of help. Notify the team leader, who may be able to administer medication to help control the nausea and vomiting.
2. Assist the patient by telling him how to reduce the nausea and vomiting.	Have the patient rest quietly and avoid sudden movement; put him on one side with his knees flexed. Remove or reduce odors that may stimulate the "gag" reflex. Instruct the patient to take short, panting breaths through his mouth when he feels the urge to vomit. Remember, it is important for you to be scrupulously clean and free from heavy perfumes, lotions, cigarette smoke, and other odors because sick people are highly sensitive to odors.
3. Help the patient who is vomiting or has vomited. 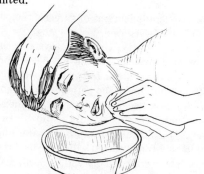 Care of vomiting patient.	Wash your hands. Position the patient's head on one side and place an emesis basin under his cheek. Use tissues to wipe vomitus from his nose or mouth in order to avoid possible inspiration of the vomitus material into his lungs (this may cause "aspiration pneumonia," which could be fatal). Provide privacy for the patient. After the patient has vomited, take the emesis basin to the bathroom or utility room. Note the color, odor, consistency, and other characteristics of the vomitus. Measure the amount before discarding it. Record the amount as output on the Intake and Output record. Wash and dry the basin, and return it to the night stand for future use.
4. Leave the patient safe and as comfortable as possible.	Vomiting leaves a foul taste in the mouth, as well as a disagreeable odor. Some patients may simply want to rinse out their mouths with tap water to avoid further nausea or vomiting. Other will want to use a mouthwash or brush their teeth.

Important Steps	Key Points
	Provide a washbasin with warm water, a washcloth, a towel, and soap. Assist the patient to wash his face and hands, or do it for him.
5. Remove soiled linen and tidy up the room.	Change all soiled linen. The odor of vomitus lingers if the immediate area is not cleaned thoroughly. This odor will often induce further nausea and vomiting. If possible, open the window to air the room for a few minutes, or use an unscented room deodorizer.
6. Record pertinent information on the nurses' notes and on the Intake and Output record.	The amount of the vomitus is recorded as output on the I & O record.

The following terms are used when charting incidents of nausea and vomiting:

a. hematemesis — blood in the vomitus

b. tarry — looks black, usually from old blood.

c. partially digested food — from a recent meal

d. odor — describe any unusual smell; sweet, fruity, sour, fecal, etc.

e. amount — the measured amount, or an estimate (i.e. small, moderate, or large).

f. projectile vomiting — sudden, forceful emesis.

Charting example:

1330. Emesis of partially digested food, approx. 100 ml. Linen changed. Still c/o nausea.
1345. Emesis — 120 ml of greenish-yellow fluid.   J. Jones, NA

Abdominal Distention and Flatus. The distention of the abdomen with flatus occurs as a result of a hypoactive bowel. Medications, anesthesia, handling of the bowel in some types of surgery, inactivity following surgery, and change in diet habits all contribute to the hypoactive bowel.

Gas in the stomach and the small intestine is mainly from swallowed air. The large intestine contains considerable amounts of flatus, or gases, produced from foods and bacteria. All but a very small amount of the flatus is reabsorbed by the healthy and active person, although decreased bowel activity causes the patient's abdomen to become swollen and painful. The discomfort from "gas pains" has been described by many patients as being the worst part of having an operation. Narcotics and other medications given for pain tend to slow down bowel activity and further contribute to the discomfort of distention.

The doctor usually prescribes a rectal tube, enema, Harris flush, or medication to stimulate the passage of flatus. As the patient passes gas, the distention is relieved, often within a matter of minutes. You can help relieve the discomforts of distention by helping the patient to turn frequently, and to get up if he is allowed to ambulate. Hot liquids and solid food help to reduce distention; but iced liquids seem to aggravate the condition. When the rectal tube is used, remove it after 30 minutes. The tube can be reinserted in an hour or so if the patient becomes uncomfortable again. Positioning can help in many cases. Sims' position and the prone position make it easier to pass the flatus. Some patients may be able to use the knee-chest position for a short time to get rid of some gas, but most postoperative patients will not be able to tolerate this position during the first few days after surgery.

Constipation. When the surgical procedure has been a minor one, the patient will probably experience no change in his bowel habits. However, some patients will not have a normal bowel movement until the third or fourth day after surgery, due to decreased intake of food and fluids, less movement and exercise, and the hypoactive bowel. Narcotics and other medications, anesthesia, and surgery all contribute to decreased bowel activity.

You can help the patient who is constipated by encouraging him to eat a diet with normal amounts of roughage, to drink large amounts of fluid, to get some form of exercise, and to walk about if able. Provide privacy and time when he is attempting to move his bowels. An enema or a suppository may be given when ordered by the doctor.

Other Discomforts. Less frequently, the patient may develop (1) *parotitis*, (2) *urinary retention*, or (3) *hiccups* (singultus) during the postoperative period, and these can be just as distressing as the problems already discussed.

Parotitis is an inflammation of one or more of the salivary glands and is seen in patients who have not eaten or taken fluids orally for a period of time, or who have not had good mouth care regularly and have thus lacked stimulation of the salivary gland. Frequent mouth care will prevent this condition.

Urinary retention is the inability to void or to empty the bladder when voiding does occur. Small, frequent voidings are often a sign of overflow from a full and distended bladder Position, privacy, a high fluid intake, and reassurance are all important when you assist the patient to empty his bladder.

Having the patient breathe into a paper bag will often relieve hiccups, but persistent hiccups require more vigorous treatment prescribed by the doctor.

Question 21.   Almost without exception, the postoperative patient will experience the

   discomfort of _____.

Question 22.   The depressing action of drugs and anesthesia causes hypoactivity of the

   bowel and contributes to the discomforts of _____ and

   _____.

Question 23.   The patient had surgery about ten hours ago and is allowed to take fluids and
   diet as tolerated, but continues to have moderate nausea. Some actions you
   might take to reduce the patient's nausea are:

   a. _____   b. _____   c. _____

   d. _____   e. _____.

ITEM 12. SHOCK AS A COMPLICATION

Every postoperative patient should be treated as though he might develop shock at any time. Shock is the body's response to inadequate circulation due to a variety of causes. In the postoperative patient, the stress of surgery, the anesthesia, the blood loss, and the injury from the incision itself can lead to shock. Progressive and prolonged shock leads to death, so the faster the state of shock can be reversed, the better are the patient's chances for recovery. Unless circulation is restored, damage may occur to the brain, kidneys, or other organs resulting from the lack of blood and oxygen. With prompt and adequate treatment, shock is reversible and the patient will recover.

The most common cause of shock in the postoperative patient is the loss of blood. Other causes of shock may be (1) faulty pumping of the heart, as in a myocardial infarction, or heart attack; (2) dilation of some blood vessels so that they become engorged and the blood does not move along rapidly enough to be part of the circulating volume; (3) insult (injury) to the nervous system; (4) severe, strong emotional response such as extreme fear of pain; and (5) infections that overwhelm the body's defenses.

The signs of shock are related to the effects of inadequate circulation. The symptoms are:

1. Skin — pale in color, clammy to the touch.

2. **Blood Pressure** — progressive, consistent fall in pressure (the earliest change to signify shock).

3. **Pulse** — rapid (often over 120 beats per minute), thready, or quivery.

4. **Respirations** — rapid and shallow, often grunting as if hungry for air.

5. **Cyanosis** — blueness of fingernail beds or lips due to lack of oxygen; use inner lip for detection in a dark-skinned person.

6. **Urine output** — scanty or absent because of decreased circulation through the kidneys.

At the onset of shock, the patient may be anxious and apprehensive. As the state of shock progresses, he becomes listless and finally, unconscious as the shock deepens. The early signs of impending shock are apprehension, a rapid and thready pulse, and air hunger. Profound shock is characterized by a change in the level of consciousness, profuse sweating, and markedly low blood pressure.

Question 24. In the postoperative patient, the cause of shock is usually _____ .

Question 25. A patient going into shock would have early signs that include a. _____ ,

b. _____ , and c. _____ .

ITEM 13. THE TREATMENT OF SHOCK

The best treatment for shock consists of prevention and early recognition. Shock can be prevented by careful physiological and psychological preparation of the patient for surgery. Postoperatively, it can be avoided by the replacement of the blood and fluid lost, careful movement of the patient, judicious (careful) use of drugs that depress circulation or respiration, and retention of body warmth through the provision of light covers and a warm room. (However, *do not* apply external heat directly to the body because this dilates superficial blood vessels in the skin and further reduces deep circulation.) Keep the patient in a flat position, and give him a sense of security through skillful care performed in a calm, quiet atmosphere. Early signals of shock are detected by carefully observing the patient and his vital signs.

If your observations indicate that the patient may be going into shock, you should *immediately* summon help and report the signs to the nurse so that the doctor can be notified. *Do not leave the room.* The team leader or the nurse in charge may instruct you to remain with the patient to calm and reassure him, or she may take care of him and ask you to collect the necessary supplies and equipment.

You can help in the treatment of shock. Keep the patient warm by providing additional blankets and help put him in Trendelenburg's (shock) position by mechanically elevating the foot of the bed or placing it on "shock blocks." *Exceptions*: Patients who are recovering from a spinal anesthesia or who have had brain surgery *must not* be placed in shock position, *but should be kept flat.* The doctor will order the replacement of blood or fluids, so that if the patient does not have an IV running, you should have the equipment ready. He may also order the use of oxygen and various drugs to treat the shock. Close observation of the patient and his vital signs is essential until he has recovered from shock.

Question 26. When you observe signs of shock in your patient, what is the first thing you

should do? _____ .

Question 27. The treatment of shock by the nurse-doctor team, in which you also participate, consists of:

a. _____ b. _____ c. _____

d. _____ e. _____ f. _____ .

ITEM 14. OTHER CIRCULATORY COMPLICATIONS

Hemorrhage. Hemorrhage can occur as a complication during the immediate post-operative period, and such loss of blood has been mentioned as one cause of shock. With external hemorrhage, the bleeding is visible. Since the volume of blood in circulation is reduced, the other symptoms of hemorrhage are the same as those for shock: pale color, anxiety or apprehension, rapid pulse, and lower blood pressure. In addition to taking the vital signs (BP, then P), the dressings, drainage, and bedding of the postoperative patient should be inspected frequently for signs of bleeding. Dark-brownish color of the blood in drainage or on dressings indicates that the bleeding occurred some time ago, while bright red blood is a sign of fresh bleeding. Report the color and the amount to the charge nurse and record it on the patient's chart.

The treatment for hemorrhage is (1) to stop the bleeding, and (2) to treat the shock. If your patient starts to hemorrhage, you should call for help immediately, notify the nurse in charge and the doctor, attempt to staunch (or stop) the bleeding if possible (some patients may have to return to surgery so that the doctor can stop internal bleeding), and treat the shock. Place the patient in a flat position or a shock position, provide additional blankets if necessary, and collect the supplies and equipment needed to replace the lost blood with IV's or transfusion.

Thrombophlebitis. Another complication is called thrombophlebitis (thrombo = blood clot, phleb = vein, itis = inflammation). It is an inflammation of the vein and commonly occurs in the leg, which has a sluggish blood flow that leads to the formation of a clot. The condition may be caused by the patient's prolonged inactivity (especially of his legs) or by pressure caused by a pillow under his knees, or a tight strap around the arm or leg that restricts venous circulation. The symptoms are pain, heat, redness, and swelling around the affected area of the leg. The treatment consists of complete bed rest, elevation of the limb, application of warm wet packs to the area, and drugs as ordered by the doctor. Thrombophlebitis is not as common a complication today because postoperative patients are encouraged to move about and ambulate early.

Embolism. The most dreaded possible consequence of thrombophlebitis occurs when the blood clot dislodges from the vein and travels through the blood stream to the heart and the lungs. This is called a cardiac or pulmonary embolism, which at its best produces pain and an extended period of illness, but at its worst causes sudden collapse and death. The symptoms are severe chest pain, cough, and difficulty in breathing. Because of the danger and possible tragedy from pulmonary embolism, all efforts should be made to prevent thrombophlebitis and embolism in the blood stream. Preventive measures include exercising the legs, using elastic stockings or wrapping them with elastic bandages, and slightly elevating the foot of the bed to improve venous return of blood. Because of the danger of dislodging possible clots, one essential rule to remember is: Avoid rubbing or massaging the legs of the postoperative patient, even as a comfort measure.

Question 28. Mr. Sloan had an operation on his stomach three hours ago. Which of the following conditions would lead you to suspect that he may be hemorrhaging? More than one answer may be correct.

    a. You notice more dark reddish-brown drainage on his abdominal dressing.

    b. He has started moving restlessly from side to side, his eyes seem to roll around, and he is moaning.

    c. In the last few minutes, the Levin tube has filled with bright red drainage.

    d. His IV fluids have slowed down to a rate of 20 drops per minute.

    e. His pulse is now 116 beats per minute, but had been around 60 to 80 in surgery.

Question 29. The day after surgery, Mr. Sloan asked you to put a pillow under his knees to ease the strain on his abdomen, and also wanted you to rub his legs because they seemed sore. What would you do and why?

Question 30. What measures can you take to prevent thrombophlebitis from become a complication for Mr. Sloan.

_____ .

ITEM 15. RESPIRATORY COMPLICATIONS

Postoperative complications of a respiratory nature occur more often than all the other problems combined. Hypoventilation is an underlying factor in most respiratory complications. In hypoventilation, the breathing is slow and shallow so that a smaller amount of air — and oxygen is taken into the lungs. Portions of the lungs do not receive enough air to expand all of the air sacs; thus the scene is set for complications to develop. The treatment of hypoventilation consists of nursing measures that increase the respiratory function: deep breathing, coughing to clear mucus from the passages, and frequent turning to relieve pressure on the lungs and to allow lung expansion. Without treatment, hypoventilation may progress to respiratory failure. This can occur several days after surgery as the patient tries to be more active and places greater demand on his poorly functioning respiratory system.

Postoperative, or hypostatic pneumonia is a common complication of hypoventilation. Air sacs in the lungs that are not expanded with air become filled with fluid, or they collapse. They become a fertile field for the growth of viruses and germs that cause inflammation of the lung (pneumonia). Decreased respiratory function and the possiblity of infection occur when the air sacs are plugged with bits of mucus in a condition called atelectasis. The treatment of both pneumonia and atelectasis includes ventilating the lungs and administering antiboiotics or other drugs.

Question 31. The underlying cause of most respiratory complications is _____ .

Question 32. To increase the postoperative patient's respiratory function, you should assist

and encourage him to a. _____ , b. _____ , and

c. _____ .

Question 33. Two complications that result from decreased respiratory functions are

a. _____ and b. _____ .

ITEM 16. WOUND COMPLICATIONS

Wound Infection. The two types of wound complications are infection and the breaking open of the incision. During recent years, some organisms have emerged that are resistant to the action of various antibiotics. It is still very important to prevent wound infections because the use of antibiotics may prove ineffective in treating the infection. Prevention of infections of the wound depends on careful handwashing, scrupulous cleaning of equipment, use of sterile supplies, and practice of aseptic techniques by the nurse.

The first sign of wound infection is increased pain in the incision. In normal recovery, pain decreases each day. The incision shows signs of infection by becoming reddened, warm, and swollen, and by draining puslike material. If a patient develops a wound infection, it is important to prevent it from spreading to others. The treatment prescribed by the doctor may include antibiotics to fight the infection, drainage of the pus, and often, application of wet or dry heat.

Wound Separation. Wound separation (the breaking apart of the edges of the incision) may occur in some patients during the sixth to eighth day after surgery. The causes of wound separation are malnutrition, which interferes with the normal healing process; defective suturing; and excessive strain on the wound from retching, coughing, and so forth. When the wound separates so completely that body organs (viscera) are exposed, the condition is called evisceration. Usually the patient will feel that something "has broken loose," or "given way." You should have the patient stay at complete bed rest, inspect the dressing for pinkish drainage, look to see if the wound has separated, relieve strain on the wound, and reassure the patient by saying that you would like the doctor to check his dressing. The nurse in charge and the doctor should be notified immediately. If there is evisceration, the nurse will cover the wound with a sterile dressing moistened with sterile saline solution to protect the exposed organ.

Question 34.   Since antibiotics have been so miraculous in curing many infections, why is it necessary to go to all the trouble of cleaning and sterilizing equipment and using aseptic technique to prevent infections?

_____.

Question 35.   Wound infections produce inflammation; the symptoms of inflammation are:

a. _____   b. _____   c. _____

d. _____   e. _____ .

Question 36.   Evisceration means the exposure of _____ .

ITEM 17.   CONCLUSION OF THE LESSON

You have now completed the lesson on postoperative care of the surgical patient. After sufficient practice in the skill laboratory, you should be able to collect the necessary equipment and prepare the patient's unit for his arrival following surgery so that there is no delay in giving him care. Your responsiblity for the patient is based on the cardinal rules of postoperative care, knowledge of ways to identify and prevent complications, and methods to reduce the patient's discomforts.

Make an appointment with your instructor and arrange to take the post-test. After that, you should be able to use your beginning skills to provide safe and effective nursing care to the post-op patient in the clinical area.

VI.   ADDITIONAL INFORMATION FOR ENRICHMENT

Postoperative care of the patient is a rich and rewarding field of study. It is complicated by the wide variety of special needs, precautions, and procedures that are used depending on the type of surgery performed and the condition of the patient. Those of you who are interested may wish to read and learn more about the nursing care of the patient after surgery has disrupted the function of a particular organ or system of the body. For instance, you may want to investigate the special nursing care requirements of the patient following a kidney transplant, a knee operation for torn cartilages, the removal of a brain tumor, or the amputation of a limb or breast. In each case, the surgery has interfered with the function of a body part or a system, and the postoperative emphasis is on assisting the patient to regain, maintain, or adapt to a change in this function. The lesson you have just completed provides the basic framework for *all* post-op care, but it has not been possible to cover every variation.

As you take care of post-op patients in the clinical setting, you may want to read more about their particular needs. Textbooks on surgical nursing are quite detailed concerning the nursing care, and articles in various journals provide sources of up-to-date information. To start you on your reading, select a few of the articles listed below, most of which are in the *American Journal of Nursing.*

1.   Transplants and replacements

Shoemaker, Rebecca: Total Knee Replacement Procedure and Results. *Nursing Clinics of North America.* 8: 117–126, March 1973.

Taylor, Karleen, Nancy Commons, and Mary Sue Jack: Liver Transplant. *American Journal of Nursing,* 69:1895–1899, September 1969.

Willy, Maxine: Care of the Patient with a Kidney Transplant. *Nursing Clinics of North America,* 8:127–136, March 1973.

2. Postoperative care, discomforts, and complications

Gardner, Arlene M.: Responsiveness as a Measure of Consciousness. *American Journal of Nursing*, 68:1034–1038, May 1968.

Blackwell, Ardith, and William Blackwell: Relieving Gas Pains. *American Journal of Nursing*, 75:66–67, January 1975.

Harrington, J.D.: Symposium on Intensive Care of the Surgical Patient. *Nursing Clinics of North America*, 10:1–146, March 1975.

Johnson, Colleen, and Richard Convery: Preventing Emboli After Total Hip Replacement. *American Journal of Nursing*, 75:804–806, May 1975.

3. Nursing care related to heart and blood vessel (cardiovascular) surgery

Betson, Carol, Patricia Valoon, and Cynthia Soika: Cardiac Surgery in Neonates: A Chance for Life. *American Journal of Nursing*, 69:69–73, January 1969.

Breslau, Roger: Intensive Care Following Vascular Surgery. *American Journal of Nursing*, 68:1670–1676, August 1968.

Hunn, Virginia K.: Cardiac Pacemakers. *American Journal of Nursing*, 69:749–754, April 1969.

Verderber, Anne: Cardiopulmonary Bypass: Postoperative Complications. *American Journal of Nursing*, 74:868–869, May 1974.

4. Nursing care related to head and neck surgery

Dison, Norma: A Mother's View of Tonsillectomy. *American Journal of Nursing*, 68:1024–1027, May 1969.

Pitorak, Elizabeth F.: Laryngectomy. *American Journal of Nursing*, 68:787–791, April 1968.

Stowe, Sharon: Hypophysectomy for Diabetic Retinopathy. *American Journal of Nursing*, 73:632–637, April 1973.

5. Nursing care related to other systems and cancer

Boegli, Emily, and Mary Steele: Scoliosis: Spinal Instrumentation and Fusion. *American Journal of Nursing*, 68:2399–2403, November 1968.

Mamaril, Aurora: Preventing Complications After Radical Mastectomy. *American Journal of Nursing*, 74:2000–2003, November 1974.

Seaman, Florence W.: Nursing Care of Glaucoma Patients. *Nursing Clinics of North America*, September 1970, pp. 489–496.

Formation of Thrombus and Embolus

You may be interested in learning how the blood forms a thrombus within the blood vessel. Without going into the complex clotting mechanisms of blood, we can consider the physical conditions that are involved.

Two physical causes of blood clotting within blood vessels are (1) a roughened surface of the vessel, (2) the slow movement of blood through the vessels. The slow movement of blood allows the clotting factors, which are always being formed, to concentrate in one area rather than disperse in the blood flow. Once the clotting begins, the clot tends to promote further clotting, so that it grows in size.

Some elements of the circulatory system need to be considered. The blood circulation is a closed system — that is, there are no normal openings between the system and the outside of the body. The heart pumps blood from its chambers by contracting, and the force increases pressure that speeds the blood along through the vessels. The heart rests for a fraction of a second, then pumps again to send out more blood under pressure. This alternating contraction–rest–contraction action causes the beat of the pulse that you can feel in various parts of the body. The action can be compared to a roller coaster. The cars approach the starting point (the heart); the first car fills with people and is given a push onto the course (contraction of the heart); it speeds down the declines, swoops around the curves, labors up the inclines (blood circulates through the body), and then returns to the starting place while other cars follow it around the course. The process is then repeated.

Now let's see what happens to the roller coaster car when the track near one of the curves is narrow and bumpy (roughened surface of the vessel). The car slows down and stops, causing the cars behind it to slow and stop (formation of a clot). Or the car runs out of energy or power and goes slowly until it comes to an incline, then travels even more slowly or stops. Cars following it are slowed, stopped, and unable to pass (formation of a clot). The formation of a blood clot in a vessel is illustrated in the following figure.

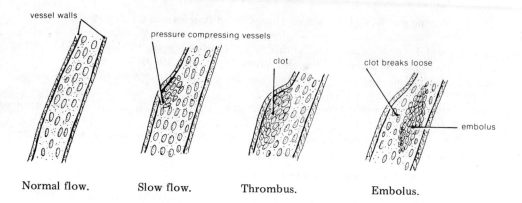

Normal flow.   Slow flow.   Thrombus.   Embolus.

The immobility of the surgical patient slows the rate of his blood flow. This sluggish flow of blood is further aggravated by bed rest and the former practice of putting pillows under the knees. Blood flowing slowly through the legs will begin the clotting process within a matter of a few hours.

Clots (thrombi) have been known to grow in size and length until they are the length of the leg itself. When a portion of the clot breaks loose from the wall of the vessel, it becomes an embolus and circulates until it reaches a vessel too small to pass through. If that vessel is a vital one, such as those in the lungs, brain, or heart, sudden death occurs. There are certain drugs available for treatment that control and retard the clotting process when thrombus or embolus formation is suspected.

WORKBOOK ANSWER SHEET

Question 1. a. a deliberate injury to the body

　　　　　b. reduced response to stimuli

　　2. a. helping

　　　　b. caring

　　3. b.

　　4. his own unit or room

　　5. when he has reacted from anesthesia and his vital signs are stable

　　6. listed in any order: tissues, emesis basin, thermometer, stethoscope, sphygmo-manometer, Intake and Output record, and IV standard

　　7. d.

　　8. a. breathes shallowly

　　　　b. has a bluish tinge to nails or skin

9. c. two

10. a. accumulated secretions

    b. tongue falling back in the throat (answers may be transposed)

11. to help secretions drain and keep the tongue from falling back into the throat

12. a. falling BP and rising pulse may be signs of shock

    b. report changes to the team leader

13. stable

14. four times a day, or every four hours until the temperature returns to normal

15. intake of fluids equals output

16. the same, or 2150 ml

17. within 8 hours

18. a. urine catheter

    b. Levin or nasogastric tube

    c. oxygen (answers may be in any order)

19. a. provide constant attention until he is fully conscious

    b. keep siderails up

    c. frequently change his position

    d. prevent infections

20. all four answers are correct

21. pain

22. abdominal distention; constipation

23. a. give sips of fluid

    b. give preferred liquids if allowed

    c. have the patient take deep breaths through his mouth

    d. have the patient rest quietly

    e. offer only the food he thinks he can eat (any order)

24. blood loss

25. a. rapid, thready pulse

    b. apprehension

    c. air hunger (any order)

26. summon help

27. a. added warmth

    b. shock position

    c. replacement of blood or fluids

    d. oxygen

    e. drugs

    f. close observation of the patient (any order)

28. c. and e.

29. I would not use a pillow under his knees or rub his legs because of the danger of thrombi and emboli. I would explain that it would be better to exercise his legs and change his position.

30. encourage movement and exercise, especially of the legs

31. hypoventilation

32. a. breathe deeply

    b. cough

    c. turn frequently (any order)

33. a. pneumonia

    b. atelectasis (any order)

34. many organisms became resistant to antibiotics

35. a. pain

    b. redness

    c. heat

    d. swelling

    e. drainage of pus (any order)

36. an organ

PERFORMANCE TEST

Your instructor will ask you to perform the following procedure in the skill laboratory without reference to other resource material.

1. Given an adult patient returning from surgery on his abdomen, collect the equipment needed, and prepare the patient's unit for his arrival in such a way that you would be able to begin his postoperative care safely and without delay. For the purpose of this exercise, the patient will have an IV running and will have a urinary catheter in place.

2. To improve your skills in charting, record the observations you would make about the patient's condition and indicate some of the ways in which you would assist the postoperative patient. Chart on the nurses' notes used by your hospital. You may use the following information as a guideline, but you will need to add more details of your own.

> Mrs. Goodwill had her gallbladder removed early this morning and has been transferred from the recovery room to her own room. She is awake and has no complaints at this time except for a dry mouth. She has a nasogastric tube, an IV is running in her left arm, and she has an indwelling catheter. You have been taking care of her since she arrived back on the unit and have taken her vital signs twice:
>
>   T — 98, P — 88, R — 16, BP — 132/82
>   15 minutes later, they were: P — 84, R — 16, BP — 130/82

PERFORMANCE CHECKLIST

POSTOPERATIVE CARE

PREPARATION OF PATIENT UNIT FOR POSTOPERATIVE CARE

1. Obtain instructions for securing special equipment (the type of equipment is dependent on patient's condition and the surgery procedure performed).

2. Collect appropriate equipment, including at least the following items:

   a. Linens

   b. Tissues

   c. Sphygmomanometer

   d. Stethoscope

   e. Intake and Output record

   f. IV standard

   g. Airway

   h. Paper and pencil

3. Prepare a postoperative bed (refer to the unit on bedmaking if necessary).

4. Arrange the equipment appropriately.

5. Ensure that the bed is accessible by stretcher.

6. Maintain the respiratory functions.

7. Connect the drainage tubes.

8. Take the vital signs as directed.

9. Observe and record fluid intake and output.

10. Check the operative site.

11. Maintain the IV (if appropriate).

12. Provide for the patient's safety.

13. Report and record the care given, as appropriate.

CHARTING OF POSTOPERATIVE CARE

1. Follow the instructions for charting for your hospital. One example of charting is shown here:

HOURS		NURSING OBSERVATIONS
A.M.	P.M.	
	1:30	From Rec. Rm. per stretcher. To bed in Rm 410. Siderails up. IV of 5% D/W running at 30 gtts/min in L. Arm. Foley catheter draining well — straw-colored urine NG tube attached to low suction. Mod. amount of green-colored fluid. Abd. dressing dry and intact. Awake and responding. T 98, P — 88, R — 16, BP — 132/82
	1:45	P — 84, R — 16, BP — 130/82 No complaints of discomfort.
		C. Allen, RN

POST-TEST

Matching Test: Select a word from List II that most accurately defines the phrase in List I. Not all of the words in List II will be used. Place the letter from List II in the space provided.

List I	List II
_____ 1. reduced amount of air inhaled into the lungs	a. unconscious
_____ 2. a device to keep the tongue from falling back into the throat	b. thrombus
	c. cannula
_____ 3. a clot circulating within the blood vessels	d. airway
_____ 4. the bluish-tinged color of the skin and nails	e. atelectasis
_____ 5. inadequate circulation of blood	f. hypoventilation
_____ 6. a blood clot formed in the inner wall of a blood vessel	g. cyanosis
_____ 7. unresponsive to all stimuli	h. antisepsis
_____ 8. state of being unaware of pain	i. shock
_____ 9. blockage of air sacs in the lungs with mucus	j. embolus
_____ 10. excessive amount of bleeding	k. apnea
	l. anesthesia
	m. hemorrhage

Multiple Choice Test: For each of the following situations, you are to select the one best answer to the question. Place the letter of the answer you select in the space provided.

_____ 11. Your patient, Mr. Blake, has gone to surgery to have an operation for a bleeding duodenal ulcer. Your team leader has assigned you to prepare Mr. Blake's unit for his return and has mentioned that he will probably have a Levin tube in place. In setting up his unit and bed for postoperative care, you would provide:

a. an Output record to keep track of all drainage from the Levin tube

b. extra blankets and hot water bottle to conserve his body heat in case of shock

c. an extra airway you could insert to keep his tongue from blocking the air passages

d. a suction machine to withdraw drainage from the stomach or upper bowel

_____ 12. After the operation, Mr. Blake is taken to the recovery room. He has had a general anesthesia and while unconscious, he:

a. needs the nurse's assistance to cough

b. is unaware of any stimuli

c. reacts to stimuli, but feels no pain

d. is unable to swallow salivary secretions

_____ 13. The nurses in the recovery room have started their post-op care of Mr. Blake. The *first* observation they make is to:

    a. see that he is breathing

    b. take the blood pressure and pulse

    c. observe the level of consciousness

    d. inspect the dressings for bleeding

_____ 14. The recovery room nurse noticed that Mr. Blake's vital signs at the end of the operation were: BP — 124/80, P — 84, and R — 16. Now, a half hour later, the vital signs are BP — 118/80, P — 92, and R — 10. From these readings, the nurse suspects that Mr. Blake may be:

    a. bleeding internally

    b. in the early stage of shock

    c. developing a thrombus

    d. underventilating his lungs

_____ 15. As part of Mr. Blake's care in the recovery room, the nurse has taken his vital signs every 15 minutes, checked the dressing, which has remained dry, and noted the dark, greenish-brown drainage from the Levin tube. Now, Mr. Blake has become more restless, moving his arms and moaning. As he groggily opens his eyes several times and starts to spit out the airway in his mouth, the nurse knows that:

    a. she should remind him to leave the airway in place

    b. he is restless because of pain and should have medication

    c. he is beginning to react from the anesthesia

    d. his restlessness is a symptom of impending shock

_____ 16. Mr. Blake is now waking up, and the nurse hastens to reassure him by saying, "Your operation is over, and you are in the recovery room. I'm Miss Jensen and I'm taking care of you." In addition, Miss Jensen also asks him:

    a. to keep his head turned to one side so secretions will drain out of his mouth

    b. to take several deep breaths, cough, and move his legs in the exercises

    c. whether he is thirsty, and what type of fluid he would prefer to drink

    d. to lie quietly so that the Levin tube and the dressing on the incision will not be disturbed.

_____ 17. Miss Jensen helps turn Mr. Blake to his side, and he dozes off. The reason she turned him was:

    a. to help make him more comfortable

    b. to relieve pressure areas on his back

    c. to promote the expansion of the lungs

    d. all of the above

_____ 18. A short time later, Mr. Blake complains of pain and is given medication for it, since he has fully reacted from the anesthesia and his vital signs are quite stable. Stable vital signs indicate that:

    a. there is no change from the previous reading

    b. there are no postop complications or discomforts

c. the readings are within the patient's normal range

d. there is rapid recovery from the general anesthesia

_____ 19. You have been notified that Mr. Blake is being transferred from the recovery room to his own unit. When he arrives, you notice that he is very relaxed from the medication and that he has an IV still running in one arm. As you help settle him in his bed, you are careful to:

a. avoid dislodging the IV needle from the vein

b. elevate the knees of the bed to prevent strain on his abdominal muscles

c. raise the siderails before leaving the bedside

d. take his vital signs every 15 minutes for one hour

e. all except b.

f. all except c.

_____ 20. Now that Mr. Blake is back in his room, it is important that you:

a. check his condition frequently

b. stay with him constantly until the IV is completed

c. help him to turn, cough, and breathe deeply every 4 hours

d. massage his back and legs as a comfort measure

_____ 21. It is now nearly 8 hours since Mr. Blake had his surgery. You offer him a urinal and ask him to void. The reason for doing this is that:

a. you need to write down the amount as output on the Intake and Output record.

b. distention of his bladder with urine causes him additional discomfort and pain

c. you want to make sure his kidneys are putting out urine following the surgery

d. the doctor needs to know how long to keep him on IV fluids

_____ 22. Since Mr. Blake returned to his room, you have assisted him to turn and encouraged him to breathe deeply, to cough, and to move his legs at least every 2 hours. By coughing, Mr. Blake will be less likely to develop the post-op complication of:

a. embolus

b. pneumonia

c. shock

d. hemorrhage

_____ 23. By moving his legs every 2 hours, he is less likely to develop the complication of:

a. pain

b. shock

c. thrombus

d. hypoventilation

_____ 24. The second day after surgery, the doctor removes Mr. Blake's Levin tube and leaves an order for fluids as tolerated and a liquid diet. Mr. Blake is eager to try taking fluids. What would you recommend that he do?

   a. wait until his liquid diet arrives at the next meal time

   b. go ahead and drink all the water he wants

   c. take at least 2000 ml of fluids daily

   d. start with small sips at first to see if it is retained

_____ 25. Later that day Mr. Blake complains of gas pains in his abdomen. The most probable reason for the gas pains would be that:

   a. his bowel is hypoactive following surgery

   b. the Levin tube was removed too soon

   c. he has not had enough solid foods

   d. his fluid intake has been too high

_____ 26. You can help relieve Mr. Blake's gas pains by which of the following nursing measures?

   a. providing a paper bag for him to breathe in

   b. assisting him to turn or to get up and walk about

   c. giving him only ice-cold fluids to drink

   d. having him breathe deeply and pant through his mouth

_____ 27. On his third postoperative day, Mr. Blake stated that he did not feel well. He had a lot more pain in his incision. You call the team leader, and both of you inspect his incision. You notice that the area around the lower end of the incision is very red. From the symptoms, you would suspect that Mr. Blake has developed:

   a. an embolus

   b. strained muscles

   c. an evisceration

   d. a wound infection

_____ 28. Suppose that Mr. Blake had been on complete bed rest for several days after surgery, that he had not moved his legs, and that he has kept a pillow under his knees. If he then complained of soreness and pain in one leg, what probably had happened?

   a. he had cramping in his leg muscles due to lack of exercise

   b. he had become weak due to the prolonged bed rest

   c. he had an inflammation and blood clot in a leg vein

   d. he had developed a contracture from flexion of the knees

_____ 29. Mr. Sloan, who is in the room next to Mr. Blake, went to surgery today and has just returned to his room from the recovery room. He had a spinal anesthesia for his operation less then 4 hours ago. If he were to develop symptoms of shock, what should you *avoid* doing when helping to treat the shock?

   a. provide warmth to his body with extra blankets

   b. lower the head of his bed in the shock, or Trendelenburg's position

c.   remain with the patient at all times and give reassurance

d.   take and record the vital signs until they have stabilized

_____ 30.   One of the doctor's post-op orders for Mr. Sloan was "Diet as tolerated." Mr. Sloan began taking some liquids by mouth in the recovery room, but now is experiencing a great deal of nausea. You have suggested that he do all but one of the following until the nauseated feeling passes. Which one does *not* apply?

a.   breathe deeply through his mouth several times

b.   cough several times and turn frequently

c.   take small sips of any liquid he chooses

d.   lie quietly in one position or on his right side

POST-TEST ANNOTATED ANSWER SHEET

1. f. (p. 482)	16. b. (p. 488)
2. d. (p. 483)	17. d. (p. 488)
3. j. (p. 482)	18. c. (p. 489)
4. g. (p. 483)	19. e. (p. 498)
5. i. (p. 483)	20. a. (p. 489)
6. b. (p. 483)	21. c. (p. 491)
7. a. (p. 483)	22. b. (p. 499)
8. l. (p. 483)	23. c. (p. 498)
9. e. (p. 482)	24. d. (p. 494)
10. m. (p. 482)	25. a. (p. 495)
11. d. (p. 485)	26. b. (p. 495)
12. b. (p. 483)	27. d. (p. 499)
13. a. (p. 487)	28. c. (p. 498)
14. d. (p. 487)	29. b. (p. 497)
15. c. (p. 488)	30. b. (p. 494)

Unit 24

ASSISTING WITH
INTRAVENOUS THERAPY

I. DIRECTIONS TO THE STUDENT

Proceed through the following lesson. In the skill laboratory in the presence of your instructor, demonstrate your ability to assist with intravenous (IV) therapy.

In the laboratory you will need:

1. Armboard.

2. Nonallergic tape.

3. IV bottle and tubing.

4. Adult mannequin in a patient gown.

5. Infant mannequin.

6. Soft restraints.

Your instructor will test you on your demonstration.

II. GENERAL PERFORMANCE OBJECTIVE

When you have completed this lesson, you will be able to give daily care to a patient who is receiving IV therapy. You will apply good safety measures throughout the procedure.

III. SPECIFIC PERFORMANCE OBJECTIVES

Following this lesson, you will be able to:

1. Give daily care (bath, dress/undress, meals, and so forth) to a patient with an IV.

2. Assist the patient to ambulate with an IV.

3. Recognize the need for professional assistance while caring for a patient receiving IV therapy.

4. Practice proper safety precautions for the patient receiving IV therapy.

IV. VOCABULARY

acidosis—a condition in which the acid-base chemistry of the body is unbalanced; acidity increases beyond normal, as in diarrhea, and diabetes.

alkalosis—a condition in which the alkalinity, or base balance, of the body tends to increase beyond normal; an excess of alkalies or decrease of acid in the blood, as in hyperventilation.

amino acids—the end products of protein digestion: there are 22 known amino acids.

bore (needle)—the inside passageway of a needle through which liquid passes.

flask—a bottle or container for liquids.

ASSISTING WITH INTRAVENOUS THERAPY   513

U
N
I
T
24

glucose (dextrose)—solution of sugar and water or saline, commonly given intravenously as a nutrient.

gtt—an abbreviation for "drops," used in the calculation of IV flow.

infusion—the act of pouring into, commonly associated with a vein, as in the introduction of liquids into a vein.

intravenous injection—a term used for the giving of a small amount of drug into the vein (5 to 20 cc).

lumen—a hollow passageway.

pH—a term used to indicate alkalinity or acidity.

parenteral—pertaining to the introduction of materials into the body by other than the intestinal tract (orally); intravenous.

saline—solution of sodium chloride (NaCl), or salt, and distilled water, frequently given intravenously; it is also used as an irrigating solution to wash tissues or wounds.

transfusion—the act of transferring blood or its component parts (plasma, serum, packed cells) from one person to another.

viscous (viscosity)—pertaining to a substance that is sticky or gummy in consistency.

V. KNOWLEDGE BASIC TO THIS LESSON

ITEM 1. WHY ARE IV'S GIVEN?

IV's are given to supply the body with needed elements that cannot be supplied as rapidly or efficiently by other means. These elements may be:

1. Blood, plasma, or other blood components.

2. Nutritional requirements in the form of glucose, amino acids, or salines, used to prevent a metabolic crisis such as acidosis or alkalosis.

3. Fluids and salts when the patient is unable to receive enough of these by mouth (orally).

4. Medications that the patient is unable to take by any other means.

ITEM 2. SCIENTIFIC PRINCIPLES OF INTRAVENOUS THERAPY

Anatomy and Physiology. Walls of veins are elastic and moveable. They contain sensory nerves. The superficial veins used for intravenous therapy are usually the basilic or median cubitus veins inside the elbow. Other veins on the back of the hand or dorsum of the foot may be used.

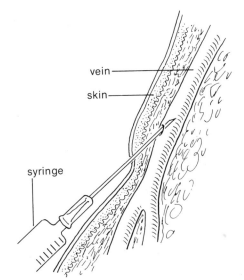

Intravenous infusion

When IV therapy is administered, fluid is deposited within the blood vessel, and enters the circulation immediately. The body can best adapt to fluids given at the rate of 20 to 60 gtts per minute. Infused solutions in large amounts increase the work of the heart; therefore, the patient should have his vital signs taken so that changes in blood pressure and pulse rate can be observed. Increased secretion of urine results from large amounts of infusion.

Microbiology. Contact with any object contaminates sterile equipment, such as the needle and tubing used to insert into the sterile IV solution. You must therefore be careful to maintain the sterility of the equipment, as well as the intravenous fluid.

Chemistry. Solutions for intravenous therapy must be constituted so that the pH value of the blood is approximately 7.4 (blood is slightly alkaline). If the pH rises above 7.8 or falls below 7.0, life is endangered. Coma usually occurs when the pH of the blood falls slightly below pH 7.0. On the other hand tetany is a danger when blood alkalinity rises to a pH of 7.7 or 7.8.

Physiologic salt solution is 0.9 per cent sodium chloride. It resembles most of the body fluids in action, density, and osmotic pressure, and combines well with blood. It may be used in conjunction with whole blood infusion.

Physics. Fluid leaves an inverted hanging flask (bottle of IV fluid) by the force of gravity. If a clamp is used on the tubing, it should be placed as near as possible to the needle in order to keep from producing negative pressure within the tubing.

Factors that influence the rate of flow of an IV solution are the size of the needle, the height of the flask, and the viscosity of the fluid. Fluids flow less rapidly through a needle with a small bore than through a needle with a larger bore. The higher the container is held, the faster is the flow of fluid. Blood is more viscous, requires a larger needle, and has a different drop size than other fluids. A small lumen makes it easier to expel air from the tubing since fluid can run through as a solid column to replace the air rather than trickle down the side as it does in larger tubing.

ITEM 3.   WHO STARTS IV'S OR BLOOD TRANSFUSIONS?

The amount and type of fluid to be given within a specific time period are *always* ordered by a physician. The agency policy dictates who is to start an IV, hang subsequent bottles, and terminate an IV. Usually, these are the responsibilities of the licensed nurse who has had special IV training, or the physician.

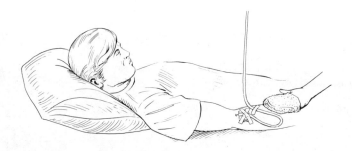

IV using median cubitus vein.

ITEM 4.   DAILY CARE OF PATIENTS WITH IV'S OR BLOOD TRANSFUSIONS

Bathing. IV needles, and special IV needles and tubing, are usually inserted in the arm at the elbow, or in the veins on the back of the hand or wrist. The most common sites are in the bend of the elbow, on the back of the hand, and in the scalp if the patient is an infant.

Gently wash around the area of the needle without dislodging the tape holding the needle secure in the vein. Do not neglect to wash the patient's fingers and give nail care according to your previous lessons.

Dressing and Undressing. (Remember, you had this procedure in the unit on assisting the patient to dress and undress.) Sleeveless nightgowns have large enough armholes to thread an IV bottle and tubing through them.

Some agencies have special gowns that have one sleeve open. It is secured on the patient's arms with ties (see the illustration at the right).

ITEM 5. SAFETY PRECAUTIONS

Although most agencies do not allow a student to adjust the rate of flow of an IV, you should be aware of this procedure as a safety precaution.

There are two kinds of drip chambers. One is called a macro-drip (macro means large) and the other is a micro-drip (micro means small). There are four micro-drips to every one macro-drip. Micro-drip chambers are used for infants in whom the amount of fluid taken must be exact. Check with your team leader for the kind of drip chamber being used and the number of drops per minute the fluid will run.

When a patient is undergoing IV therapy or a blood transfusion, he should be checked every 15 or 20 minutes. Watch:

1. *The rate of flow*, or drops per minute; if it is not what was ordered, call your team leader to make the necessary adjustments.

2. *The amount* of fluid left in the bottle. When fluid is as low as the neck of the bottle, report it to the team leader so that she may prepare either to hang a continuing bottle of fluid or to discontinue the IV.

3. The needle *injection site*; an infiltrated IV is one in which the needle has come out of the vein, and the IV fluid leaks (infiltrates) into the surrounding tissue, causing swelling. If this occurs, report it to the team leader *immediately* because this is painful to the patient, and the IV should be restarted in another vein.

4. The *patient's reaction* to the IV therapy. You must be alert to any unusual reaction by the patient receiving IV therapy, such as twitching, increased respiration, or flushing. If you notice any of these changes, call your team leader *at once*.

5. The *patient's restraints*. The older patient who is confused often requires

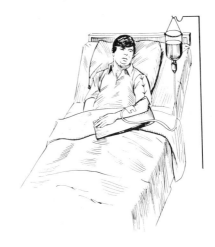

Arm is placed on armboard.

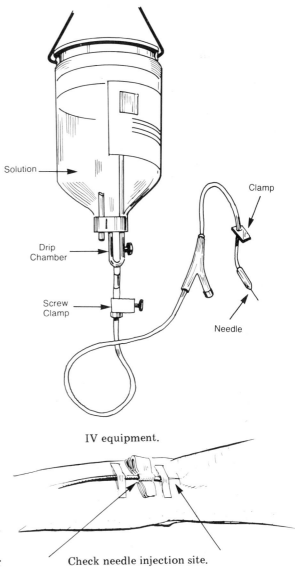

Solution

Clamp

Drip Chamber

Screw Clamp

Needle

IV equipment.

Check needle injection site.

soft restraints on the extremity that has the IV. Follow your agency's policy regarding restraints. If restraints are used, be sure that they are not so tight as to occlude (block) the vein and prohibit the fluid from entering the vein.

In infants, the veins in the arms and legs are frequently too small to receive fluids. In these cases, fluids are often infused into the scalp vein. To restrain the infant with a scalp vein infusion, wrap him in a "mummy restraint." A child is "mummied" by wrapping a sheet folded in fourths (or a receiving blanket) around the body so that the arms are bound lightly to the sides of the body. Only the head, neck and feet are free. Movement of the entire body is minimal when this type of restraint is used.

If the child is receiving an IV in an arm, be sure that both arms are restrained to prevent him from pulling the IV out. If the IV is given in the child's leg, care should be used in restraining the leg. Children receiving IV therapy should *never* be left unattended.

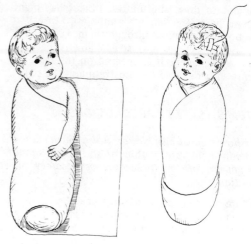

Restrain infant for IV.

ITEM 6. CARING FOR A PATIENT RECEIVING IV THERAPY

Important Steps	Key Points
1. Remove the patient's hospital gown.	Slip the gown off by removing the sleeve from the arm without the IV. Keep the patient covered with a bath blanket to avoid exposure and chilling. Remember to protect his modesty at all times. Carefully remove the IV bottle from the stand or hanger. Holding the bottle with one hand, pull the gown over the patient's arm and tubing, and over the bottle. *Do not* lower the IV bottle below needle level; if you do, the patient's blood will flow back into the needle and into the tubing. We want the fluid to run into the vein, not the blood to run out of the vein. Rehang bottle on the IV stand.
2. Bathe the patient.	Proceed according to the unit on Baths. Wash gently around the area where the needle is inserted. Be sure not to loosen the tape that holds the needle secure. When drying the patient, do not rub over the vein; pat it gently to avoid dislodging the needly.
3. Dress the patient.	Remove the IV bottle from the hanger. With the sleeve of the gown (to be put on the arm with IV) in one hand, pull the sleeve over the bottle with the other hand. Rehang the bottle on the IV stand. Continue carefully to thread the sleeve of the gown over the tubing and arm. Then finish dressing the patient as you would any other

Important Steps	Key Points

patient. Remember: to *undress* a patient, the IV arm is *last*; to *dress* a patient, the IV arm is *first*.

U
N
I
T
24

4. Assist the patient to eat.

If the IV is infusing in the hand or arm that the patient uses to eat, you will have to assist him to cut his food and prepare his liquids. You may need to feed the patient; if so, use the techniques prescribed in the lesson on nutrition.

Even if the IV is attached to the arm that the patient does not use to eat, you will cut his meats and prepare his drinks. The food and utensils should be nearby for his convenience. Assist him as required; usually after the food is cut up, he can manage for himself.

5. Ambulate the patient who is receiving IV therapy.

Provide a portable IV standard on wheels. Assist the patient out of bed as you were taught. Observe him closely for weakness or dizziness. Support the IV arm to assure a continuous flow from the IV. A sling may be used for the patient to rest his arm in.

If the patient is able, have him grasp the IV pole with the hand that has the IV in it. This provides support for the arm, enables the patient to move the pole at his own pace, and leaves his other arm free to help him balance by holding onto the railing along the hall corridor.

Tell the patient to walk along one side of the corridor to keep people from bumping into him and to avoid blocking the corridor.

6. Maintain safety precautions.

Check the patient's IV every 15 to 20 minutes. Know how many drops per minute he is to receive. You should have this information in your patient report.

Report *immediately* to your team leader the following:

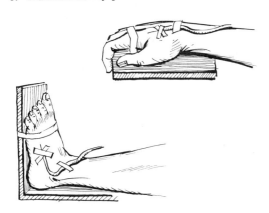

a. Drops running too fast or too slow.

b. Low fluid level left in bottle.

c. Swelling around the needle site.

d. Patient reaction to the IV fluid such as twitching, flushing, or blanching of skin, and increased respiration or pulse.

Hand and foot support for IV.

When reporting to the team leader, check the label on the IV bottle, the medication name (if added), and the stated amount. Check the time it was started and the time it will be completed.

7. Apply the patient's restraints if ordered.

Follow your agency policies regarding the use of restraints, the type, and their application. Check the restraints frequently to see that circulation is not inhibited and that the fluid is running in correctly.

Important Steps	Key Points

8. Chart on the nurses' notes and the I & O Record (if it is being used).

Charting example:

0815. Fed all food on general tray. Taken eagerly.   J. Jones LVN

0945. Bed bath given. In good spirits this A.M. Ambulated in hall for 15 minutes. Returned to bed quite tired. IV running well. 200 cc solution left in bottle.   J. Jones LVN

If hospital policy requires you to be responsible for maintaining the number of gtts per minute, then note the information as follows:

0945. Bed bath given. Ambulated in hall for 15 minutes. Returned to bed fatigued. IV gtts running at 20 gtts/min. Needle site in good condition. 200 ml solution remaining in bottle.

ITEM 7. IV DRIP RATES

If your hospital policy requires you to be responsibile for regulating the amount of fluids the patient is to have by IV during a given period of time, you must know how to calculate and regulate the drip rate.

The physician generally orders IV fluids, 1000 ml, to be run in during an 8-, 10-, or 12-hour period. This amount should infuse at an even rate so that equal amounts are given each hour. If the IV is running behind the hourly scheduled amounts, it should not be run wide open to catch up. Large amounts of IV fluids infused in a short period of time (an hour or less) can overload the patient's circulatory system and can cause a damaged heart to fail. Keep the IV on time by regulating the drip rate. If the IV fluids are infusing behind schedule, recalculate or reschedule the time in consultation with your team leader or the physician.

The flow of IV fluids from the bottle, through the tubing, and into the vein is by drops. The size of the drop varies according to the drip chamber opening on the tubing that is used. By knowing the number of drops that are contained in a ml or cc of fluid, and by controlling the drops released per minute, you can control the amount infused each hour and for the total period.

1. A regular IV drip chamber releases 15 gtts for each ml or cc

2. A blood transfusion drip chamber releases 10 gtts for each ml

3. A pediatric micro-drip chamber releases 60 gtts for each ml

How To Calculate. If you have questions about how to calculate the IV drop rate, check with your instructor. There are charts available that have already calculated the rates for the various drip chambers and for the period of time ordered to run in standard amounts, such as 1000 ml. If you do not have one of these charts, it is necessary to solve the problem mathematically.

Calculation of Rate Using the Regular IV Drip Chamber

Problem: How many drops per minute are required for the physician's order of "1000 ml 5% dextrose in water in 12 hours"?

Known Facts: 15 gtts are released by the drip chamber for each ml.

60 minutes = one hour.

IV to run for 12 hours.

Amount is 1000 ml.

Solution: 12 hours × 60 minutes = 720 minutes to run IV.

1000 ml × 15 gtts/ml = 15,000 gtts to be given.

Divide 15,000 gtts by 720 minutes = 21 gtts/minute.

Rate is 21 gtts per minute.

Calculation of Rate Using the Micro-drip Chamber

Problem: How many drops per minute are required for an order of "500 ml 5% dextrose in normal saline in 10 hours" for a child?

Known Facts: 60 gtts are released by the drip chamber for each ml.

60 minutes = one hour.

Since there are 60 drops in a ml and there are 60 minutes in an hour, the micro-drip will deliver drops on a ratio of 60:60, or 1:1.

Solution: Divide 500 ml by 10 hours = 50 ml per hour.

The ratio of gtts per ml and minutes per hour is 1:1.

Therefore, the rate is 50 gtts per minute.

Calculation of Rate Using the Blood Transfusion Drip Chamber

Problem: How many drops per minute are required when the physician's order states: "Give 500 ml whole blood in 4 hours"?

Known Facts: 10 gtts are released by the drip chamber for each ml.

500 ml are to be given in 4 hours.

60 minutes = one hour.

Solution: 500 ml × 10 gtts/ml = 5000 gtts.

4 hours × 60 minutes = 240 minutes.

Divide 5000 gtts by 240 minutes = 21 gtts/minute.

Rate is 21 gtts per minute.

RATE OF IV SOLUTION FOR REGULAR DRIP

125 gtts/min = 500 cc/hr — Run 2 hrs.
100 gtts/min = 400 cc/hr — Run 2 1/2 hrs.
 90 gtts/min = 333 cc/hr — Run 3 hr.
 75 gtts/min = 300 cc/hr — Run 3 1/2 hrs.
 63 gtts/min = 250 cc/hr — Run 4 hrs.
 50 gtts/min = 200 cc/hr — Run 5 hrs.
 42 gtts/min = 167 cc/hr — Run 6 hrs.
 38 gtts/min = 150 cc/hr — Run 6 1/2 hrs.
 36 gtts/min = 143 cc/hr — Run 7 hrs
 31 gtts/min = 125 cc/hr — Run 8 hrs.
 28 gtts/min = 111 cc/hr — Run 9 hrs.
 25 gtts/min = 100 cc/hr — Run 10 hrs.
 23 gtts/min = 91 cc/hr — Run 11 hrs.
 21 gtts/min = 85 cc/hr — Run 12 hrs.
 19 gtts/min = 75 cc/hr — Run 13 hrs.
 17 gtts/min = 67 cc/hr — Run 15 hrs.
 13 gtts/min = 50 cc/hr — Run 20 hrs.
 11 gtts/min = 42 cc/hr — Run 24 hrs.

PERFORMANCE TEST

In the skill laboratory, bathe, feed, and ambulate a patient receiving IV therapy in his right arm. Maintain constant safety checks as outline in the unit of instruction.

When you have finished this part, complete the Intravenous Therapy Worksheet.

PERFORMANCE CHECKLIST

INTRAVENOUS THERAPY

1. Dress and undress a patient receiving IV therapy without dislodging the needle. (For additional detail, refer to the checklist in the unit Dressing and Undressing.)

2. Give assistance with meals when needed. (For additional details, refer to the unit on nutrition.)

3. Bathe the IV site during the regular bath without causing pain to the patient or dislodging the needle. (Refer to the unit on Baths, if required.)

4. Assist the patient with an IV to ambulate. (Refer to the unit on Mechanical Aids for Ambulation, if required.)

5. Check safety hazards often.

     a. The IV fluid level.

     b. Swelling around the needle.

     c. The patient's reaction to the IV.

     d. The rate of flow.

INTRAVENOUS THERAPY WORKSHEET

Directions: Proceed through the following items. After each situation, answer the questions on this worksheet and record the appropriate information on the nurses' notes.

Item I

Situation: Mrs. Rowe, the patient in Room 333, has a continuous intravenous drip going into the right forearm. A bed bath was given at 9:30 A.M. The nurse aide then assisted Mrs. Rowe to walk in the corridor for 15 minutes. When getting into bed, Mrs. Rowe slipped and was assisted to the floor by the nurse aide. Mrs. Rowe incurred no apparent injuries. The IV drip slowed down but continued to drip. The area around the insertion of the needle appeared slightly swollen.

Question: What action should the nurse aide take?

What will the nurse aide chart? Record the appropriate information in your nurses' notes.

Item II

Situation: Mr. Budd, in Room 624, is on continuous bed rest because of extreme weakness. He has been getting blood transfusions daily. Miss Wood, RN, started his blood transfusion (500 cc) at 11:00 A.M. in the left elbow. At 11:40 A.M. he rang his call light.

When the nurse aide answered, she found Mr. Budd's face extremely flushed. He said he was chilled and needed more covers. She observed tremors around his lips. The blood transfusion was dripping rapidly and approximately 300 cc had been absorbed. Mr. Budd complained that he ached all over.

Question: What action should the nurse aide take?

What will the nurse aide chart? Record the appropriate information in your nurses' notes.

Item III

Situation: Baby Vincent had brain surgery and has an intravenous running in his left inner angle. His left leg is securely restrained. The intravenous drip has been ordered to drip at a rate of 10 gtts per minute. When the nurse aide had given 2 oz of Baby Vincent's formula, she noted that the IV bottle was empty and had blood coming back in the IV tubing near the needle.

Question: What action should the nurse aide take?

What will the nurse aide chart? Record the appropriate information in your nurses' notes.

Item IV

Situation: Mr. James, a 38-year-old healthy male was hospitalized after fracturing his right femur. An open reduction was done and Mr. James was received on the Orthopedic Ward with an IV running. The doctor ordered the present IV to be followed with 1000 ml 5% dextrose and water to be run during a period of 12 hours.

Question: At how many gtts per minute would the IV be set to complete in 12 hours?

Question: How many gtts per minute would be required to complete the IV in 8 hours?

Question: At how many gtts per minute would the IV be set to complete in 6 hours?

Item V

Situation: Mr. George suffered a severe laceration on his left arm. The doctor ordered 500 ml of whole blood Type O to be infused at 30 ml per hour.

Question: How many gtts per minute would be given?

POST-TEST

1. Give two reasons for intravenous therapy.

   a. _____

   b. _____ .

2. Name the three most common sites for giving an intravenous infusion.

   a. _____ , b. _____ , and c. _____ .

3. What are the five most important items to be checked when an IV is running?

   a. _____ d. _____

   b. _____ e. _____

   c. _____

4. Define micro-drip: _____

   _____

   _____ .

5. Define macro-drip: _____

   _____

   _____ .

6. What are your responsibilities in intravenous therapy? Name two.

   a. _____

   b. _____ .

POST-TEST ANNOTATED ANSWER SHEET

1. a. Replace the nutrients rapidly (p. 513)

   b. When the patient is unable to take nutrients orally

2. a. Leg (usually the foot) (p. 514)

   b. Arm (usually the elbow or hant)

   c. Scalp (in infants)

3. a. Rate of flow (p. 515)

   b. Amount of fluid left in the bottle

   c. Injection site for swelling

   d. Patient's reaction

   e. Patient's restraints

4. Micro-drip: Drip chamber that is usually used for infants where the amount of fluid taken in must be exact (p. 518)

5. Macro-dip: Larger drip chamber of the two; the micro-drip drips four to every one macro-drip (p. 518)

6. a. Observe (p. 517)

   b. Report to the team leader

OXYGEN THERAPY

I. DIRECTIONS TO THE STUDENT

Read the introduction and procedures in this lesson carefully. They will tell you what you need to know regarding the nursing care of patients receiving oxygen therapy. Arrange with your instructor to practice using the various types of oxygen apparatus in your skill laboratory.

II. GENERAL PERFORMANCE OBJECTIVE

You will be able to demonstrate your knowledge of the various oxygen therapies as well as the nursing care indicated when caring for patients who are receiving oxygen therapy.

III. SPECIFIC PERFORMANCE OBJECTIVES

Upon completion of this lesson and your laboratory practice, you will be able to correctly:

1. Describe and identify the methods of oxygen therapy administered to patients.

2. Show how to regulate oxygen flow and how to care for a patient with an oxygen tent, nasal cannula, nasal catheter, oxygen mask, Venturi mask, or IPPB (intermittent positive pressure breathing apparatus), and properly record your activities.

3. Demonstrate and discuss safety precautions that must be observed when patients are receiving oxygen therapies.

IV. VOCABULARY

anoxia—a deficiency of oxygen.
atelectasis—lack of air in the lungs due to blockage of small bronchial tubes.
bronchioles—the terminal ends of the bronchi.
bronchus (plural, bronchi)—one of two branches of the trachea.
complication—a secondary disease or condition developing in the course of a primary disease.
cough—an explosive expiratory effort to rid the respiratory track of an obstruction.
diaphragm—the musculomembranous wall separating the abdominal and thoracic cavities.
diffusion—a chemical process whereby a liquid or gas mixes its chemical components.
dyspnea—difficult or labored respiration.
epiglottis—the small pedicle over the larynx (voice box) that closes when swallowing to permit food to go down the esophagus and to shunt air to the trachea.
expiration—breathing air from the lungs.
hiccough (hiccup)—spasmodic contraction of the diaphragm caused by an irritation of the respiratory or digestive system.
humidifier—an apparatus used to increase the moisture content of the air.

hypoxemia—low oxygen content in the blood.
hypoxia—low oxygen content in the tissues.
inspiration—the act of breathing air into the lungs.
medulla—the enlarged portion of the spinal cord just inside the cranium.
nasal catheter—a tube of rubber or plastic used to give oxygen through the nose.
nebulizer—an atomizer or sprayer.
pharynx—the throat, a common passageway for food and air.
pleura—the covering of the lung.
respiration—the act of breathing (inspiration and expiration).
sneeze—similar to a cough except that the explosive expiratory effort is through the nose.
spirometer—an apparatus used to measure lung volumes of inspired and expired air.
syncope—fainting.
therapeutic—pertaining to treatment given for the purpose of healing.
trachea—the windpipe, a 4½-inch-long tube from the larynx to the bronchial tree.
trauma—injury.
vertigo—dizziness.

V. INTRODUCTION

Respiration is essential to life. The breathing rate is regulated by the respiratory centers in the brain as well as in some peripheral centers that are composed of clusters of chemosensitive cells known as carotid bodies and aortic bodies. Normal respiratory rates are: newborn, 40 respirations per minute; infant, 30 respirations per minute; adult, 14 to 18 respirations per minute. Through the act of breathing in and out (inspiration and expiration), we take in air, which is about 20 per cent oxygen (O_2); it is carried to the lungs by way of the nose, pharynx, larynx, trachea, and bronchi. Gas exchange takes place within the lungs where the oxygen is absorbed into the circulatory system and excess carbon dioxide molecules are removed. The oxygen content in the blood is a necessary chemical component upon which all tissues and living cells exist. Without oxygen, some cells begin to die in 30 seconds.

A constant balance of oxygen and carbon dioxide is essential for health. When either of these is out of balance, some type of respiratory therapy may be required. Disease or obstruction in some part of the respiratory tract may constitute the factors causing this imbalance.

Oxygen is carried by the hemoglobin in the red blood cells. It is a clear, odorless, tasteless gas that is heavier than air. It is a component of all living tissue and it supports the metabolism of foods by combustion (the act of burning, or fire).

In the Additional Information for Enrichment segment of this unit, you will learn more about the anatomy and physiology of the respiratory system. Some signs and symptoms you may observe in the patient who is not getting enough oxygen are as follows:

1. He may comment that he "can't breathe" or that he "feels as though he were suffocating."

2. He may become dyspneic (have difficulty breathing) and use all his energy trying to get enough oxygen for his body needs.

3. He will have decreased muscle coordination and slowed mental capacities. All living tissue must have oxygen in order to continue proper functioning.

4. He will appear restless and irritable, anxious or frightened (he won't know why).

5. He may become cyanotic (bluish in color) because of diminished oxygen content in the blood.

6. He may increase the rate and depth of respirations to try to get enough oxygen from the air to supply the needs of his body.

7. He may faint (syncope) or complain of vertigo (dizziness), which is caused by a lack of oxygen in the brain.

Whenever your patient complains of breathing problems or exhibits behaviors indicating decreased oxygen intake, notify your team leader or the doctor promptly. Continuous oxygen therapy for the patient is usually initiated and supervised by the nurses. Most hospitals have respiratory therapists who carry out more complex treatments using a variety of drugs, respirators, and other equipment.

Treatment of patients with respiratory diseases can take one of several forms:

1. The maintenance of an open breathing passage:

   a. You can suction (a method of sucking up obstructing material by changing air pressure) if the patient can't cough up mucus and obstructions.

   b. An airway may be used for easier breathing. The airway keeps the tongue from falling into the back of the throat and obstructing the passage of air. (Recall the procedure from the unit on Postoperative care.)

   c. Another method of keeping an open air passage is to thin out the mucus secretions so that they can easily be removed by coughing or suction. This can be done by giving the patient steam inhalation treatments, nebulizers with or without medication, and intermittent positive pressure breathing (IPPB) with an aerosol attachment.

2. The increasing of oxygen content. Oxygen can be given directly to the patient via one of several methods, for example, nasal catheter, nasal cannula, mask, Venturi mask, or hyperbaric oxygen chamber.

Because of the combustive characteristic of oxygen as a gas, special precautions must be taken by the patient, staff, and visitors to prevent a fire or explosion during oxygen treatments. Cautionary "No Smoking" signs must be placed in strategic places around the patient—on the oxygen equipment, at the head of the bed, and on the door to the patient's room. Most fires and explosions connected with oxygen therapy are caused by matches lit in the immediate vicinity of the oxygen. Sparks from improperly working electrical equipment (electrical connections, electric shavers, radios, and TV's) or from static electricity, which can be generated by wool blankets and synthetic clothing and may produce a fire or explosion when in the presence of a high oxygen concentration. Most health agencies, therefore, use cotton blankets and request personnel to wear cotton clothing.

ITEM 1. ADMINISTRATION OF OXYGEN BY NASAL CATHETER

Oxygen is given by nasal catheter when high concentrations of oxygen are required (up to 35 per cent). This method is the most frequently used because it is efficient, it is not frightening to most patients, it permits easy observation of the patient by nursing personnel, and it gives the patient freedom to move about in bed. The catheter may cause some irritation to the nasal passages if it is left in for a long period of time; therefore, a humidifier is always used with this type of administration to keep the passageways moist. Although as a beginning nurse practitioner, you will not initiate the use of the various nasal oxygen techniques, you may be responsible for starting and stopping the oxygen flow per doctor's or patient's orders. Oxygen therapy is given only on a doctor's order except in certain emergency situations established by the agency (in the coronary care units, intensive care units, recovery room, emergency room, or other special care units within the agency).

You should be aware of the techniques for beginning administration so that you can assist the nurse or doctor and the patient. You must know how to regulate the oxygen flowmeters.

In the skill laboratory, given an emergency patient who is having severe breathing problems, assist in obtaining, assembling, and initiating oxygen by using a nasal catheter.

U
N
I
T
25

Important Steps	Key Points
1. Wash your hands, approach and identify the patient, and explain what is to be done.	Check his identification band. In this way it will be easier to obtain his cooperation. The patient may be frightened, anxious, irritable, and somewhat slow to understand your explanations because of insufficient oxygen intake. Speak slowly, kindly, and with patience. Instruct him on safety precautions, such as the no smoking rule and the restricted use of electrical appliances.
2. Assemble the necessary equipment.	You will need an oxygen flowmeter and humidifier with connecting tubing and a nasal catheter, a glass of water, a lubricant, a piece of gauze, and "No Smoking" signs. (Equipment can be obtained from storage, from the supply department, or the respiratory therapy department.) The nasal catheter may be rubber or plastic. It is about 16 inches long, with several small holes in the tip of the catheter so that the oxygen can come out of the tube in several places. The type and size of the catheter for an adult is usually a #14 French. Always check the equipment to see that it is in good working order.
3. Connect the apparatus. 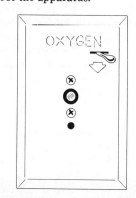 Wall-mounted oxygen outlet. 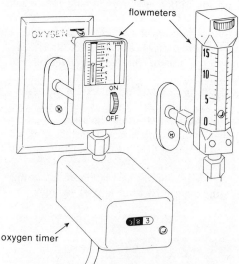 oxygen timer	Usually the bottle will come to you with distilled water in it, filled to the level marked on the outside of the bottle—about $2/3$ full. To fill an empty humidifier bottle, unscrew and remove the bottle cap. Fill the bottle with distilled water (tap water may be used with some equipment). Replace the bottle cap. Attach the top of the humidifier to the oxygen *flowmeter*. Attach the flowmeter to the piped-in oxygen outlet on the wall by pressing it firmly into the outlet. Attach connector tubing to the humidifier and the nasal catheter. Set the wall-mounted oxygen flow at 3 liters per minute. This is done by turning the flow adjustment valve toward the "on" position (see the diagram). Flowmeter "on" valves are either at the top or side of the meter, depending on which manufacturer's product it is. Continue turning the valve until the desired flow level is reached. This level is recorded on the gauge just above the flow adjustment valve. The flow is prescribed by the physician and is recorded in liters. Test the oxygen flow by inserting the tip of the nasal catheter in a glass of water. The oxygen will bubble out through the holes in the catheter. If it does not, check to see if the holes are plugged.

Important Steps	Key Points

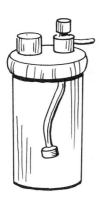

Humidifier bottles

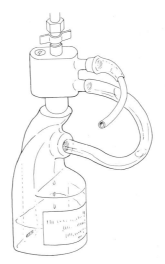

4. Pick up the catheter and measure the length for insertion.

The depth to which the catheter is to be inserted is determined by holding the catheter near the patient's face and measuring the distance from the tip of his nose to his ear lobe. Mark the length with the thumb of your left hand (you can use a piece of tape if you prefer). (Reverse hand positions if you are left-handed.)

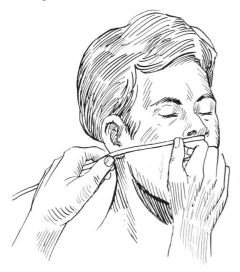

5. Squeeze some lubricant onto a gauze square.

The nasal catheter needs to be well-lubricated for ease of insertion. The easier the insertion, the less trauma (or injury) there is to the delicate mucous membrane lining the nasal cavity. (Mineral oil and vaseline are not used because they may cause lipoid pneumonia.) Lubricate the tip end of the nasal catheter in a *water* soluble lubricant.

6. Insert the nasal catheter with the oxygen on.

Holding the catheter at the level marked on it for insertion, gently introduce it into one side

Important Steps   **Key Points**

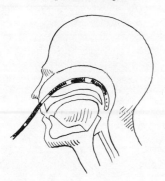

and along the floor of the nasal passageway. It should go straight toward the ear instead of arching upward. Do not use force to get the catheter in. If you hit an obstruction, remove the catheter and insert it into the other nostril.

7. Check the level of the catheter in the back of throat.

Have the patient open his mouth wide. You may need a tongue blade to hold his tongue flat and a flashlight to see at the back of his throat. The tip of the catheter should be seen slightly to one side of the uvula (the small pedicle of tissue hanging down from the roof of the mouth at the back).

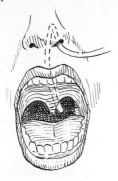

Avoid activating the gag reflex with the catheter. Be aware that serious stomach distention can be caused if the oxygen flow is directed into the esophagus.

8. Adjust the oxygen flow.

Set it at the rate prescribed by the physician. (You may have done this under step 3.)

9. Secure the nasal catheter to the patient's face with tape.

Split a 2-inch piece of tape in half to about the center of the strip. Wrap one split end around the catheter and attach the other to the patient's face. The catheter can be placed in one of two positions: (1) brought to the side of the nose and fastened to the face, or (2) brought back up over the bridge of the nose and fastened to the forehead. Make the patient comfortable in good body alignment, with the call light and bedside stand conveniently located, and fresh water at hand.

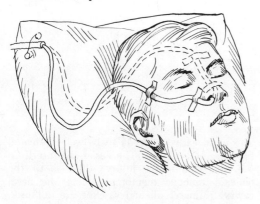

10. Place a "No Smoking" sign strategically.

Put signs on the head of the bed, on the oxygen equipment, and on the patient's door. Warn visitors against smoking. Although oxygen does not burn, it provides the climate for fires to start. Fire, like living tissue, needs oxygen to burn.

11. Record the initiation of oxygen by the RN.

Note the method, time, flow rate, and any observations about the patient's condition, such as improved color and less labored breathing.

Important Steps	Key Points
	(Remember the *Initiation* of the oxygen treatment is usually done by the nurse.) However the oxygen may be ordered p.r.n. and you may be responsible for turning the flowmeter on or off as the patient requrests. Be sure to record each administration. Charting example:

Nasal oxygen started at 3 L per minute. Respirations seem less labored, color is pink. Seems less apprehensive.   R. Olsen, SN

ITEM 2. SPECIAL CARE FOR PATIENTS RECEIVING NASAL OXYGEN

General nursing care for patients with oxygen therapy is part of your nursing routine and will not be ordered by the doctor (in most instances).

1. The main consideration is to keep the breathing passageways open. The conscious patient can tell you if he is having difficulty; if mucus accumulates in the passageways, he can usually cough it up. If he is unconscious, however, you must be alert to his wet, gurgling respirations. When this occurs, you must see that he is suctioned immediately (either by doing it yourself if possible, or obtaining assistance at once). If the patient is unconscious, place him in Sims' position so that the secretions can run out of his mouth.

2. For the unconscious patient, Sims' position keeps the tongue from falling back into the throat (remember that the head is held high and straight in this position). Also, throat secretions (mucus) can easily drain out of his mouth. However, Fowler's position for the conscious patient permits fullest lung expansion. Change your patient's position frequently to prevent decubitus ulcers from occurring, and also to expand the lungs fully (the exertion of moving will make him breathe more deeply).

3. Be familiar with the operation of the various types of oxygen equipment. This will tend to give the patient confidence in what you are doing and make him less likely to be frightened. Replace any defective working equipment immediately.

4. Give good general nursing care to your patient. Keep him clean, dry, and warm. Change his position frequently. Give frequent oral fluids (unless limited) to keep his breathing passages moist; give frequent oral hygiene throughout the day and night.

5. Observe safety precautions and notify the patient and his family to observe them also.

   a. No smoking is permitted because of the danger of fire or explosion.

   b. Wool blankets are not permitted because sparks from static electricity may start a fire or explosion in the highly concentrated oxygen environment.

   c. Do not give oil or alcohol backrubs to patients in oxygen tents. If this must be done, turn off the oxygen flow.

   d. Do not use electrical equipment (call bells, electric razors, radios, hearing aids, suction equipment) inside the oxygen tent. Electrical sparks may be generated when you turn the equipment on that could ignite the high oxygen concentration and set off an explosion.

   e. Secure the oxygen tank to a cylinder cart or stand with a restraining strap in order to keep the cylinder from falling.

   f. Use no lighted candles (which may be required in religious activity). (This would be an extreme explosion hazard.)

6. Take the patient's temperature rectally.

7. You may have to wrap a lightweight cotton blanket around the patient's shoulders while he is in an oxygen tent if he gets too cold. This is particularly necessary for elderly patients.

In addition to these considerations, you will need to pay special attention to a number of details:

1. The nasal catheter should probably be exchanged for a clean one every 8 hours (or follow your agency procedure). Applying fresh lubrication and alternating between the right and left nostril each time the catheter is inserted will keep the nasal passageway moist and will be less irritating for the patient.

2. Observe the water level in the humidifier bottle several times during your tour of duty. Keep the water at the prescribed level ($^2/_3$ full). Turn off the oxygen supply while you unscrew the top of the water bottle for refilling. Fill the bottle to the prescribed level with distilled water, replace the cap, and reattach it to the flowmeter. Turn on the oxygen and adjust the flow rate. Remember, oxygen is extremely drying to tissue when given in this manner, and moisturization is very important for the comfort of the patient.

3. Be sure that the tubing is not kinked (this stops the O_2 flow) and has enough slack to permit the patient to move freely in bed.

4. Check the oxygen liter flow; be sure that it is maintained at the designated rate. Become accustomed to checking the oxygen flow rate each time you enter the patient's room, so that any reduction in the oxygen level in the central oxygen system can be noted and corrected immediately.

5. Some agencies use oxygen labels to indicate the following information: the patient's name, his room number, the liters used per minute, the duration of treatment, the order date, and the initials of the responsible nurse.

6. Observe the skin where the tape is attached to the patient's face. Watch for any marked irritation. Some patients may be allergic to the tape and you will have to fasten the catheter in some other way. (For example, tie gauze around the catheter and attach it with a pin to the sheet. Care must be taken not to puncture the catheter with the pin.)

7. Oxygen dries tissue and makes the mouth dry and stale-tasting. To remedy this, give frequent oral hygiene to the patient throughout the 24-hour period.

ITEM 3. USING THE OXYGEN CYLINDER

Obtain the oxygen cylinder (tank) and accessory equipment from central service or the respiration therapy department (as designated by your agency). Observe and maintain the following safety measures before the first step of the procedure is begun.

1. Stand the cylinder in its carrier or with a steel cylinder brace placed securely around it in order to keep it from falling.

2. Put the cylinder beside the head of the bed, away from doors, doorways, heaters, and areas that have continuous, concentrated traffic.

3. Check the oxygen cylinder tag, which has a perforated design to indicate the following information: "Full," "In Use," "Empty." When the cylinder is turned on for the patient, remove the "Full" segment, leaving the "In Use" marker visible. When the tank is empty, remove the In Use segment, leaving the "Empty" marker visible. At this point notify the respiratory therapy department to remove or replace the cylinder.

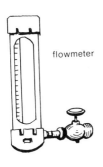

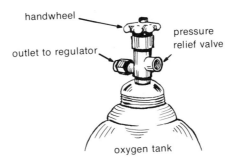

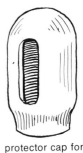

handwheel

outlet to regulator

pressure relief valve

flowmeter

oxygen tank

protector cap for oxygen tank (cylinder)

U
N
I
T
25

Important Steps	Key Points
1. Stand at the side of the cylinder.	Direct the oxygen outlet away from people and warn the patient of the impending noise.
2. Slowly turn the handwheel clockwise to slightly open the cylinder.	The handwheel is on the top of the cylinder. The slight opening removes dust particles and is known as "cracking the valve." The slow motion prevents combustion.
3. Close the handwheel immediately (counterclockwise).	
4. Attach the regulator to the valve outlet connection.	Using a wrench, tighten the regulator nut onto the outlet valve until the nut is tight and holds the regulator firmly.
5. Attach the top of the humidifier to the oxygen regulator flow gauge or flowmeter.	Refer to step 3 in the foregoing procedure on the wall oxygen outlet (water in the humidifier).
6. Open the handwheel slowly and adjust the flow gauge or flowmeter to the prescribed liter flow.	This turns on the cylinder regulators.
7. Proceed to utilize the oxygen equipment prescribed for the patient (nasal catheter-mask, nasal cannula-test).	Refer to the application and safety steps in Items 1 and 6.

ITEM 4. SPECIAL CARE FOR PATIENTS RECEIVING OXYGEN BY NASAL CANNULA

The nasal cannula is used when the desired concentration of oxygen is 27 to 35 per cent (3 to 7 L). The cannula consists of a rubber or plastic tube with short curved prongs that extend into the nostril about 1/4 to 1/2 inch. The cannula is held in place with an elastic band that fits snugly around the head and attaches to the cannula, and can be easily adjusted for the patient's comfort. There is no need to fasten the cannula to the patient's face with tape; therefore, with this method of oxygen therapy the skin will not become irritated. This may be useful for patients requiring oxygen during meals.

Follow the same precautions in caring for the patient receiving oxygen by nasal cannula as those learned in the previous section.

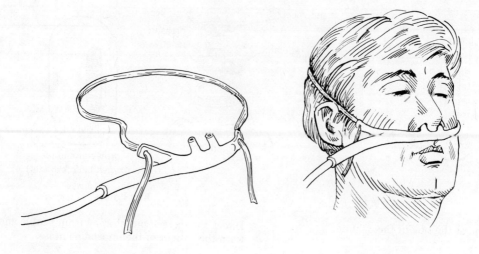

Nasal cannula.   Cannula in place.

ITEM 5.   ADMINISTRATION OF OXYGEN BY MASK

Various types of masks are available for the administration of oxygen in concentrations ranging from 24 to 55 per cent at flows of 3 to 7 liters per minute. Oxygen concentrations above 60 per cent are rarely used because of the danger of oxygen toxicity. Some patients may dislike this method of oxygen administration since the mask must be placed over their face and they feel that the mask will suffocate them.

In the skill laboratory, given a middle-aged woman who is having an asthma attack, obtain and assemble the equipment, and assist in the initiation of oxygen via mask.

Important Steps	Key Points
1. Wash your hands, approach and identify the patient, and explain what you will be doing.	Check the patient's identification. Explain in detail what you are going to do. Answer all the patient's questions thoughtfully and correctly. If you are unable to answer the questions, refer them to the nurse or doctor. All of the patient's questions should be answered if possible.
2. Assemble the equipment and demonstrate its use	Obtain a mask in the proper size (either for an adult or a child) and an oxygen flowmeter. Show the patient the correct placement of the mask and retaining strap by holding it near his face.

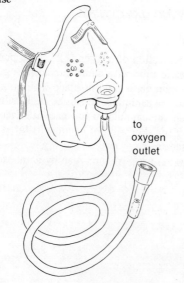

to
oxygen
outlet

Important Steps	Key Points
3. Attach the humidifier to the oxygen flowmeter, then attach the mask tubing to the humidifier.	Start the oxygen at the prescribed liter flow, as most patients seem less apprehensive if they feel the oxygen coming through the mask.
4. Place the mask on the patient's face.	Ask him to breathe naturally as you apply and adjust the mask to fit comfortably over his nose and mouth. Adjust the retaining strap around his head and around his ears so they will not be pinched. Talk quietly to him during the application so that he will relax and breathe normally. Stay by his side until he has adjusted his breathing into the mask.

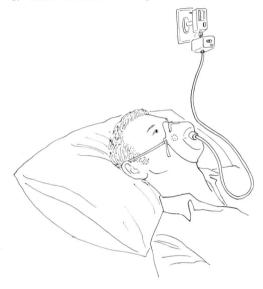

U
N
I
T
25

Important Steps	Key Points
5. Secure the head band.	Adjust it so that it is comfortable for the patient and holds the mask securely in place.
6. Leave the patient comfortable.	Semi-Fowler's or high Fowler's position is usually the choice position for patients requiring oxygen therapy. Tell your patient when you will return (in 15 to 30 minutes). Be sure that you return within the promised time; keeping hourly checks on him will help alleviate his apprehension. Leave the call light and bedside stand within easy reach.
Note: When the inside of the face mask becomes excessively moist, clean and dry it, and immediately return it to the patient.
7. Record the procedure.	Record the initiation of the treatment, the time, method, rate of flow, and patient's response. Sometimes oxygen is ordered p.r.n. The oxygen will therefore be turned off and on at the patient's request. You may be responsible for regulating the flowmeter on these occasions. Again, remember that the initiation of the treatment is done by the nurse. Charting example:

Important Steps	Key Points
	1000. O_2 mask initiated at 8 L. Very apprehensive at onset. Quieted quickly after initiation of treatment. Pulse and respirations became slower. Color good. A. Turno, RN

ITEM 6.   THE OXYGEN VENTURI MASK

There are various types of Venturi mask to deliver oxygen concentrations—24, 28, 35 and 40 per cent. The manufacturer's recommendation regarding liter flow should be followed; however, most masks are relatively accurate at one-half or twice the recommended flow.

The Venturi mask is made to provide oxygen mixed with room air in precise proportions to deliver a known oxygen concentration to the patient. Usually the respiratory therapist performs and supervises its use.

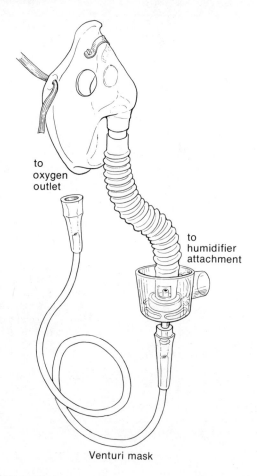

to oxygen outlet

to humidifier attachment

Venturi mask

Important Steps	Key Points
1. Wash your hands, approach and identify the patient, and explain what you will be doing.	Refer to step 1 of the oxygen mask procedure.
2. Assemble the equipment.	Obtain the mask sized to give the desired per cent. Refer to step 2 of the oxygen mask procedure.

Important Steps	Key Points
3. Attach the mask tubing to the flowmeter. (*Do not use a humidifier.*)	Start the oxygen at the recommended liter flow for the desired oxygen concentration. The humidifier causes inaccurate oxygen concentration.
Follow steps 4 through 7 of Item 5, Oxygen by Mask.	Charting example: 1000. 24 per cent oxygen initiated by Venturi mask. B. Olsen, SN

U
N
I
T
25

ITEM 7.   ADMINISTRATION OF OXYGEN BY TENT

Oxygen tents are used less frequently than they were 25 years ago. They supply a relatively high concentration of oxygen (50 to 60 per cent) and provide a means of circulating the moist air around the patient. The temperature of the air can be somewhat controlled and it provides comfortable air-conditioning for the patient. The oxygen tent is not economically efficient because of the high volume of oxygen needed to maintain the designated concentration, as well as loss of concentration when the oxygen tent is raised to permit working with the patient. Also, the equipment is hard to maintain and clean.

The concentration of oxygen is lost each time a part of the oxygen tent is raised. There should therefore be a minimal amount of disturbance to the patient. You must plan your work so that you do not have to loosen the oxygen tent frequently; on those occasions that you do loosen the tent, do several things for the patient.

While many patients like the oxygen tent because they can move about freely, they sometimes have a feeling of isolation. You must therefore talk with these patients frequently. If you speak loudly and clearly, they can hear you without your disturbing the tent.

Most oxygen tents now in use are electrically cooled models. When taking care of children in pediatrics, an apparatus is used similar to the oxygen tent. Called a mistogen tent, or Croupette, it provides both oxygen and very high humidity (moisture content). The Croupettes are commonly used for children who have respiratory congestion or disease process.

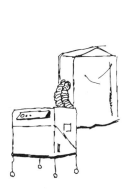

One type of
oxygen tent.

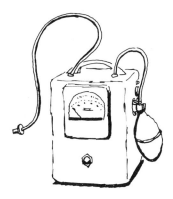

Oxygen analyzer
(records oxygen
concentration).

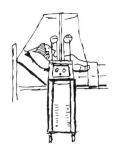

Oxygen tent
in operation.

In the skill laboratory, given a young male patient who has pneumonia, you will assist in setting up and regulating the oxygen tent.

Important Steps	Key Points
1. Wash your hands, approach and identify the patient, and explain what you are going to do.	Identify the patient. Answer all his questions. Speak audibly, clearly, kindly, and knowledgeably. (If you are unable to answer a question, ask your team leader immediately.)
2. Obtain the equipment.	Get the oxygen tent. (The tent may be set up by someone from the central service department, or the inhalation therapy department, or by someone in nursing.)
3. Assemble the oxygen tent. 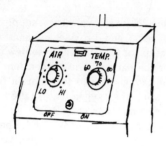	Move the tent to the head of the bed. Place it along one side of the bed with the regulating dials facing away from the patient. Extend the canopy arm to a horizontal position. Plug the cord into the electrical outlet. Check the cord to be sure it is not frayed. (If frayed, it could be a fire hazard; replace it with a new cord.) Turn the motor on and set the control knobs on the control panel. Set the temperature at 70°F. Set the circulation dial halfway between low and high. Attach the oxygen flowmeter to the wall outlet; then connect the oxygen outlet from the tent to the flowmeter and start the oxygen at 15 meters per liter. Check the water tray at the back of the machine often and empty the accumulated water. (Not all units have a water tray.) Arrange the canopy over the patient (do not drag it over the patient's face). Secure the edges in place by folding a drawsheet in half lengthwise and laying it across the patient's abdomen, then placing the bottom edge of the tent canopy securely under the mattress at both sides of the bed and at the head of the mattress. Be sure that zippered openings in the sides of the canopy are tightly closed.
4. Check the oxygen concentration in the tent.	Utilize the oxygen analyzer routinely at 2- to 4-hour intervals to determine the concentration (per cent) of oxygen in the tent. Allow 15 minutes for oxygen concentration to increase and stabilize after the tent has been opened. After the initial analysis the flow rate may be reduced to maintain the desired concentration but should never be below 10 liters (*flow below 10 liters does not allow for adequate removal of CO_2*).
5. Leave the patient comfortable.	Place the patient in good body alignment. Put a *manual call bell* within his reach. (The conventional electric call bell is not used because it could provide an electric spark when activated in the high oxygen concentration and start a fire or explosion.) Raise siderails if appropriate.
6. Check the patient frequently.	This will provide reassurance to the frightened patient and will also give you an opportunity to check the patient's condition and the function-

Important Steps	Key Points

ing of the equipment. Empty water trays as needed (if there are any); check the oxygen level.

7. Record the procedure.

Make a note concerning the initiation of the treatment including the time, method, liter flow, oxygen concentration (analysis check), and response of the patient. Charting example:

2030. Oxygen tent initiated 50% oxygen maintained with 15 liters per minute (LPM), BP 150/90, pulse 110, respirations 22, dyspnea and restlessness decreased, color good.

2100. Sleeping quietly, no coughing.
M. Mann, RN

ITEM 8.   USE OF HYPERBARIC OXYGEN CHAMBERS

Hyperbaric oxygen chambers are a recent innovation. They are especially constructed rooms that provide for very high oxygen concentration; they are used to treat patients who have anaerobic (without oxygen) infections, or patients whose hemoglobin is not carrying enough oxygen to the tissues. Inasmuch as these units are installed in few health agencies at this time, we will not describe their opration. If you are assigned to this type of patient, you will undoubtedly receive some training in working with a hyperbaric chamber before your assignment.

ITEM 9.   INTERMITTENT POSITIVE PRESSURE (IPPB) THERAPY

Generally you will not be given IPPB treatments; they will be administered by the respiratory therapy department or by the nurse. You will, however, be required to observe these patients carefully as you would any patient receiving oxygen therapy. Give frequent oral hygiene and maintain the previously stated safety precautions. If you do give IPPB treatments in your agency, you will undoubtedly be given a special training program.

IPPB is a method of inflating the lungs with air or oxygen given under slight pressure on an intermittent basis. The best positive pressure ventilators can be adjusted to the requirements of the individual patient. IPPB treatments are given for 15 to 20 minutes three or four times a day and are utilized for:

1. Preoperative familiarization of the patient in anticipation of postoperative use.

2. Preventing atelectasis by increasing the depth of respiration.

3. Promoting the clearing of bronchial secretions in pulmonary edema, pneumonia, asthma, bronchitis, and emphysema.

4. Delivering aerosol medications to dilate the bronchi and relieve bronchospasm.

5. Lessening the effort of breathing for patients who have certain respiratory diseases.

6. Facilitating the exchange of oxygen and carbon dioxide, and improving alveolar ventilation.

IPPB treatment can be given on a p.r.n. (as needed) basis or continuously, depending on the needs of the patient. Some types of positive pressure ventilators are used on a continuous basis for patients who have had severe head injuries, or whose respirations are critically reduced by drugs, disease, or surgery. In these cases, an interruption of the regular respiratory rate for more than 2 minutes can lead to death. Most patient's needing mechanical ventilation on a continuing basis are cared for in medical or surgical intensive care units during the acute period of their illness. Since an artificial airway is needed, constant supervision of these patients is mandatory.

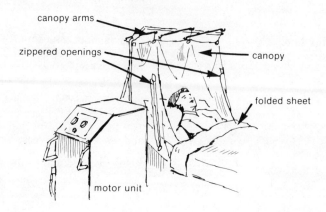

VI. ENRICHMENT

Attend any additional classes that your employing agency may offer on the care of patients receiving oxygen therapy.

Take a few minutes to review the components of the respiratory tract.

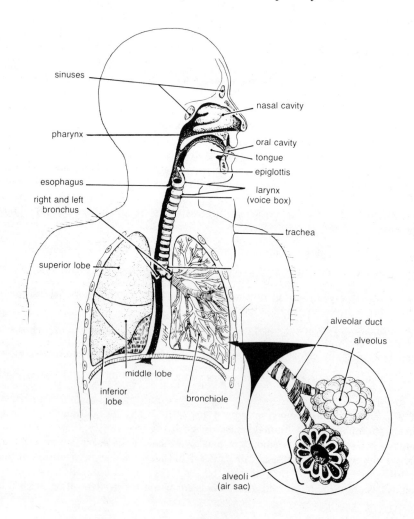

The first organ of respiration is the nose. As air is brought into the respiratory system through the nose, the air is warmed, moistened (by flow over the mucous membranes), and filtered or cleaned by the action of the fine hairs (cilia) in the nasal cavity. Thus, as air passes down the throat and the trachea to the lungs, it is warmed, moistened, and cleaned.

The air then goes down to the throat (pharynx), which is a common passageway for both food and oxygen, and then to the larynx or voice box. At this juncture a small pedicle (epiglottis) protects the opening of the larynx when one is swallowing: food is shunted into the esophagus, and air into the trachea. (An inflammation of the larynx is called laryngitis.)

The trachea (windpipe) is a 4½ inch tube extending from the larynx to the bronchial tubes. It, too, is lined with a mucous membrane and cilia for continuing moistening and cleaning of the air. (An inflammation of the trachea is called tracheitis.)

From here the air goes to the bronchus, which leads directly into the lungs. The right bronchus is short and vertical. (For this reason when foreign objects [peanuts, bones] get into the respiratory tract they go into the right branches and lung.) The left bronchus is double branched and is more horizontal in direction. The bronchi (plural for bronchus) branch into many small tubes called the bronchioles. This part of the respiratory tract is commonly called the bronchial tree because it looks like the trunk of a tree with two limbs and many small branches. (Inflammation of the bronchus is called bronchitis.)

These tiny bronchioles lead to air sacs in the lung tissue. The alveoli are surrounded by a network of tiny blood capillaries. Because of the closeness of these tissues (alveoli and capillaries), gas (O_2) passes into the circulatory system by a process called diffusion. (CO_2 from the blood passes back into the pulmonary alveoli to be exhaled into the air.)

Diffusion is a chemical process whereby a liquid or gas mixes its chemical components. The O_2 and CO_2 from the air mix with the components of the blood; the O_2 and CO_2 tend to distribute themselves equally between the alveoli and the capillaries.

The bronchi, bronchioles, and alveoli are imbedded in tissue called lung (pulmonary). There are two lungs (right and left) located in the chest cavity (thorax). The lungs are encased in a covering called pleura, which is separated from the lungs by a small amount of liquid. (An inflammation of the pleura is called pleurisy or pleuritis.)

The process of the O_2 entering the blood through the pulmonary capillaries is called oxygenation of the blood.

The lungs work with several muscles to bring air into the body. The diaphragm is a large, flat muscle separating the chest and abdominal cavities. During inspiration, which is an active process, the diaphragm moves down and out to enlarge the thoracic cavity from top to bottom. The intercostal muscles (between the ribs) move up and out to enlarge the thoracic cavity from front to back and side to side. During expiration the diaphragm and intercostal muscles relax and help to push the air out of the lungs. However, this is usually passive because of the elasticity of the lungs.

The volume of air in the lung is measured by the use of an instrument called a spirometer. Patients with pulmonary diseases may have a spirometry examination to determine how the lungs are functioning. When a newborn infant takes his first breath, there is already some air in the lungs.

The respiratory regulating center is located in the part of the brain called the medulla and is activated by nerve impulses which respond to the chemical composition of the blood. The cells in the respiratory center are particularly sensitive to CO_2 (carbon dioxide). If there is excess CO_2 in the blood, the respirations become more rapid and deep in order to facilitate the removal of excess CO_2.

The cough is nature's mechanism for ridding ourselves of a respiratory tract obstruction or blocking. It is an abrupt expiration with the mouth open. A sneeze is a similar action to relieve the respiratory tract of a foreign object; however, the expiration of air is through the nose. Hiccough (singultus) is a spasmodic contraction of the diaphragm caused by irritation of the stomach. Yawning is a deep, long inspiration usually due to mental or physical fatigue (tiredness). A sigh is a prolonged inspiration followed by a long expiration.

All of these mechanisms may be observed as you care for patients with respiratory diseases or conditions. The symptoms may be significant clues in the progress of the disease and should be observed and recorded.

PERFORMANCE TEST

1. Regulate the oxygen flowmeter to give (1) 4 liters of oxygen per minute, and (2) 10 liters of oxygen per minute. Be sure to have your instructor check you at each point. Practice recording the activity in the nurses' notes.

2. Demonstrate the equipment used and discuss the purpose of the four major methods of oxygen administration.

PERFORMANCE CHECKLIST

OXYGEN THERAPY

USE OF OXYGEN THERAPY EQUIPMENT

1. Wash your hands, identify the patient, and explain the procedure.

2. Assemble the appropriate equipment and position the bed to a comfortable working height.

3. For the catheter:

    a. Measure the catheter length for insertion (from the nose to the ear lobe).

    b. Lubricate the tip with water soluble lubricant.

    c. Insert the catheter and check the length by looking into the patient's mouth.

    d. Secure the catheter with tape.

4. To prepare the oxygen cylinder:

    a. Obtain equipment from the respiratory therapy department or from Central Service. Take it to the patient's room utilizing all known safety measures.

    b. Direct the oxygen outlet away from people.

    c. Warn the patient of the impending noise.

    d. Turn the handwheel clockwise to slightly open the cylinder.

    e. Close the handwheel.

    f. Attach the regulator to the valve outlet connection.

    g. Open the handwheel slowly and adjust the flowmeter to the prescribed liter flow.

5. For the cannula and mask:

    a. Place the equipment in or over the patient's nose.

    b. Adjust the head strap for comfort.

6. For the tent:

    a. Place the tent along the top side of the bed with the regulating dials away from the patient.

    b. Extend the canopy arm.

    c. Plug in the electrical cord (be sure your hands are dry, and use no frayed cords).

d. Turn on the motor and set the dials.

e. Set the temperature at $70°$ F.

f. Connect the O_2 to a wall outlet or O_2 tank.

g. Arrange the canopy over the tent and secure the bottom edge in the cuff of the drawsheet.

h. Close all zippered openings.

7. Regulate O_2 flow per the physician's order.

8. Leave the patient comfortable and in good body alignment.

9. Offer water and tell the patient the time of your return.

10. Raise the siderails if indicated and put the hand call bell within reach.

11. Record the activity on the patient's chart.

REGULATION OF FLOWMETER

1. Wash your hands.

2. Approach and identify the patient, and explain the procedure.

3. Check the flowmeter to be sure that the humidifier bottle is $2/3$ filled with water. If it is not filled, turn off the O_2, remove the jar, fill to $2/3$ level, and replace the jar on the flowmeter.

4. Adjust the flow by opening the flow valve until the gauge reads 4 LPM (to be checked by your instructor).

5. Continue adjusting the flow valve until the gauge reads 10 LPM.

6. Adjust the flow to read 4 LPM.

7. Record the activity on nurses' notes.

POST-TEST

Directions: Choose the answer that will make the statement complete.

1. Common methods of delivering oxygen to patients are all of the following except:

    a. the nasal cannula

    b. a mask

    c. an oxygen tent

    d. the bronchioles

2. The respiratory system consists of all of the following except:

    a. the nose

    b. the larynx

    c. the bronchi and trachea

    d. carbon dioxide

3. The following symptoms of a cyanotic patient are correct except:

    a. diminished coordination

    b. pink skin

    c. slowed mental capacities

    d. increased respiratory rate

4. Oxygen given by nasal catheter may have safe concentrations of:

    a. 27–35 per cent

    b. 10–20 per cent

    c. 15–30 per cent

    d. 5–18 per cent

5. The following steps are included in the initial procedure of nasal catheter insertion except:

    a. wash your hands

    b. identify the patient

    c. obtain the mask

    d. place no smoking sign

6. The equipment needed for the oxygen set-up includes all except:

    a. an oxygen flow meter

    b. a nasal catheter

    c. a connecting tube

    d. an oil-based lubricant

7. The water level in the humidifier should be at:

    a. $2/3$ capacity

    b. $1/2$ capacity

    c. $1/4$ capacity

    d. $5/8$ capacity

8. The oxygen liter flow is prescribed by the:

   a. inhalation therapist

   b. supervisor

   c. head nurse

   d. physician

9. The tip of the nasal catheter should be placed:

   a. to one side of the uvula

   b. at the top of the bronchi

   c. at the trachea

   d. at the front of the nose

10. Secure the nasal catheter to the patient's face by:

    a. taping the catheter up and over the bridge of the nose

    b. taping the catheter to the chin

    c. taping the catheter to the jaw

    d. bringing the catheter up and over the bridge of the nose, and taping it to the forehead

11. When nasal catheters are needed for a long period of time, they should be lubricated and inserted alternately in the right and left nostrils to prevent:

    a. hemorrhage

    b. itching

    c. marked irritation

    d. bruising

12. Oxygen is drying to the tissues, and therefore it is necessary to give:

    a. oral hygiene every 12 hours

    b. oral hygiene every 24 hours

    c. frequent oral hygiene

    d. oral hygiene every 6 hours

13. Masks used to give oxygen may frequently cause the patient to complain of:

    a. skin irritation

    b. a feeling of smothering

    c. face pain

    d. a feeling that the mask is too small

14. The patient usually finds that the most comfortable position is:

    a. prone

    b. Sims'

    c. Trendelenburg's

    d. semi-Fowler's

15. When you use any oxygen, important safety factors include all of the following except:

    a. "No Smoking" signs

   b. nonfrayed electric cords

   c. high caloric diet

   d. water in the humidifier

16. 15 minutes after the oxygen tent has been opened and closed, accurate oxygen concentration must be determined by using:

   a. an oxygen analyzer

   b. an IPPB machine

   c. hyperbaric chambers

   d. a flowmeter

17. The IPPB treatment is utilized for all of the following except:

   a. the prevention of atelectasis

   b. delivery of aerosol medications to constrict the bronchi

   c. the improvement of alveolar ventilation

   d. the promoting of clearance of the bronchial secretions in pulmonary edema

18. The important safety measures used when setting up the oxygen tank are all of the following except:

   a. a safety brace at the tank base

   b. "FULL," "IN USE," "EMPTY" tags

   c. "No smoking" signs

   d. Cleaning the tank with alcohol

19. Important nursing care measures to consider for the patient who is getting oxygen therapy are all of the following except:

   a. frequent oral hygiene

   b. vigorous exercises

   c. frequent fluid intake unless contraindicated

   d. constant awareness of respiratory and pulse rate changes

POST-TEST ANNOTATED ANSWER SHEET

1. d. (p. 525)   11. c. (p. 530)

2. d. (p. 524)   12. c. (p. 530)

3. b. (p. 524)   13. b. (p. 532)

4. a. (p. 525)   14. d. (p. 533)

5. c. (pp. 526–528)   15. d. (pp. 529–530 and 536)

6. d. (p. 526)   16. a. (p. 536)

7. a. (p. 526)   17. b. (p. 537)

8. d. (p. 526)   18. d. (p. 529)

9. a. (p. 528)   19. b. (pp. 529–530)

10. d. (p. 528)

THE PATIENT WITH GASTROINTESTINAL TUBES

I. DIRECTIONS TO THE STUDENT

Please read the following paragraphs carefully. They will tell you what you will be expected to do and know with respect to the collection of sputum and gastric content specimens, and the care of patients who require the use of gastrointestinal (GI) tubes of various types.

Proceed through the lesson. Practice the steps of the procedures on the laboratory mannequin (Mrs. Chase). It will not be necessary at this point to obtain an actual specimen of sputum or gastric contents, or to actually insert a GI tube.

After you have practiced the steps of the procedures, arrange with your instructor to take the post-test. You will be expected to perform the activities accurately.

II. GENERAL PERFORMANCE OBJECTIVE

At the completion of this unit you will be able to employ the correct techniques for obtaining a sputum or gastric specimen, and taking care of patients with various gastrointestinal tubes—tubes with and without suction, and tubes for special feedings and special laboratory tests.

III. SPECIFIC PERFORMANCE OBJECTIVES

When you have finished this unit, you will be able to:

1. Instruct and assist the patient to produce sputum without undue discomfort and distress, and collect the sputum specimen correctly for delivery to the laboratory.

2. Identify four kinds of tubes used in the gastric analysis procedure.

3. Assemble equipment and assist with the insertion of the various GI tubes.

4. Collect a gastric content specimen and prepare it correctly for delivery to the laboratory.

5. Feed a patient with a gastrostomy tube, or through the proctoclysis procedure.

6. Identify and describe the action of the four common types of suction apparatus: portable electric suction, wall-outlet suction, a Gomco Thermotic Pump, and a water displacement system with or without suction and with intermittent or continuous action.

7. Describe and give major nursing care activities to patients with various types of gastrointestinal tubes: testing, drainage, suction, and feeding.

8. Describe and record correctly and accurately the color, amount, and consistency of the intake and output of patients with the GI tubes discussed in this unit.

IV. VOCABULARY

aspiration—the act of drawing in or out of a cavity of the body by suction; withdrawal of fluid from a body cavity by suction with an instrument called an aspirator.

Cantor tube—a single long tube used for intestinal decompression; it has a mercury-weighted balloon at its distal tip to assist in stimulating peristalsis and moving the tube into the intestine; it is inserted through the nose and down the digestive tract to the intestine; the proximal end of the tube is connected to a suction machine.

decompression—the removal of air or drainage from a wound, cavity, or passageway.

distention—the state of being stretched out or bloated, as the abdominal cavity may be with gas or fluid.

emesis—vomiting.

esophagus—the muscular tube in the digestive tract that connects the oral cavity with the stomach; it is located directly behind the trachea (windpipe).

Ewald tube—a specific rubber tube with a large lumen that is passed through the mouth into the stomach to withdraw stomach contents for various laboratory examinations.

expectorate—to spit out or expel mucus or phlegm from the throat or lungs.

flatus—gas that is expelled rectally; expelling gas orally is called burping or eructating.

gag reflex—an involuntary (not controlled by the will) retching or vomiting action caused by stimulation of certain nerve endings in the back of the throat that in turn stimulate the vomiting center in the brain.

gastric—refers to the stomach.

gastrostomy (gastro- = stomach; -ostomy = mouth)—a surgical operation making a temporary or permanent opening through the abdominal wall into the stomach; a tube is inserted into the opening and the patient may be fed in this manner; this procedure may be done for a carcinoma in the upper digestive tract.

gavage—feeding through a tube inserted through the nose and down the esophagus into the stomach.

Gomco Thermotic Pump—a special electric suction machine commonly used with various gastrointestinal tubes.

lavage—the washing out of a cavity; gastric lavage is the washing out of the stomach contents, which is done in emergency cases such as that of a child who has swallowed a poisonous fluid.

Levin tube—a long plastic or rubber single-lumen tube that is inserted through the nose or mouth to the stomach and used to drain off stomach fluids and to keep the stomach decompressed.

lumen—an opening.

Miller-Abbott tube—the most common double-lumen GI rubber tube used to drain or decompress the small intestine; it has an inflatable rubber bag on the distal end that helps stimulate peristalsis (the involuntary, wavelike motion of the digestive tract) when in the small intestine; it is inserted through the nose, down the esophagus, through the stomach, and into the intestine; the proximal end is connected to a suction machine.

nasogastric tube—a rubber or plastic tube that is inserted through the nose (naso) down to the stomach (gastric).

nausea—the inclination or desire to vomit.

peristalsis—the involuntary, wavelike motion of the digestive tract that moves food through the alimentary canal.

projectile vomiting—the forceful and sudden ejection of stomach contents, usually without preliminary nausea.

sputum—a substance from the lungs that is coughed up and spit out of the mouth; it contains saliva, mucus, and sometimes, pus.

suction—the act of sucking up (or drawing up) by reducing air pressure and creating a partial vacuum.

vomitus—gastric contents ejected through the mouth during the act of vomiting.

Wangensteen suction—an early type of water displacement suction apparatus used with various gastrointestinal tubes for drainage.

ITEM 1. COLLECTION OF THE SPUTUM SPECIMEN

In this section, we will be considering primarily the patient with a possible respiratory problem and a cough. It may be necessary to obtain specimens of sputum from the coughing patient to aid in the diagnosis and determination of his disease. It is important to know that the patient may be encouraged to cough (in certain medical and postoperative situations) in order to clear mucus from the respiratory tract and from the lungs. This promotes adequate expansion and ventilation of the lungs. However, in other postoperative conditions, such as eye surgery or hernia repair, it is advisable to inhibit (prevent) coughing. Sputum specimens are requested most often from patients who are suspected of having a respiratory disease such as pneumonia, tuberculosis, or bronchitis. Obtaining the specimen may be difficult, painful, or unpleasant for the patient, and so you must know how you can best assist him.

There are times when it is very painful for the patient to cough. If the patient has pain in the abdominal or chest area when he coughs, obtain a drawsheet or a folded large sheet and wrap it around the painful area of his body. Hold the sheet securely with minimal pressure so that the body walls of the affected area are supported. This gives the patient the external pressure necessary to equalize the internal pressure occurring during the coughing period, and it minimizes the pain and discomfort. *Do not hold the sheet too tightly* or you will defeat your purpose by causing pain and increased difficulty in breathing.

In the classroom or skill laboratory, you should practice the steps of the procedure until you are familiar with them and can carry them out skillfully.

Important Steps	Key Points
1. Wash your hands.	

2. Obtain the materials required for the specimen.
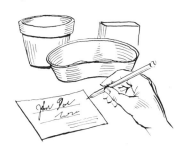
	You will need a container and cover for the specimen, a small paper bag, tissues, a label for the container, and the laboratory requisition slip.
	    The label should have the patient's full name and room number, the hospital unit or floor number, the date, and the time of collection. The laboratory slip should be properly marked with the patient's identifying information, the tests to be done, and your or the doctor's signature. Most hospitals now have a mechanical recorder (Addressograph) that imprints a patient's identifying information from a metal or plastic card.
	    Take all items except the laboratory slip to the patient's room.

3. Approach and identify the patient.	Check his identification band, read his name aloud, and have him confirm it.
4. Tell the patient how to collect the sputum specimen. 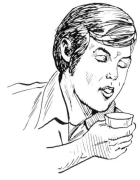	Explain that sputum is the mucus coughed up from his lungs, and *not* the saliva in his mouth. Ask him to cover his mouth with tissues when coughing. (This will keep him from coughing germs into the air that you and others breathe.) Have him hold the sputum container close to his mouth and spit the coughed-up sputum into the container.

Important Steps	Key Points
5. Assist the patient to produce an immediate specimen if possible.	Provide privacy for the patient. If he is able, he may go to the bathroom while trying to produce the sputum. If he is not able to get up and if other patients are in the room, pull the curtain. Although the curtain will not shut out the sound of coughing, it keeps others from seeing the effort involved. Ask the patient to breathe deeply and cough in order to bring up the sputum from his lungs, and not merely from the back of his throat. Collect at least 1 to 2 tablespoons of sputum unless directed otherwise. Observe the patient carefully and assist him when necessary; offer him encouragement. Avoid contamination by his sputum. Keep the outside of the container and your hands free of the sputum when you are collecting it and transporting it to the laboratory. After the patient coughs the sputum into the container, seal it with the lid. Wash and dry the outside of the container (paper towels from the patient's bathroom may be used). Put the labeled container in the paper bag for delivery to the laboratory with the lab requisition slip. (Some agencies do not require that the specimen be enclosed in a paper bag. Follow your agency procedure for transporting sputum specimens to the laboratory.)
6. Give the patient instructions again if he is unable to produce an immediate specimen, and ask him to notify the nurse when he is able to provide the specimen.	It may be easier for the patient to produce the specimen early in the morning. Mucus that collected in the lungs during the night is more apt to be coughed up at this time. Have the patient notify the nurse who will pick up the specimen.
7. Provide for the patient's safety and comfort.	
8. Arrange for delivery of the specimen to the laboratory.	Use the appropriate method designated by the hospital. If there is any delay in delivering the specimen, put it in the refrigerator used for specimens.

9. Record all pertinent information concerning this task in the nurses' notes of the patient's chart.	Include statements on the color, amount, odor, consistency, date, and time. The following descriptive terms are used in charting the sputum specimen collection procedure:
	
	  a. hemoptysis—blood in the sputum.
	
	  b. clear, gray, yellow, red, brown, green, black—color variations.
	
	  c. liquid, thick and sticky (tenacious), mucuslike (mucoid)—consistency.
	
	  d. profuse—large amount.
	
	  e. scanty—small amount.

ITEM 2.   INSERTION OF A GASTRIC TUBE FOR DRAINAGE PURPOSES

Gastrointestinal intubation is the insertion of a specified tube through the nose (naso) or throat into the stomach (gastro) or the intestine. The primary reasons for this relatively common procedure are:

1. To drain the stomach or intestinal tract by means of some kind of suction apparatus. It is used to prevent postoperative vomiting, postoperative obstruction (blocking) of the intestinal tract, and gas formation in the stomach or intestine after an operation.

2. To diagnose a disease (to identify a disease, to determine the cause of a pathological condition).

3. To wash out the stomach contents, such as in the case of a person who has taken a poison.

4. To provide a route for feeding one who is unable to take food by mouth.

There are usually three markers (black rings) on the distal end of each of the tubes to indicate how far the tube has been inserted: 1 band = stomach, 2 bands = pylorus, and 3 bands = duodenum.

U
N
I
T
26

The Levin Tube. The Levin tube is the most commonly used tube for gastric (stomach) intubation and suction. It is designed to empty (decompress) the stomach of its contents (food, blood, gas, or other drainage). The Levin tube is about 3 feet long with a number of holes along its side approximately 6 to 9 inches from the solid tip. The opposite end of the tube is open and is usually connected to one of several types of suction equipment, which will be discussed later in this unit.

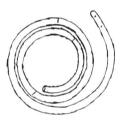

At this time you will not be expected to insert the gastric tube; however, you will need to practice getting the patient and supplies ready, and you should know the steps of the procedure so you can assist the nurse, lab technician, or physician as necessary.

Important Steps	Key Points
1. Prepare the equipment.	Wash your hands and clear a place for the equipment on the bedside stand. If the rubber or plastic Levin tube needs added stiffness when it is to be inserted, immerse it in a pan of ice (15 to 30 minutes) until the degree of stiffness is obtained. Assemble an emesis basin, tissues, a water-base lubricant, a 20- to 50-cc aspirating syringe, adhesive tape, and a glass of water. In some agencies, you will obtain these items separately for the patient; in other agencies a special tray may be ordered that includes the tube, lubricant, and aspirating syringe.
2. Approach the patient, explain what you are going to do, and enlist his cooperation. Wash your hands.	Check his identification bracelet to be sure that you have the correct patient. The patient may be in pain and very frightened. You need to reassure him that the

Important Steps

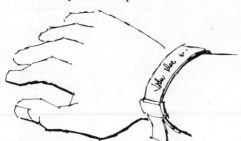

3. Position the patient.

4. Give the patient a basin and some tissues.

5. Measure the tube for insertion distance.

6. Take the correct working position and lubricate the tip of the tube.

7. Instruct the patient to open his mouth and to hold a glass of water.

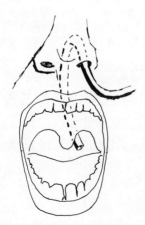

Key Points

nurse or doctor will be gentle with him and that you will tell him exactly what is being done.

Once you learn the purpose of the procedure from the charge nurse, explain it to the patient. Tell him that passing the tube down the back of the throat is painless, but could cause gagging. Tell him to breathe deeply so that he will be less likely to become nauseated and vomit.

Fowler's position is usually assumed because it enables the tube to move by gravity down the digestive tract. This makes it easier for the patient to spit out vomitus if necessary. However, the patient can be in the supine position if his condition warrants it.

If he is able to hold them, hand the emesis basin and the tissues to the patient. Otherwise, place the emesis basin close beside his face with the tissues near the pillow.

The person who is inserting the tube measures the distance from the patient's nose to the proximal earlobe and then down to the umbilicus (navel). This is roughly the distance from the lips to the stomach. Mark this distance on the tube by placing a piece of tape at that point.

The person who is inserting the tube stands at the right side of the patient; the tip end of the tube is grasped in the right hand; and the left hand holds the remaining tube. (Reverse hand positions if left-handed.)

For easier insertion, use water or a water-base lubricant to moisten the tip of the tube. *Do not use an oil-base lubricant*; the possibility of lipoid aspirational pneumonia is to be avoided.

Tell the patient to swallow a mouthful of water as the tube is passed down the esophagus to the stomach (bend his head forward so that his chin rests on his neck). Assist the patient as necessary.

The tube is passed in one of two ways:

Through the mouth: Pass the tube over the top and middle of the tongue toward the back of the throat.

Through the nose: Pass the tube up one nostril and down the back of the throat, rotating it gently and slowly between your index finger and thumb. (Test each side of the nose for obstructions, to ensure free passage of the tube.) Check the position of the tube as it passes down the back of the patient's throat by having him open his mouth and holding down his tongue with a tongue depressor. (See the diagram.)

Important Steps	Key Points

8. Push the tube slowly, firmly, and gently into the stomach.

Pushing the tube too fast stimulates the nerve endings in the back of the throat, which in turn stimulates the vomiting center in the medulla of the brain, causing the patient to vomit. Continue to have the patient swallow water or ice chips as the tube is passed; the esophageal peristalsis and the fact that you work in a quiet, reassuring manner will help the patient tolerate the procedure without undue apprehension.

9. Test to see if the tube is in the stomach.

Attach the aspirating syringe to the open end of the tube. Pull the plunger back. This action should pull the gastric juice through the tube into the syringe. (Discard the gastric content into the proper receptacle.)

10. Test to see if the tube is in the trachea.

The following observations and procedures are often used to determine whether the tube is in the trachea:

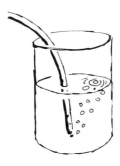

   a. Observe the patient for cyanosis (bluish tinge to the skin) or dyspnea (difficult breathing).

   b. Put the free end of the tube in a glass of water and observe for air bubbles.

   c. Hold the free end of the tube near your ear and listen for a crackling sound.

   d. Instruct the patient to hum; if he is unable to do this, the tube is properly placed. If the above procedures bring positive responses, *remove the tube immediately; it is in the trachea.*

11. Secure the tube to the patient's face with adhesive tape.

When the tube is in his stomach, tape the outside end to the bridge of the patient's nose and to his forehead. This will keep it out of the patient's way as he moves.

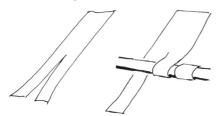

12. Attach the free end of the tube to the suction machine.

The physician orders the kind of suction machine used to remove gas and drainage from the stomach. He states the degree of "pressure pull" and whether continuous or intermittent (off–on) suction is indicated. *If there is no suction action, call the charge nurse so that appropriate action can be taken to correct it.*

   Note: As the patient's condition improves, the physician may test his tolerance for gastric content by clamping the tube for a few hours. During this time, loosely loop the tubing in a circle, secure it with adhesive tape, and pin it to the patient's gown. This will help prevent pulling that would be uncomfortable for the patient.

Gastric Tube Irrigation

The process for clearing the blocked or plugged passageway of the gastric tube is called irrigation. If the tube becomes plugged, the physician orders an irrigation to be done at stated intervals or p.r.n. (Remember: the doctor or nurse does the irrigation while you do assist and comfort the patient.)

13. Assemble the equipment.

Obtain an aspirating syringe, irrigating solution (usually normal saline), and a receptacle for the returned solution (emesis basin). This is a clean procedure, but not a sterile one.

14. Disconnect the gastric tube from the drain tube on the machine.

Turn off the suction power. Secure the drain tube to the holder on the machine. Hold the gastric tube in a fistlike grasp with the last three fingers of your left hand.

15. Fill the syringe with the irrigating solution.

Hold the syringe between your index finger and thumb. Place the tip of the syringe in the solution, using your right hand to pull the plunger up to obtain 15 to 30 cc of solution.

16. Attach the filled syringe to the free end of the gastric tube, and irrigate.

Inject 10 to 15 cc of solution gently and slowly into the tube. Pull back on the plunger to withdraw. Repeat this process until the passageway is clear. Do not injure the mucous lining of the stomach.
Note: If fresh bleeding is apparent, stop the procedure and notify the physician immediately.

17. Observe the contents of the irrigating solution.

The color, odor, consistency, and amount (absence or excess) must be noted and accurately recorded on the patient's chart.

18. When the irrigation is completed, attach the gastric tube to the drain tube of the suction machine.

Turn the power of the machine on. Check to see whether there is an NPO sign.
Note: The continuous loss of gastric content dictates the need for intravenous fluid replacement. Therefore, if it is not dripping at the designated rate, or if there is swelling at the needle site, notify the nurse so that appropriate corrective action can be taken.

Other means can be utilized to unplug the tubing:

a. Change the position of the tube by gently pushing it in and pulling it out.

Occasionally an eyelet opening of the tube adheres to the wall of the stomach, preventing drainage. Pulling the tubing from the lining of the stomach permits full drainage to occur.

b. Use a gentle "milking action" on the tube to free blockage. (Hold the tube securely in place while milking).

Thick material may plug the passageway of the tube between the patient's nose and the drainage bottle. Gently squeeze the tubing between your palm and fingers. Move carefully along the tubing in this manner until suction is restored.

19. Leave the patient comfortable.

Wash the equipment and store it in a convenient place. (Replace it p.r.n.) Tidy the bedside unit and place the call light within easy reach of the patient.

20. Report and record the procedure.

Completion of treatment with description of stomach contents. Charting example:

Important Steps	Key Points
	1030. Levin tube inserted. Tubing irrigated with NaCl solution, solution returned clear. Many gas bubbles noted. Felt relief immediately. Attached to low suction. A. Brown, RN

One of the most uncomfortable aspects of this procedure is the constant irritation by the tube of the back of the throat. Therefore, the doctor may permit the patient to suck on ice chips, throat lozenges, or hard candy to keep his throat as well as the tube slightly moist.

The nose may also become tender, sore, and cracked; good hygiene must be given not only to the patient's nose but also to his throat. Frequently cleansing of his mouth is comforting to the patient, and it is an excellent way to prevent infections caused by the tube's continuing irritation.

Because the patient is usually very ill and apprehensive, you must keep his environment quiet, clean, tidy, and well-ventilated. The patient often is supersensitive to odors, thus his room and belongings must be kept immaculately clean and sanitary. Unsavory stimuli in his environment can cause him to become nauseated and vomit.

Answer his light promptly. Check on him frequently.

U
N
I
T
26

ITEM 3.   COLLECTION OF A GASTRIC CONTENT SPECIMEN FOR ANALYSIS

A sample of the gastric contents can be obtained for analysis (1) from the emesis produced by a vomiting patient; and (2) by aspirating the necessary amount from an inserted gastric tube, which is described in the following steps.

Important Steps	Key Points
Insert the gastric tube: refer to steps 1 through 9 of Item 2.	Obtain a gastric analysis tray from Central Supply. Assemble the equipment conveniently near the patient's head on the bedside stand. *Note:* Each agency has a gastric analysis tray available, which is usually obtained from the supply department. Items found on the tray include a stomach tube (Levin, Rehfuss, Jutte, or Ewald), a tube clamp, a lubricant towel, an aspirating syringe, and several specimen bottles. The various tubes mentioned are shown in the adjacent illustrations.

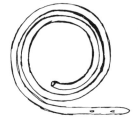

Levin tube.

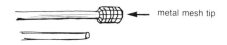
← metal mesh tip

Jutte tube.

Important Steps   Key Points

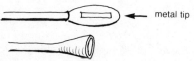 ← metal tip

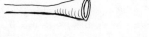

Rehfuss tube.   Ewald tube.

10. Withdraw a sample of the gastric contents.

Use an irrigating syringe to obtain at least 10 cc of fluid.

11. Place the specimen in the designated containers and put on the lids.

If test tubes are used, apply stopper lids. Avoid contaminating the outside of the container; if it has been soiled, use paper towels to wash and dry it. Label each specimen container with the patient's name and room number, the hospital number, the time, the date, and the number of the specimen (specimens are numbered in the sequence they were obtained). The number and times for specimen collections are determined by the purpose of the test. Check the laboratory manual for the specific requirements of your agency.

12. Remove the tube.

When all of the specimens have been collected, pinch the tube near the patient's nostril or mouth and slowly pull it out. (Pinching the tube prevents gastric fluid that is left inside the tube from dripping down the patient's throat and causing aspirational pneumonia.)

13. Leave the patient comfortable. Wash his hands and face, and give oral hygiene.

Place the bedside stand at a convenient location. Adjust the bed in a comfortable position. Leave the call light within easy reach.

14. Wash and dry the equipment, and return it to its proper place.

Paper towels are convenient for drying equipment; they are clean and disposable. Use them but don't waste them.

15. Record the pertinent information on the patient's chart.

Note the time, amount, color, and consistency of the specimen. Charting example:

0630. Gastric specimen obtained via the Ewald tube. Specimen 1 10 cc foul-smelling, dark brown liquid. Odor somewhat like feces. Specimen to laboratory stat.   D. Brown, RN

16. Send or take the specimen to laboratory.

Include the laboratory requisition slip. Some hospitals require that the specimen and the lab slip be put in a paper bag for delivery to the laboratory. Some agencies use other methods; check with the nurse. Take the specimens to the laboratory yourself or arrange to have them taken by a messenger service.

ITEM 4. INSERTION OF INTESTINAL TUBES FOR DRAINAGE PURPOSES

In the procedure, you will again be assisting the doctor or nurse to insert the tube. However, you need to know the procedure and be ready to help as needed. Stand opposite the doctor or nurse; talk reassuringly to the patient.

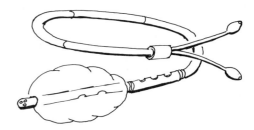

Miller-Abbott Tube. This is a long double-lumen rubber tube used for draining the small intestine. One of the lumens supplies the drainage passageway; the other supplies an air passage to inflate the balloon at the distal end of the tube. The inflated balloon in the small intestine stimulates peristalsis (the wavelike movement of the digestive tract).

The procedure for inserting this tube is as follows:

Important Steps	Key Points

Refer to steps 1 through 9 of Item 2.

10. After the tube reaches the stomach, inflate the balloon.

The doctor or nurse will use a sterile syringe and needle to inject 5 to 10 cc of air (or mercury) into the outlet connecting the air passageway to the balloon. The inflated (and weighted if mercury is used) tube then passes into the small intestine.

11. Place the patient in *right Sims'* position.

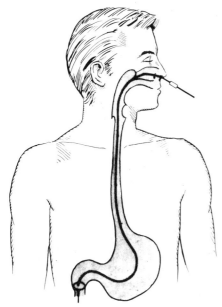

This makes the passage of the tube faster and easier by helping the peristaltic action and gravity to move the tube from the stomach to the small intestine.

The tube should not be secured until it is finally inserted into the small intestine. This can be determined by the ring markings on the outside of the tubing as well as by the appearance of the drainage. When the tube reaches the intestines, it is attached to a suction machine. The outside tip of the tube is secured to the patient's face with adhesive tape and pinned to his gown to permit freedom of movement.

Remove the tubing as follows:

a. Deflate the balloon; use an appropriately sized syringe to remove the air or mercury.

b. Pinch and slowly pull the tubing a few inches every 5 minutes or so.

c. Avoid stimulating the gag reflex and causing the patient to vomit.

U
N
I
T
26

Important Steps	Key Points

Cantor Tube. This is another type of intestinal drainage tube. It has a small inflatable bag sealed to the distal end of the tube. Before insertion of this tube through the nose, the inflatable (balloon) bag is injected (use a needle and syringe) with 5 to 10 cc of mercury. This will make the tip end of the tube bulky for insertion and therefore it must be well-lubricated. The principle of operation is the same as for the Miller-Abbott tube. The proximal end of the tube is attached to a suction machine. The drainage holes in the tube are proximal to the balloon bag.

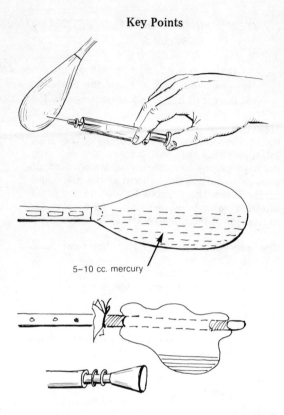

5-10 cc. mercury

Harris Tube. A long, single tube used for intestinal suction and drainage, it is similar to the Cantor tube, except that the inflatable balloon is tied to the distal end of the tube (it has 4 cc of mercury in it). The holes that allow the drainage to be sucked into the tubing are proximal to the balloon bag. The well-lubricated tube is inserted through the nose, using the Levin tube procedure.

The nursing care and observation of the equipment and drainage are the same as for other patients with gastrointestinal suction and drainage.

ITEM 5.   SPECIAL FEEDING METHODS: GASTRIC GAVAGE, AND GASTROSTOMY AND ENTEROSTOMY FEEDINGS

Gastric gavage is a feeding given via a tube inserted through either the mouth or nose into the stomach. Patients who receive this type of feeding are unable to take foods orally (by mouth). Patients of any age may be fed in this manner, from the very small infant to the elderly geriatric patient.

The feeding can be given continuously over a 24-hour period by means of a special Murphy drip method, or it can be given at prescribed intervals, such as q.i.d. (four times a day) or q.4 h. (every four hours).

Gavage feedings are special formulas prepared commercially or in the diet kitchen. They vary in nutritive value. The physician prescribes the caloric value, the volume, and the frequency of fluids to be given in a 24-hour period. The patient's disease, age, and weight are the determining factors.

The *gastrostomy* feeding may also be used. In this case a small incision is made in the upper left abdominal wall directly into the stomach. A gastrostomy tube (catheter with a large lumen) is inserted into the opening. The area is sutured (sewn) to close the surgical wound and also to secure the catheter to prevent it from slipping out of the incision. In about 10 days the wound is healed and the tube can be taken out and reinserted p.r.n.

Although you will not be inserting the tube, you probably will be responsible for giving the periodic feedings if you are assigned to the patient. You must understand the procedure and demonstrate concern, support, and the ability to perform the task easily, correctly, and quickly.

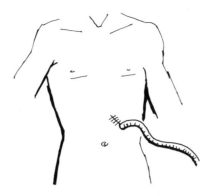

A gastrostomy or enterostomy
tube in place.

Important Steps	Key Points
1. Wash your hands and prepare the equipment.	The tray for the feeding procedure can be obtained from the supply department. The formula (feeding) is obtained from the diet kitchen. It is then usually stored in the refrigerator on the nursing unit, although it is ordered daily like any other diet. Take the equipment to the bedside and place it conveniently on the bedside stand or overbed table.
2. Approach and identify the patient, explain what you are going to do, and enlist his cooperation.	Some patients receiving this type of feeding may be unconscious and therefore will not be able to cooperate. Check your patient's identification bracelet to be sure you have the correct person.
3. Position the patient.	Use the same position as that used for the gastric tube insertion procedure in Item 2. However, for enterostomy and gastrostomy feedings, the patient should be in a dorsal recumbent position.
4. Hand the basin and tissues to the patient.	See step 4, Item 2.
5. Measure the tube for insertion.	This is the same as step 5 of Item 2. However, the gastrostomy and enterostomy tubes are inserted directly into the special openings in the abdomen. These tubes are usually 12 to 18 inches long.
6. Insert the tube and check for correct location.	Follow steps 9 and 10 of Item 2. If the tube is already in place, check before you begin feeding to make sure the tube is in the stomach, not in the trachea or lung.
7. Pour an ounce of water into the funnel or syringe.	The syringe or funnel is attached to the free end of the tube. Room-temperature water is used to see that the tube is patent (open). *Note:* If the tube is inserted each time it is used, this step is omitted.

Important Steps	Key Points
8. Pour warmed formula (105°F) into the equipment.	Formula should be given slowly; gravity pull will draw it in. You can regulate flow by raising and lowering the receptacle as demonstrated in the adjacent diagram.

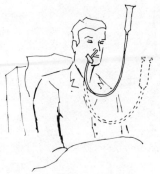

Regulating formula flow.

9. Keep the level of the formula no lower than the neck of the syringe.	If you allow the formula level to fall below the neck of the syringe, air will enter the tubing and the stomach, causing great discomfort due to distention of the stomach. Continue adding formula to the syringe until the prescribed amount is given.

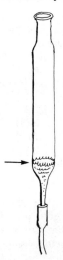

10. Pour 1 to 2 ounces of water into the syringe to clear the tube.	When the formula feeding is finished, pour in fresh water to clear the tube. Again, be sure to keep the liquid above the neck of the syringe to prevent air bubbles from collecting in the system or in the patient's stomach. (This step is eliminated if the tube is removed after each feeding.)
11. Clamp the tubing	If the tubing is removed, clamp it tightly between your right index finger and thumb to prevent the tube from dripping as it is removed. If the tubing is left in, close it (with a clamp or medicine dropper that comes on your tray) before removing the funnel or syringe to prevent backflow of the formula.

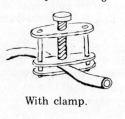

With clamp.

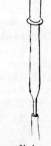

With medicine dropper.

Important Steps	Key Points

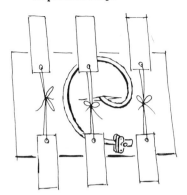

Secure under bandage.

For gavage: Secure the end of the tube with tape to the patient's forehead. Be sure to avoid irritating the skin area and keep it clean and dry.

For gastrostomy and enterostomy: Secure the end of the tube under the dressing on the abdomen.

12. Give oral hygiene and nose care (for gavage only).

If tubing is left in the patient's mouth, be sure that the nose is kept moist, clean, and free from crusts. Sometimes the tubing is left connected to a large flask that may be hung on an IV pole at the head of the bed.

13. Make the patient comfortable.

A person undergoing this procedure needs extra reassurance, kindness, and patience. It is possible that he will have to be fed by this means for a long period of time. You may need to teach the patient and his family how to accomplish this feeding procedure. Be sure to stress the *safety* technique of checking to make sure that his tube is not in the lung. Stress the importance of cleanliness of the equipment, the patient, and the environment for his peace of mind and as a preventive measure against infection.

Be sure to tell the patient when you expect to return, and keep your word.

14. Record the procedure on the patient's chart.

Note the amount of formula, the way it was taken, and any other comments about the patient's reaction. Charting example:

0800. Gastric feeding given. 200 cc formula taken without difficulty.   A. Brown, RN

ITEM 6.   PROCTOCLYSIS OR FEEDING OF FLUIDS OR NOURISHMENT INTO THE COLON

This method, although seldom used now, is a way of giving patients fluids and nourishment when the previously described methods are inappropriate. The fluids are given slowly, drop by drop, over a long period of time through a special drip tube (Murphy drip) attached to the catheter or tubing. The tubing and Murphy drip can be connected to the gastrostomy or enterostomy stoma, or they can be attached to a rectal tube and the feeding given rectally. If the nourishment is given rectally, the treatment should be preceded by an enema to cleanse the colon in preparation for the proctoclysis.

The procedure for giving the proctoclysis is similar to other tube feedings. The rectal tube (18 to 22 French catheter) is lubricated and then inserted about 4 to 5 inches into the rectum. It is taped in place by looping tape around the tube once and attaching the tape to each side of the buttocks. The flask for holding the feeding is attached to the tubing and the Murphy drip, and then attached to the free end of the rectal tube. The flask is hung on an IV pole adjusted to a height of 12 inches above the mattress. (See the following diagram.)

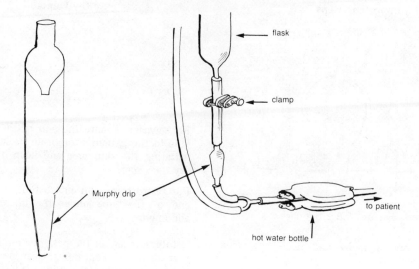

Since the feeding must be at a temperature of 105°F to facilitate absorption, place hot water bottles around the tubing (near the rectal area). Hold them in place by wrapping a bath towel around the hot water bottles and securing it with tape or safety pins. It would not help to place the hot water bottles around the flask (and not in the tubing) because the fluids would then cool as they passed through the tubing. The rate of flow of the fluid is adjusted to the doctor's order, depending on the amount of feeding the patient is to receive over the stated period of time.

ITEM 7. GASTROINTESTINAL DRAINAGE WITH AND WITHOUT SUCTION

A. Drainage Without Suction

Let us discuss common methods of draining secretions from incisions without suction.

The *Penrose drain*, a tube frequently employed, is a flat, soft rubber drain available in various widths from 1/4 inch to 2 inches. The physician inserts one end of the drain into the wound in the designated site, using strict aseptic technique. The free end of the tube resting on the skin may be held securely in place with a stitch of surgical suture or a safety pin. The tube is covered with sterile padding (dressing) to catch the drainage. The dressing is changed p.r.n. Care must be taken not to dislodge the tube when changing the dressing (usually done by the doctor or nurse, using strict aseptic technique to prevent infection). Careful observation of the amount, color, odor, and consistency of the drainage is vital to the physician's planning of the medical care for his patient. Therefore, the observations and recordings must be accurate.

A *cigarette drain* is a Penrose drain with a gauze bandage pulled through the lumen acting as a wick, like tobacco in a cigarette. It may be used as the doctor deems necessary. The same precautions are to be taken in placing, caring for, and removing the cigarette drain as those described for the Penrose drain.

A *T-tube rubber drain* is commonly used to drain bile from the liver into the intestine—often following a cholecystectomy (surgical excision of the gallbladder). Care must be taken not to dislodge the catheter. Since a large amount of bile may be excreted in 24 hours, the T-tube may be attached to an external tubing system that empties into a drainage bag or bottle attached to the patient's bedside. T-tubes can be used any time the physician indicates the need.

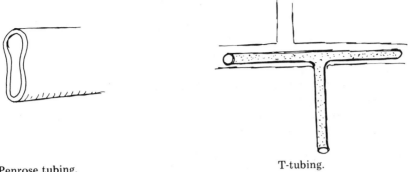

Penrose tubing.　　　　　　　　　　　　　T-tubing.

Urethral catheters may also be used to drain surgical incisions. The size of the lumen must be large enough to accommodate the drainage (a large lumen is used if a large amount of thick fluid is to be drained). Since catheters come in varying sizes, the actual size is selected on the basis of need. The choice is usually made by the physician.

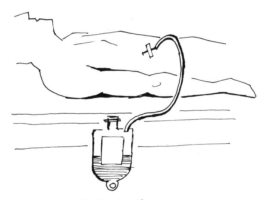

Urethral catheter
in abdominal incision.

B. Drainage With Suction

The portable wound suction unit is a commercially made plastic apparatus used to drain pus-filled wounds. It is composed of a needle, needle protector, wound tube, connector tube, bellows (container), and belt strap.

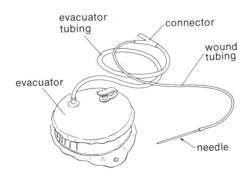

The wound suction tube is generally inserted in the wound by the physician. The implantation is usually done in surgery, but it can be accomplished elsewhere as long as a sterile field and technique are maintained.

The wound tube has an attached 5-inch needle, approximately 25 holes along the midsection, and 12 inches of closed tubing extending beyond the midsection. The end of this extension is inserted into one of the open ends of the double-ended connector tube. The connector tube is attached to the port side of the bellows. The drain plug (on top of the bellows) is opened, and pressure is applied to depress the bellows. At this step, the drain plug is reinserted and a vacuum then exists.

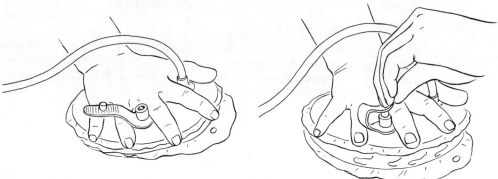

Compressing bellows unit to form vacuum.   Placing plug in outlet to retain suction.

This vacuum pressure causes the drainage from the wound to flow into the bellows where it will remain until the nurse opens the bellows, empties it, and measures and records the amount of drainage on the Intake and Output sheet of the patient's records. The discarding of the drainage is a procedure that must be repeated until drainage no longer exists and the unit is removed from the wound.

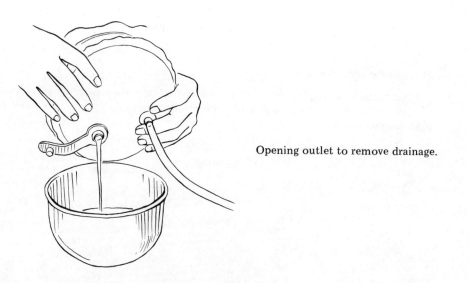

Opening outlet to remove drainage.

Wound drainage can also be accomplished by connecting various tubes to different types of suction machines (special machines that suck or withdraw contents from a cavity by means of decreasing air pressure). Suction can be maintained on a continuous basis or intermittently (on and off) as the doctor orders. There are four general types of suction apparatus that you should know about:

1. A *portable electric suction machine* is a common piece of equipment. It has a gauge on it that permits regulation of the amount of suction. It is particularly useful when the drainage becomes thick and viscous.

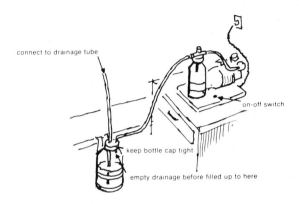

connect to drainage tube

on-off switch

keep bottle cap tight

empty drainage before filled up to here

Your main responsibility will be to see that the drainage bottle does not overflow: it would back up into the vacuum bottle and when that became full, into the motor. The repair in such a case is costly and sometimes, impossible. Therefore, you must check it frequently to ascertain the amount of drainage and the working order of the suction, and to ensure the general comfort of your patient.

2. Most health agencies now have suction outlets in the wall at the head of the patient's bed. This avoids having to clutter the patient's room with extra equipment. Wall suction units are particularly useful in special care units (ICU, CCU, and others). Occasionally there is a problem of maintaining enough suction in the entire system (supplying all patients). Some physicians are therefore reluctant to use this system. Again, your responsibility will be to see that the drainage bottle does not overflow.

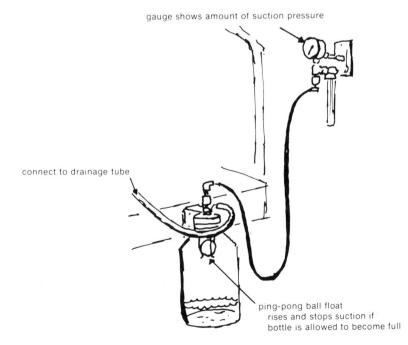

gauge shows amount of suction pressure

connect to drainage tube

ping-pong ball float
rises and stops suction if
bottle is allowed to become full

3. Another type of suction machine often used is the *Gomco Thermotic Pump*. This is an electric pump (without a motor) that provides intermittent suction through alternating air pressure by expanding and contracting the air. The Gomco suction can be regulated by a "low" or "high" pressure button (the amount of pressure will be ordered by the physician). You will see this type of machine used most often with patients who have either gastric or intestinal suction tubes.

Again, close observation of the drainage bottle contents is important to prevent overflow. Check the workings of the machine frequently to be sure it is pulling the drainage from the cavity (stomach or intestine). As the pressure alternates, the red light and the green light alternate on the operating unit.

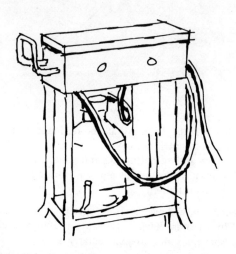

4. The fourth type is a *two-bottle water displacement system* designed to create suction (an early type of suction apparatus). One of the first models was the Wangensteen suction machine. There have been several adaptations made to the basic system, but most hospital personnel still continue to use the term Wangensteen suction when they refer to a water displacement system of suction. The figure below illustrates a modification but demonstrates the main principles. When the top water bottle is empty, the bottom bottle is rotated in the frame to the top position. The two water bottles are supported in the metal frame, and the entire frame is rotated so that the bottles exchange positions. It is vital that you check frequently to make sure that the water level in the top bottle never goes below the neck of the bottle; if it did, the suction would be lost and the draining stopped.

The water drains to the bottom much as the sand drains in a 3-minute egg timer. The draining water produces a suction in the drainage bottle that in turn causes the drainage to be drawn into it. Because of the nature of this suction operation, all bottles must be absolutely airtight to assure enough constant suction to withdraw the drainage fluids. Of course, airtight connections are essential for proper operation of any and all suction systems.

The water displacement system is an excellent example of Bernoulli's Principle: as a gas or liquid flows, it enters a contricted area, and the velocity increases. As it moves out the other end of the constriction, the velocity decreases. This raises the pressure in the lower bottle on the frame, creating a vacuum in the suction bottle.

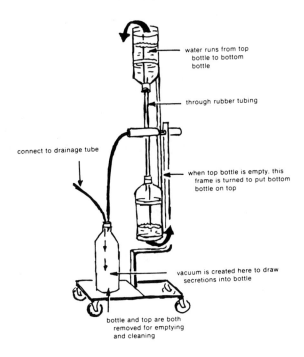

water runs from top
bottle to bottom
bottle

through rubber tubing

connect to drainage tube

when top bottle is empty, this
frame is turned to put bottom
bottle on top

vacuum is created here to draw
secretions into bottle

bottle and top are both
removed for emptying
and cleaning

Emptying and Measuring the Contents of Drainage Bottles

Important Steps	Key Points
1. Wash your hands, approach and identify the patient, explain the procedure to the patient, and turn off the suction momentarily.	This will break the suction in the system, allowing easy removal of the rubber stopper on the drainage bottle.
2. Remove the rubber stopper from the bottle top.	Unclamp the holding bracket if there is one.
3. Pour the contents into a graduate.	Measure the contents and record the time, amount, color, odor, and consistency after reassembling the system.
4. Rinse the graduate and the drainage bottle.	Dry the outside of the drainage bottle with paper towels and then discard them in the wastebasket.
5. Clean and replace the rubber stopper on top of the cleaned drainage bottle.	Make sure that it is airtight and held in place with the clamps securely tightened.
6. Turn the switch back to the "on" position on the suction machine.	This will reestablish the suction system. Observe the flow of drainage for a few minutes. Tell the patient when you will return.
7. Make the patient comfortable and record the amount of drainage on the chart of the I & O sheet.	

ITEM 8. NURSING CARE

The nursing measures that must be observed include frequent special mouth care for these patients. Since they are NPO, the mouth becomes very dry and tastes bad, and the lips may become cracked. (These are ideal locations for pathogens to set up housekeeping.) To keep the mouth and lips moist, swab the oral cavity with a cotton swab that has been moistened in equal parts of glycerin and lemon juice. This liquid comes prepackaged for use in most agencies; if not, you can mix the solution, which is very refreshing to the patient. Mouthwash may also be used if the patient is able to spit the liquid out; he must not swallow it.

The nostrils often become dry and tender. When you take care of patients with the various gastrointestinal tubes, you should remember the following:

1. Demonstrate kindness, gentleness, and quiet concern for their comfort.

2. Give meticulous and frequent oral hygiene and nose care.

3. Provide for freedom of movement as much as possible by securing the suction tubing to the patient's clothing or skin to permit maximum activity.

4. See that the patient does not lie on the tubing; do not permit the tubing to be kinked because the suction will stop, as well as the fluid drainage.

5. When you are checking to see if the suction machine is operating satisfactorily, first check to see that it is properly attached to the patient and the wall outlet, that the machine is turned on, and that the tubes are not kinked. If you have checked all of these points and made sure that the drainage bottle is not overflowing, but you see that the machine is *not* working, report at once (stat.) to your team leader. This situation can be crucial to the well-being of your patient because there may be a plugged tube.

6. Observe, report, and record the contents of the drainage bottles accurately. Report and record any unusual contents promptly to your charge nurse.

These patients will provide a challenge to nursing care. They often relax if you give an extra backrub or straighten or change bed linens p.r.n. Your quiet attention to details when caring for these patients can hasten their recovery.

ITEM 9. CONCLUSION OF THE UNIT

You have now learned about drainage systems with and without suction. You have also learned about continuous and intermittent suction equipment, and you have become acquainted with four common types of suction apparatus and the emptying of the drainage bottles. Arrange to take the post-test.

PERFORMANCE TEST

In the classroom or the skill laboratory, your instructor will ask you to demonstrate the following procedures. You should be able to do so accurately without reference to your study guide, notes, or other source material.

1. Given a patient with a suspected respiratory disease who is allowed bathroom privileges, you are to instruct and assist the patient to produce a specimen of sputum, and prepare the specimen for delivery to the laboratory.

2. Given a patient who has had some gastric contents aspirated by the physician, you are to prepare the specimen correctly for delivery to the laboratory.

3. Given a patient with a feeding tube, you will assemble the equipment, prepare the patient (or the mannequin, Mrs. Chase), and give a feeding of 50 cc of water following the procedure outlined in the lesson, maintaining safety precautions. You will practice recording the activity on the nurses' notes.

4. Given a patient with a gastric suction apparatus and a three-fourths full drainage bottle, you will empty the bottle and reattach it to the suction machine using the procedure you have just learned. Upon completion of the bottle change, you will record the output on the appropriate records.

PERFORMANCE CHECKLIST

THE PATIENT WITH GASTROINTESTINAL TUBES

COLLECTION OF A SPUTUM SPECIMEN

1. Wash your hands.

2. Obtain the necessary items and prepare the labels correctly.

3. Identify the patient.

4. Instruct the patient on how to collect a specimen.

5. Provide for the patient's privacy.

6. Assist the patient as needed.

7. Avoid contamination of your hands, your uniform, and the container by the patient's sputum.

8. Seal the container, wash and dry the outside of the container.

9. Apply a label to the container.

10. Put the labeled container and laboratory slip in a paper bag for delivery to the laboratory.

11. Provide for the patient's safety and comfort.

12. Arrange for delivery of the specimen to the laboratory.

13. Record the pertinent information on the patient's chart.

COLLECTION AND PREPARATION OF A GASTRIC SPECIMEN

1. Obtain the necessary items and prepare the labels after washing your hands.
2. Identify the patient as the one who produced the specimen.
3. Put 10 cc of gastric contents into the specimen container or test tube.
4. Put the lid or stopper on the container, clean the outer surfaces, and attach the label.
5. Arrange for delivery of the specimen and laboratory slip to the laboratory.
6. Wash, dry, and return all the equipment to the proper place.
7. Record the pertinent information on the patient's chart.

GAVAGE

1. Wash your hands and prepare the equipment.
2. Approach and identify the patient.
3. Position the patient (Fowler's).
4. Hand an emesis basin and tissue to the patient.
5. Test the location of the tube in the stomach, and pour 1 ounce water at room temperature into a funnel to check that the tubing is *patent*.
6. Pour the warmed formula (105°F) into the syringe.
7. Regulate the flow by raising and lowering the feeding tube.
8. Keep the level of the formula above the neck of the syringe to prevent air from entering the stomach.
9. Continue giving the formula until the prescribed amount has been given.
10. Pour in 1 to 2 ounces of water to clear the tube.
11. Clamp the tube; remove the funnel from the tube.
12. Secure the distal end of the tube.
13. Give oral hygiene and nose care.
14. Leave the patient comfortable (position him in good alignment and put the call cord and bedside stand nearby; tell the patient when you will return).
15. Chart the activity.

REMOVAL AND REPLACEMENT OF THE DRAINAGE BOTTLE

1. Wash your hands.
2. Identify the patient.
3. Explain the procedure to the patient.
4. Turn off the suction.
5. Remove the stopper from the bottle.
6. Pour the contents of the jar into a graduate cylinder.
7. Attach a new drainage jar to the apparatus.

8. Replace the rubber stopper.

9. Turn on the suction machine (put it in operation for several minutes).

10. Measure and record the volume, color, odor, and consistency of the drainage.

11. Rinse and dry the materials used.

12. Provide for the patient's comfort and safety.

13. Inform the patient of the time of your return.

U
N
I
T
26

POST-TEST

Directions: Choose the answer that will make the statement complete.

1. Gastric suction is used for the following reasons except:

    a. to prevent postoperative vomiting

    b. to prevent postoperative obstruction of the intestinal tract

    c. to prevent postoperative pneumonia

    d. to prevent gas formation in the stomach or intestine

2. The most commonly used tube for gastric intubation and suction is called:

    a. Miller-Abbot tube   c. Cantor tube

    b. Levin tube   d. Harris tube

3. When the Levin tube needs added stiffness for insertion, the following is done:

    a. it is immersed in a pan of water at $105°F$

    b. it is immersed in a pan of ice for 15–30 minutes

    c. it is immersed in water at $212°F$

    d. it is placed under cold, running tap water

4. Patients are uncomfortable during this procedure and will probably:

    a. sneeze   c. gag

    b. cough   d. have an itching throat

5. During the procedure, the patient is usually placed in:

    a. Sims' position   c. prone position

    b. Trendelenburg's position   d. Fowler's position

6. The tube is measured for insertion distance from the:

    a. patient's ear to his umbilicus

    b. patient's nose to his proximal earlobe to his umbilicus

    c. patient's mouth to his nose to his proximal earlobe to his umbilicus

    d. patient's nose to his umbilicus

7. The tube should be lubricated with:

    a. a water-base lubricant   c. glycerin and lemon juice

    b. petrolatum   d. mineral oil

8. While the tube is being inserted, the patient should:

    a. keep his mouth closed   c. swallow sips of water or ice chips

    b. close his eyes and mouth   d. swallow warm coffee

9. When inserting a gastric tube, one can do all of the following except:

    a. to pass the tube over the top and middle of the tongue to the back of the throat

    b. to pass the tube up the nose and down the back of the throat

    c. to push the tube slowly, gently, and firmly into the stomach

    d. if one nostril is obstructed, to place the tube in the other one

10. Which one of these is not a true test for checking the tube in the stomach and the trachea?

   a. if gastric content returns in the aspirating syringe, the tube is in the esophagus

   b. if the free end of the tube placed in water causes bubbles, the tube is in the trachea

   c. if the patient can hum, the tube is in the trachea

   d. if the patient becomes cyanotic, the tube is in the esophagus

11. Plugged gastric tubes should be irrigated:

   a. 3 to 4 hours per day

   b. twice a day

   c. as ordered by the physician

   d. at 12 noon and 12 midnight

12. Which of the following is not true regarding the suction machine?

   a. Suction is intermittent

   b. The physician indicates the amount of pull pressure

   c. Suction is continuous

   d. It is necessary to check flow drainage only once a day

13. It is important to note and record the following observations on the nurses' notes when gastric irrigations are done:

   a. color, odor, and amount

   b. color and odor

   c. color, odor, and consistency

   d. color, odor, amount, and consistency

14. An acceptable method of clearing the gastric tube without saline irrigation is to:

   a. use a gentle "milking action"

   b. blow air through the tubing

   c. irrigate the tubing with oxygen

   d. pull the tube in and out approximately 3 to 4 inches

15. The most important nursing care measure for this patient will be:

   a. frequent oral hygiene and facial skin care

   b. a daily bed bath

   c. daily oral hygiene

   d. special skin care daily

16. The intestinal tube used for drainage is called a:

   a. Jutte

   b. Miller-Abbott

   c. Levin

   d. Rehfuss

17. The differentiating factor in the intestinal and gastric tube is that:

   a. one is made of rubber

   b. one is inflated with mercury, the other with air

   c. one has a balloon on the end that is in the patient

   d. one is called Jutte, the other Miller-Abbott

18. Which of the following is not true when one sends a gastric specimen to the laboratory?

     a. it is labeled with the patient's name, his room number, the hospital number, the time, the date, and the sequence of numbered specimens

     b. it is sent with the laboratory requisition

     c. all gastric analysis tests require at least 50 cc of fluid

     d. the outside of the container must be washed if it is soiled by gastric content

19. The difference between gavage feeding and gastrostomy feeding is:

     a. the place of insertion for the tube

     b. only formula is used in gavage feeding

     c. gavage feeding is kept at a temperature of $110°F$

     d. gastrostomy feeding is given twice a day

20. Deep breathing and coughing are important for the patient to practice when you are obtaining:

     a. gastric specimens   c. saliva

     b. sputum specimens   d. histamines

POST-TEST ANNOTATED ANSWER SHEET

1. c. (p. 549)	11. c. (p. 552)	
2. b. (p. 549)	12. d. (pp. 551 and 553)	
3. b. (p. 549)	13. d. (p. 552)	
4. c. (p. 550)	14. a. (p. 552)	
5. d. (p. 550)	15. a. (p. 553)	
6. b. (p. 550)	16. b. (p. 555)	
7. a. (p. 550)	17. c. (pp. 555 and 556)	
8. c. (p. 551)	18. c. (p. 554)	
9. d. (p. 550)	19. a. (p. 556)	
10. d. (p. 551)	20. b. (p. 548)	

HOT AND COLD APPLICATIONS

I. DIRECTIONS TO THE STUDENT

Proceed through the lesson using this workbook as your guide. You will need to practice the tasks and procedures using the different types of equipment with the mannequin (Mrs. Chase) or student partners in the skill laboratory. After you have completed the lesson and practiced the procedures, arrange with your instructor to take the post-test.

For this lesson you will need the following items:

1. Pen or pencil.

2. Hot water bottle and cover.

3. Ice bag and cover.

4. Heat cradle.

5. Mannequin (Mrs. Chase).

6. Electric heating pad.

If at all possible, the following equipment should be available for demonstration and practice purposes:

1. Hypothermia machine.

2. Aquathermia machine.

Please read the following paragraphs carefully. They will tell you what you will be expected to know and how you will be expected to assist in giving the heat or cold treatment that is ordered for the patient. If you feel that you already have the necessary skills, discuss this with your instructor and then arrange to take the performance test. All students are expected to demonstrate accurately the skills required in the performance test and to know the material in the written post-test.

II. GENERAL PERFORMANCE OBJECTIVE

Upon the completion of this lesson, you will be able to apply heat and cold as treatments for the patient's condition accurately, effectively, and safely.

III. SPECIFIC PERFORMANCE OBJECTIVES

Upon the completion of this unit, you will be able to:

1. Apply heat locally to a portion of the patient's body efficiently and safely, using a hot water bottle, heating pad, heat cradle, or aquathermia pad.

2. Apply cold locally to a portion of the patient's body efficiently and safely, using an ice bag, cold pack, or hypothermia machine.

3. Assist in setting up and operating the hypothermia/hyperthermia machine for the general application of heat or cold to the patient's body correctly, efficiently, and safely.

IV. VOCABULARY

aquathermia—a small, electric, jarlike container that is used to hold an alcohol/distilled water solution; it has outlets to permit circulation of the fluid through tubes and a hollow vinyl pad (K-pad).

autonomic nervous system—the part of the nervous system not under voluntary control that governs the heart, glands, and smooth muscle in the body.

Central Service (CS)—a supply area in the hospital that provides sterile and unsterile equipment and supplies used in the care of patients.

cornea—a clear and transparent tissue of the eye that covers the iris and the pupil and permits light to enter the eye.

electrolyte—a charged particle (ion) capable of conducting an electrical charge; electrolytes are essential for normal body functioning.

hypothermia—body temperature below the normal range (hypo- = less, below; -thermia = temperature).

hyperthermia—body temperature above the normal range (hyper- = more, above).

infrared lamp—a special device that has light rays beyond the red end of the visible light spectrum.

light spectrum—light is the sensation produced by electromagnetic radiation that strikes the retina of the eye; spectrum refers to the length of the light ray.

metabolism—the entire process by which the body is nourished, maintained, and provided with energy.

suppuration—the formation of pus.

systemic—relating to the whole system; the whole body.

toxin—a poisonous or noxious substance.

ultraviolet lamp—a special lamp that emits light rays outside the visible spectrum at the violet end.

V. INTRODUCTION

The application of heat or cold to the skin surface is important in treating certain infections and traumatic conditions. Usually a physician's order is necessary before one uses any of these treatments because of the related and opposing effects produced elsewhere in the body.

In order to understand the use of heat and cold applications, and their effect on the body, you need to know about some of the principles involved:

1. Heat causes dilation of blood vessels and increases the supply of blood to the area.

2. Heat stimulates metabolism, and the growth of new cells and tissues.

3. Cold causes contraction of blood vessels and decreases the supply of blood to the area.

4. Cold retards metabolism and decreases cell activity or growth.

5. Applications of heat and cold to portions of the body cause autonomic nervous system responses throughout the body.

6. Because the blood volume of the body is constant within a closed system, an increase in the blood supply to the skin causes a decrease in the blood supply of other portions of the body; conversely, a decrease in the blood supply to the skin increases the blood supply elsewhere in the body.

7. As a conductor of heat and cold, water is more effective than air.

The dilation of blood vessels caused by heat application and the constriction of vessels resulting from application of cold are shown in the figures below.

These principles explain the effects of heat and cold on the body. Let us consider heat first. Heat is applied to the skin surfaces to provide general comfort and to speed up the healing process. The elevated temperature or fever that so often accompanies an illness or infection is the body's way of combating the illness and promoting the healing process.

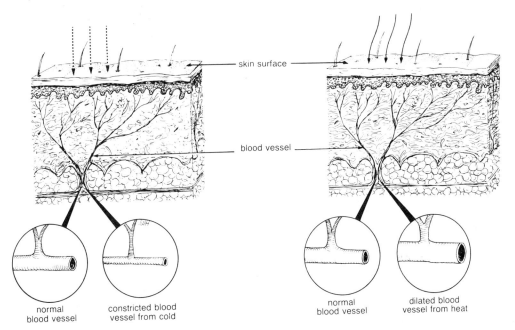

skin surface

blood vessel

| normal blood vessel | constricted blood vessel from cold | normal blood vessel | dilated blood vessel from heat |

Effect of cold application.   Effect of heat application.

Heat dilates the blood vessels in the area of application. This increases the blood supply, adds nutrients and oxygen to the tissue, removes toxins and excess tissue fluid, and reduces pain caused by pressure on the nerve endings. The dilated blood vessels and the increased blood supply in the area of heat application cause the skin to appear pinkish or reddened, although this color is more difficult to detect in dark-skinned or black patients. Heat is used to decrease inflammation and to promote the formation of pus (suppuration).

Cold applications are used to prevent or reduce swelling, to stop bleeding, and to decrease suppuration. When cold is applied to the skin surface, it contracts the muscles, which in turn squeeze the blood vessels to reduce the blood supply further. The blood vessels themselves contract, the diminished blood supply reduces the nutrients and oxygen to the cells, and cell activity is cut down. Since cold applications slow the metabolism of the body, the body can be cooled for prolonged surgery to decrease the stress of trauma and blood loss.

Prolonged cold reduces sensation and therefore lessens pain. However, if cold continues to interrupt the circulation, it can lead to necrosis (death of tissue), as seen in severe frostbite. When a cold application is removed from the skin, there occurs a secondary reaction as the circulation returns to normal. The blood vessels dilate and give the skin a warm, glowing pink color.

Heat and cold treatments can be either dry, as with hot water bottles, heating pads, and ice caps, or they can be moist, as with baths, soaks, and compresses. Moist applications have a more effective action because water is better than air as a conductor of heat and cold. Dry heat is tolerated better than a moist heat application of the same temperature, which may cause pain or burning.

Applications of heat and cold to the skin activate the autonomic nervous system. The nerve endings in the skin send a message to the control center in the brain, for example, that heat has been applied. In an effort to maintain the body temperature at an even level, the control center acts to dilate the blood vessels and increase the circulation to the area. Other blood vessels to the internal organs are constricted so that the temperature of those organs is maintained to prevent disturbance of other delicately balanced body functions. Although the procedure of applying heat or cold to the body is relatively simple, the effect on the body is much more complex.

Heat and cold can be applied to large or small body areas. A general application is one that is applied to the entire body; a local application is one that is used on a specific part of the body. The following figures show some examples of general and local applications.

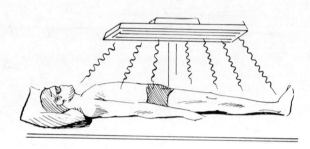

Example of general temperature application.

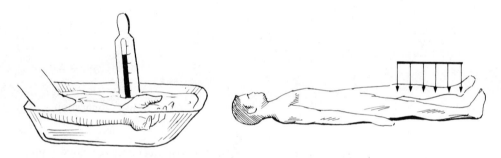

Examples of local temperature applications.

ITEM 1.   IMPORTANT CONSIDERATIONS

1. Physician's Orders

When electric or nonelectric appliances are used for heat or cold in patient care, an order must be written by the physician on the patient's chart before any appliance can be used. The order must state the kind of appliance, and the frequency and length of its application for the designated treatment.

2. Safety to the Patient

When electric or nonelectric appliances are used for heat or cold in patient care, the patient's safety is of utmost importance. Do not use electric appliances close to open oxygen unless they are well-insulated, and the electric outlets and plugs are far enough away so that it is impossible for electric sparks to ignite the oxygen and cause a fire. Do not permit the patient to put the plug in the electric outlet. Do not permit the patient to handle the temperature control. Do not permit the heat or cold pad to be used without a cloth cover. When heat or cold is applied to the *unconscious* patient, remember to be doubly aware of inadvertently burning or causing numbness to the patient. He *cannot* tell you whether the pad is too hot or if he is in pain or discomfort.

3. Safety to the Worker

When an electric appliance is used, be aware that it is dangerous to put the plug in the electric outlet in a dark room. Use a light to find the outlet; do not try to locate the outlet using your hand as a guide. Do not handle the plug or put it in the electric outlet when you have wet hands. Do not remove the plug from the outlet by pulling at the cord. Be aware of the cord; it may be stretched across a walking area on the floor. Do *not* trip over it and hurt yourself.

4. Cost to the Patient

All appliances obtained from Central Service are rented for the patient in most agencies. Some agencies have a daily treatment rate that includes the cost of all treatments and equipment the patient needs. A requisition slip is usually sent to Central Service requesting the item; it is dated and stamped with the patient's name and hospital number. When the appliance is no longer needed, the requisition slip may be returned with it to Central Service. (Check your agency for specific procedure.) When the patient's needs have been met, the appliance must be returned to Central Service so that it can be reprocessed for the next patient. Do not keep it longer than necessary; the patient may be charged for something that he is not using.

5. Care of the Equipment

Initial care of the equipment is usually accomplished by the health workers in Central Service. When it is being used by the patient, it is maintained by the health worker who is responsible for the patient's care. It must be kept clean and in good working order. When necessary, report needed repairs to the proper person, and replace it immediately (send to Central Service). If equipment is faulty, do not express your concern or annoyance verbally in the presence of the patient or his family. This will only cause unnecessary apprehension or fear.

ITEM 2. AQUATHERMIA PAD (K-PAD)

The Aquamatic K control unit is a small, jarlike, plastic unit operated by electricity. There is a temperature gauge on one side and two coupling outlets at the base. The top has a wide mouth with a lid on it so that distilled water can be poured into it. The vinyl Aquamatic K-pad (called K-pad for short) is attached to the coupling outlets at the base of the control unit. The water is heated and circulated through the unit and the pads in a manner similar to that of the hypothermia body unit. The pad is placed directly on the patient's injured area for a continuous heat treatment.

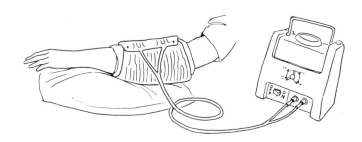

Important Steps	Key Points
1. Obtain the Aquamatic K-pad and control unit, and take it to the patient's bedside.	Bring it from the supply area (it will include the jarlike container, control unit, vinyl K-pad, and

Important Steps	Key Points
	bottle of distilled water), and place these articles on the patient's bedside stand.
2. Wash your hands; approach and identify the patient.	Explain what you will be doing.
3. Explain the task to the patient.	When you think he understands, proceed with the task.
4. Check the operation of the unit; set the temperature of 105°F.	The pad should feel warm within 1 to 2 minutes. This is a delicate instrument; be sure it is not dropped or bumped.
5. Place the pad on the patient's injured area.	Secure the pad with sheeting or a bath towel if necessary. Wrap it around the outside of the pad and the injured extremity firmly, evenly, and securely. Fasten it with a safety pin or tape. Be sure not to puncture the K-pad with a pin because the fluid will leak out. Be very careful when you use this pad for diabetics, infants, and patients who have circulatory problems. The temperature should never be set in the red area (105° to 115°F). If oxygen is used at the same time, keep it at least 3 feet from the unit to prevent possible fire or explosion from a spark generated by the electric motor.
6. Check the injured area at frequent intervals.	Note any increased or decreased swelling, redness, circulation, pain, or numbness. Record on the patient's chart as necessary.
7. Remove the equipment.	Remove the electric plug from the electric outlet in the room. *Do not yank or pull the cord; put your hand on the plug and pull the plug.* Unwrap and remove the sheeting and K-pad.
8. Take the equipment to a sink or utility area, and wash it with soap and water or a disinfectant solution.	*Do not immerse the electric jarlike unit in water. Do not autoclave it.*
9. Return the equipment to the supply area.	Return all the equipment to the supply area or to the proper storage place.
10. Leave the patient comfortable and safe.	Place the bedside stand, fresh water, and the call signal so that the patient can reach them. Adjust the bed to the low position and raise the siderails.
11. Record on the nurses' notes.	Charting example: 1930. K-pad applied to Rt. shoulder. States pain is relieved by heat. P. Shaw, SN.

To Refill and Adjust the K-pad

If you are required by your agency to make adjustments of the temperature setting or to refill the aquathermia unit, refer to the manufacturer's operating manual for instructions, or use the following steps as a guideline.

Important Steps	Key Points
1. Unscrew the reservoir cap on the top of the control unit.	All parts are easily visible. Review the equipment operations manual before proceeding. This unit works like the hypothermia machine except that the temperature equipment is applied to a local area for treatment.

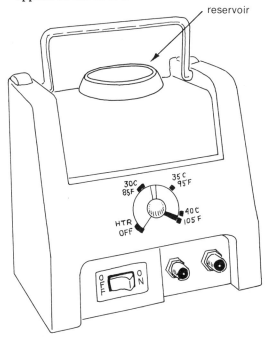

reservoir

2. Fill the unit 2/3 full with distilled water.

3. Tilt the control unit slowly from the side to let air bubbles escape.

4. Plug the unit into the electrical outlet.

Important Steps	Key Points
5. Fill the K-pad with water by sliding the switch on the right to the "on" position.	Allow it to run at least 2 minutes.
6. Switch the unit off and tilt the control unit again to let air bubbles escape.	
7. Refill the reservoir to the cap level.	
8. Replace the cap, but loosen it 1/4 turn.	
9. Set the desired temperature by inserting a special key into the center of the dial.	Turn the dial until the indicator points to the desired temperature on the dial. Keep the key attached to the machine for p.r.n. changes in temperature.

ITEM 3. ELECTRIC HEATING PAD

Important Steps	Key Points
1. Wash your hands; approach and identify the patient.	Explain what you will be doing.
2. Obtain the electric heating pad from the storage area.	The pad is usually made of rubber or plastic asbestos. If the patient's own personal electric pad is used, it must be checked by your agency maintenance department to assure that it meets agency safety standards.
3. Obtain a protective cover.	It should encase the entire pad.

Important Steps	Key Points
4. Check the pad. 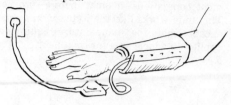 Heating pad.	Put the plug into an electric outlet. Turn the regulating button to "high" so that the heating mechanism can be checked. The pad should become hot immediately. *Caution*: Do not abuse electrical appliances or you will cause a dangerous short circuit that could result in fire or electrocution. *Do not use* heating pads if the cords are frayed, worn, or haphazardly repaired.
5. Take the electric pad to the patient's bedside.	Give a detailed explanation to the patient, stressing all the safety measures to observe while the electric pad is being used. Tell him that excess heat may lead to burns and that a protective covering prevents blistering of the skin.
6. Place the covered electric pad on the patient's injured area.	Turn the control button to *"low."* *A low degree of heat should always be used when the electric pad is used for the patient.* Immobilize the pad if necessary by using sheeting wrapped around the pad and the injured area firmly, securely, and with an even pressure.
7. Return to the patient at frequent intervals.	Check to see that the appliance is effective. Observe the skin area for increased or decreased redness, pain, or blood circulation. Remove the heating pad and report all unusual changes immediately to the charge nurse.
8. Remove the electric heating pad when the treatment is completed.	Place your hand on the *plug* and pull it from the electric outlet. Remove the protective cover from the heating pad and put it in the soiled laundry hamper or chute, or discard it into the wastebasket.
9. Leave the patient comfortable and safe.	Make sure that the call light and bedside stand are nearby.
10. Obtain the chart.	Record all pertinent information on the nurses' notes. Charting example: 1610. Electric heating pad applied at low temperature on anterior aspect of lower left leg. P. Shaw, SN

ITEM 4. APPLICATION OF THE HOT WATER BOTTLE

Hot water bottles may be used to provide heat to a localized area of the body. Care must be used to avoid using hot water that will cause a burn on the patient's skin. Patients with certain conditions such as emaciation, malnutrition, and circulatory problems are less able to tolerate warm water that may be comfortable to your skin. Some agencies may limit the use of hot water bottles for this reason. Given a patient with an inflamed area on the knee, apply a hot water bottle safely.

Important Steps	Key Points
1. Wash your hands; approach and identify the patient.	Explain the reason for using this treatment.

Important Steps	Key Points
2. Obtain the hot water bottle from the supply area.	The location may vary from agency to agency; it could be the Central Service, utility room, nurseserver or some other area.
3. Obtain the protective cover from the supply closet.	If a cover is not available, use a pillowcase. Some agencies use disposable protective covers so follow your agency procedure.
4. Fill the hot water bottle 1/3 to 1/2 full with hot water (some agencies recommend filling it 1/2 to 2/3).	Do not fill it so full that it is cumbersome and heavy. Lay the bottle on a flat surface and press on the outside to remove the excess air. Expel excess air until the water comes to the mouth of the water bottle, and then put on the screw-top (or clamp the bottle shut with special closure tab). Use a paper towel to wipe any water drops from the outside of the bottle. (Check for leakage; if leakage is evident, return the bottle to Central Service and obtain a new one.) Check the temperature of the bottle by placing it against the inner aspect of your forearm. If it feels comfortable to you, it will be safe and comfortable for the patient. Put the bottle in the flannel cover or the pillowcase. Fold the pillowcase around the bottle so that it appears as a neatly wrapped package. This will give added thickness to the cover and avoid an accidental burn to the patient.

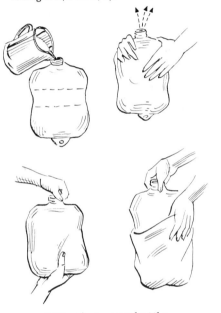

Filling hot water bottle.

5. Put the hot water bottle on the affected area.	Explain the importance of its use in relation to his injury or infection. Refer any questions that you are unable to answer to the charge nurse. To ensure effective immobilization, wrap a piece of sheeting or towel firmly and securely around the area. (Fasten the ends with safety pins or tape.)
6. Return to the patient at frequent intervals.	Check to see that the hot water bottle is effective. Observe the skin for an increase or decrease in redness, heat, swelling, pain, and blood circulation. As the treatment continues, empty the cool water from the bottle and refill it with hot water. (Repeat steps 4 through 7.)
7. Remove the hot water bottle.	When the treatment is completed, or if redness, swelling, or pain increases, report immediately to the charge nurse. Put the cover in the soiled laundry bag. Discard the disposable cover into the wastebasket.
8. Return the hot water bottle to the central processing department for cleaning.	Most agencies no longer clean equipment on the unit. If this is done in your agency, follow the procedure for cleaning the hot water bottle with germicidal solution.

U
N
I
T
27

Important Steps	Key Points
9. Return it to the proper storage place.	You may take it to Central Service or to the designated storage area on the unit.
10. Leave the patient comfortable and safe.	Make sure that he is settled in good body alignment. Raise the siderails if indicated. Attach the call signal within his reach. Arrange the bedside table for his convenience.
11. Record all pertinent information on the nurses' notes.	Charting example: 0900. Hot water bottle applied to right knee. J. Lang, SN

ITEM 5.   ADMINISTRATION OF A DISPOSABLE HOT PACK

The disposable hot pack eliminates the inconvenience of the reusable hot water bottle. Equally important advantages are that its one-time use reduces the probability of cross-infection, and that its scientifically controlled temperature minimizes the danger of burning the patient.

The lightweight hot pack is a prefilled plastic package containing an exact amount of interreacting ingredients that, when mixed by striking, squeezing, or kneading, produce a sustained temperature. Most of the manufacturers color-code the hot packs by using a red package.

The packages come in a variety of sizes and shapes. They are made to conform to the body contour (shape) when applied. Sizes range from 4½ to 11½ inches for perineal applications to 6¼ × 7½ inches and 7½ × 9½ inches for applications to reduce general swelling and pain. The temperature ranges from $101°F$ to $114°F$; the action lasts from 20 to 60 minutes, depending on the size of the pack and the manufacturer's instructions. You must therefore check the specific directions on the product used by your agency.

Like the cold packs, most of these hot packs are applied directly to the skin surface. If the package is punctured and the contents leak onto the patient's skin, wash the area thoroughly and quickly with water to remove the chemical from the skin. Dispose of the punctured bag and obtain a new pack.

Important Steps	Key Points
1. Obtain a hot pack from the storage area. 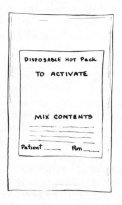	Select the size according to the body area to be treated (small or large). The prepared packet is a single-use, self-contained unit containing a precise amount of chemical compound and solution that, when mixed in the package, create a controlled heat.
2. Wash your hands.	
3. Approach and identify the patient.	Check his identification band. This step is particularly important here since heat treatments may be contraindicated for some conditions.

Important Steps	Key Points
4. Explain the procedure.	Gain the cooperation of the patient.
5. Mix the contents of the package.	This is done by a striking, squeezing, or kneading motion. The action breaks the internal chambers to permit the contents to mix. Knead until the chemical contents are mixed.

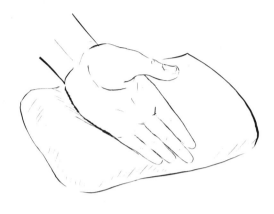

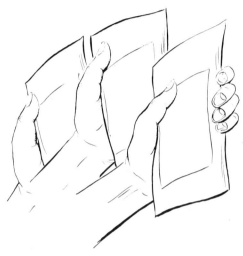

| 6. Apply the pack to the designated area. | The pack can be applied directly to the area of treatment, e.g., over an abscess on the inner aspect of the right arm. To ensure effective immobilization, wrap a piece of sheeting or towel firmly and securely around the area. (Fasten the ends with safety pins or tape.) |

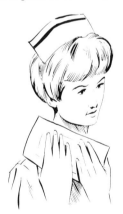

| 7. Return to the patient at frequent intervals. | See that the pack is producing heat. Observe the patient's skin for an increase or decrease in redness, swelling, pain, and blood circulation. The same general principles and safety precautions for using heat applications apply for this disposable pack as those you learned in the introduction to this unit. |

Important Steps	Key Points
8. Replace as needed.	The heat effect should be produced by the packet for 20 to 60 minutes. Dispose of the packet when it becomes cold. Replace it with a new one p.r.n.

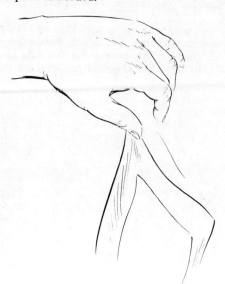

9. Record the treatment on the patient's chart.	Charting example: 1010. Disposable hot pack applied on the inner aspect of the right forearm. J. Lang, SN

ITEM 6.   HEAT CRADLE

The heat cradle is made of metal bands, soldered and shaped in a half-moon form like the cradle used to keep the bedding off the patient's legs. An electric socket with a cord is attached to the center top band at the highest point. A 25-watt electric bulb is used, and the heat from the bulb produces the warmth necessary for the treatment. When in use, the cradle is covered by a sheet or the top bedding so that the heat is kept within the area. The size of the cradle permits air to circulate, and there is no weight on the patient's body to cause discomfort. This method of heat application is generally used on the lower trunk and extremities to promote healing of wounds and to increase the circulation.

Important Steps	Key Points
1. Obtain the heat cradle from Central Service.	
2. Wash your hands; approach and identify the patient.	Explain what you plan to do.
3. Take the cradle to the patient's bedside and place it on the bed over the area requiring the treatment.	Pull the curtains around the bed to provide for privacy while setting up the heat cradle. Fold back the top covers, but avoid undue exposure of the patient. For heat treatment of the lower extremities, place the cradle over the feet and legs. Plug the cord into an outlet near the bed. Make sure that the cord does not droop or lie on the floor where someone may trip over it or pull the cradle off the bed. Turn on the light. Use only a 25-watt bulb.

Important Steps	Key Points
4. Prepare the patient for the treatment. 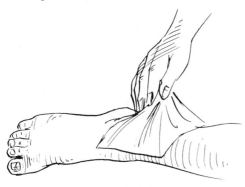 Check for dressing.	The heat cradle treatment may be ordered for a specified period of time or on a continuous basis. Check the physician's order for length of treatment. Also check the area for need of dressings. For dry heat and no dressings, the body part is exposed. If dry or moist dressings are required, apply them. Moist dressing should be wrapped with plastic sheeting and covered with a towel. Replace the top covers. *Make sure that the sheets do not come near or in direct contact with the light bulb.* The heat from the bulb could burn a hole in the sheets and start a fire. Position the patient in good alignment, and adjust the position of the bed for his comfort.
5. Return to the patient at frequent intervals.	Observe the condition of the skin, noting decreased or increased circulation, swelling, temperature, or pain. Note the condition of the dressings. It may be necessary to add saline (a weak salt solution) or water to keep the dressing moist. (Usually this is done with a basin of water and an irrigating syringe.) Leave the heat cradle in place for the *ordered* length of time.
6. Remove the cradle. 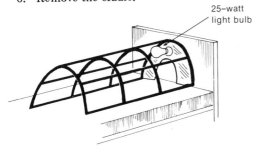 25–watt light bulb	If treatment is to be continued at intervals during the day, put the cradle in a safe place in the patient's room. *Do not* set it on the floor. Organisms from the floor could adhere to the cradle and become the source of a secondary infection to the patient.
7. Leave the patient comfortable and safe.	Offer the bedpan/urinal. Adjust the bed and siderails. Attach call light within easy reach. Position the patient in good body alignment.
8. Wash, rinse, and dry the cradle per agency procedure when the treatment is completed, and return it to Central Service for cleaning and storage.	
9. Record all pertinent information in the nurses' notes.	Include the time, duration, type of treatment, and results. Charting example: 1900. Heat cradle applied to legs for 30 minutes. P. Shaw, SN 1930. Heat cradle removed. Skin looks pink, swelling and pain have decreased. P. Shaw, SN

U
N
I
T
27

ITEM 7. ADMINISTRATION OF A DISPOSABLE COLD PACK

The disposable lightweight cold pack is a prefilled plastic package containing an exact amount of interreacting ingredients. When these ingredients are mixed by striking, squeezing, or kneading (depending on the manufacturer's instructions), they produce a sustained, controlled temperature. Most of the manufacturers color-code the cold packs by use of a blue package.

The packages are manufactured in many sizes and shapes, and conform readily to the body contour when applied. Sizes range from 4½ × 11 inches for tonsillectomies or perineal packs to 6¼ × 7½ inches for small areas needed for emergency room treatment of burns, sprains, epistaxis, fractures, etc. The larger pack (7½ × 9 inches) can be used to reduce swelling in IV infiltrations, following dental extractions, and postoperatively to reduce swelling at a surgical site.

The temperature of these packs ranges from 50°F to 80°F. Because of the controlled temperature, there is almost no possibility of a freeze burn to the patient. The action lasts from 30 minutes to 4 hours, depending on the size of the pack and the specific product used. Therefore, extreme caution must be taken to *read* the directions for the product used in your agency. There are variations in size, temperature control, length of action, and method used to initiate the reacting ingredients.

Some cold packs may be reused by placing them in the freezer section of the refrigerator. However, disposable packs are generally designed for one-time use.

Most of the packs are intended to be applied directly to the skin surface. The outer covering of the pack is a special material that absorbs perspiration and prevents the cold, damp feel of plastic. Again, there may be a slight variation in this procedure, depending on the manufacturer.

The fact that the pack is usually meant for one-time use serves to prevent cross-infection. If the pack is punctured and the contents leak out, thoroughly and quickly wash the patient's skin with water to remove any of the harmful chemical ingredients. Dispose of the punctured bag and replace it with a new pack.

Important Steps	Key Points
1. Obtain the cold pack from the storage area. 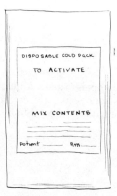	Select the size according to the patient's needs (the area to be treated, small or large). The prepared package is a single-use, self-contained unit that contains a combination of precise ingredients within an insulated wrap that delivers a controlled cold temperature after being altered by a special procedure.
2. Wash your hands.	
3. Approach and identify the patient.	Check his identification band to assure that you are treating the right patient. Cold applications may be contraindicated in some conditions.
4. Explain the procedure.	This is done to gain the patient's cooperation and to keep him from being apprehensive.
5. Mix the contents of the package.	This is done by striking, squeezing, or kneading the package. (The method varies, depending on

Important Steps   **Key Points**

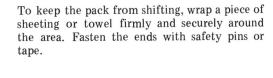

the specific manufacturer's product used in your agency.) The force will break the internal chambers and cause the chemicals to mix and create the cold temperature. Make sure that the chemical contents are well-mixed.

6. Apply the package directly to the designated area.

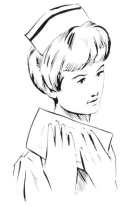

To keep the pack from shifting, wrap a piece of sheeting or towel firmly and securely around the area. Fasten the ends with safety pins or tape.

7. Return to the patient frequently.

Check to see that the cold pack is working properly. Observe the patient's skin for an increase or decrease in redness, swelling, pain, or blood circulation. The general principles for use and safety for cold applications should be followed for this disposable pack. (Report all apparent changes immediately to the charge nurse.)

Important Steps	Key Points
8. Replace the cold pack as needed.	The cold effect should continue for 30 minutes to 4 hours, depending on the size of the pack and its manufacturer. Dispose of the pack in a waste container when it becomes warm.

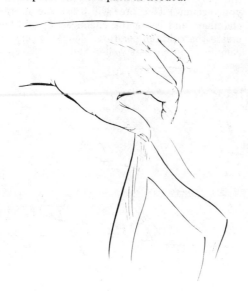

Important Steps	Key Points
9. Record the treatment.	Charting example: 0210. Cold pack applied to perineum. <div align="right">P. Shaw, SN</div>

ITEM 8.   ICE BAG OR ICE COLLAR

Another common method used for the local application of cold is the reusable ice bag or ice collar. Made of rubber or plastic, they can be filled with ice.

Some agencies have ice bags that are pneumatically sealed with a liquid solution inside. They are stored in the freezing unit of a special refrigerator. When the ice melts, the ice bag is returned to the refrigerator for refreezing.

Important Steps	Key Points
1. Wash your hands; identify the patient.	Explain what you are going to do.
2. Obtain the ice bag from storage area.	Select the appropriate size of the pneumatically sealed or open-necked vinyl-covered ice bag.
3. Obtain a protective cover from the storage area.	If a cover is not available, use a pillowcase (some agencies use disposable covers).
4. Take the open-necked vinyl-covered ice bag to the utility working area. 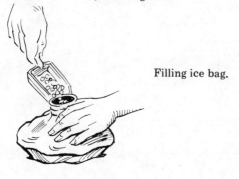 Filling ice bag.	Get a pan of ice cubes or crushed ice from the ice maker. Many hospitals have an ice machine either on the unit or in a centrally located area. If you use ice cubes, make sure that the edges of the cubes are not sharp. If sharp-edged ice is used, it may puncture the ice bag. Fill the ice bag 3/4 full. Lay it on a flat surface and press on the outside to expel the air from it, so that the bag will be flexible and will easily fit the contour of the affected area. Seal or close the bag. Water may cling to the outside of the bag; use paper towels to wipe it off. Check the bag for leakage. (If there is a leak, return the bag to

Important Steps

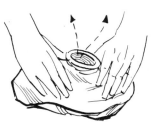

Expressing air from bag.

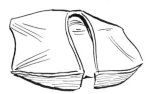

Ice bag with cover.

Key Points

the supply room for repair, and obtain a new one.) Wrap the bag with the special cover; this is done to protect the patient's skin. When the ice melts, droplets of water appear on the outside of the bag. If the bag is wrapped in a plastic cover, the cloth cover underneath will not become wet.

5. Take the ice bag to the patient and put it on the affected area.

Explain the importance of its use for his injury or infection. Refer questions that you are unable to answer to the charge nurse. To ensure that the bag will remain in place, wrap a piece of sheeting or towel firmly and securely around the area, and fasten the ends with safety pins or tape.

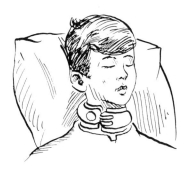

Ice collar.

6. Return to the patient at frequent intervals.

Check to see if the ice bag is effective. Observe the skin area for increased or decreased redness, swelling, pain, numbness, and blood circulation. Report all unusual changes in the patient's condition immediately to the charge nurse.

7. Remove the ice bag when the treatment is completed or if the skin becomes more red or painful.

Put the linen cover in the soiled laundry hamper (or down the linen chute). Discard the plastic and disposable covers in the wastebasket.

8. Wash, rinse, and dry the ice bag, or return it to the central processing room.

If you must clean the ice bag on your unit, follow your agency procedure for cleaning, disinfecting, drying, and then returning it to storage.

9. Leave the patient comfortable and safe.

Remember the safe, comfortable bed positions. Raise the siderails if indicated. Attach the call signal within reach. Leave the bedside stand conveniently close.

Important Steps	Key Points
10. Obtain the chart.	Record all pertinent information on the nurses' notes. Charting example: 1100. Ice collar applied to throat. J. Lang, SN

ITEM 9. HYPOTHERMIA AND HYPERTHERMIA TREATMENT (FULL-BODY)

Hypothermia, or the lowering of body temperature below the normal range, is a useful technique to decrease the rate of metabolic processes in the body. It is used to reduce high fevers, to control gastrointestinal hemorrhages, and to prevent cerebral edema (swelling of the brain) in head injuries or surgeries, and for certain types of surgery. Usually the body temperature is reduced only a few degrees by cooling the body surface, but for surgical operations it may be reduced to $25°C$ ($77°F$) or even lower. Cooling may be achieved by cooling the body surface, or by cooling the blood directly.

Hyperthermia may be used to increase the body temperature after it has been lowered by hypothermia. It may also be used to increase the metabolic rate in the body.

The Aquamatic K Thermia Machine, a refrigerated unit with cooling blankets (or pads) attached to it, is used to raise or lower body temperature in a safe, simple, but precise manner. It controls body temperature in neurological (nervous system), cardiovascular (heart and circulatory), and thoracic (chest) surgical procedures. It is also used as a quick means to lower and regulate fevers or high temperatures due to infections, and postoperative and traumatic conditions. It is both a labor- and time-saving device in caring for adult and child patients.

The machine, an electronically controlled freezing and heating unit, contains a 20 per cent ethyl alcohol and distilled water solution. This solution circulates through the freezing or heating unit to produce the desired temperature (automatic or manually operated). The hollow, cordlike vinyl Aquamatic K-pads, containing the circulating solution, are placed in direct contact with the patient's skin to maintain the body temperature at the desired degree.

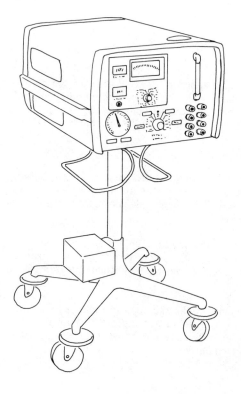

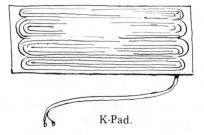

K-Pad.

To Initiate Use of Hypothermia Machine

Important Steps	Key Points
1. Obtain the Aquamatic K Thermia Machine and take it to the patient's bedside.	Bring the equipment from the supply area, including all its parts: the main refrigeration unit on a stand, the temperature control box, the thermistor probe, a gallon of 20 per cent ethyl alcohol and distilled water solution, vinyl body-sized or small-sized K-pads, and the manufacturer's complete instructional manual. (Size will depend on usage, the size of the patient, and the area to be treated.)
2. Wash your hands; approach and identify the patient.	Explain the procedure to him.
3. Prepare the unit.	
a. Plug the electric cord into a wall outlet.	All Roman numerals in the following instructions refer to the two sets of sketches appearing on the next two pages.
b. Select the number and size of K-pads to be used.	This depends on the size of the patient and whether treatment is local or general.
c. Attach the pads to the unit (I).	There are eight plugs for the pads clearly marked on the machine. Protective couplings remain on any plug not used. Coupling caps may or may not dangle on a chain when not attached to outlets, depending on the model.

U
N
I
T
27

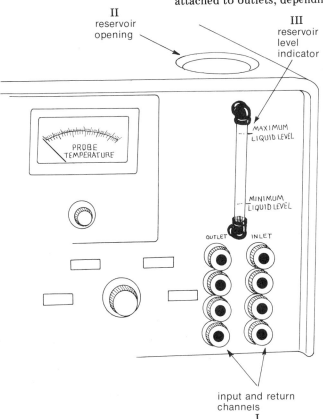

Couplings and plugs of machine.

Important Steps	Key Points
d. Fill tne reservoir (II) with distilled water and denatured alcohol. (Remove the cap on top of the machine before filling.)	See your equipment operating instructions; there are minor variations among manufacturers.
e. Observe the reservoir level indicator (III) as a guide to how much fluid is needed, and fill it at least half full.	
f. Turn on the pump by setting the cool and heat dials at 80° F (IV).	This will pump fluid from the reservoir into the pads.
g. After a few minutes, check the reservoir level indicator (III).	More fluid may be added because some was used in filling the pads.

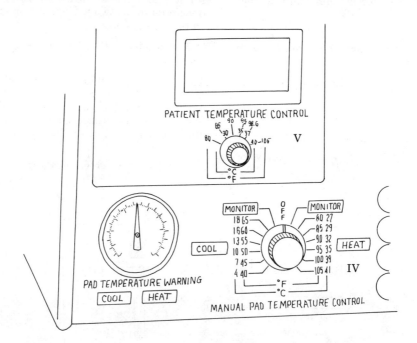

h. Turn off the pump before adding fluid.	It may be necessary to turn the machine off and on several times until the pads are filled.
i. Tighten reservoir cap (II) when the pump is turned off.	Loosen the reservoir cap (II) 1/4 of a turn when the pump is running to prevent a vacuum from developing.
j. To cool the water, set the "Cool" dial to the desired temperature.	The blanket temperature will be adjusted from 40° to 50°F, initially, then adjusted to the patient's temperature. Remember, this 40° to 50°F is the temperature in the blanket, not the patient's temperature.
	Note: The patient's body can be warmed and his body temperature raised. Set the "Heat" dial to the desired temperature.

Important Steps	Key Points

4. Place the pads on the patient (for fullbody cooling).

   a. Put one body-sized vinyl pad under the patient so that the pad comes in direct skin and body contact.

Some agencies may recommend placing a sheet between the pad and the patient's skin. Check your agency procedure.

   b. As you remove the patient's gown, put the second body-sized vinyl pad on top of the patient.

Be sure to keep him covered with a blanket or the top bedding to protect his modesty.

   c. Do not expose the patient unnecessarily.

   d. Put a sheet over the top of the patient and the pad.

This will prevent the cooled or heated air from escaping.

   e. Optimum body temperature control is maintained by having as much of the body covered with the pads as possible.

Once the patient is on the cooling blankets, his temperature will begin to drop. It may take several hours to reduce the temperature as low as necessary; the doctor prescribes the temperature he wants and the length of time the temperature is to remain at that level. Check the reservoir fluid level frequently. Refill p.r.n.

5. Attach the thermometer unit to the hypothermia unit at the marked connection.

The thermometer unit may be separate from the hypothermia unit. Check your agency equipment. Remove the thermistor probe from its plastic container. Insert the thermistor probe into the appropriate outlet in the control box shown below.

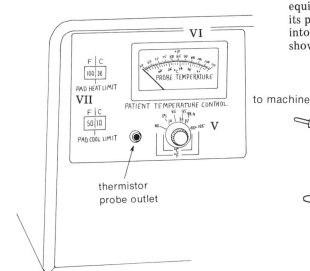

to machine

Temperature control unit.

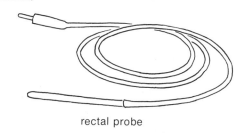

rectal probe

Thermistor probe.

6. Place the thermistor probe into the patient.

Insert the free end of the thermistor probe into the patient's rectum. (It is most often used rectally, but check with the physician for the proper place of insertion.) *Remember, the thermometer machine will not work if the probe is not in the patient.* (The continuous, automatic temperature of the patient is recorded on the patient temperature indicator scale shown above [VI].)

Important Steps	Key Points
7. Set the dial (see VII in foregoing sketch) for temperature limits between 40° and 100°F.	
8. Set the automatic temperature control (V in the sketch) at the desired temperature for the patient.	When the unit is working, the indicator light will go on. The electronic control device will automatically provide the heating and cooling control within the safety limits set on the temperature dial. The patient's temperature is indicated by the patient temperature indicator scale (VI). Check the patient's skin condition at frequent intervals. Observe for circulation problems: increase or decrease in redness, numbness, swelling, or pain. If the patient's temperature must be reduced more rapidly than the machine alone can do it, place an alcohol-soaked sheet between the patient and the top vinyl pad, and the cooling process will then speed up. Place the small K-pads in specific arterial areas of the body, such as the groin, armpits, and neck.
9. Ensure safety.	
a. Keep the 20 per cent alcohol and distilled water mixture above the minimal level on the gauge.	Check the liquid level gauge at frequent intervals. (Refer to equipment manual for specifics.)
b. Keep the unit on a stand in an open area so that air in and around the unit circulates freely.	
c. If oxygen is used, keep it at least 3 feet away from the unit.	
d. Use heavy extension cords.	
e. Remember that other electrical appliances may cause interference.	Refer to the manufacturer's instruction manual for other safety factors.
f. Keep the patient from shivering during the cooling process.	Report any shivering to the team leader or nurse in charge. The shivering action increases the metabolic rate, which produces heat. Shivering can be controlled by various medications. Charting example: 2330. Placed on hypothermia pad for full-body cooling. Machine set at 60°F. T 103.4, P 112, R 24. No shivering. P. Shaw, SN

To Remove the Hypothermia/Hyperthermia Equipment

Important Steps	Key Points
1. Remove the electric cord plug from the room outlet.	
2. Remove the thermistor probe from the patient and wipe it clean with a tissue and an appropriate germicidal solution.	
3. Disconnect the thermistor probe plug from the unit.	Put it in a safe place, to be returned with the rest of the equipment to the storage area for

Important Steps	Key Points

cleaning. These probes are frequently lost in the linens. They are costly, so be careful.

4. Disconnect the vinyl pads from the coupling outlets in the unit.

5. Replace the caps to the coupling outlets in the unit.

6. Remove the pads from the patient.

7. Take the equipment to a sink or utility area, and wash it with soap and water or a germicidal solution, or return it to the central processing area for cleaning and storage.

Return *all* the equipment to the supply area or the proper storage place. Be sure that all parts of the hypothermia unit are returned. This is an expensive piece of equipment that will not operate effectively without all of its parts.

8. Leave the patient comfortable and safe.

Place the bedside stand, fresh water (if permitted), and call signal within easy reach. Adjust the bed to the low position and raise the siderails. Remember: Utilize proper body alignment and movement for yourself and the patient. Provide for the general comfort of the patient. Take and record his vital signs frequently. If the patient has an indwelling catheter, record an accurate I & O. Reassure the patient by your quiet presence, conversation, and gentle touch.

10. Obtain the patient's chart.

Record all pertinent information concerning this task in the nurses' notes; include the time treatment ended, the vital signs, and the patient's general condition. Charting example:

2330. Hypothermia unit removed. Patient comfortable and quiet. Temperature $97°$F.

P. Shaw, SN

UNIT 27

CONCLUSION OF THE UNIT

You have now concluded the lesson on Hot and Cold Applications. When you have practiced the procedures so that you know them, arrange with your instructor to take the post-tests. You will be expected to demonstrate your skills in carrying out the required tasks, as well as knowledge of the effects of heat and cold on the body.

VI. ADDITIONAL INFORMATION FOR ENRICHMENT

Other types of heat appliances that may be used are the ultraviolet and infrared lamps. Usually these treatments are given by the physical therapy staff, but you should know about them. The ultraviolet lamp projects heat rays and produces some chemical reactions that inhibit the growth of bacteria; it is also used for the heat it produces. The ultraviolet light seems to be effective in stopping rickets (a vitamin D deficiency disease).

The infrared lamp projects invisible heat rays beyond the red end of the light spectrum. The wavelength is below 477 billion vibrations per second, or longer than those at the other end of the spectrum. These rays are readily absorbed by the tissues. Infrared lamps are used for the relief of pain caused by arthritis and rheumatic conditions. Other heat sources are the sun, the electric arc, and the incandescent lamp.

Use of these two types of lamps is usually reserved for the professional health workers in the physical therapy department. Great caution must be observed when these lamps are used and the patient must be under constant supervision to avoid severe burns. The heat rays from the lamps are like the rays of the sun, but the heating method is subtle (quietly active) because the light rays convert to heat in the tissue.

Like sun rays, the lamps act on the skin and tissue. If you have experienced a sunburn, you can understand the possible dangers from these lamps. When the ultraviolet lamp is used, specially fitted dark glasses or protective eye coverings are worn by the patient to protect his eyes, particularly the cornea. When the light rays turn to heat rays, the corneal tissue could be destroyed. (The eye tissue would be coagulated like the white of an egg when it is cooked.)

The lamps can be and are used for superficial and deep heat therapy under the supervision of the physical therapist. If the patient is overexposed to the lamp rays, tissue damage can be extreme — a third-degree burn will result. The skin area first becomes red, blistered, swollen, and burned so that the tissue eventually sloughs off. When this happens, there is danger of a systemic (general, throughout body) infection and an electrolyte imbalance due to the loss of fluid through the open wound. Symptoms to be noted accompanying the burn are nausea, headache, vomiting, and possible kidney malfunctions (anuria). For these reasons, the lamps are used only in the physical therapy department or by specially trained personnel.

Several precautions must be taken when one gives these treatments:

1. Apply to the local area only.

2. Observe the time elements very rigidly. The time of the treatment may be as limited as 1 to 2 minutes.

3. Know the heat method you are using, its expected results, and the complications that could arise from improper use.

4. Follow directions explicitly for applying the procedure (time, location, distance from light to skin surface).

5. Stay with the patient and observe his reactions closely.

PERFORMANCE TEST

In the classroom or your skill laboratory, your instructor will ask you to perform the following activities without reference to any source material. You will need the mannequin or another student to take the part of the patient.

1. Given a patient who has a swollen, stiff, and painful right shoulder, apply a hot water bottle (or disposable hot pack) to the part without danger of burning the patient even if the bottle should leak or break.

2. Given a patient with a circulatory disease of both legs, apply a heat cradle that will be used indefinitely in a manner that will provide for his comfort and safety.

3. Given a patient who has just had his tonsils removed, apply an ice collar (or disposable cold pack) to his throat in a manner that will provide for his comfort and safety.

4. Given a patient who is suspected to have cerebral edema (swelling of the brain), set up the hypothermia machine to control his body temperature at $95°$ F.

U
N
I
T
27

If the machine is not available in your agency, describe the steps of the procedure that you would use.

PERFORMANCE CHECKLIST

ASSISTING WITH HOT AND COLD APPLICATIONS

APPLICATION OF A HOT WATER BOTTLE TO THE RIGHT SHOULDER

1. Wash your hands.
2. Approach and identify the patient.
3. Obtain a hot water bottle and cover from storage.
4. Fill the hot water bottle 1/3 to 1/2 full with hot water.
5. Expel the excess air from the bottle before securing the top.
6. Test the temperature of the bottle against the inner aspect of your arm.
7. Put a cover on the bottle.
8. Take the hot water bottle to the patient and explain why it is being used.
9. Place the bottle snugly against the patient's right shoulder.
10. Make sure that the patient is comfortable.
11. Record pertinent information on the patient's chart.

USE OF A HEAT CRADLE OVER THE EXTREMITIES

1. Wash your hands.
2. Approach and identify the patient.
3. Obtain a heat cradle and bring it to the bedside.
4. Provide for the patient's privacy by pulling the curtain.

5. Fold back the top covers without undue exposure of the patient.

6. Place the heat cradle over the patient's legs.

7. Plug in the cord and turn on the light.

8. Check the wattage of the light, and the length and position of the cord.

9. Inspect the patient's legs for need of dressings.

10. Replace the top covers over the heat cradle but away from the light itself.

11. Position the patient in good alignment.

12. Adjust the bed for the patient's comfort.

13. Tell the patient that he will be checked at frequent intervals.

14. Record all pertinent information on the patient's chart.

APPLICATION OF ICE COLLAR TO THE THROAT

1. Wash your hands

2. Approach and identify the patient.

3. Obtain an ice collar and cover from storage.

4. If a freeze pack is available, put a cover on it, or fill the ice pack about 3/4 full with ice.

5. Expel air from the pack and wipe the outside dry after closing the top.

6. Wrap the ice collar in a cover or towel.

7. Apply the ice collar securely to the patient's throat.

8. Inform the patient that the pack will be checked frequently.

9. Make sure that the patient is comfortable.

10. Record all pertinent information on the patient's chart.

SET UP HYPOTHERMIA MACHINE AND CONTROL TEMPERATURE OF 95°F

1. Wash your hands.

2. Approach and identify the patient, and explain the procedure.

3. Obtain a hypothermia machine with all its parts and take it to the bedside.

4. Prepare the hypothermia unit:

    a. Plug in the cord.

    b. Select two large K-pads and attach them to the unit.

    c. Fill the reservoir with fluid.

    d. Then turn the machine on by turning the temperature dial to 80°F.

    e. Turn the machine off before adding more fluids.

    f. Tighten the cap on the reservoir.

    g. Set the dial between 40° and 50°F for the pad cooling limit and 100° for the pad heating limit.

5. Prepare the patient:

    a. Place one large K-pad under the patient.

    b. Place a second large K-pad over him, and remove his gown.

    c. Place a sheet over the upper pad on the patient.

6. Attach a thermometer unit to the hypothermia unit.

7. Insert the thermistor probe into the patient's rectum.

8. Set the desired temperature of 95°F on the patient temperature control.

9. Provide for the patient's comfort and report any shivering.

10. Inform the patient that his temperature and the adjustment of the blanket temperature will be checked frequently.

11. Record all pertinent information on the patient's chart.

POST-TEST

Multiple Choice: Select the best answer for each of the questions and place an X before your choice.

1. A local application of heat to the upper back would cause:

_____ a. a numbness or loss of sensation

_____ b. a bluish, mottled color of the skin

_____ c. dilation of blood vessels elsewhere in the body

_____ d. increased circulation of blood in the area

2. Metabolism and growth of new cells are stimulated by:

_____ a. oxygen

_____ b. cold

_____ c. heat

_____ d. light

3. A hot water bottle is filled only 1/3 to 1/2 in order to:

_____ a. make the bottle lighter and less cumbersome to use

_____ b. keep it from getting too hot and burning the patient

_____ c. assure that it is refilled frequently as it cools

_____ d. make it easier to expel the air from the bottle

4. Heat makes the blood vessels:

_____ a. dilate

_____ b. contract

_____ c. increase

_____ d. decrease

5. Hypothermia can be defined as:

_____ a. decreased blood supply to a part of the body

_____ b. a decrease in the temperature of the blood

_____ c. an increase in the temperature of the body

_____ d. freezing of a part or all of the body

6. Infrared and ultraviolet lamps are used under the supervision of the physical therapist because:

_____ a. heat from the light rays produced can cause serious burns

_____ b. someone must observe the patient frequently

_____ c. the rays can coagulate albumin, or the white of an egg

_____ d. the lamps must be a certain distance from the patient's skin

7. A patient can tolerate the dry cold of an ice bag for a longer period of time than a local bath of ice-cold water because:

_____ a. the nerve endings are numbed by the ice bag

_____ b. the intensity of dry cold is greater than wet cold

_____ c. dry cold reduces the contraction of muscles

_____ d. water is a better conductor of cold than air

8. The temperature indicated by the "Cool" dial or button (IV) on the hypothermia machine is used to regulate the temperature of:

_____ a. the fluid in the reservoir

_____ b. the patient's body

_____ c. the fluid in the K-pads

_____ d. the air in the room

9. When you are working with electrical equipment, such as the electric heating pad or the hypothermia machines, you should always avoid:

_____ a. using the equipment when oxygen is being used in the same room

_____ b. touching the controls without an order from the doctor

_____ c. using a cover between the electrical pad or machine and the patient's skin

_____ d. plugging the cord into an outlet with wet hands

10. A cold application causes which of the following effects:

_____ a. an increase in the metabolic rate of the body

_____ b. a decrease in the blood supply to the area

_____ c. a reduction in excess tissue fluid, or swelling

_____ d. more rapid removal of toxins and waste products

POST-TEST ANNOTATED ANSWER SHEET

1. d. (p. 574)
2. c. (p. 574)
3. a. (p. 581)
4. a. (p. 574)
5. b. (p. 575)

6. a. (p. 596)
7. d. (p. 575)
8. c. (p. 592)
9. d. (p. 577)
10. b. (p. 574)

Unit 28

PATIENT TURNING FRAMES

I. DIRECTIONS TO THE STUDENT

Proceed through this unit using the workbook as your guide. You will need to practice setting up and operating various patient turning frames in the classroom or the skill laboratory, using the mannequin (Mrs. Chase) or a student partner in the role of the patient. After you have completed the lesson and your practice of the procedures, arrange with your instructor to take the performance test.

For this unit you will need the following items:

1. Foster or Stryker turning frame and accessory parts.

2. Circ-O-lectric bed and accessory parts.

3. Sheets, bath blanket, and safety pins.

Please read the following paragraphs carefully. They will tell you what you will be expected to know and how you will be expected to set up and operate the turning frames in order to care for the patient. If you feel that you have the necessary skills, discuss this with your instructor and arrange to take the performance test. All students are expected to demonstrate their skill in setting up and operating the turning frames safely and efficiently.

II. GENERAL PERFORMANCE OBJECTIVE

Upon completion of this unit, you will be able to set and operate the Circ-O-lectric bed and the Foster or Stryker turning frame correctly, efficiently, and safely.

III. SPECIFIC PERFORMANCE OBJECTIVES

When you have finished this lesson, you will be able to:

1. Set up a Stryker (or Foster) frame and assist in transferring the patient onto the frame in an accurate, efficient, and safe manner without causing additional apprehension or injury to the patient.

2. Turn the patient on a Stryker (or Foster) frame from the supine to the prone position with the use of the anterior frame so that the patient is held securely and safely during the movement.

3. Set up and operate the Circ-O-lectric bed and assist in transferring the patient onto the bed in an accurate, efficient, and safe manner that does not cause additional apprehension or injury to the patient.

4. Operate the Circ-O-lectric bed correctly and rotate the patient from a supine to a vertical standing position and then to a prone position, using the anterior frame so that the patient is held securely and safely during the movement.

IV. VOCABULARY

immobilize—to secure or fix a part of the body so that it cannot move.

orthopedics—the prevention or correction of deformities and the treatment of diseases of the bones and joints.

paraplegia—paralysis of the lower portion of the body and both legs.

perineal—refers to the perineum, located between the vulva and the anus of the female, and between the scrotum and the anus of the male.

pubis—the lower anterior part of the innominate bone in the pelvis.

quadriplegia—paralysis of all four extremities (arms and legs).

vertigo—dizziness.

INTRODUCTION TO SPECIAL TURNING FRAMES

In the hospital, certain patients with orthopedic conditions (disease, surgery, or fracture of bones or joints) must be kept immobilized in order that healing may take place. Other patients may be immobilized or unable to move because of their disease or physical condition. For example, the patient with a fracture or injury to his spinal column may need to be immobilized so that his spine can heal. At the same time, the patient needs to change position at frequent intervals to relieve pressure, to promote circulation, and to make himself comfortable. As you know, any position that is maintained for a long time becomes unbearable. In order to maintain the immobilization of part of the patient's body and yet provide for turning, various types of turning frames or beds may be used. The more common types that you may see or use are the Stryker frame, the Foster frame, or the Circ-O-lectric bed.

Patients who may need to use these special turning frames include those who have paraplegia, quadriplegia, spinal fusion, multiple fractures of the spine or long bones, acute arthritis, severe dermatitis, genitourinary disorders, and other diseases that cause immobility or paralysis.

In this unit, you will become familiar with the various types of turning frames, and the way to set them up and operate them in order to provide care for the patient.

ITEM 1.   THE PSYCHOLOGICAL NEEDS OF THE IMMOBILIZED PATIENT

How would you feel if you were unable to turn yourself and had to be confined to a narrow bed for days, weeks, or even longer? How, do you think, might you express your feelings, and what would these emotions be? What fears, do you think, might you have? The immobilized patient has many apprehensions in addition to his great need for physical care. His behavior and his willingness to cooperate in the treatment are related to the manner in which his psychological needs are met, as well as to the physical care that he receives. Let's consider some of these psychological needs.

He has a need to express his feelings. The immobilized patient should be encouraged to discuss his immobilization and how it affects him. He must have someone to listen to him. His emotional response can be varied — ranging from fear, anger, and hostility to depression or withdrawal. When the patient expresses his emotions, you should accept his right to do so and yet not take this expression personally, even when it seems to be directed toward you.

The patient has a need to know. He should be told the reason for the use of the equipment. It is no longer adequate to say that it has been ordered by the doctor or some other authority figure; people want to know "why" as well. Just because we know that a treatment is beneficial or good for a patient does not mean that he knows it or is willing to accept our word for it. The patient must understand why a turning frame is being used for him. Some of these reasons might be as follows:

U
N
I
T
28

1. To change his position at frequent intervals with minimum pain or discomfort.

2. To relieve pressure on parts of his body.

3. To increase his circulation.

4. To maintain the immobility of the affected part so that healing can occur.

5. To increase his comfort, well-being, and activities.

He must be considered as a whole person. Even though he may be greatly restricted in his physical activities and dependent on others for his care, his mind is usually not impaired. He should be encouraged to use his intellectual abilities. He is not just a body lying on a turning frame, but a person who belongs to a family and to a community, and who has a purpose in life.

He also needs safety and protection. The immobilized patient must be sure that those who care for him know how to use the equipment correctly and safely. His apprehension and fear for his own safety are greatly increased by the fumbling and groping of workers who do not know how to operate the turning frames.

And finally, the patient has a need to make decisions, to determine what is to happen to him. He even has the right to refuse to be put on the turning frame. Whenever possible, the patient should be involved in planning for his care and allowed to make decisions about many things, such as the time of his bath, the foods he wants to eat, his bedtime, and other activities within allowable and recognized boundaries.

The psychological needs of the immobilized patient or the patient who may have to use a turning frame, are very important. Usually this patient has a serious injury or illness that might leave him greatly impaired and that requires a longer period of hospitalization than that required for most other patients. So, in addition to knowing how to set up and operate the equipment, you should understand how the patient might respond to these activities.

ITEM 2.   THE STRYKER FRAME AND THE FOSTER FRAME

The Stryker frame consists of a canvas-covered frame on which the patient lies. It is attached to a metal frame on wheels. The canvas-covered frame is connected at a pivot joint, so that the entire frame turns when the patient is turned from his back to his abdomen and vice versa. When turning the patient, a second canvas-covered frame is placed on top of the patient and the two frames are secured with the patient between them like a sandwich. Safety belts are used to hold them together.

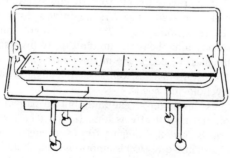

Stryker frame.

The posterior frame on which the patient lies when he is in a supine position is prepared by covering it with canvas sections: one that extends from the top of the frame to the pubis, a small middle section that can be removed for the use of the bedpan, and one that extends from mid-thigh to the foot end of the frame. The canvas sections are covered with folded bath towels and drawsheets, which are pinned on the underside.

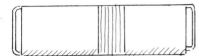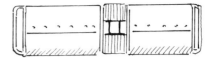

Preparation of turning frame.

The anterior frame is usually prepared in a similar manner except that one section extends from the shoulders to the pubis in order to allow space for the head. A narrow section is used to support the forehead. The lower section extends only to the ankles so that the feet can be properly aligned when the patient is lying on his abdomen.

With the patient strapped securely between the anterior and posterior frames, one nurse can safely turn the patient in the Stryker frame by loosening a spring lock at either end of the frame. The frame will automatically trip the lock when it is turned, and again be locked in place. After the patient has been turned, the upper frame is removed. Armrests can be attached to the sides of the frame when the patient is in a prone position. The sketch below shows the patient being turned to and in a prone position.

When the bedpan is needed, the small canvas section across the middle of the frame is detached and the bedpan is placed as shown in the bottom illustration.

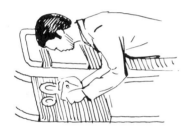

Patient in prone position.

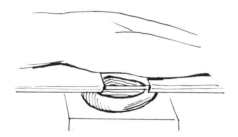

Perineal section
detached for bedpan use.

The fracture pan can be used for elimination if the lifting of the patient's hips is not contraindicated. (Refer to the unit on Urine Elimination.)

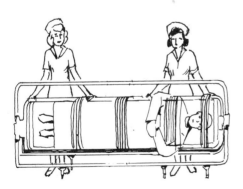

Turning patient.

The Foster frame is similar to the Stryker frame except that it is bigger, more stable, and more expensive. It is used for the same purposes and the procedure for setting it up and operating it is almost the same as for the Stryker frame.

U
N
I
T
28

*ITEM 3.   PROCEDURE FOR SETTING UP AND USING THE STRYKER
              FRAME*

Important Steps	Key Points
1. Obtain the frame.	It is usually kept in a supply area, and personnel from that area are usually responsible for assembling the equipment and bringing it to the patient's room.
2. Check to see that you have all the parts.	You should have the following parts:

a. basic frame

b. anterior and posterior frames

c. four long-stem pins

d. canvas sections: two long, two short, and two narrow

e. sponge pads: two long, two short, two narrow, two shoulder pads, and one abdominal pad

f. footboard and two armrests

g. tray table

h. bedpan support

i. two safety straps (webbed) with airplane buckles

j. forehead strap or face mask

k. cover for forehead strap or face mask

l. spring clamps

m. covers for sponge pads, or linen and safety pins to secure it

Important Steps	Key Points
3. Prepare the posterior frame.	
a. Attach the canvas sections across the posterior frame and secure them with spring clamps.	Measure the canvas sections to fit the patient and fold the unneeded portion underneath.
	Top section—from the top of patient's head to the pubis.
	Middle section—(perineal section) from the pubis to the upper third of the thigh.
	Lower section—from the upper third of the thigh to the bottom of the frame.
b. Place sponge pads on the canvas sections and cover them with bath blankets or sheets.	Make sure that all ends of the linen coverings are secured (pinned) so they won't catch or interfere when the frame is turned.
c. Place the posterior frame on the basic frame.	Tightly latch or screw the nuts in place at the pivoting joint.
d. Attach the footboard in the slat at the bottom of the posterior frame.	
4. Take the Stryker frame and its parts to the patient's room.	
5. Wash your hands.	

Important Steps	Key Points
6. Approach and identify the patient, explain what is to be done, and enlist his cooperation.	Be sure to explain to the patient and his family the reasons why the turning frame is used and how it will benefit the patient.
7. Transfer the patient to the frame.	A physician may be required to be present when a patient is transferred to the frame. Lock the wheels of the frame so that it will not move.
	Leave a folded bath blanket or sheet covering the patient to avoid exposing him.
	Move all furniture and equipment away to provide a clear path from the patient's bed to the frame. Reassure the patient during the transfer.
a. Ask for additional help.	At least three or four people will be needed. Use at least a three-man carry, and another to support the head if needed. Use good body alignment and smooth, coordinated movements. Lift and move the patient on signal.
8. Position the patient in correct body alignment on the frame.	
a. Head and neck are straight in line with the rest of the spine.	Usually no pillow is used, or a small one may be allowed. Avoid flexion of the neck.
b. The shoulders should be relaxed and flat against the frame.	
c. The back should be straight and flat against the frame.	A small pillow or pad may be used to support the small of the back if it is needed. A cloth restraint (approximately 12 inches wide and 6 inches long) should be secured around the patient's waist and the frame at all times as a safety precaution.
d. The buttocks are supported by the perineal section except when the bedpan is used.	
e. The arms should be alongside the body, or supported on the armrests attached to the sides of the frame.	
f. The knees should be slightly flexed.	A small pillow or pad can be used under the knees unless contraindicated by the patient's condition.
g. The feet should be in good alignment, placed against the footboard, and supported laterally.	
9. Place the top covers over the patient.	These covers may have to be folded so that they do not drag on the floor. Make sure that they cause no pressure on the toes or feet.
10. Provide for the patient's comfort and care.	Leave the call light within his reach. The immobilized patient on the Stryker frame needs highly skilled and attentive nursing care. Unless acutely ill, he also needs diversional activities to help pass the time, such as reading or TV.

UNIT 28

Important Steps	Key Points
11. Move the regular hospital bed and tidy the room.	The regular bed may be moved out of the way in the room, or it may be taken out of the room by the housekeeping department in order to provide more space for the Stryker equipment. (Follow your agency procedure.)
12. Record the pertinent information on the patient's chart.	Charting example:

1015. Transferred onto the Stryker frame under the direction of Dr. Jensen. Color good. Cardinal signs stable. No complaints.

P. Shaw, RN

ITEM 4.   TURNING THE PATIENT ON THE STRYKER FRAME

Important Steps	Key Points
1. Wash your hands; approach and identify the patient.	Read his name from his identification band so that he can confirm it.
2. Explain that you are going to turn him to the prone position.	The patient should be involved in planning a schedule in which he is turned every 1 to 3 hours.
3. Provide privacy.	Pull the curtain around the Stryker frame or close the door of the room.
4. Check or prepare the anterior frame for use.	The anterior frame should have its three canvas sections padded and covered. There should be space at the top for the head and the forehead support, and space at the bottom for the feet.
5. Remove the top covers and restraint or safety belt.	Pull the patient's gown down over his body to avoid undue exposure.
6. Ensure secure body alignment and comfort.	Use padding such as rolled sheets, rolled pads, and pillows under the neck, and under, between, and along the side of the legs.
7. Attach the anterior frame in place over the patient.	Explain to the patient what you are doing as you go along.
a. Latch or screw the ends of the frame to the basic frame.	
b. Remove the armrests and place his arms along his sides.	
c. Adjust the forehead support or face mask to the proper position.	
d. Wrap the safety belts around both frames and the patient: one around his chest and the other around his thighs.	
8. Turn the patient to a prone position.	*For the patient's safety, always have two people turn the frame.* (The policy in many agencies requires that two people turn the frame; check for confirmation.)
a. One worker stands at the head and the other at the foot of the frame.	

Important Steps	Key Points
b. Each worker will unlock the safety locks at each end of the frame with one hand, and with the other hand will hold the same side of the frame.	Explain to the patient and your assistant that you will be turning the frame to the right on the count of three.
c. On a signal, such as "1, 2, 3, turn," quickly and smoothly turn the frame clockwise until it locks in position.	The patient will now be facing the floor, or in the prone position. Wait a few moments for him to become oriented. Stay close beside him, talking, comforting, and reassuring him.
9. Remove the posterior frame.	Place the frame so that it will be out of the way, and will not tip over or interfere with work in the area.
10. Adjust the patient's body alignment.	Check for alignment as in step 8 of Item 3. Also check for pressure, particularly around the ankles, when the patient is in the prone position.
11. Provide for the patient's comfort and welfare.	Put the top covers over him again. Leave the call signal within his reach. Provide other assistance and diversional activities as may be needed.
12. Report and record on the patient's chart.	In some hospitals or agencies, turning the patient on a schedule is recorded as a treatment: "Turn q 2 h ~~10~~ MD ~~12~~ BN ~~2~~ MD 4, 6, etc." (The hours are marked through and initialed by the worker turning the patient.)

Note: To turn the patient from the prone to the supine position, the same procedure would be used as above except that the posterior frame would be placed over the patient, and the turn would be made in the direction preferred by the patient (the frame turns 360°).

ITEM 5. PLACING THE PATIENT ON THE BEDPAN

Important Steps	Key Points
1. Wash your hands, approach and identify the patient, and explain what you will do.	Usually the patient will request the bedpan when he needs it.
2. Place the patient in a supine position.	Both male and female patients may be able to urinate while in the prone position, but need to be in the supine position for a bowel movement. (Some women patients find it difficult to urinate while in a prone position.)
3. Put the bedpan support on the proper inserts of the basic frame, and place the bedpan on the support.	When the fracture pan is used, delete steps 3 and 4; continue with steps 5 through 8.
4. Detach the perineal (middle canvas section) support and put it out of the way to prevent soiling.	
5. Clean and dry the patient's perineum after use of the bedpan.	The immobilized patient is unable to do this for himself. You will therefore wipe him with

Important Steps	Key Points
	tissue, and use soap, water, a washcloth and a towel if the patient is soiled. Leave him clean and dry. Return supplies to storage.
6. Empty and clean the bedpan, then store it for later use.	The bedpan support may be left in place for future use, but should be clean.
7. Reattach the perineal section to the frame.	
8. Provide for the patient's comfort and welfare.	

ITEM 6. THE CIRC–O–LECTRIC BED

The Circ-O-lectric bed is an electrically operated circular frame used to turn and position a patient who has restricted or limited body movement. The turning movement is in a vertical direction rather than from side to side as in the Stryker frame. It is used for patients who have any of the following: severe circulatory conditions, orthopedic problems, or other conditions requiring specific treatment.

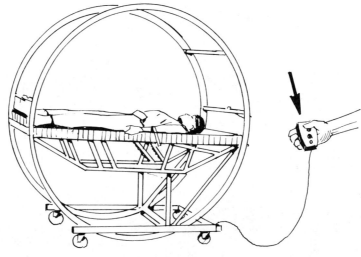

Circ-O-lectric bed.

The bed is operated by an electric motor that has hand controls that can be used by the patient when he is well enough. The worker can operate the bed by using a push-button on the control switch. The patient lies on a posterior frame that generally forms the diameter of the circular frame. Before the patient is turned from his back (supine position), the anterior frame is placed over the patient's body and attached in place. The bed is then rotated forward to the "face" position until the patient is in a prone position. The posterior frame can then be raised in the frame so that it is not resting on the patient, as shown in the sketch on the opposite page.

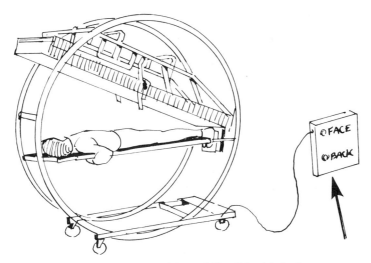

Face or prone position of Circ-O-lectric bed.

*ITEM 7. PROCEDURE FOR SETTING UP AND OPERATING THE
CIRC–O–LECTRIC BED*

Important Steps	Key Points
1. Order the Circ-O-lectric bed.	The bed is usually obtained from the storage area and delivered by the housekeeping department. The bed is set up before the patient is admitted to the room in order to lessen the number of times the patient is moved. The regular bed can be stored until it is needed.
2. Check the parts and accessories for the bed.	Follow the manufacturer's instructional manual. The parts of the Circ-O-lectric bed that should be checked are the basic frame, anterior frame, foam mattress, special sheet, safety or restraining straps, footboard attached to the frame, adjustable siderails, forehead and chin straps, and accessory parts such as traction bars, suspension, and exercise apparatus.
3. Prepare the bed.	Place the plastic cover over the posterior frame and use spring clamps to hold it in place. Place the foam mattress on the frame. (Note that the mattress has a circular section that can be removed when the bedpan is in place.) Use the special sheet that fastens to the mattress with elastic bands. Lock the wheels to stabilize the bed during the transfer. *Note:* The nursing team may require practice in manipulating the bed, since it may have been some time since it was used.
4. Wash your hands.	
5. Approach and identify the patient.	He may be one who is to be transferred from a regular bed, or one who is admitted from Emergency, Surgery, or a special care unit. Read the patient's name aloud and have him or a co-worker verify it.

Important Steps	Key Points
6. Explain the task to the patient and his family.	If at all possible, demonstrating the use of the bed before the patient is placed in it is helpful.
7. Transfer the patient to the Circ-O-lectric bed.	You will need additional help. The presence of a doctor may be required. You will need at least three or four people.
a. Move all furniture and equipment away to provide a clear path to move the patient onto the frame of the bed.	
b. Transfer the patient by using at least a three-man carry.	Use good body alignment and smooth, coordinated movements. Lift and move the patient on signal.
8. Position the patient in correct body alignment on the frame.	Follow steps 8 through 12 in Item 3, the Stryker frame procedure.

ITEM 8.   TURNING THE PATIENT TO A PRONE POSITION IN A CIRC–O–LECTRIC BED

Important Steps	Key Points
Follow steps 1 through 7 in Item 4, the Stryker frame procedure.	
8. Turn the patient to the prone position.	Set or press the "face" position button on the control and put the bed in motion. Turn the patient gradually and slowly to prevent vertigo and loss of consciousness.
9. Remove the posterior frame.	Release the locks on the posterior frame and push the frame upward at the head end until it locks in position above the patient (see the sketch on page 611).
	Place the safety or restraining belts over the patient and hook them into the underside of the frame. These are used to prevent a possible fall because the siderails cannot be used in the prone position.

Follow steps 10 through 12 of Item 4.

To turn the patient from the prone to the supine position, the same procedure is used except that the posterior frame is placed over the patient and secured in place, and the "back" button is pressed on the control.

ITEM 9.   USE OF THE BEDPAN IN THE CIRC–O–LECTRIC BED

Follow the same procedure as described in Item 5 for use of the bedpan on the Stryker frame except:

1. Remove the circular metal plate and the circular mattress section under the perineal area.

2. Place the bedpan on the Evertaut fasteners so that it is held in place under the patient's buttocks.

3. The bed may be tilted slightly or the head gatch elevated if the patient's condition permits.

4. The circular sections are replaced after the bedpan has been used.

5. Use the fracture pan for urine or bowel elimination unless it is contraindicated by the patient's condition.

ITEM 10. ADJUSTING THE POSITIONS OF THE CIRC-O-LECTRIC BED

When the patient is permitted unrestricted movements, the bed can be put in a sitting position. His hips should be centered over the point where the bed "breaks" for best body alignment when sitting.

Manual Gatching. The posterior frame has a lever on each side within easy reach of the patient. When one or both levers are pulled, the head and foot sections adjust in relation to the amount of effort exerted to sit up when the levers are depressed. This action is similar to that of adjusting seats in a bus or an airplane. Releasing the pressure on the lever locks the posterior section to the desired degree of gatch.

Electrical Tilting. After the bed is gatched, other positions can be obtained by tilting the bed forward or backward on the basic circular frame. When the bed is moving in the head-down position, automatic stops prevent it from going too far. The forward or "face" adjustments must be controlled by the patient or an attendant.

U
N
I
T
28

ITEM 11. PREOPERATIVE INFORMATION

When the use of the Circ-O-lectric bed, or the Foster or Stryker frame is necessary for scheduled surgical patients, it is extremely important that the following aspects of patient care be included in the preoperative preparation:

1. Measurement and adjustment of the canvas sections to fit the patient's body.

2. A detailed explanation of the working parts of the frames.

3. Assistance and supervision of the patient so that he can safely be on the Circ-O-lectric bed to learn how the motion will make him feel as he turns the bed.

4. Assistance and supervision of the patient so that he can safely be on the Foster or Stryker frame to learn how the motion will make him feel, as it is turned by 2 persons on the nursing staff.

ITEM 12. CONCLUSION OF THE UNIT

You have now completed the lesson on the operation of patient turning frames. After you have had sufficient practice with the equipment to become familiar with it and learn some skills in performing the procedures, you should arrange with your instructor to take the performance test.

PERFORMANCE TEST

In your classroom or the skill laboratory, your instructor will ask you to perform the following skills accurately without any use of reference or source materials. You may need the assistance of other students in the procedures, and you may use the mannequin (Mrs. Chase) or another student to play the part of the patient.

1. Given a patient who is quadriplegic and paralyzed from the neck down, set up a Stryker frame and assist in transferring him onto the frame as he arrives on the unit from Emergency so that the transfer is achieved safely and without injury to the patient or the workers.

2. Given a patient who has had surgery on his spine and who is lying in a supine position on a Stryker frame, turn him to a prone position safely and without increasing his apprehension.

3. Given a patient in a Circ–O–lectric bed, turn him from a supine (back position) to a prone position accurately and safely and align his body properly. (If a Circ–O–lectric bed is not available for your use, describe the steps of the procedure to your instructor.)

PERFORMANCE CHECKLIST

OPERATION OF PATIENT TURNING FRAMES

SET UP AND TRANSFER A PATIENT TO A STRYKER FRAME

1. Obtain a Stryker frame.

2. Check to see if all the parts are present.

3. Prepare the posterior frame.

   a. Measure and attach the upper, middle, and lower canvas sections to the frame.

   b. Place the sponge pads on the sections and cover them with linen so that all the ends are secure.

   c. Place the posterior frame on the basic frame.

4. Attach the footboard.

5. Take the frame to the patient's unit.

6. Wash your hands.

7. Approach and identify the patient.

8. Explain the reasons for using the Stryker frame.

9. Obtain assistance to help transfer the patient.

10. Lock the wheels of the frame so that it will not move.

11. Clear the furniture and equipment away between the bed and frame.

12. Put a bath blanket or sheet over the patient during the transfer.

13. Use at least a three-man carry, lift on signal, and move the patient to the frame.

14. Position the patient in good alignment on the frame.

    a. Make sure his head and neck are straight, his shoulders flat, his spine straight, his arms supported, his knees slightly flexed, and his feet against the footboard and supported laterally.

15. Replace the top covers on the patient.

16. Provide for the patient's comfort by giving him the signal cord and so forth.

17. Tidy the room.

18. Record the pertinent information on the patient's chart.

TURNING A PATIENT TO PRONE POSITION ON STRYKER FRAME

1. Approach and identify the patient.

2. Explain what is going to be done.

3. Provide for the patient's privacy by pulling the curtains.

4. Check or prepare the anterior frame for use.

    a. Provide space for the patient's face.

    b. Provide support for the patient's forehead.

    c. Provide space for the bottom of the frame and the patient's feet.

5. Remove the top covers and the 12-inch cloth safety restraint and smooth down the patient's gown.

6. Add the necessary padding for maximum body support.

7. Place the anterior frame correctly over the patient's body.

8. Secure the ends of the frame to the basic frame.

9. Remove the arm supports if these have been used.

10. Apply at least two safety belts — one around the chest, another around the thighs; secure them snugly.

11. Have an assistant help to turn patient.

    a. One worker stands at the head and the other at the foot.

    b. Unlock the safety locks with one hand, hold the frame with the other.

    c. Both persons must turn in a clockwise direction smoothly until the frame is locked in place.

12. Remove the posterior frame.

13. Adjust the alignment of the patient's body.

    a. His head and neck must be straight, his shoulders flat, his spine straight, his arms supported, his knees slightly flexed, his feet against the footboard, and the anterior of his foot protected from pressure.

14. Provide for the patient's comfort; leave the call signal within reach, and so forth.

15. Report or record the turning procedure.

UNIT 28

TURNING THE PATIENT IN THE CIRC–O–LECTRIC BED TO PRONE POSITION AND ALIGNING HIM

1. Approach and identify the patient.

2. Explain what is going to be done.

3. Provide for the patient's privacy by pulling the curtain and closing the door.

4. Check or prepare the anterior frame for use.

   a. Provide space for the patient's face.

   b. Provide support for the patient's forehead.

   c. Provide space for the bottom of the frame and the patient's feet.

5. Remove top covers, the 12-inch cloth safety restraint, and smooth down the patient's gown.

6. Add the necessary padding for maximum body support.

7. Place the anterior frame correctly over the patient's body.

8. Secure the ends of the frame to the basic circular frame.

9. Apply safety belts and secure them snugly around the patient and both frames.

10. Turn the patient slowly by pressing the "face" button on the control.

11. Remove the posterior frame by pushing the head end up until it is locked in place on the frame.

12. Adjust alignment of the patient's body.

    a. His head and neck should be straight, his shoulders flat, his spine straight, his arms supported, his knees slightly flexed, and his feet against the footboard with the anterior of the foot protected from pressure.

13. Provide for the patient's comfort; leave the call signal in reach, and so forth.

14. Report or record the turning procedure.

POST-TEST

Directions: Mark the answer that will make the statement complete.

1. The immobilized patient should be encouraged to discuss his immobility and how it affects him. His emotional response will be varied. All of the following will probably be true except:

   a. joy

   b. fear

   c. anger

   d. withdrawal

2. The following reasons for using the turning frames are all true except:

   a. to relieve pressure on parts of the body

   b. to increase circulation

   c. to decrease respiratory intake

   d. to maintain immobility of the affected part so that healing can occur

3. The patient's needs should be considered within the realm of a whole person. These include all of the following except:

   a. encouragement to use his intellectual abilities

   b. assurance that his safety and protection needs are met

   c. permission to make a decision

   d. decisions made for him as to what to eat, when to sleep, or when to take a bath

4. The Stryker frame consists of all the following parts except:

   a. a canvas-covered frame for the patient to lie on

   b. a second canvas frame placed on the top of the patient

   c. safety belts used to keep the patient safe

   d. attachment to a metal frame that is secured to the wall

5. The utensils used for bowel and urine elimination include all of the following except:

   a. fracture pan

   b. bedpan

   c. urinal

   d. sterile basin

6. When you are transferring the patient from the bed to the frame, all of the following are true except:

   a. only two people are needed to make the transfer

   b. a physician may be required to be present

   c. at least three or four people will be needed

   d. the patient is lifted and moved on signal

7. When the patient is on the frame, the most important safety measure to be taken is:

   a. keeping the floor clean and dry

   b. keeping the 12-inch restraint around the patient's waist and frame at all times

   c. keeping the patient on a very high protein diet

   d. keeping visitors out

8. When the patient on the frame is turned from the supine to the prone position, the number of people required is:

   a. three

   b. four

   c. two

   d. one

U
N
I
T
28

9. The turning of the Circ–O–lectric bed is done slowly and gradually to prevent:

     a.   nausea and vomiting   c.   vertigo and loss of consciousness

     b.   diarrhea and incontinence   d.   distention and flatulence

10. When the bed or frames are turned, the patient's safety usually requires all of the following except:

     a.   added padding under body crevices

     b.   safety straps around the patient and frame

     c.   two people to turn the frame

     d.   turning the patient and frame without a signal

POST-TEST ANNOTATED ANSWER SHEET

1. a.   (p. 603)   6. a.   (p. 607)

2. c.   (p. 604)   7. b.   (p. 607)

3. d.   (p. 604)   8. c.   (p. 608)

4. d.   (p. 604)   9. c.   (p. 612)

5. d.   (p. 605)   10. d.   (p. 608)

USE OF RESTRAINTS

I. DIRECTIONS TO THE STUDENT

Please read the following paragraphs carefully. They will tell you what you will be expected to know and how you will be expected to use restraints when caring for patients in your agency. You are to proceed through the lesson using this workbook as your guide. You will need to practice the procedures in the skill laboratory, using the mannequin (Mrs. Chase) or another student as the patient.

For this lesson, you will need the following items:

1. Cloth limb-holder or wrist restraint.

2. Restraint belt, or safety belt with buckle, 5 or 6 feet long.

3. Body or jacket restraint.

4. Roller gauze.

5. ABD pads or washcloth.

After you have completed the lesson and your practice of the procedures, arrange with your instructor to take the post-test. If you feel that you have the necessary skills, talk with your instructor; then arrange to take the post-test, during which you will be expected to demonstrate accurately the required skills.

II. GENERAL PERFORMANCE OBJECTIVE

Upon completing this lesson, you will be able to apply various types of restraints that will help to immobilize or support a part of the body.

III. SPECIFIC PERFORMANCE OBJECTIVES

When you have finished this unit, you will be able to:

1. Apply a wrist restraint or limb-holder to partially immobilize a patient's arm or leg in such a way that it does not interfere with his circulation or cause him injury.

2. Apply a body or jacket restraint to partially immobilize a patient who is in bed, or to support a patient in a chair or wheelchair, in a manner that provides for his safety and comfort.

3. Apply an elbow restraint safely and effectively on an infant or young child to prevent flexion of the elbow.

4. Apply a belt restraint or safety belt around a patient's waist in such a way as to give him a feeling of safety and security.

IV. VOCABULARY

discipline—training that corrects, molds, or perfects the behavior or moral character; to correct or train.

619

limb-holder—a cloth tie or restraint that keeps a limb (arm or leg) in a certain position or limits its full range of motion (sometimes called a soft restraint).

Posey belt—a commercially made restraint belt or strap.

punishment—act of subjecting to penalty, pain, loss, or other affliction for some offense or transgression.

restrain—to hold back from action, to check or keep under control, to repress, to deprive of liberty.

V. INTRODUCTION

In the field of health, restraints are used only as a safety measure. The most common safety needs of the patient are those to immobilize a part of his body wholly or partially, to assist in the support of part of his body, or to prevent possible harm to himself or to others. There are legal restrictions concerning the use of restraints that forcibly interfere with the patient's right to liberty, and these must be observed. Restraining a person (or patient) in a locked room, for instance, is subject to certain legal requirements.

Restraints may be indicated in the care of patients based on the patient's need for safety, or on the doctor's judgment of a need to limit the patient's movements for medical reasons. You must know the principles involved in the use of restraints, and the correct method of applying them. In this unit, you will learn procedures for using restraints on an extremity or on the body.

ITEM 1. PRINCIPLES RELATED TO THE USE OF RESTRAINTS

There are certain principles involved in the use of restraints for patient care in any health facility. These principles and the attitudes about restraints as described in this unit may differ from those taught or practiced by other workers in nursing. The emphasis here is on the patient and his needs, and how the use of the restraint will benefit him.

Principle 1. *The use of restraints must meet some need or help the patient.*

The patient must have some safety need involving total or partial immobilization of a part of his body, support of part of his body, or prevention of harm to himself or others. If he is unable to handle these safety needs himself because of his mental or physical condition, and if other methods have been tried without effect, then the use of restraints may be indicated.

As an example, a patient may be receiving an IV in his left arm, which is supported on a board. After he has had a medication for pain that dulls his awareness, he tries to pull out the IV with his other hand. As a safety measure, a loose wrist restraint might be applied to the right wrist that would allow some movement, yet not enough to reach the IV.

Another example is the patient who has periods of mental confusion (often seen in the elderly). He may require a body jacket or safety belt when in bed or sitting in a wheelchair. Without the reminder of the jacket or belt, he might try to get up without assistance and suffer further injury.

Principle 2. *All restraints that limit movement or immobilize must be ordered by a physician.*

Most agencies have specific policies and regulations about the use of restraints. You should check these. In every state there are legal requirements and regulations about providing for the safety of patients, and limiting the patient's liberty or movements by forcible means. When the patient's movements must be limited for medical reasons, there has to be an order for the restraint, either a specific written order or an agency policy statement that stipulates when and what kind of restraints may be used.

Principle 3. *Restraints must not be used as a means of punishing or disciplining the patient for his behavior.*

The use of restraints or the threat of tying the patient down as a method of coercing, threatening, punishing, or disciplining should not be tolerated in any health agency. If a bossy, dictatorial, "Do as I say, or else" approach is taken with the patient, it often leads to anger on both the part of the patient and the worker, and the probable use of force and restraints. The "caring for" and "caring about" approach to the patient would be more effective in understanding his need for our help.

Perhaps it would be better if health workers referred to restraints as "safety belts." The very word "restraint" conveys a sense of punishment or discipline.

Principle 4. *Restraints are applied snugly to a body part, but not tightly enough to interfere with blood circulation.*

Care must be taken when applying safety belts or restraints so that the patient's restless movement or tugging does not close off the circulation. Impaired circulation to the part will cause the following symptoms: coolness of the skin, pallor or bluish color, numbness, and loss of sensation or movement. The restraint should be loosened or removed immediately, and the part gently massaged to restore the circulation.

Principle 5. *The patient's position should be changed every 2 hours when restrained, and active or passive exercise should be given; the restrained part is released unless contraindicated.*

The change of position for the patient is necessary to relieve pressure, to increase circulation, to improve body functioning, and to make him more comfortable. Positioning, changing, and exercising the restrained part help to reassure the patient that the restraint is truly a safety measure and not a punishment.

ITEM 2. TYPES OF RESTRAINTS AND SAFETY BELTS

Restraints come in many sizes and shapes. Increasingly, hospitals and health facilities are using commercially made restraints made of a strong cloth or canvas; the belts are usually webbing or tightly woven strong twill. Some agencies use folded sheets, bathrobe belts, woven strips of material or webbing, or gauze as a means of immobilizing a part of the body. A few examples of the commercial type of safety belt or restraint are described below.

Safety belt or restaint — made of webbing or twill with a buckle on one end. It is available in a variety of lengths, but is often 5 or 6 feet in length. Longer lengths are used to secure the patient on stretchers, when turning a patient on a Stryker frame, or on a Circ-O-lectric bed, and for other purposes. It is often used for patients in wheelchairs to provide safety. See the sketch below for the safety belt.

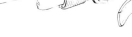

Safety belts.

Limb-holder or
wrist restraint.

Limb-holder or wrist-type restraint (also called a soft restraint) — made of strong cloth about 3 inches wide with an 8- to 10-inch soft flannel padded end that is wrapped around

U
N
I
T
29

the wrist or ankle. The padded end has a slit in it so the longer belt part can be drawn through it to encircle the wrist or leg. Some people may refer to it as a Posey, which is the name of one of the leading manufacturers of restraints.

Body restraint — made of canvas or strong material; it has a short belt that buckles around the patient's body and is attached to the middle of a much longer belt that can be tied to the bed or around a wheelchair. (See the following sketch.)

Jacket restraint — made of canvas or strong material; it has a portion that fits over the patient's chest with straps or belts that go over the shoulders and others that go around the waist. The straps or belts may be crossed or tied behind the patient's back. It is generally used as a safety measure and to support the patient's trunk in an upright position while he is in a wheelchair. (See the sketch below.)

Elbow restraint — made of a folded, thick cotton or flannel material. It is approximately 12 inches long, 10 inches wide with six or eight slots in which are inserted tongue blades or plastic slats, and three or four double ties along one edge used to secure the restraint around the elbow. One double tie at the top of the restraint is used to secure the restraint onto the child by crossing the back and tying under the opposite arm. If the ties for securing the restraint under the arm are missing, use safety pins to attach the restraint to the infant's shirt. This is used to restrain infants and small children from flexing their elbows to reach their face in cases of severe skin rashes or surgery of the face, such as the repair of a harelip. (An example of an elbow restraint is shown below.)

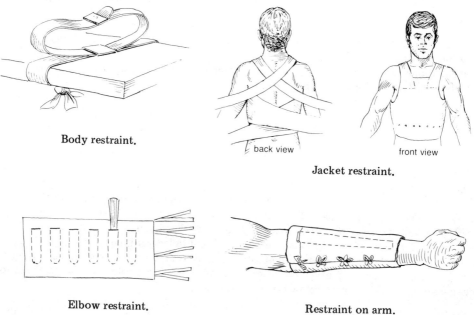

Body restraint.

back view   front view

Jacket restraint.

Elbow restraint.   Restraint on arm.

Leather restraint — made of leather with a buckle that has a locking device. A key must be used to unlock the buckle to remove the restraint. This is used only as a last resort when a patient is so disoriented that he becomes dangerous to himself, to other patients, or to the health workers. This type is being used less and less today, and always requires a doctor's written order when it is employed.

ITEM 3.   PRECAUTIONS TO BE USED IN APPLYING RESTRAINTS

You should avoid tying unnecessary knots in restraints. In case of danger to the patient (such as a fire) or when emergency treatment is needed, restraints may have to be removed in a hurry. In such cases, you may have to cut the restraint if there are numerous knots, or if the knots are tied so tightly that it is difficult and time-consuming to untie them. A word or two about knots is therefore important.

Clove hitch — may be used to apply a wrist-type restraint to an extremity. The advantage of this type of knot is that it permits the patient some mobility while it will not cut off the circulation to the extremity. The clove hitch is made as shown. Your observational skills are needed when you have any patient in restraints to assure that circulation in the extremity is maintained.

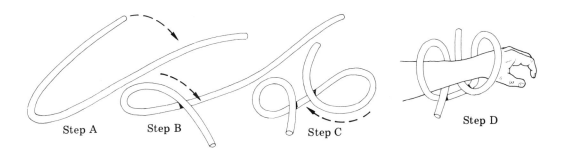

Step A   Step B   Step C   Step D

Square knot — may be used to secure the restraint to an extremity, or to secure the ends to the bed frame or the wheelchair. The advantage of the square knot is that it does not slip and will not tighten if pulled on. It also will not loosen when the stress or pull on the ties is released. The square knot is made as follows and as shown below. Take the left tie and pass it over, under, and across the right tie. It is now on the right side. Take the original right tie, pass it under, over, and across the other tie. Place the first crossover where you want the knot to be located, and tighten the second crossover to form the square knot. (*Note:* the two crossovers form a partial loop at each end, and the ties on each side of the loop are in the same position; see step C.)

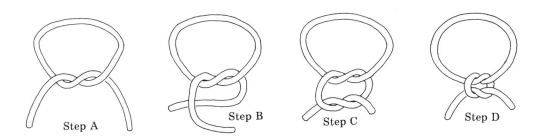

Step A   Step B   Step C   Step D

Half-bow knot — used to secure the restraint to the bed frame or the wheelchair. It is much easier to untie than the square knot, because you merely pull the loose tie end to remove the bow portion, and then loosen the crossover tie. It also will not slip even when stress or pull is exerted on the secured portion of the tie. You already know how to make the half-bow knot because you use it when tying your shoelaces, except that for a restraint you make only one loop in the bow.

These types of knots are likely to be the ones you will use to apply and secure restraints.

One final precaution should be noted before you begin practicing the procedures. When a restraint is secured to the bed frame, *do not tie* it to the *moveable siderails* or to the *immoveable portion* of the bed. If the siderails are lowered, it may pull the restraint too tightly or cause strain on the patient's body where it is being immobilized. Raising or lowering the head of the bed may produce the same effects if the restraint is tied to the immovable portion of the bed frame.

U
N
I
T
29

ITEM 4. APPLY A LIMB-HOLDER OR WRIST-TYPE RESTRAINT

Important Steps	Key Points
1. Check for a doctor's order or agency policy before restraints are applied.	This is a legal requirement when a patient's movement is to be restricted.
2. Wash your hands.	
3. Obtain the cloth restraint that is to be used: a limb-holder or Posey wrist restraint.	A charge may be made for the use of a restraint, depending on the policies of your agency.
4. Approach and identify the patient.	Read the patient's name aloud so he can confirm it.
5. Explain to the patient what you plan to do and why.	The manner in which you approach him and explain the procedure may determine whether the patient will accept or resist all efforts to apply it. Stress that the limb-holder or tie is used for his safety and as a reminder not to move his arms (or legs).
6. Apply the limb-holder to the wrist (or leg). Take the padded end and wrap it around the wrist. Pull the tie through the slit in the wrist portion. Attach the loose end to the spring frame of the bed, tying a half-bow or a square knot.	If a commercially made limb-holder is not available, you can improvise: use roller gauze, preferably 2 or 3 inches wide and at least 3 to 4 feet long. Use a washcloth or ABD pad to wrap around the wrist. Tie the gauze around the wrist using a square knot, or fold the gauze in half and make a slipknot. Secure the loose ends to the spring frame of the bed.
7. Check the extremity distal to the restraint for adequate circulation.	Good circulation in hands and feet is indicated by warmth, normal color, and capability of movement.
8. Provide for the patient's comfort and welfare.	Place the signal cord where he can reach it even with his restrained hand. *Do not leave your patient unable to signal for you.* Adjust the position of the bed as allowed or desired. Make sure he is in good body alignment.
9. Assure the patient that you will return soon to check on the restraint and to change his position.	The patient needs assurance that you will not avoid him or neglect him. *Note:* If the patient were receiving an IV, you would be checking on him every 15 to 30 minutes to make sure that the IV has not infiltrated.
10. Provide care for the patient who has one or more extremity in restraint: Remove one restraint at a time; give active or passive exercise to the joints, and then replace the restraint. Change the patient's position every 2 hours. He can be placed on his side and the restraint attached to the other side of the bed, or the tie can be lengthened so that good alignment of shoulders and arms (or hip and leg) is maintained.	If his behavior is unpredictable because of confusion, mental illness, or disease of the brain, you should have an assistant to help you care for the patient when you release the restraint.
11. Remove the restraints when the time specified by the doctor has elapsed, or the need to immobilize has passed.	

Important Steps	Key Points
12. Record the pertinent information on the patient's chart, including the time the restraint was applied, the type, the reason, and the time removed.	Charting example: 0930. Soft wrist restraint applied to right wrist per doctor's order while IV running in other arm. M. Dolan, NA

ITEM 5. APPLYING A JACKET RESTRAINT

The following procedure is used to apply a jacket restraint to a patient who is in a wheelchair. It could also be used for the patient who is in bed, although he would have to be turned from side to side, and the wrinkles in the bed would have to be smoothed out.

Important Steps	Key Points
Follow steps 1 through 5 in Item 4.	

6. Apply the jacket support or restraint to a patient in a wheelchair.	Be sure that the wheelchair brakes are locked.
	    Place the front portion of the jacket over the patient's chest with the shoulder straps and side straps in place. Have the patient lean forward slightly while you stand behind the chair. You may need an assistant to help hold the patient so he won't fall if the jacket is being used to support his trunk in an upright position in the wheelchair.
	    Reach for the lower side ties, cross them behind his back, (smooth out wrinkles in his clothing) and tie them in a half-bow knot or square knot at the back of the wheelchair. Reach for the upper ties, cross them behind this shoulders (avoid wrinkles), and tie them in a half-bow or square knot behind the wheelchair.

Follow Steps 8 through 12 in Item 4.	Charting example: 1000. Up in wheelchair. Jacket restraint applied for safety. M. Dolan, NA

U
N
I
T
29

ITEM 6. APPLYING AN ELBOW RESTRAINT ON AN INFANT

Important Steps	Key Points
Follow steps 1 through 4 in Item 4.	
5. If necessary, prepare the elbow restraint.	You may have to slip a tongue blade into each of the insert pockets unless the restraint has built-in rigid supports.

6. Apply the elbow restraint, one on each of the infant's arms.
    Wrap the restraint snugly around the arm with the ties on the outer edge. Tie the ties around the arm, using a half-bow knot. Use the double tie at the top of the restraint to secure it on the infant.
	Start at shoulder top, place one tie across the back, and one tie across the chest; use a bow knot to secure the ties under the opposite arm.
	    When pins are used to secure the restraint to the infant's shirt, keep your fingers between the area being pinned and the baby's skin to avoid sticking him.

Follow steps 7 through 12 of Item 4.

Even though the baby will not know enough to expect you, you must return frequently to turn him, exercise his elbows, and provide care. Charting example:

1300. Elbow restraints applied to both arms. Incision on upper lip dry and clean.

M. Dolan, NA

ITEM 7.   APPLYING A SAFETY BELT OR RESTRAINT STRAP

Important Steps	Key Points

Follow steps 1 through 5 in Item 4.

6. Apply the safety belt or restraint strap around the patient's waist.

   With the patient sitting in a chair, place the strap around his waist, bringing both ends behind the chair and tying them in a half-bow or square knot, or fasten the buckle if there is one;

   or

   place the strap or belt completely around the patient's waist, cross the ends in the back, then bring both ends behind the chair and tie them in a half-bow or square knot (or fasten the buckle);

   or

   place the strap around the patient's waist, tie it at one side in a square knot, bring the ties to the back of the chair, and fasten them with a half-bow or square knot.

This can be done for the patient who is lying in bed, sitting in a wheelchair, or lying on a stretcher. It is not commonly used, however, for the bed patient because siderails are generally adequate to protect the patient from falling out of bed.

There are several ways to apply the safety belt or strap. You may find that one method works well for one patient and another method is better for a different patient.

Follow steps 8 through 12, Item 4.

Even though the patient is sitting up, his position must be changed or his weight shifted frequently to relieve pressure. Charting example:

1015. Up in wheelchair. Safety belt applied around waist.   M. Dolan, NA

ITEM 8.   CONCLUSION OF UNIT

You have now completed the lesson on application of restraints. After you have practiced the procedures to become familiar with them and gain some skills, arrange with your instructor to take the performance post-test. You will be expected to demonstrate correctly the procedures involved in providing for the patient's safety in a reassuring manner.

PERFORMANCE TEST

In the classroom or your skill laboratory, your instructor will ask you to perform the following activities to demonstrate your skill without referring to any source material. You may use Mrs. Chase (the mannequin) or another student in the role of the patient.

1. Given a patient receiving an IV in the left arm who tries to remove the needle from the vein, apply a limb-holder, or similar soft restraint, to the right wrist. Tie the restraint at the wrist with a knot so that the patient's tugging on it will not cut off circulation to the hand.

2. Given a patient with a muscular disease involving the muscles of the trunk, apply a jacket restraint to support his body while he is sitting in a wheelchair, using the method that provides the most safety for the patient.

3. Given a 4-month-old child who has a severe rash on his face and neck, apply elbow restraints to both arms and describe the care you would give the child during the time the restraints are used. The care referred to would be in addition to bathing, diapering, feeding, or holding the child.

4. Given an elderly, slightly confused patient in a wheelchair who is not to bear any weight on the left leg, place a safety belt or restraint strap around his waist and fasten the ends of it behind the wheelchair, using the method and knots of your choice from those described in the procedure.

UNIT 29

PERFORMANCE CHECKLIST

APPLICATION OF RESTRAINTS

APPLYING LIMB–HOLDER TO RIGHT WRIST

1. Check for the doctor's order.

2. Wash your hands.

3. Obtain a limb-holder or similar soft cloth restraint.

4. Approach and identify the patient.

5. Explain what you are going to do and why.

6. Apply the limb-holder or wrist restraint to the right wrist correctly.

   a. Place a padded end around the wrist, or pad it.

   b. Pull the tie through the slit, or make a clove hitch or square knot in gauze or another cloth strap.

   c. Tie the loose end to the spring portion of the bed.

   d. Make clove hitch, square, or half-bow knots correctly.

7. Check the wrist and hand to see if circulation is good.

8. Provide for the patient's comfort and welfare.

   a. Adjust the bed to the allowed position.

   b. Leave the signal cord within reach.

   c. Make sure that the patient is in good body alignment.

9. Explain to the patient that he will be checked in 2 hours or sooner.

10. Record pertinent information on the patient's chart.

APPLYING A JACKET RESTRAINT FOR SUPPORT OF PATIENT IN WHEELCHAIR

1. Check for the doctor's order. (Some agencies may not require an order for support, but it would be better to have one.)

2. Wash your hands.

3. Obtain a jacket support or restraint.

4. Approach and identify the patient.

5. Explain what is to be done and why.

6. Apply the jacket restraint to the patient in a wheelchair.

   a. Lock the wheels of the wheelchair.

   b. Have an assistant support the patient while the jacket is being applied.

   c. Place a large portion of jacket correctly over patient's chest with the shoulder straps at the top.

   d. Stand behind the chair while your assistant supports the patients, cross the lower side ties behind the patient, and tie them behind the wheelchair.

   e. Take the shoulder straps, cross them behind the patient's shoulders, and tie them behind the wheelchair.

   f. Make a square or half-bow knot correctly.

7. Provide for the patient's comfort and welfare.

8. Tell the patient that he will be checked at a specified time.

9. Record pertinent information on the patient's chart.

APPLYING ELBOW RESTRAINTS TO A CHILD AND GIVING CARE WHILE RESTRAINED

1. Check for the doctor's order.

2. Wash your hands.

3. Obtain elbow restraints, and tongue blades if needed.

4. Approach and identify the patient.

5. Prepare the elbow restraints by inserting tongue blades.

6. Apply the elbow restraints, one on each arm.

   a. Wrap it around the arm, leaving the tie edge outermost.

   b. Wrap the ties around the arm and tie them in half-bow knots.

   c. Pin the restraint to the baby's shirt without sticking him.

7. Check the circulation in his hand.

8. Provide for the child's comfort.

   a. Adjust the bed if necessary

   b. Check for good alignment of his body.

APPLYING A SAFETY BELT OR RESTRAINT STRAP AROUND WAIST

1. Check for the doctor's order.

2. Wash your hands.

3. Obtain a safety belt or restraint strap.

4. Approach and identify the patient.

5. Explain what you are going to do and why.

6. Apply the safety belt or restraint strap around the patient's waist while he is sitting in a chair.

    a. Place a strap around the patient's waist and back of the chair, then tie or buckle it; *or*

    b. place the strap around his waist, cross the straps behind him, and tie the ends behind the chair or buckle them; *or*

    c. encircle the strap about his waist, tie it to one side in a square knot, and then tie it behind the chair.

    d. Make a square or half-bow knot correctly.

7. Provide for the patient's comfort and welfare.

8. Tell the patient that he will be checked in 2 hours or sooner.

9. Record pertinent information on the patient's chart.

U
N
I
T
29

POST-TEST

Directions: Mark the answer that makes the statement complete:

1. The use of restraints must meet some need or help the patient. They are used in all of the following cases except:

    a. for the elderly, confused wheelchair patient

    b. when the patient attempts to pull an IV out of arm

    c. to discipline the patient

    d. when the disoriented patient becomes combative

2. All restraints that limit movement or immobilize the patient must be ordered by a physician. All of the following statements are true except:

    a. the order is written by the physician

    b. there are legal requirements and regulations about providing for the safety of patients

    c. the agency policy may determine restraint use

    d. restraints are used to coerce the patient

3. To eliminate the patient's feeling of being threatened when he is restrained, use the following phrase:

    a. these are safety belts

    b. these are restraints

    c. these are belts to keep you in bed

    d. these straps are used to keep you immobilized

4. Restraints are applied snugly to a body part, but not tightly enough to interfere with circulation. All of the following are symptoms of circulation impairment except:

    a. pallor or bluish color

    b. numbness

    c. blanching

    d. loss of sensation or movement

5. The patient's position should be changed when restraints are utilized. The restrained part should be exercised unless contraindicated (choose the one correct answer):

    a. at least every 1 to 2 hours

    b. at least every 3 to 4 hours

    c. at least every 2 to 5 hours

    d. at least every 3 to 6 hours

6. The change of position for the patient is necessary for all of the following reasons except:

    a. to relieve pressure

    b. to increase circulation

    c. to improve body functioning

    d. in contraindication of the physician's orders

7. Restraints come in all sizes and shapes. The following are examples of commercial restraints except:

    a. folded sheets

    b. a jacket restraint

    c. a limb-holder

    d. a leather restraint

8. The following knots are used when applying restraints except:

    a. clove hitch

    b. half-bow knot

    c. double knot

    d. square knot

9. Restraints should be tied to the following part of the bed:

   a. the siderails

   b. the moveable part of the bed frame (spring attachment)

   c. the immoveable part of the bed frame

   d. the head and foot board

10. When restraints are attached to the bed frame, the safest knot used is:

   a. the half-bow knot

   b. the double knot

   c. the square knot

   d. the plain knot

POST-TEST ANNOTATED ANSWER SHEET

1. c. (p. 620)

2. d. (p. 621)

3. a. (p. 621)

4. c. (p. 621)

5. a. (p. 621)

6. d. (p. 621)

7. a. (pp. 621–622)

8. c. (p. 623)

9. b. (p. 623)

10. a. (p. 623)

UNIT 29

Unit 30

BANDAGES AND BINDERS

I. DIRECTIONS TO THE STUDENT

Proceed through this lesson and practice in the skill laboratory. After you have finished, demonstrate the application of common bandages and binders for your instructor, and take the post-test.

II. GENERAL PERFORMANCE OBJECTIVE

Following this lesson, you will be able to apply bandages and binders to achieve the purpose for which they are being used.

III. SPECIFIC PERFORMANCE OBJECTIVES

When you are through with this lesson, you will be able correctly to:

1. Discuss with the instructor the reasons for which bandages and binders are applied.

2. Check for impaired circulation in an area that is wrapped with a binder or a bandage, and take correct steps to remove the impairment as soon as discovered.

3. Apply circular, figure-8, spiral, spiral reverse, and recurrent bandages.

4. Apply a scultetus, straight abdominal, T-binder, double-T-binder, breast binders, and Ace bandage.

IV. VOCABULARY

1. Bandages

bandage—a piece of soft material, like gauze, used to wrap, bind, support, provide warmth for, protect, or immobilize a part.

circular bandage—a bandage that is wrapped around and around a part; each turn covers the preceding turn and holds it securely in place; it is fastened with tape, a special holding clip, or a safety pin.

elastic bandage—a bandage that is stretchable; when pulled tightly, it causes compression (a commonly used elastic bandage is called the Ace bandage).

figure-8 bandage—a bandage in which the turns cross each other like a figure-8; generally used over joints to retain dressings or to exert pressure in the case of sprains or hemorrhage.

recurrent bandage—used over the end of a stump of an amputated extremity, such as a leg or a finger.

reverse spiral bandage—special technique used in which a part of the bandage is folded back on itself to make it fit more uniformly (evenly); the reverse, or folding back, method may be used as a part of each complete spiral or circular turn to make the bandage fit neatly over a difficult area (wrist, fingers or ankles).

roller bandage—a continuous strip of soft material (commonly gauze or elastic material) used to bind up injured parts. It comes in widths of ½ inch to 6 inches, and lengths of 2 to 6 yards. The length and width you will use depend on the area to be bandaged.

spiral bandage—a bandage that consists of a series of circular turns ascending (going up) a part, such as from the fingers to the wrist; each turn is higher than the preceding one and overlaps the previous turn about half the width of the bandage.

triangular bandage—a bandage that is three-cornered; it holds dressings in place; it is called a *sling* when used as a swinging bandage to support the forearm or elbow; it is most often used in this way.

2. Binders

binder—a bandage generally used to provide encircling support of the chest or abdomen, although it can be used in other situations.

abdominal binders—a single width of soft material (18 to 24 inches and 3 to 5 feet long) used to provide strong abdominal support.

breast binder—usually a sleeveless, jacket-type, soft muslin binder used to hold breast dressings in place, support the breasts, or compress the breast as in the case of a new mother who is trying to dry up the milk in her breasts.

scultetus binder (many-tailed)—a succession of interlocking, overlapping bands used to enclose a part with rigid support, such as an abdominal girdle-like support following an abdominal operation.

T-binder (sanitary belt)—shaped like a letter "T," it is used to hold in place perineal pads (peri-pads) as well as rectal or perineal dressings.

T-binder, double—shaped like a letter T except that it has two tails TT ; commonly used for male patients who have had rectal or perineal surgery to hold the dressings in place.

V. INTRODUCTION

Bandages and binders are used for the following purposes:

1. To apply pressure (compression) in order to stop bleeding or swelling, and to assist in absorbing tissue fluids.

2. To provide for immobilization of an injured part, such as a fractured (broken) arm.

3. To hold dressings in place.

4. To protect open wounds from contaminants.

5. To apply warmth to a joint, as for persons suffering from painful joints due to arthritis.

6. To provide support and aid in venous (return blood flow) circulation, as when bandaging the leg of a patient suffering from varicose veins or limited circulation in the extremities (arms or legs).

Bandages and binders are made from many kinds of soft materials such as muslin, gauze, flannel, rubber, and elastic fabric. There are a number of commonly used bandages and binders; you should be familiar with their names and know how to apply them correctly. These bandages, and combinations of them as described in this unit, represent the most generally applied types. The specific method used will not only depend on the part to be bandaged, but on the purpose of the bandage, for example, support, immobilization, and so forth.

Bandages and binders should be applied so that pressure is evenly distributed to the area. If a joint is involved in bandaging, it should be supported in its normal position with a slight flexion of the joint. Both the bandage and binder should be attached securely to avoid friction or rubbing of the underlying tissue, which could cause severe irritation. However, great care must be taken not to make it too tight so that circulation is cut off. It must be tight enough to stay in place, but *not so tight as to cut off circulation!* Do you remember the signs and symptoms of impaired circulation from the unit on Special Skin Care?

Signs of impaired circulation are _____ , _____ , _____ , and _____ . It is helpful if you can leave the tips of the fingers and toes visible on a bandaged extremity so that you can watch for possible darkening of the nailbeds in order to determine if the circulation is impaired.

A bandage or binder should be applied over a clean, dry area. Remember that microorganisms grow in warm, damp areas. Be sure that skin surfaces are not bandaged directly together — they will sweat and provide a moist environment in which microorganisms can grow. Always put some kind of padding (4 × 4 or ABD bandage) between adjoining skin surfaces before bandaging or binding. It is also wise to pad over a bony prominence before bandaging to avoid friction, which could lead to excoriation of the skin. If left unattended for several days, such an irritation could become a decubitus ulcer.

If a bandage or binder is applied to the dressing of a draining wound, it must be changed frequently to keep it as clean and dry as possible. This reduces the chance of pathogenic organisms getting into the wound and setting up an infection. Discard the soiled dressing, and return the binders to the laundry for washing and reprocessing, or discard them if your agency uses disposable items.

General rules for determining length and width of roller bandages:

Type	Length	Width
head bandaging	6 yards	2 inch
body bandaging	10 yards	3 to 6 inch
leg bandaging	9 yards	2 to 4 inch
foot bandaging	4 yards	1½ to 3 inch
arm bandaging	7 to 9 yards	2 to 2½ inch
hand bandaging	3 yards	1 to 2 inch
finger bandaging	1 to 3 yards	½ to 1 inch

You will be expected to apply the following bandages and binders safely and correctly. With your partner in the skill laboratory, practice the following procedures.

ITEM 1.   THE APPLICATION OF A CIRCULAR BANDAGE

Apply a circular bandage to secure a clean dressing on the posterior aspect of the right middle arm.

Important Steps	Key Points
1. Obtain your supplies.	Get the type and amount of bandage needed to complete the procedure. Select the proper width of bandage. Wash your hands.
2. Approach the patient and explain what you are going to do.	Check his identification band. Gain his cooperation by explaining that you will be applying, or changing, his bandage. Tell him why it is being done — for support or immobilization, to hold a dressing in place. You can get this information from your team leader.
3. Wash the area to be wrapped if it is soiled.	Remember that microorganisms grow in dark, moist, dirty places. You may use soap and water or an antiseptic cleansing solution to wash the skin. Apply a dressing if needed. (Check your agency rules).

Important Steps	Key Points
4. Elevate the area to be wrapped.	Raise the arm so that it is at the same level as the heart. It should be elevated in this manner at least *15 minutes before* applying the bandage. This will restore equal circulation in the arm. If a limb is wrapped while edematous, the bandage will be too loose when the edema subsides. To prevent this from happening, place the limb comfortably in a horizontal position for at least 15 minutes. Note: To bandage a leg, have the patient in the supine position.
5. Place the patient in a comfortable position. Stand directly in front of the patient.	The position should also be convenient for you when you work with him. The patient may be sitting or prone, depending on where the bandage is required. Adjust the patient to your comfortable working height (remember your body alignment). Standing will make it easier for you to see what you are doing.
6. Begin applying the bandage on the right arm.	Stand near the working edge of the bed with the patient lying close to the right side of the bed. Ask him to raise his right arm slightly (about 6 to 12 inches) from the bed, palm upward, so that you can wrap the arm. If the patient is unable to lift his arm, you may need some assistance. Be sure that the area of application is dry and clean.

U
N
I
T
30

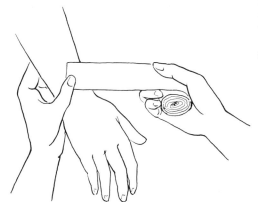

7. Unroll the bandage and anchor it in place.	Unwind it toward the right, around the patient's arm. Hold the roll of bandage in your right hand so that it unwinds from the top (reverse hand positions if you are left-handed). Hold the bandage in place with your left thumb with moderate tension. If you hold the bandage too loosely while wrapping, it will come off easily. If the bandage is wrapped too tightly, it will cut off the patient's circulation. You will have to practice wrapping until you judge the proper tension to use.

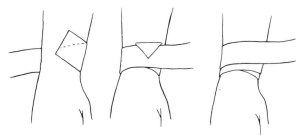

Anchoring bandage in place.

8. Make two initial circular turns to secure the bandage in place.	Secure the proximal (free) end to the arm directly over the site. Hold the bandage in place with your left thumb on top of the bandage and the anterior surface of the arm, and your left index finger on the posterior side of the

Important Steps	Key Points

arm. For the patient's comfort, the beginning (initial) and terminal end of the bandage are not to be placed directly over the wound, a bony prominence, the inner aspect of a limb, or a part that the patient will lie on.

9. Each circular turn goes directly over the preceding turn.

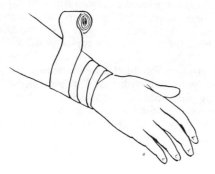

Each successive turn anchors (hold in place) the underlying layer of bandage. Continue unrolling the bandage from right to left around the arm. (Reverse hand positions if you are left-handed.) Use only as many circular turns as needed to hold the dressing in place or to immobilize the part. You may need to cut off a portion of the bandage with your scissors. (The remaining portion may be used for later changes.)

10. Secure the terminal end of the bandage.

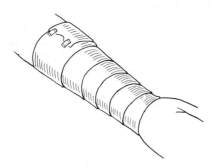

Circular bandage.

You can use tape, special metal clips, or a safety pin. Usually the circular bandage is used to keep a dressing in place. Place the patient's arm in a comfortable position.

11. Tidy the work area.

Return unused supplies to the storage area. Dispose of soiled bandages in a waste container. Place the call light, bed controls, and bedside stand conveniently for the patient (check every 30 minutes for an hour and a half after application; if circulation is impaired, remove the bandage immediately and rewrap).

12. Record the procedure on the patient's chart.

Chart the time, and the type and location of the bandage applied. Charting example.

1010. Dressing changed on right arm. Large amount of purulent, foul-smelling discharge.
J. Jones, RN

To remove a roller gauze bandage from a patient's arm or leg, cut the bandage off with your scissors. Be careful not to injure the tissue under the dressing with the tip of the scissors; to prevent this from happening, insert your left index finger under the bandage and elevate it slightly. With the scissors in your right hand, cut the bandage free slightly to the side of your left finger. (Cutting the bandages off will usually save time and avoid fatigue for the patient.) If it is not soiled, carefully unwind the bandage from left to right for reuse. Roll it as you unwind; this will prevent it from becoming soiled and tangled as it is removed.

The Ace bandage or elastic bandage can be laundered and reused. The cling-type bandage may also be reused as an outer bandage.

ITEM 2.   THE APPLICATION OF A SPIRAL BANDAGE

This procedure is used to apply an Ace bandage to an arm or leg.

Important Steps	Key Points

Follow steps 1 through 5 for the circular bandage procedure in Item 1.

6. Begin applying the bandage on the patient's ankle.

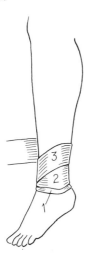

Anchor the bandage at the ankle with two circular turns. Start as you did for the circular bandage. Hold the roll in your right hand to unwind it downward from right to left around the leg. Secure the bandage on the back of the leg with your left index finger, and on the front of the leg with your left thumb. (Reverse hand positions if you are left-handed.)

7. With each succeding turn of the bandage, angle slightly upward around the leg.

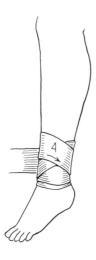

The direction is downward, around, upward, and around, like a spiral staircase, in the same direction as the blood that is returning to the heart. Each turn is parallel to the preceding turn and overlaps about 1/2 to 2/3 the width of the bandage. The spiral bandage is usually applied on the legs, arms, and fingers.

U
N
I
T
30

Important Steps	Key Points

8. Wrap the bandage evenly and smoothly.

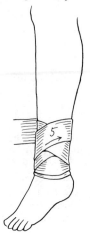

Hold the limb firmly and wrap it securely. Take care not to wrap it so tightly that you cut off the patient's return circulation. As you wrap, ask the patient how it feels. Loosen it immediately if he says it is too tight. Signs of impaired circulation are cyanosis or pallor, a cold, tingling sensation, and swelling. If you are applying the bandage over a wet dressing, you must wrap loosely to allow for shrinkage of the bandage as it dries.

9. Continue wrapping in the spiral fashion.

Wrap until the part is thoroughly covered. Do not use excessive bandage. Do not waste motions or material while wrapping.

10. Secure the terminal end of the bandage.

Use tape, clips, or safety pins. As before, do not start or finish the bandage over wounds, bony prominences, and so forth.

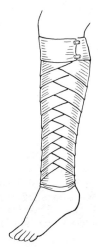

Turns of spiral bandage form a neat
sawtooth pattern

11. Make the patient comfortable.

Check the circulation flow by looking at the color of his toes and toenails, and feeling the temperature of the toes. They should feel as warm as the toes on the other foot.

Note: Ace bandages are rewrapped at least every 8 hours.

12. Tidy the work area.

Dispose of waste materials. Return unused supplies to the storage area.

13. Record the procedure on the patient's chart.

Chart the time and the type and location of the bandage. Charting example:

0800. Right leg rewrapped with Ace bandage. Toes warm and pink.   J. Jones, SN

Note: When the leg is involved, an elastic stocking may be ordered instead of the Ace bandage. Read the directions on the package before applying. Frequently observe the circulation in the toes after application. Refer to Unit 12 for general instructions.

ITEM 3. THE APPLICATION OF A SPIRAL REVERSE BANDAGE

This bandage is used to wrap an extremity that has varying thicknesses (such as the thin ankle portion which rises to a thick area like the calf of the leg). This method of bandaging provides a means to make a secure, smooth, even-fitting bandage on an extremity.

Important Steps	Key Points

Follow steps 1 through 8 of the spiral bandage procedure (Item 2) as though you were wrapping the left leg. Always start a bandage with at least two circular rounds to fasten the initial end securely.

9.   Make a spiral reverse turn.

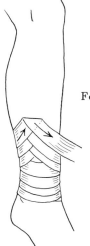

Folding bandage over to make spiral reverse turn.

This is done at the place on the leg where the bandage will no longer lie smoothly as you continue around the leg. Place your left thumb on the upper edge of the anterior turn; hold the bandage firmly. Unwind the roll of bandage about 4 to 6 inches; turn your hand downward (pronated) so that the bandage is now folded over your thumb in a downward direction toward the lower edge of the previous layer. Continue unrolling the bandage to the right and then to the left on the underside of the leg, covering about 1/2 to 2/3 of the previous lap.

U
N
I
T
30

10.   Continue making spiral reverse turns.

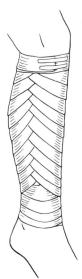

Spiral reverse bandage fits contours of extremity.

Wind the bandage in the same manner, and place it like the previous layers until the bandage will once again lie smoothly as you unroll it in a spiral direction. Then follow Steps 10 through 13 of the procedure in Item 2. Charting example:

0925. Spiral reverse bandage changed on right foot. Patient states less discomfort when up walking.   J. Jones, RN

ITEM 4. THE APPLICATION OF A FIGURE-8 BANDAGE

The figure-8 bandage may be used by itself or with the circular, spiral, or spiral reverse bandage whenever a joint is included in the wrapping. The figure-8 bandage turns around the joint serve to protect dressings and keep them in place, to support and limit the movement of the joint, and to promote the venous blood return, which reduces swelling, or edema. The advantage of the figure-8 bandage is that it can support the joint in a position of flexion, or allow limited movement when this is necessary.

To apply a figure-8 bandage to the ankle, follow these steps.

Important Steps

Key Points

Follow steps 1 through 8 in Item 1.

To bandage the ankle, place the initial anchoring turns around the foot, beginning near the toes. The anchoring turns generally are placed distal to the joint being wrapped.

9. Make a circular turn over the foot and around the ankle.

For purposes of support, the first turn may be placed at the upper part of the ankle, and each successive turn placed lower over the ankle and heel.

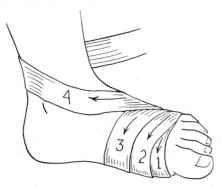

Anchoring turns for figure-8 bandage.

10. Continue to make a spiral turn down over the ankle and around the foot.

For promoting venous blood return, the first turn is placed lower on the heel, and each successive turn overlaps higher onto the ankle. The rest of the leg is also wrapped.

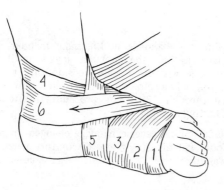

Continue alternate turns around ankle and foot.

Important Steps	Key Points
11. Alternate the upward and downward spiral turns about the joint.	Overlap each layer all but ½ to 1 inch, and make at least three complete turns. Continue bandaging the lower leg as necessary.

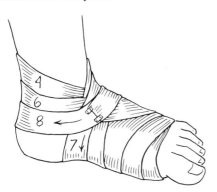

One type of figure-8 bandage.

Proceed to carry out steps 10 through 13 of Item 1, the circular bandage procedure.	Charting example: 1515. Ace bandage applied to right ankle. Slight swelling of foot. Toes pink and warm. J. Jones, RN

ITEM 5.   APPLICATION OF THE RECURRENT BANDAGE

This type of bandage is applied to hold pressure dressings in place over the tip end of a finger, toe, fist, or stump of an amputated extremity.

This is the type of bandage used on the stump of an *above-the-knee (AK) amputation. Below the knee amputation is identified as BK amputation.*

Important Steps	Key Points
Follow steps 1 through 7 of the circular bandage procedure, Item 1.	
8. Turn the bandage roll and bring forward over the tip. Bring bandage over tip.	Hold the top layer of bandage securely on the anterior leg with your left thumb at the highest (proximal) edge of the circular bandage. Continue unrolling the bandage downward over the tip of the stump toward the back. Continue to the highest point of the circular bandage layer at the center of the posterior aspect of the leg. Hold the bandage firmly at this spot with the left index finger.
9. Bring the roller bandage downward over the tip of the stump and forward up to the same level as the previous layer. Bring bandage up to level of previous layer.	Move each successive turn alternately to the left, then to the right of the first layer over the tip of the stump (in a somewhat spiral manner). Continue wrapping until the stump end is well covered, overlapping each layer about 1/2 to 2/3 the width of the previous layer. Continue to hold succeeding layers securely in place with your left thumb and index finger. (Reverse hand positions if you are left-handed.)

Important Steps	Key Points
10. Secure the ends with several circular turns. Secure ends with several circular turns. Complete the procedure by following steps 9 and 11 of the circular bandaging procedure.	When the stump is smoothly, evenly, and totally covered, once more reverse the direction of the roller bandage and make at least two circular turns to cover the gathered ends that you have been holding securely between your left thumb and index finger. Secure the final end with tape, a clip, or a safety pin. Charting example: 1100. Right AK stump bandage removed. Wound cleansed with antiseptic. Wound appears to be healing well. No drainage noted. Bandage replaced. J. Jones, SN

ITEM 6.   THE APPLICATION OF A SCULTETUS (MANY–TAILED) BINDER

The scultetus binder is designed to provide abdominal support after an abdominal operation, post-delivery, or post-paracentesis. The binder is made by sewing heavy flannel strips 3 to 4 inches wide and 4 feet long in overlapping layers of 1/2 inch. The middle third section of the strips is sewed together, leaving about 20 inches free on each end.

Important Steps	Key Points
Follow steps 1 through 3 in the circular bandage procedure.	
4. Move the patient to the proximal side of the bed.	This makes it easier for you to work. To avoid straining your back muscles, you must stand close to the bed facing the patient at his hip level. The height of the bed should be comfortable for your work. Fold back the top bedding, exposing only the portion of the body you are working on. Remember the patient's modesty and his need for privacy. (Siderails should be in place if you have to roll the patient.)
5. Ask the patient to raise his hips.	Quickly slip the scultetus binder under the hips, the top edge at waist level. The solid portion of the binder should be centered under the patient's body, the many-tailed ends lying flat on the bed extending straight out from the patient. If the patient is unable to raise his hips, have him roll to his side away from you. Place the solid portion of the binder on the bed, centered on the area on which his hips will rest. Return him to the supine position.
6. Begin application by bringing the *bottom tail* across the abdomen.	You will begin in the direction in which the tail is going, to provide for smooth, successive spiral-type layers with a 1/2-inch overlap of each layer. Pull tightly. If the end is too long, you may need to fold the free end back on itself, just far enough so it fits smoothly. *Note:* Incorrect placement of the overlaps causes pressure and discomfort for the patient.

Important Steps   Key Points

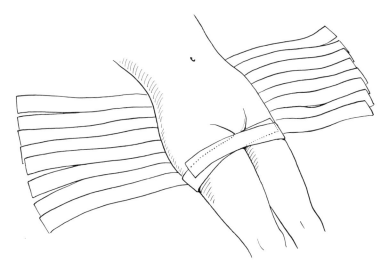

Start applying scultetus binder at the level
of the pubic region, or lower hip.

7. Proceed toward the waist, slanting each succeeding tail slightly upward.

Alternate strips (tails) first from one side of the abdomen, then the other side.

8. Secure the final tail with a safety pin.

This type of abdominal bandage provides good support for the patient. If you have pulled it securely enough as you criss-crossed each strip and then firmly pinned it, the patient will be able to move freely about (even walk) without having the bandage come undone.

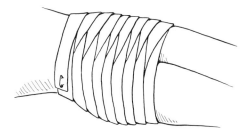

Scultetus binder secured firmly at the waist.

Follow steps 10 and 11 in the circular bandaging procedure to complete the action.

Charting example:

0800. Scultetus binder reapplied after bath. The additional support is comforting, the patient states.   J. Jones, SN

ITEM 7. THE APPLICATION OF A STRAIGHT ABDOMINAL OR CHEST BINDER

The exact type of binder (scultetus or straight) will depend on what is available, the purpose for which it is intended, and possibly the size and shape of the abdomen or chest. Breast binders may not be used in your agency. Check your agency procedure.

Important Steps   Key Points

Follow steps 1 through 4 in the scultetus binder procedure. Pull back the top bedding to expose only the area with which you are working. Remember the patient's modesty.

Important Steps	Key Points
5. Ask the patient to raise his hips or chest.	Quickly slip the binder under the hips, or chest if you are applying a breast binder. Center it under the patient's body. The lower edge of the abdominal binder should come well below the curve of the buttocks (rump). (If it is a breast binder, the lower edge comes to the waistline.) For the breast, fold the binder so that it laps well over the largest part of the breast.

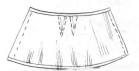

Straight binder.

Important Steps	Key Points
6. Fasten the lower edge first with a safety pin.	Pull the binder very tightly. Keep your hand between the patient's skin and the binder to prevent sticking the patient with the pin.
7. Continue pinning straight up the midline.	Pull the edges tightly with about a 3-inch overlap. Secure every 3 to 4 inches with a safety pin.
8. Make darts in the binder.	Because of the contour (shape) of the chest or abdomen, it is often difficult to make the binder lie flat without puckering; therefore, a few darts at the waistline will help to make the binder fit more snugly. With safety pins, take up the slack in the material and secure the tuck with a safety pin. Pin perpendicularly. Make a "V" dart, starting with a large tuck at the midline, and decreasing the size a few inches inward to make the binder fit neatly. You may need a tuck on each side of the midline. The darts in these binders serve the same purpose as darts when you are sewing a blouse. If the breasts are very large, be sure to pad under the breasts before applying the chest binder. This will prevent perspiration resulting from the two skin surfaces being held tightly together. Some physicians may specify that the abdominal binder be applied in the female by securing it downward from the waistline so that the abdominal organs are pushed against the uterus (womb) to control uterine bleeding. Check with your agency.

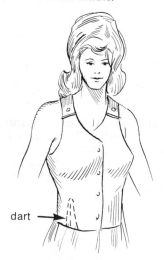

dart

Breast binder.

Follow steps 10 and 11 in the circular bandaging process to complete this procedure.

Charting example:

1640. Breast binder changed. No drainage noted. No complaints of pain or discomfort.

J. Jones, SN

ITEM 8.   APPLICATION OF A T–BINDER OR A DOUBLE T–BINDER

These binders are primarily used to keep peri-pads or rectal and perineal dressings in place. (The double T-binder is used for the male patient.)

Important Steps	Key Points
1. Obtain the supplies.	Select a binder, peri-pad, and dressings. Wash your hands.

Important Steps	Key Points
2. Approach the patient and explain what you are going to do.	Identify him by the identification band. Explain why you are using this type of binder. Fold back the top bedding to expose the area you are working with. Avoid undue exposure or chilling of the patient. The male patient may be somewhat embarrassed and may wish to apply the binder himself. If able, permit him to do so. Stand by to give assistance if needed, however.

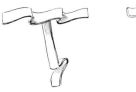

T-binder.   Double T-binder.

3. Ask the patient to raise his hips.	Quickly center the binder under the patient's back at waist level. Be sure the tail (or tails) lie smoothly under the patient toward the bottom of the bed. Secure the band around his waist firmly with a safety pin.
4. Apply the peri-pad or dressing to the rectal or perineal area.	Avoid touching the side of the pad or dressing that will come in contact with the patient's skin.
5. Secure the pad in place.	Fasten by bringing the free end of the T forward between the legs and securing it snugly at the waist with a safety pin. The double-tailed binder is usually used for the male patient. Bring each tail or strip forward between the legs. Extend the right tail to the right of the external male organs and secure it snugly to the waistband just to the right of the midline with a safety pin. Bring the left tail forward up between the legs to the left of the external male organs, and attach it snugly to the waistband slightly to the left of the midline with a safety pin.
6. Leave the patient comfortable.	Adjust the top linen neatly over the patient. Make sure that he is in a comfortable, well-aligned position. Place the call light, bed controls, and bedside stand conveniently within his reach. Tidy the room. Dispose of waste materials. Return unused supplies to the storage area. Wash your hands.
7. Record the procedure on the patient's chart.	Chart the time, type, and location of the dressing; describe drainage if any was present (sanguineous—bloody, or serous—thin, watery). Charting example: 0945. Peri-pad changed. Large amount of foul-smelling sanguineous drainage present. J. Jones, SN

U
N
I
T
30

ITEM 9. APPLICATION OF A SLING (TRIANGULAR) BANDAGE

This bandage is commonly used to support an injured arm. It can be made from a piece of cloth 30 to 40 inches square. Fold diagonally in half to make a double triangle. You can cut it across the diagonal fold if you want a single thickness.

Important Steps	Key Points
1. Obtain the supplies from the storeroom.	Wash your hands.
2. Approach the patient and explain what you are going to do to enlist his cooperation.	Identify him by checking his identification band. Quickly demonstrate how you will be applying the sling. Adjust his bed to working height. Have him sit on the edge of the bed facing you.
3. Put one end of the triangle over the shoulder on the uninjured side (1).	For this lesson, we will say it is the right arm that is injured. Therefore, the end of the triangle will be placed over the patient's left shoulder.

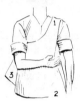

Place sling against body and under injured arm.

4. Place the point (apex) (3) of the triangle toward the elbow.	Ask the patient to bend his injured arm horizontally across his body with his thumb up. Place the bandage under his arm flat against his chest.
5. Bring the other end of the triangle (2) around his injured arm and up over his right shoulder (injured side).	Have the patient keep his elbow bent at right angles across his lower chest.

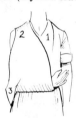

Secure sling by tying it at neck.

6. Tie the two ends of the triangle together with a square knot.	Make the knot to one side of the neck so that it will not be uncomfortable if the patient lies down (or will not cause continuing pull on the back of the neck when the arm is in the sling). Tie the knot securely so it will not come loose from the weight of the arm in the sling.
7. Fold the apex (or point) of the triangle neatly over the elbow toward the front.	Secure it with a safety pin.

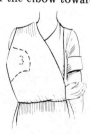

Injured arm supported by sling.

Important Steps	Key Points
8. Adjust the height of the sling by adjusting the knot at the neck.	The hand should be slightly higher than the elbow (about 4 inches). This will prevent the fingers from swelling.
9. Check the circulation in the fingers frequently.	Observe the color of the fingernail beds; they should be pink. Feel the fingers; they should be the same temperature as the fingers on the good hand. If the fingers are cold and pale, report immediately to the charge nurse.
10. Tidy the work area.	Dispose of waste materials in the wastebasket. Return unused supplies to the storage area.
11. Record the procedure on the patient's chart.	Chart the time and type of bandage. Comment about the appearance of the extremity. Charting example:

1510. Sling applied to right arm. Fingers warm and nailbeds pink. No pain reported by patient.
J. Jones, SN

UNIT
30

PERFORMANCE TEST

In the skill laboratory with a partner, you will correctly apply two of the following types of binders or bandages:

1. Scultetus binder.

2. Breast binder.

3. Triangular bandage.

4. Figure 8 bandage.

PERFORMANCE CHECKLIST

APPLICATION OF BANDAGES

1. Identify the patient.

2. Wash your hands.

3. Explain the procedure to the patient.

4. Identify the proper bandage for use.

5. Obtain the proper materials.

6. Identify the proper location.

7. Anchor the bandage properly.

8. Follow the specific sequential wrapping procedures.

    a. Wrap to achieve smoothness.

    b. Overlap correctly.

    c. Check for tension indicators.

        (1) Pain.

        (2) Decreased temperature.

        (3) Color change.

        (4) Wrap falling off due to insufficient tension.

9. Secure (anchor) the tail of the bandage.

10. Chart appropriately.

POST-TEST

1. List three purposes for which bandages and binders are used.

   a. _____

   b. _____

   c. _____.

2. The skin should be _____ and _____ before applying bandages or binders. Why? _____
_____.

3. Circulation of the extremity distal to the bandage or binder should be checked every _____ minutes.

4. _____ and _____ are good indicators of impaired circulation.

5. Describe a scultetus or many-tailed binder as to its shape and where and why it is applied.

_____

_____

_____.

6. Describe the usage of a triangular bandage. _____
_____.

7. Describe the use of the T-binder and double T-binder. _____
_____
_____.

POST-TEST ANNOTATED ANSWER SHEET

1. any three of the following: to apply pressure, provide immobilization, hold dressings in place, protect open wounds from infection, apply warmth to a joint, provide support, and aid circulation (p. 633)

2. clean; dry; to prevent pathogenic organisms from getting into the wound and setting up an infection (p. 634)

3. Every 30 minutes, for 3 times (p. 636)

4. Fingers; toes (634)

5. A many-tailed abdominal girdle-like support; provides support through a succession of overlapping bands (p. 642)

6. Triangular in shape and used to hold dressings in place; it is called a sling when used to support the forearm (pp. 645–646)

7. Binder-shaped like a single or double T used to hold rectal or perineal dressings in place (p. 644)

Unit 31

I. DIRECTIONS TO THE STUDENT

Obtain a sample packet of consent, release, and incident report forms from your instructor. Proceed through this lesson. When you are through, complete the post-test.

II. GENERAL PERFORMANCE OBJECTIVE

You will know how to obtain consents and releases and complete incident reports according to legal requirements.

III. SPECIFIC PERFORMANCE OBJECTIVES

Upon the completion of this unit, you will be able to:

1. Describe the circumstances that require consents and releases, and the factors that constitute an informed consent.

2. Explain the different consents and releases commonly used in hospitals and other similar agencies, including the admission agreement and the operative permit.

3. Explain the release from use of siderails form to the patient or his family, and obtain a valid signature.

4. State at least five types of events that are reported as patient incidents.

5. Prepare a patient incident form for submission to the hospital administration.

IV. VOCABULARY

biopsy—the excision of a small piece of tissue for the purpose of examination and diagnosis.

bone marrow—the soft (spongy) tissue in the hollow of long bones; the center bone marrow is yellow and is chiefly fat; the surrounding tissue is called the red bone marrow because it manufactures red blood cells.

informed consent—sufficient information about the advantages and disadvantages is given to the person to permit him to decide what action to take.

lumbar puncture—the procedure of inserting a needle into the lumbar spine in order to withdraw spinal fluid or inject a drug.

radiology—a branch of medicine that deals with X-rays and other radiations for the purpose of diagnosis or treatment.

V. INTRODUCTION

Purposes of Consents and Releases

Consents and releases are legal records of agreements between two parties, for our purposes, those between the patient and the hospital. The hospital provides printed documents that state the services that will be provided and the general treatment that the patient can expect. By signing the consent, the patient indicates that he agrees to what has been specified, and to the limits set for him and for the hospital. Both parties are protected legally. The patient who signs an operative permit for the repair of a hernia authorizes a specific operation performed on him. The doctor and the hospital staff in the operating room agree to repair the hernia, and do only the procedures necessary to achieve this.

ITEM 1. COMMON TYPES OF CONSENTS

Patients are required to sign a number of consents and forms when entering a hospital or nursing care facility. In some agencies, you may be expected to help secure the patient's signature on these forms. Usually, this will be done by the admission clerk or the nurse. However, you will need to know about the types of consents, and be able to explain them to the patients and their families.

The Admission Agreement. Hospitals routinely require that patients or their legal representatives sign the admission agreement. This document describes the type of care and services the patient can expect the hospital to provide, and in return, the patient assumes responsibility for the costs. The admission agreement states that the hospital will provide general staff nursing care and the usual medical treatment prescribed by the physician, and also states the limits of responsibility for the patient's personal property kept at the bedside, and for valuables. The agreement outlines the patient's financial obligation for the care rendered and provides for the release of certain information to insurance companies, worker's compensation, or other similar agencies for payment purposes.

The medical care that is covered in the admission agreement includes obtaining specimens for examinations in the clinical laboratory, X-rays that may have been ordered, and other medications and treatments commonly used in the treatment of disease.

Often the admission agreement form consists of several copies, one that is given to the patient, and another copy that is placed in the patient's chart.

The Operative Consent. The operative consent is called by a variety of names including the *Consent to Operation and Administration of Anesthesia*, and the surgical permit. The operative consent is prepared and the patient's signature is obtained when the physician operates on the patient's body with his hands or instruments. Most people know about the operations that are done in surgery and involve some sort of incision or cutting into body tissue. All surgical procedures and biopsies require that an operative consent be signed preoperatively to authorize the surgery, the giving of the anesthesia, and the services of pathology or other departments when needed. An operative consent form is pictured on the following page:

U
N
I
T
31

**CONSENT TO OPERATION, ADMINISTRATION OF
ANESTHETICS, AND THE RENDERING OF OTHER
MEDICAL SERVICES**

....

Name of Patient

Date ....

Hour ....M.

1. I authorize and direct.. M.D.

my surgeon and/or associates or assistants of his choice to perform the following operation upon me

....

and/or to do any other therapeutic procedure that (his) (their) judgment may dictate to be advisable for the patient's well-being. I have been informed by my Doctor, of the nature and intended result of this operation, as well as its foreseeable risks and possible alternatives. I further understand that no warranty or guarantee has been made as to the result or cure.

2. I hereby authorize and direct the above named surgeon and/or his associates or assistants to provide such additional services for me as he or they may deem reasonable and necessary, including, but not limited to, the administration and maintenance of the anesthesia, and the performance of services involving pathology and radiology, and I hereby consent thereto.

3. I understand that the above named surgeon and his associates or assistants will be occupied solely with performing such operation, and the persons in attendance at such operation for the purpose of administering anesthesia, and the person or persons performing services involving pathology and radiology, are not the agents, servants or employees of the above named hospital nor of any surgeon, but are independent contractors and as such are the agents, servants, or employees of myself.

4. I hereby authorize the hospital pathologist to use his discretion in the disposal of any severed tissue or member, except ....

                     Patient's Signature ....

                                Witness ....

                                Witness ....

(If patient is a minor or unable to sign, complete the following:)

Patient is a minor, or is unable to sign, because ....

....
           Father   Guardian

....
           Mother   Other Person and Relationship

The operative consent, or a similar form specified by your agency's policies, is used for procedures and examinations of an "invasive" nature when the physician uses an instrument or introduces a substance into one of the patient's body spaces or cavities. The procedures that need an operative consent vary so you should consult your agency's policies. Generally the list would include, but should not be limited to the following:

1. Arteriogram

2. Bone marrow puncture

3. Bronchoscopy

4. Cardiac catheterization

5. Cystoscopy

6. Encephalogram

7. Lumbar puncture

8. Myelogram

9. Paracentesis

10. Pneumoencephalogram

11. Thoracentesis

"Informed Consents". The law requires that any person who signs a consent for any purpose must know enough about the matter to make a reasonable decision. This means that patients asked to sign an operative consent must know the need for the surgery or procedure, basically what is involved, the expected results, the disadvantages, and the risks involved. Generally, the doctors who will perform the surgery or the procedure explain it to the patient and his family. It is the physician's responsibility to provide this information.

When you are requested to obtain the patient's signature on the consent form, you should be sure that the patient understands what it is he is signing, and that he is able to make a decision based on information given by the doctor or the nurse. The patient should read the consent form, or it should be read to him. A question such as "What has the doctor told you about your surgery (or this procedure)?" will give you an idea about what the patient does understand about the operation. If the patient does not understand, postpone getting his signature on the consent form until the patient has been given full information. Avoid rushing the patient to sign a consent form or appearing to force him to complete the form. Some patients may ask to wait until they can discuss the matter with others in their family. Decisions are not always easy to make when the procedure may be painful, pose a high risk, or result in alterations or changes in the body.

In an emergency situation where surgery is indicated to save the patient's life, the surgeon may operate without a consent form signed by the patient. However, every effort must be made to obtain permission from a responsible family member by telegram or telephone, or by an order from the court.

Other Types of Consents. You may be asked to prepare other types of consents and obtain the signatures on them. Others may be more appropriately obtained by the nurse or the physician.

1. Autopsy Permit. The nurse or physician fills out the form and obtains the signature of the next of kin for a postmortem examination of a body to determine the cause of death.

2. Authorization for Treatment of a Minor. The nurse prepares the agency form and obtains the signature of the parent or legal guardian to authorize care for the minor.

3. Consent for Photographs. The agency form is used and the patient's signature is obtained. The consent also states the purpose for the photographs.

4. Consent for Use of Experimental Drugs or Treatment. The agency form is used and is initiated by the physician or the nurse. The physician prescribing the experimental

drugs must follow guidelines set by federal agencies. The patients must give an "informed consent" for experimental drugs or treatments.

5. **Permit to Use Personal Electrical Appliances.** Some agencies require that the patient sign a request to use his own electrical appliances such as a radio, shaver, or television set. The agency form is initiated by the nurse.

ITEM 2. COMMON TYPES OF RELEASES

A release is another type of legal record that is used to excuse one party from responsibility or liability. The release is an administrative form and is usually made out in duplicate with one copy going to the administration and one copy on the patient's chart. However, you should follow instructions provided by your agency. The release forms are simple to prepare: stamp the form with the addressograph card and fill in the date and any other information requested.

Common releases you may encounter include the following:

1. **Release from Use of Siderails.** Hospitals frequently require that siderails on the beds be used for patients whenever they are in bed as a safety measure. Some patients oppose the use of siderails, refuse to cooperate or follow the agency policy, or believe that there is no need to use siderails; therefore, they sign a release. The form indicates that they are aware of the possible hazard of not using the siderails and will not hold the hospital responsible for any harm that might occur as a result of not using them.

2. **Discharge Against Medical Advice.** This form is prepared whenever a patient demands to leave the hospital without an order from his doctor authorizing his discharge. The doctor or the nurse should talk with the patient and explain the reasons that continued hospital care is needed. However, if the patient insists on leaving, make out the discharge against medical advice (also abbreviated to AMA) in duplicate, and offer it to the patient to sign. The form states that the hospital is released from responsibility for the patient's conditions as a result of his leaving the hospital AMA. If the patient refuses to sign the form, this should be noted and witnessed. Discharge of a patient AMA is reported immediately to the attending physician, the nursing supervisor, and the administration. One copy of the form remains on the patient's chart.

3. Other releases may be used for a number of conditions, including the release of information, the relase of responsibility for personal property, and so forth.

ITEM 3. WHO MAY SIGN CONSENTS OR RELEASES?

Generally, any *adult* may sign a consent or release if he is not under a guardianship (as in the case of incompetency). An adult is any person, male or female, who has reached the age of 18 years, who has contracted a valid marriage, or in some states, who has been designated as an emancipated minor.

Minors are persons below the age of 18, or who are not included in the groups described above. Minors may be treated when the authorization to treat the minor has been signed by his parent or *legal* guardian. An emergency situation, e.g., life or death, may be handled differently as prescribed by agency policy. Every parent of a minor child left in the care of babysitters, in school, or at home when the parent is on vacation should give written permission for treatment of the child in case of illness or injury at a time when the parent cannot be reached. This would avoid the many hours spent by treatment facilities trying to obtain a legal authorization to treat.

All dates, times, and signatures must be in ink, including witnesses' signatures. Follow your agency policy regarding the witnessing of consents. Usually there are specific regulations as to who may sign documents as a witness, e.g., the RN only, the admitting clerk, the notary public.

ITEM 4. PROCEDURE FOR GETTING SIGNATURES

Given a patient scheduled to have surgery, you are to prepare the operative consent and obtain the patient's informed consent.

Important Steps	Key Points
1. Obtain the form and equipment: consent, pen, and surface (e.g., clipboard) to write on.	If you are responsible for securing consents, make sure that the patient's name, age, sex, room number, physician, and type of surgery or procedure are correct before you take it to the patient. This preliminary information can be completed on the form before taking it to him for his signature. Forms are usually stored in a designated place in the nurse's station.
2. Wash your hands, identify the patient, and explain the procedure.	If he's unable to read it himself, read it to him. Make sure he understands the form. Ask him to explain what he understands the form to say. Clarify if he does not understand.
3. Give the consent form to the patient to read.	
4. Obtain the patient's signature.	Ask him to sign his full name in ink in the appropriate space. You write the date and time in the space provided. If the patient refuses to sign the consent, refer to your charge nurse. She will notify the physician and await his order. The final determination about the consent is the responsibility of the physician. *Note:* If the patient cannot sign his name, two people are required to witness him make an "X." The patient's name and the words "his mark" are written at the side of the "X" to identify the mark. If you obtained the patient's signature, you *must* witness his signature. Sign your full name and title with a pen. This form becomes a part of the patient's chart or record.
5. Place the completed consent or release on the patient's chart.	See the sample forms in your packet.

U
N
I
T
31

ITEM 5. PATIENT INCIDENT REPORTS

Patient incident reports are made out if there is an error in treatment or if a patient accident occurs. They are not part of the patient's chart as are consents and releases but are intended for the hospital administration and attorneys. They alert the hospital administration to the possibility of litigation (law suits).

What Constitutes a "Patient Incident"?

The following generally constitute incidents that are reportable:

1. Falls or injuries to the patient.

2. Burns resulting from treatment.

3. Personal articles lost or damaged.

4. Medication errors.

5. Errors in patient identification, e.g., giving the treatment to the wrong patient.

6. Injection injuries, e.g., needle injury to a nerve during medication injection.

7. Treatment injuries.

8. Thermometers broken in the patient's mouth, rectum, bed, and so forth.

9. Fights and assaults.

Who Completes Incident Reports?

The nursing personnel who are most familiar with the incident, or who observed its happening, should complete the account of the incident according to the agency policy.

If an incident occurs, provide emergency and safety measures for the patient; call for help, either verbally or by patient call bell. Your team leader will notify a house physician or the patient's own physician.

After the patient's comfort and safety are provided, try to obtain his account of the incident. You will need this to complete the report. Carry out the doctor's order for care if the incident necessitates follow-through; for example, the patient falls and breaks an arm — the doctor orders an X-ray.

ITEM 6. PROCEDURE FOR PREPARING INCIDENT REPORTS

Given a patient who has fallen in his room, provide assistance and prepare the patient incident report for the hospital administration.

Important Steps	Key Points
1. Provide for the patient's safety and comfort.	Call for help verbally or by signaling with the patient's call bell. Do not try to move him by yourself because you may hurt the patient and yourself. Remove any safety hazards such as broken glass. Provide warmth for the patient.
2. Return the patient to bed.	Do this as soon as possible. Get assistance as needed. Make him comfortable. Follow the doctor's orders if given; for example, call for an X-ray or discontinue a blood transfusion.
3. Complete an incident report form.	Ask your team leader for assistance in completing your history of the incident and other patient information. Charting should be clear, concise, and accurate.
4. Get the patient's account of the incident.	After he is calmed or has been seen by a physician, you may ask him to relate what happened to cause the incident, if he is aware that there was an incident. Write this information in the space provided in the report. It is desirable (when appropriate) to quote the patient's own words. You will start the comment on the form: "The patient states that . . ."
5. Distribute copies of the completed form according to instructions.	The physician will sign in the appropriate place; one section is forwarded to the nursing office, and one to the administration. It is an administrative form and does not become part of the patient's chart.

VI. ADDITIONAL INFORMATION FOR ENRICHMENT

Consents, releases and incident reports provide important safety aspects for the patient, for you, and for your agency. Follow the agency's established policies.

PERFORMANCE TEST

1. Complete a patient incident report form from the following information:

   At 3:45 A.M. Mrs. Mary Volk, 223^2, fractured hip, 87 years old, patient of Dr. G. Marshall, fell out of bed while trying to get up to the bathroom. Siderails were down, and the bed was in the low position. Patient had received her nembutal gr lss h.s.

2. Complete a Surgical Consent form for Mr. Victor Welk, 257^1, patient of Dr. S. First, for a right inguinal herniotomy. He is scheduled for surgery at 9:00 A.M. on Thursday, December 1.

3. Complete a Release of Siderails Form for Mr. V. Welk in Question #2.

PERFORMANCE CHECKLIST

CONSENTS, RELEASES, INCIDENTS

COMPLETION OF A PATIENT INCIDENT FORM

1. Obtain the proper form.
2. Fill in the preliminary information.
3. Wash your hands.
4. Identify the patient.
5. Explain the procedure to the patient.
6. Verify the patient's understanding of the form.
7. Complete the history of the incident as related by the patient, for example: "The patient states that _____ ."
8. Document the report if possible, i.e., list all individuals familiar with the incident.
9. Transmit the form to the appropriate departments.

COMPLETION OF CONSENT OR RELEASE FORM

1. Obtain the proper form and the necessary equipment.
2. Fill in all preliminary information.
3. Wash your hands.
4. Identify the patient, and explain the procedure to him.
5. Permit the patient to read the form, and clarify his understanding of the form.
6. Ask the patient to sign the form.
7. Write in the date and time that the form is signed.
8. Witness the form as required.
9. Place the completed form with the patient's chart.
10. In the event that the patient will not sign, you sign the form, annotating the record appropriately.

11. In the event that the patient cannot write his name, obtain the signature of two witnesses.

12. In the event that the patient is a minor, obtain his parent's or guardian's signature.

COMPLETION OF CONSENT OR RELEASE FORM

1. Obtain the proper form and necessary equipment.

2. Fill in all preliminary information.

3. Wash your hands.

4. Identify the patient, and explain the procedure to him.

5. Permit the patient to read the form, and clarify his understanding of the form.

6. Ask the patient to sign the form.

7. Write in the date and time that the form is signed.

8. Witness the form as required.

9. Place the completed form with the patient's chart.

10. In the event that the patient cannot write his name but can make an "X" or mark, obtain the signatures of two witnesses.

11. In the event that the patient is a minor, obtain his parent's or guardian's signature.

POST-TEST

Directions: Check all of the following statements that are *true*.

_____ 1. A new consent must be obtained before an operation can be performed by a physician other than the one originally named in the consent for the operation.

_____ 2. A consent usually is not required when a patient is admitted to a hospital only for observation.

_____ 3. A consent for treatment of a married woman who is under 21 years of age must be obtained from her husband.

_____ 4. A minor may legally consent to his own treatment if an emergency exists and his parent or guardian is not available.

_____ 5. A physician does not incur liability if he performs emergency surgery on an unconscious patient without a consent other than the general admission agreement.

_____ 6. A specific consent must be obtained for a blood transfusion.

_____ 7. A specific consent must be obtained for photographing a patient.

_____ 8. A patient must sign a release before he can leave a hospital against the advice of his physician.

_____ 9. When a patient signs a release from the use of siderails, this relieves the nurse of responsibility for his safety in bed.

_____10. An occurrence is classed as an incident only if it involves actual or possible injury to a patient or other person.

_____11. When an incident involves a patient, a copy of the incident report must be entered in his records.

12.   What is the purpose of a consent or release? _____

_____.

13.   Suppose a patient fails to understand the form. You try to explain, but he says he still does not understand. What do you do?

_____

_____

_____.

14.   If the patient refuses to sign the form even though he understands, how far should you go in trying to persuade him? What do you do when his guardian or relative refuses to sign?

_____

_____

_____

_____.

15.   Name two common types of consents.

     a. _____ b. _____.

16.   Name two common types of releases.

     a. _____ b. _____.

17. Define an adult (relative to signing consents and releases).

_____

_____

_____.

18. List four instances that constitute a patient incident.

a. _____

b. _____

c. _____

d. _____.

POST-TEST ANNOTATED ANSWER SHEET

1. T (p. 651)   7. T (p. 653)

2. F (p. 651)   8. F (p. 654)

3. F (p. 654)   9. F (p. 654)

4. F (p. 654)   10. F (p. 655)

5. F (p. 653)   11. F (p. 656)

6. F (p. 651)

12. To protect the patient's and the hospital's rights (p. 651)

13. Refer to his doctor for clarification and withhold signing of the consent until the patient understands (p. 653)

14. You do not need to persuade the patient, family, or guardian. Refer to the nurse and she will notify the physician. He will then determine what action to take. The final responsibility rests with the physician (p. 653)

15. Any of these: admission agreement; surgical consent, consent for use of experimental drugs; consent to photograph; autopsy permit, etc. (pp. 651 and 653)

16. Any of these: AMA; release from use of siderails; release of body to mortuary, etc. (p. 654)

17. Any person who has reached the age of 18 years or who has a valid marriage contract and is mentally competent (p. 654)

18. Any of these: patient fall; patient burn; medication or treatment error; error in patient identification; broken thermometer; damaged or lost personal articles, etc. (pp. 655–656)

UNIT 31

Unit 32

I. DIRECTIONS TO THE STUDENT

You will proceed through the lesson using this workbook as your guide. You will need to practice the skills on the class mannequin or a student partner in the skill laboratory. After completing the lesson and practicing the skills, arrange with your instructor to take the post-test.

II. GENERAL PERFORMANCE OBJECTIVES

When you have finished this unit, you will be able to demonstrate satisfactorily how to brush, comb, and shampoo a patient's hair without causing discomfort to the patient.

III. SPECIFIC PERFORMANCE OBJECTIVES

In the clinical setting or in the skill laboratory, you will be able to:

1. Brush, comb, braid, and arrange a patient's hair in accordance with recommended procedure.

2. Prepare a patient for a shampoo in bed (or at the sink in the bathroom or utility room) using principles of safety, good body alignment, and patient comfort.

3. Determine when the patient's hair is clean by using the "squeaking clean" technique.

4. Improvise a trough to keep the patient dry and provide for water drainage when giving a shampoo in bed or on a stretcher.

IV. VOCABULARY

braiding (plaiting)—a method of hair styling frequently used for the hospitalized patient with long hair to keep the hair neat.

dandruff—fungus infection of the scalp in which the scalp becomes dry and scaly; daily hair care and frequent shampoos help prevent this condition; dandruff infections may be transmitted from one person to another by sharing a comb or brush.

nits—eggs (ova) of the louse (plural, lice)

pediculosis—the presence of the parasitic louse on the body, in the hair of the scalp, or in the hair of the pubic area.

ITEM 1. THE IMPORTANCE OF HAIR CARE

Authorities believe that the condition of the hair is affected by the general health of the individual. In some cases it is easy to note disease conditions by the appearance of the shaft of the hair. For example, coarse, dry hair may be associated with an underactive thyroid gland (hypothyroidism); hair falling out may be associated with the incidence of high temperatures lasting long periods of time.

The visible portion of the hair (shaft) is supplied with nutrients (food) through the roots, which are anchored in the scalp. The supply of nutrients is therefore very important to the health of the hair. It is important to brush and comb the hair because this stimulates the circulation of the scalp, cleans the hair shafts of dirt particles and dead skin cells, and brings nutrients to the roots.

Hair care should be given regularly during illness just as it would be normally, usually with the morning care activities and throughout the day as needed. The morale of the patient is improved when his appearance is tidy. Neat, clean hair is particularly important to the female patient's sense of well-being.

ITEM 2. DAILY HAIR CARE: COMBING AND BRUSHING

Given a female bed patient with long hair, you are to comb, brush, and arrange her hair in a becoming manner.

Important Steps	Key Points
1. Approach and identify the patient, explain the procedure, and gain her cooperation.	The best time to give hair care is after the morning bath or with the early A.M. care. Explain to the patient the need to keep the hair healthy and clean, and the scalp stimulated. Encourage her to comb or brush her own hair. Since this is a daily procedure, patients are encouraged by their progress when they can do this for themselves. However, you must help the patient with this task until she can manage it.
2. *Wash your hands* and assemble the necessary equipment.	Be sure that a clean comb, brush, and mirror are placed conveniently on the bedside stand or overbed table. Hair cream or sprays may be used if the patient wishes.
3. Place a towel over the pillow.	Put a clean towel over the patient's pillow to keep it from becoming soiled. Be sure that the patient is well covered with a bath blanket to keep warm during the procedure. (Since hair care is part of the daily patient care, the bath blanket will already be in place.)
4. Turn the patient's head away from you.	This will make it easier for you to comb and brush the back of the hair. It will also keep the hair from getting in the patient's face and eyes.
5. Part the hair.	It will be easier to handle if you part the hair from the front to the back. The hair is thinner in front and it will eliminate some of the pulling of the hair, thus making it more comfortable for your patient. The teeth of the comb should be dull so that they will not scratch the scalp. Stiff bristles on the brush are best for hair care. Brushes which have widely separated tufts (clumps) of bristles are the easiest to clean. Public Health regulations require sterilization (killing of germs by submitting the item to various heating methods) of brushes made of animal bristles before they are sold in stores, to prevent the transmission of anthrax from possibly infected bristles.

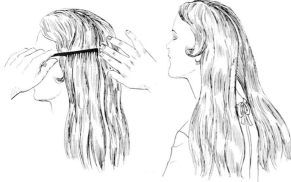

Important Steps	Key Points
6. First divide the hair into three main sections, and then as you work, handle it in smaller subsections.	This will make it simpler for you to proceed in a systematic way as you comb or brush. You will reach every portion of the scalp if you proceed in this manner.
7. Brush or comb the hair starting at the base (near the scalp) in an upward manner. 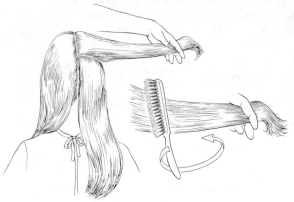	Grasp a small section of hair between your index and middle fingers (use your left hand if you are right-handed, or your right hand if you are left-handed). Place the brush or comb near the scalp and use a rotating semicircular wrist movement to push the brush or comb through the hair. This motion will not scratch the scalp or split the shaft of the hair. It stimulates circulation, massages the scalp, and loosens dry scales and dirt from the scalp and the hair. (Remember that some people have very sensitive scalps and that during an illness the scalp becomes more sensitive to pressure; therefore, make every effort not to hurt the patient.)
8. Keep the hair between your fingers when brushing or combing matted or tangled hair. 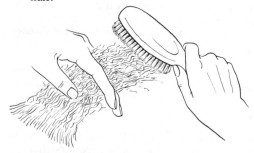	This provides a counterforce to prevent undue pulling on the scalp when you are brushing or combing matted or tangled hair. Alcohol, astringents, or water can be used to loosen hair strands when they are tangled or matted. *Do not cut* the hair to remove them. Daily and frequent brushing or combing prevents tangling and matting of the hair. Talk with the patient in a warm, concerned manner. Answer all of her questions if you can; those that you cannot, refer to the nurse or doctor. Observe the patient's condition as you work. If she becomes unusually tired, complete the hair care later in the day.
9. Continue brushing or combing.	Finish all the sections on one side.
10. Arrange the hair attractively.	The style should be simple and neat. You are not expected to be a professional hair stylist. The patient will probably tell you what is most comfortable. Short hair is the easiest to care for when a person must remain in bed for a long period of time.
11. Move to the other side of bed.	Have the patient turn her head away from you toward the opposite side. Proceed in the above method (see steps 6 through 10). When you are finished with all sections, style this side of the hair to match the first side. If the hair is long, you may want to braid it. The procedure for braiding is described later in this unit.
12. Spray the hair or apply hair cream.	Use as desired by the patient to keep the hair neat and in place.
13. Remove the towel.	Discard it into the soiled-linen hamper.

Important Steps	Key Points
14. Clean the comb and brush.	Remove the excess hair from the comb or brush, and discard it into a wastebasket. Wash the comb or brush.
15. Return the items to the bedside stand.	Leave the room tidy. Arrange items (water pitcher, books, and so forth) on the bedside stand for the patient's easy reach.
16. Record the activity on the nurses' notes.	Record any unusual observations about the condition of the scalp or hair. Usually the entry will be included as a part of the morning care. Specific entry of hair combing is made only when unusual conditions are observed. Charting example: 0800. Scalp noted to be very red and crusty when hair was combed. Complaining of severe itching. Dr. Smith was notified when he visited during bath procedure. R. Ryan, LVN

ITEM 3. BRAIDING

Braiding is a method of weaving, entwining, or interlacing together three strands of hair, which is sometimes used as a hair style for youngsters or for patients with long hair. This style is easy to maintain and comfortable for the patient; it is for the latter reason that this style is recommended during hospitalization. Braided hair helps to keep the long hair from becoming matted or tangled. Both of these conditions are uncomfortable to the patient and are particularly painful when the hair is being combed. Braiding helps keep the hair off the patient's neck, allows greater comfort by keeping her cooler, and prevents heat rash on the back of the neck.

Proceed through this lesson. You may practice braiding in the skill lab with three strands of heavy knitting yarn (or similar materials), or on a classmate who has long hair and is a willing subject. When you are sure you can braid, ask your instructor to observe you in a test situation. You will be checked on the neatness of your finished product. The hair should be firmly anchored to prevent the braids from coming apart. It can be tied with a ribbon or a rubber band.

Important Steps	Key Points
1. Explain the procedure to the patient.	You will be using this method as a part of the basic hair care procedure. Tell the patient that you will be braiding her hair to provide for her comfort by keeping her hair from becoming matted or tangled. Give her a neat, simple hair style. Your patient will already be positioned on the towel-covered pillow with her face turned away from you. The hair will be parted in the center (from front to back) and you will be working with the hair on the exposed half of the head.
2. Brush or comb the hair and then divide it into three even sections on each side of the head.	Usually the hair can be handled in three large sections for the weaving process. Proceed with each of the sections in the following manner.

UNIT 32

Important Steps   **Key Points**

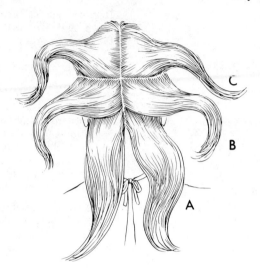

3. Hold the left (A) strand of hair in three closed fingers (fist) of your left hand. (See the accompanying illustration.)

Bring the hair to the side of the patient's head, near the ear. As you entwine the hair, hold the strands taut so that the braid will be firm and will not loosen when the patient moves around.

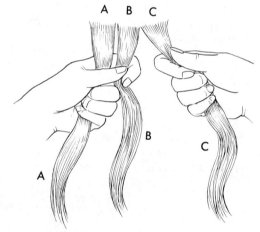

4. Hold the center (B) strand between the index finger and thumb of your left hand.

5. Hold the right (C) strand in your right hand.

Keep all the strands taut; do not pull the hair too hard because you will hurt the patient's scalp. After practice you will learn the correct amount of "pull" that is needed to keep the strands taut.

6. Cross the right strand (C) over the center strand (B).

Strand C becomes the new middle strand, and will be transferred to the left hand. The center strand (B) is transferred to the right hand.

Important Steps   **Key Points**

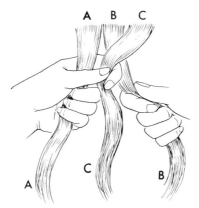

7. Cross the left strand (A) over the center strand (C).

Strand A now becomes the middle strand. Move it to your right hand.

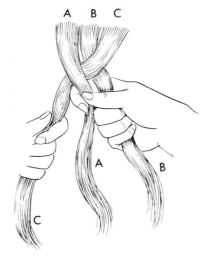

8. Cross the right strand (B) over the center strand (A).

Step 6 can start with the left strand over; step 7 would then be the right strand over the center, and so on. The important point is the crossover of the alternate outside strands.

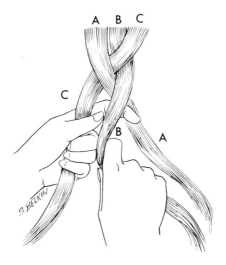

Important Steps	Key Points
9. Continue, repeating steps 6, 7, and 8.	Repeat until all the strands of hair are completely braided. Remember: the alternate outside strands cross over the center strand.

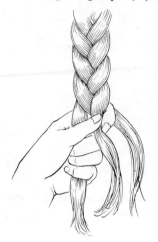

10. Secure the end of the braid.	Bind it with a rubber band looped several times around the tip end of the braid. This will keep the braid from becoming unwound. *Note:* Wind the rubber band loosely. If applied too tightly, if will injure the hair shaft. If a bright-colored ribbon is available, it can be tied at the tip end (covering the rubber band). This provides a touch of gaiety for the patient and will often raise her spirits.

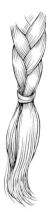

11. Move to the other side of the bed.	Proceed with the other side of the hair, as in steps 2 through 10.

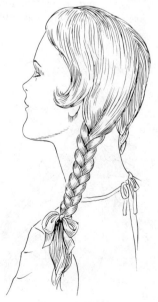

ITEM 4. SHAMPOO FOR THE BED PATIENT

Shampooing of the hair is done only upon the order of the physician, so that you may have to ask for permission if the patient requests a shampoo and it has not been ordered. Shampoos may be given in bed with the patient in a sitting position or in a recumbent position (lying on his back, or supine). It may also be given in the utility room on a stretcher, or in the shower. The supine position is preferred for some patients and by some nurses. However, patients with disease conditions such as asthma, certain heart diseases, and some lung diseases have difficulty breathing unless the head and chest are elevated as in Fowler's position. Thus, the sitting position must be maintained for these patients throughout your care for them.

Today, however, many patient rooms are equipped with showers, and the procedure of choice may be to assist the patient with the shampoo while he or she is in the shower. This, of course, will depend entirely on the patient's general condition. Your charge nurse will be able to help you make the correct decision.

Shampoos are given to keep the hair clean, to prevent or remove dandruff, to remove lice (pediculosis), to improve appearance and therefore assist in cheering the patient, and to increase the circulation of the patient's scalp.

To Prepare a Trough:

The trough is a shallow piece of equipment (metal, plastic, paper, or rubber) used to protect the bedding from becoming wet by guiding the flow of water from the patient's head to the side of the bed and into the waste receptacle.

Important Steps	Key Points
1. Spread a section of newspaper on a flat surface.	A paper, rubber, or plastic trough is improvised if a metal drain tray or trough is not available. Use several thicknesses of paper (6 to 8 sheets), spread out to the length of 3 feet (36 inches) on the bed or a table top in the utility room.
2. Place plastic (or rubber) sheeting on top of the papers.	Sheeting should be about 36 inches long and 24 inches wide.
3. Roll the long sides of the paper and plastic sheeting toward the center.	Roll each side toward the center of the sheet, leaving the center third flat. This will form two rolled edges.
4. Place one end of the trough under the patient's head.	Place the center flat surface under her head, allowing the rolled edges to provide a channel for the water to run through.
5. Place the other end of the trough in a waste pail (basin) on the chair.	Put a rolled bath towel or small pillow under the trough so that it tilts in a gradual slope, causing the water to run from the patient's head to the side of the bed and into the waste pail (basin).

To Give a Bed Shampoo:

1. Approach the patient and check her identity; explain procedure and enlist her cooperation.	Be sure that your patient is well-rested. Shampooing is a lengthy procedure that tires the patient a great deal. It is wise to consider a rest period for the patient after the completion of the shampoo. Timing is therefore important for this procedure. Usually your patient will be told about the shampoo; perhaps she has requested it.

U
N
I
T
32

Important Steps	Key Points
2. Check the room for temperature and "work" space.	Make sure that the room is warm and free of drafts and that you have space to move about easily during the procedure. *Wash your hands.*
3. Assemble the equipment conveniently at the site of the shampoo (bed, shower, or utility room).	You will need the following articles: a. Pitcher of warm water (105°F). b. Second pitcher of hot water (115°F) to add to the first pitcher in order to maintain its warmth throughout the procedure. c. Bath thermometer if available; if not, a few drops of water on the inner surface of your wrist will indicate when the water in the pitcher is comfortably warm. d. Liquid shampoo, soap, or cream provided by your agency or the patient. If shampooing is being done to remove lice, a special shampoo such as "Cuprex" may be used. e. Cup of lemon juice, vinegar, or commercial rinse. f. Pail or basin to catch drainage. g. Rubber or plastic sheet for bed protection. h. Bath towels (at least two). i. Face towel and safety pin, to protect the patient's neck and shoulders. j. Bath blanket. k. Pad, or trough made of rubber, plastic, paper, or metal. l. Plastic cover for chair. m. Hair dryer if available.

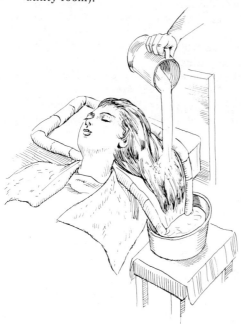

Important Steps	Key Points
4. Prepare the patient for the shampoo.	Remove the pillow and move the patient toward the proximal (near) side of the bed. Have the bed at a convenient working height. Cover her with a bath blanket to keep her warm and to protect the bed linens from becoming wet. Fan-fold the top linen to the bottom of the bed. Put a towel around the patient's shoulders.
5. Prepare the equipment.	Place the chair at the head of the bed and cover it with plastic sheeting. Put a basin or pail on the chair to collect the water. Protect the head of the bed with a plastic sheet covered with a drawsheet. Place a trough made of rubber, plastic, metal, or paper under the patient's head with one end in the drainage pail.
6. Moisten the hair with water (105°F) and apply the shampoo.	Pour a small amount of water through the patient's hair from the front hairline to the

Important Steps	Key Points
	back to moisten the hair thoroughly. A folded washcloth placed over the patient's eyes will help to protect them from soap and water.
	Work the shampoo into a good lather, using your finger tips to firmly massage all portions of the scalp. The patient will tell you if the massage is uncomfortable. Start from the front hairline and proceed toward the back of the head, just as you shampoo your own hair. Add water as needed to keep the lather going.
7. Pour water through the hair.	Rinse thoroughly.
8. Repeat steps 6 and 7.	Remember to work quickly so that your patient does not become excessively tired. Pour the water carefully as you rinse the shampoo out of the hair. Apply one more soaping if the hair is not "squeaking clean," and if your patient can tolerate the procedure.
9. Test for clean, well-rinsed hair.	Continue rinsing the hair until strands pulled between your index finger and thumb produce a squeaking sound.
10. Apply the rinse solution.	It may be necessary to use a commercial rinse, lemon juice, or vinegar solution (1 ounce to 1 quart of water) to easily rinse the shampoo from the hair.
11. Dry the hair, ears, and neck.	Use a heavy bath towel to rub the hair between the folds of the towel. Dry the hair as thoroughly as possible. Keep your patient warm and dry throughout the procedure. Avoid drafts.
12. Arrange the hair.	Comb and brush the hair using a clean comb and brush. Follow the procedure used for combing and brushing, steps 4 through 9. You may need to secure the hair with hairpins; you may be asked to set the patient's hair with rollers. If you do not know how to do this, see if someone can assist you. If no one is available, simply arrange the hair in a neat, attractive way and allow it to dry. (An electric hair dryer may be used if one is available in your agency.)
	Note: If the patient brings her hair dryer to the hospital, have it checked for safety by the maintenance department in your agency. This safety procedure is to be followed without exception for all electrical appliances that belong to patients.
13. Remove the wet towels, trough, and pail.	Place them in the appropriate area. Clean the pail and trough so that they are ready for the next patient.
14. Provide for the patient's comfort.	Remove the bath blanket and store it in the designated area. If it is soiled, put it in the soiled-linen hamper. Raise the siderails if indicated. Leave the patient dry, neat, clean, and comfortable, but check on her at frequent intervals. After such a tiring procedure for the

UNIT 32

Important Steps	Key Points
	patient, make sure that she is not overly exhausted; assist her in relaxing and resting for a brief period.
15. Record the shampoo procedure on the nurses' notes.	Report the time, the method, and any unusual reactions you observed about the patient, her scalp, or her hair. Charting example:
	1030. Bed shampoo given. Became very tired and weak. Stated it "felt very good to have clean hair again." Prepared for nap. R. Ryan, LVN

ITEM 5. STRETCHER SHAMPOO

Important Steps	Key Points
1. Approach the patient as in the procedure for the bed shampoo.	Explain that you will be taking her to the bathroom or utility room on a stretcher for her shampoo.
2. Check conditions of the room where shampooing will be done.	Be sure that it is warm and free of drafts, and that there is enough space for you to move easily around the stretcher.
3. Wash your hands. Assemble the equipment at the side where you will give the shampoo in the bathroom or utility room.	Proceed as in step 3 of the bed shampoo; choose only the necessary equipment and include a shampoo spray attachment for the faucet.
4. Prepare the patient for transfer.	Place a bath blanket over the patient, and fan-fold the top linens to the bottom of the bed.
5. Bring the stretcher (guerney) to the bedside.	Lock the wheels of the stretcher and the bed to prevent them from rolling as the patient moves onto the stretcher.

6. Move the patient to the stretcher.	Follow the procedure used in Unit 10, Item 3. Stand with your body bracing the stretcher against the bed. Ask the patient to move onto the stretcher, first her head and shoulders, then her hips and legs. Assist her as necessary while keeping her covered with the bath blanket.
	    Secure the safety belts firmly, one over the chest and one over the thighs, to prevent the patient from falling off the stretcher.
	    Place the back wheels in the swivel position (labeled on the wheels) so you can control the stretcher as you move it down the corridor.

7. Transport the patient to the shampoo area.	Push the stretcher from the head end.
8. Place the head end of the stretcher against the sink.	Lock the wheels so that the stretcher will not move during the shampoo procedure.
9. Wrap a towel around the patient's shoulders and neck.	Secure the ends with a safety pin at the patient's chest to keep her warm and dry.

Important Steps	Key Points
10. Slip the trough (metal, rubber, or plastic and newspaper) under the patient's head.	Adjust the patient's head on the trough placed at the top edge of the stretcher. The other end of the trough will extend into the sink. The patient's head will hang slightly over the end of the stretcher. A small plastic-protected pillow may be placed under her shoulders if she is uncomfortable.

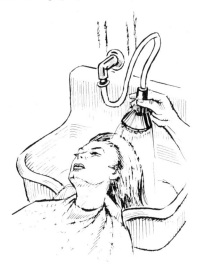

11. Attach the shampoo spray to the faucet and regulate a gentle flow of water until it is warm (105° F).	If a bath thermometer is not available, test the warmth of the water by running it over your wrist. Avoid splashing.
12. Shampoo the hair.	Use the procedure described for the bed shampoo, steps 6 through 11.
13. Comb or brush the hair.	Arrange it in a neat style. Be careful not to injure the scalp during this procedure because it may be tender after the washing. Wrap the hair with a clean, dry towel to keep from chilling the patient when you transport her back to her room.
14. Return the patient to her room.	Check that the safety belts are securely fastened. Unlock the stretcher wheels, adjust the back wheels to the swivel position, push the stretcher from the head end so that you can see where you are going, and utilize coordinated body movement as you transport the patient to her room.
15. Transfer the patient from the stretcher and provide for her comfort.	Lock the wheels. Brace the stretcher against the bed with your body while the patient moves to the bed. Pull the top covers up over the patient. Remove the bath blanket and store it in the designated place (bedside stand or closet). Remove the towel from around her hair, and discard it. Tighten the bed linens and put the call light within her reach. Move the bedside stand close to her. Be sure that she has fresh drinking water. Leave her comfortably resting.
16. Take the stretcher back to the storage area.	Remove the soiled linen. Wash and dry the mattress and make it up with a clean sheet, ready for the next patient.

U
N
I
T
32

Important Steps	Key Points
17. Return the utility room or bathroom.	Remove the articles used for the shampoo (towels, trough, shampoo, rinse). Tidy the room, remove the shampoo spray from the faucet, and return it to the storage area.
18. Go back to the patient's room.	Check on your patient's condition. After you are assured that her needs have been met, tell her to rest. Tell her that you will come in at a later time to check her condition. If you tell her when you will return (15 minutes, 30 minutes, or 1 hour), she will not disturb you from your other duties at frequent intervals.
19. Record the shampoo procedure on the nurses' notes.	Report and record the time, the method, and any unusual observations noted about the patient, her hair, and her scalp. Record her response to the procedure—"very tired," "with no apparent ill effects," and so forth. Charting example:
	1030. Taken to bathroom for shampoo. Tolerated procedure very well. Clean hair seemed to improve her spirits greatly. Returned to bed with no apparent ill effects. R. Ryans, LVN

ITEM 6. GENERAL INFORMATION

In your hair care experiences, you may encounter individual differences in hair texture and styling. Hair is considered an appendage of the skin. Just as skin textures vary, so do hair textures. Hair may be thick, coarse, straight, or very tightly curled (kinky, as it is sometimes known). Or, when hair is wet after a new permanent, it often becomes very curly after it dries—this is usually described as kinky. Another type of hair is thin, fine or wispy, and smooth, and must be handled differently from the coarse-textured kind.

If the hair is tightly curled as in the Afro style, or in a fresh, tightly curled permanent, use a wide-toothed comb to comb the hair carefully and gently. This will prevent unnecessary pulling as you try to comb out tangles and snarls. Tightly curled hair frequently needs special conditioners or sprays. Your patient can give you this information. Hair should be combed straight out from the scalp; always keep your hand between the section being combed or brushed and the patient's scalp.

Since wigs and wiglets are worn by many people today, you must see that they also are cared for with daily combing or brushing. However, shampooing wigs should be left to the professional hairdresser because some wigs and wiglets are very expensive and are easily damaged from improper shampooing. (You may have to pay for a replacement wig for the patient if you damage it!).

If you feel that you are now ready for your post-test on this lesson, see your instructor and set up a time for your test. Both a written test and a demonstration are required. You will not be permitted to have your workbook or notes with you during the testing.

PERFORMANCE TEST

In the skill laboratory your instructor will ask you to perform three of the five activities listed below without reference to any of the source materials. For some of the activities you migh have to ask another person to take the place of a patient.

1. Given a patient who has suffered a stroke and is unable to lift her arms to comb and brush her hair, explain and demonstrate how you give this patient daily hair care.

2. Given a female patient who has very long hair and is unable to braid it herself because the exertion would be too strenuous for her condition, proceed to braid the hair after the daily brushing and combing.

3. Given a person who is conscious but unable to leave the bed because of recent abdominal surgery, set her up for and demonstrate a shampoo in bed.

4. Given a convalescing patient who is still on partial bed rest, who is ready to be transferred to an extended-care facility, and who would like her hair washed before going, explain and demonstrate how to wash her hair in the bathroom, and explain and demonstrate how to transport her there on a guerney.

5. Given a patient who is to have a shampoo in bed, demonstrate and successfully make a newspaper trough, install it correctly, and then wash the patient's hair.

PERFORMANCE CHECKLIST

HAIR CARE SKILL

BRUSHING HAIR FOR ROUTINE DAILY CARE

U
N
I
T
32

1. Wash your hands.

2. Identify the patient.

3. Explain the procedure.

4. Assemble the correct equipment (Items 5 through 11).

5. Prepare the patient properly with the bath blanket in place, a towel over the pillow, and the patient's head turned away.

6. Part the hair in the center from the front to the back, and divide it into three sections on each side.

7. Grasp a small section of hair between your index and middle finger, place the brush near the patient's scalp, and use an upward rotating semicircular wrist movement to push the brush through the hair.

8. Apply alcohol-soaked pads to matted or tangled hair.

9. Hold the matted section between your index and middle finger, and in an upward motion, comb the loosened hair strands from the matted areas.

10. Perform all brushing and combing without pulling at the patient's scalp or otherwise causing her discomfort.

11. Finish the procedure by arranging the hair neatly and symmetrically.

12. Apply hair spray avoiding the patient's face.

13. Hold up a mirror for the patient to see her hair.

14. Remove the towel and dispose of it in a receptacle.

15. Remove the bath blanket and restore the bed linen properly.

16. Remove and dispose of hair in the brush and comb.

17. Tidy the area, returning all items to their proper places.

18. Complete the procedure within the time limit of _____ minutes.

BRAIDING HAIR

1. Wash your hands.

2. Identify the patient.

3. Give an adequate explanation of the reasons for braiding the patient's hair (comfort, neatness, and the prevention of matted hair).

4. Divide the hair into three sections on each side.

5. Begin braiding with the left strand in your left hand and the right strand in your right hand.

6. Proceed by crossing the right and left strands alternately over the center strand.

7. Complete the braiding without losing hold of the strands or causing them to become partly unraveled.

8. Exert sufficient tension on the strands to form neat braids without pulling at the patient's scalp.

9. Bind the tips of the braids with ribbon.

10. Arrange the braids so that they fall at each side of the head.

11. Make braids that are neat and firm, without gaps between the intertwined strands

12. Complete the procedure within the time limit of _____ minutes.

BED SHAMPOO

1. Assemble all material needed for the shampoo.

2. Identify the patient.

3. Explain the procedure.

4. Construct a trough with the edges properly rolled.

5. Place a chair at the head of the bed, protect it with a plastic cover, and put a pail on the chair.

6. Fill two pitchers with warm water, one at 105° and the other at 115°F.

7. Place a drawsheet at the head of the bed to protect the linen.

8. Prepare the patient in the correct position near the side of the bed with the pillow removed, bath blanket in place, and linen folded toward the foot of the bed.

9. Place a towel securely around the patient's shoulders.

10. Adjust the bed to a comfortable working position.

11. Slip the trough under the patient's head, providing it with sufficient slope for drainage into the pail.

12. Check the temperature of the water before beginning the shampoo; add water from the warmer pitcher if necessary.

13. Complete all preparations before beginning the shampoo.

14. Moisten the patient's hair with water before applying the shampoo.

15. Apply the shampoo in the quantity indicated by the directions on container.

16. Work the shampoo into the hair from the front hairline to the back of the head, massaging the scalp firmly with your fingertips.

17. Rinse the hair, removing all shampoo and taking care that the water drains properly into the trough.

18. Repeat the cycle (steps 15 through 17) until the hair is clean, testing for a squeaky sound after each rinse.

19. Check the water temperature and adjust it as necessary to keep it at about $105°F$.

20. Carry out the procedure without getting shampoo or water in the patient's eyes or face, and without undue wetting of other areas.

21. Dry the patient's ears, neck, and hair thoroughly with the bath towel.

22. Brush the hair and comb out tangles holding the strands correctly and not pulling at the patient's scalp.

23. Hold up a mirror for the patient to see her hair.

24. Remove the towel and other materials from the bed, and dispose of all soiled materials.

25. Restore the linen and bed to their original positions, put back the pillow, and remove the bath blanket, leaving the patient dry and comfortable.

26. Remove and dispose of hair from the brush and comb.

27. Tidy the area, returning all articles to their proper places.

28. Record the time and method of the shampoo in nurses' notes.

29. Complete the procedure within the time limit of _____ minutes.

UNIT
32

STRETCHER SHAMPOO

1. Assemble all materials in the utility room before moving the patient.

2. Identify the patient.

3. Explain the procedure to the patient.

4. Place a bath blanket over the patient.

5. Fan-fold the top linens to the bottom of the bed.

6. Adjust the bed to the high position and lower the siderail.

7. Place a stretcher in the correct position beside the bed.

8. Lock the stretcher and bed wheels before moving the patient.

9. Use the correct body position when moving the patient, standing with your body bracing the stretcher tightly against the bed.

10. Direct and assist the patient in moving (head and shoulders first, then hips and legs) onto the stretcher without undue strain on the patient or yourself.

11. Keep the patient properly covered by the bath blanket while moving the stretcher.

12. Secure the safety belts firmly before unlocking the stretcher wheels.

13. Transport the patient without bumping or jolting, pushing the stretcher from the head end.

14. Place the stretcher correctly, with the head end toward the sink, and lock the wheels.

15. Secure a towel in place around the patient's neck and shoulders.

16. Slip a trough under the patient's head, arranging it for sufficient slope to allow the water to drain into the sink.

17. Adjust the patient's head in a comfortable position, placing a pillow under her shoulders if necessary.

18. Attach a spray to the faucet and adjust it to obtain a gentle flow of water at about 105°F.

19. Indicate your readiness to proceed with the shampoo at this point by telling the patient, and then proceed.

20. Wrap the patient's hair in a clean, dry towel.

21. Remove the trough, take the towel from the patient's shoulders.

22. Transport the patient back to her room without bumping or jolting, pushing the stretcher from the head end.

POST-TEST

Multiple choice: Choose one answer.

1. The reasons for daily brushing and combing of the hair include all of the following except:

    a. to stimulate circulation of the scalp   c. to stimulate the hair to curl

    b. to clean her hair shafts   d. to bring nutrients to the roots

2. Water temperature for shampoos should be approximately:

    a. 120°F   c. 125°F

    b. 140°F   d. 105°F

3. The length of the plastic paper trough is approximately:

    a. 4 feet   c. 6 feet

    b. 3 feet   d. 24 inches

4. A style that is often used for keeping a patient's long hair neat and tidy is called:

    a. braiding   c. Afro

    b. a finger-wave   d. a shag

5. A common fungus infection on the scalp is:

    a. impetigo   c. eczema

    b. dandruff   d. herpes simplex

6. Parasites of the scalp are called:

    a. impetigo   c. pediculosis

    b. ascaris   d. ringworm

7. Matted hair may be loosened with the use of all except:

    a. astringent   c. alcohol

    b. water   d. hair spray

8. A lemon juice rinse is made of:

    a. 1 ounce of juice and 1 quart of water

    b. 3 ounces of juice and 1 quart of water

    c. 1 ounce of juice and 1½ quarts of water

    d. 4 ounces of juice and 1 quart of water

9. The room environment for giving a patient a shampoo in bed should be:

    a. Warm and free of drafts   c. Temperature of 100°F

    b. Temperature of 68°F   d. Temperature of 95°F

10. Illness often causes the scalp to become very:

    a. sensitive   c. colorful

    b. shiny   d. coarse

UNIT
32

11. Braided hair does not easily become:

   a. damaged   c. matted

   b. stiff   d. loose

12. The hair should always be brushed with:

   a. an upward motion   c. oil

   b. water   d. A & D ointment

13. Dandruff causes the scalp to become:

   a. oily and scaly   c. discolored

   b. dry or scaly   d. very sore

14. Brushing the hair and scalp stimulates:

   a. the hair shafts to grow

   b. dandruff cells to grow

   c. circulation

   d. molecular cells to become rapid-growing

15. When giving a bed shampoo, an important improvised piece of equipment can be the:

   a. stretcher   c. bath cover

   b. comb and brush   d. trough

16. When moving the patient from bed to stretcher for a shampoo at the sink the following safety measures are taken:

   a. the bed is moved close to the stretcher

   b. the wheels are unlocked

   c. the stretcher is moved against the bed, and its wheels are locked

   d. the wheels are kept straight.

17. A patient's hair should be shampooed only on the order of the:

   a. patient   c. physician

   b. head nurse   d. patient's family

18. Each time a shampoo is given, it should be recorded in the:

   a. progress sheet   c. nurses' notes

   b. physician's order sheet   d. Intake and Output sheet.

19. After giving a shampoo in the utility room, you should make sure that the area is cleaned:

   a. before you return the patient to her room.

   b. after you return the patient to her room

   c. before you put the patient to bed

   d. after you put the patient to bed

20. Wigs should be shampooed by the:

   a. patient's family   c. professional hairdresser

   b. nurse   d. orderly

POST-TEST ANNOTATED ANSWER SHEET

1. c. (p. 663)
2. d. (p. 670)
3. b   (p. 669)
4. a. (p. 665)
5. b. (p. 662)
6. c. (pp. 662 and 669)
7. d. (p. 664)
8. a. (p. 671)
9. a. (p. 670)
10. a. (p. 664)

11. c. (p. 665)
12. a. (p. 664)
13. b. (p. 662)
14. c. (p. 664)
15. d. (p. 669)
16. c. (p. 672)
17. c. (p. 669)
18. c. (p. 672)
19. d. (p. 674)
20. c. (p. 674)

UNIT
32

Unit 33

PERINEAL CARE

I. DIRECTIONS TO THE STUDENT

Please read the following paragraphs carefully. They will tell you what you are expected to know about perineal care. Practice the procedure in your classroom or laboratory until you feel confident of your ability and skills. You will need the following items for the procedure:

1. A perineal care tray containing:

   a. Graduate pitcher or a 250 cc plastic bottle with a lid modified for squirting.

   b. Cotton balls or gauze squares.

   c. Dressing—sanitary pad, ABD, or 4 X 4's.

   d. T-binder for male or female.

   e. Chux pads.

   f. Dressing forceps—optional.

   g. Paper (newspaper, paper bag, was paper, etc.).

   h. Disposable gloves.

2. Bedpan.

3. Mrs. Chase, or a similar type of mannequin.

4. Bath blanket.

When you have had sufficient practice in the procedure, arrange with your instructor to take the performance test. You will be expected to perform the procedure to demonstrate your knowledge and skill.

II. GENERAL PERFORMANCE OBJECTIVE

As a health worker, you will be able to assist the patient with the care and cleansing of his perineal area, and to give perineal care as required. You will perform this task skillfully, effectively, and in a reassuring manner to reduce or avoid embarrassment to the patient.

III. SPECIFIC PERFORMANCE OBJECTIVES

Upon completion of this lesson you will be able to:

1. Provide perineal care for the female patient by pouring warm solution over the perineal area, cleansing and drying the area properly, applying a dressing or pad, if required, and securing it in place.

2. Give perineal care to the male patient by pouring warm solution over the perineal area, cleansing and drying the area properly, applying a pad or dressing if required, and securing the dressing in place.

3. Approach the patient, explain the procedure in an objective and matter-of-fact way, and give reassurance in a nonjudgmental way in order to avoid embarrassing the patient.

IV. VOCABULARY

A-P repair—corrective surgery of the female perineum that includes repair of anterior and posterior muscle defects, tears, or weakness usually occurring after the birth of a baby.

genitalia—the reproductive organs of the male and the female.

hysterectomy—surgical removal of the uterus (womb).

perineal—refers to the perineum.

perineum—the area between the vulva and the anus in the female, and between the scrotum and the anus in the male.

lochia—the discharge from the uterus consisting of blood, mucus, and tissue during the period immediately after the delivery of a baby.

scrotum—the double pouch containing the testicles and part of the spermatic cord in the male.

uterus—the muscular, hollow, pear-shaped organ of the female, located within the abdomen; the womb.

vulva—the external female genitalia.

vaginal hysterectomy—surgical removal of the uterus (womb) through the vaginal opening.

V. INTRODUCTION

Perineal care (often referred to in the hospital as "peri care") is necessary for the health and well-being of the patient. It is the term usually applied to the external irrigation or cleansing of the vulva and perineum following voiding or defecation. The procedure is performed to prevent contamination or infection in the genital area, and to remove drainage or odors through cleansing. The procedure is used following the birth of a child, or following an operation involving surgery on the perineum, the vagina, the lower urinary tract, or the anus. Although the procedure is more commonly performed for the woman patient, it may be required for the male patient following surgery on the perineum or the anus.

You will find that some health workers use the term "peri care" to refer to the portion of the patient's bath when the genital area is washed and dried. Usually the patient is able to perform this part of his bath, but you may need to assist certain patients who are helpless. The use of the term "peri care" is correct in such a situation, but this lesson will be concerned with cleaning the perineal area by external irrigation, or the pouring of a solution.

ITEM 1. DEALING WITH PATIENT EMBARRASSMENT

The procedure of giving perineal care to the patient may cause him or her embarrassment as a result of the nurse's close contact with his or her genitals. Most patients will accept the nurse's assistance and make very little fuss about having the procedure done. A few, however, may find it very difficult to overcome their feelings of embarrassment and will try to avoid the perineal care even when they know it might be necessary.

Why do patients become embarrassed and reluctant about using the bedpan or having perineal care? We all know some of the reasons. In this country, until very recent changes of attitude, our cultural and social customs were such that certain parts of the body and its functions were not seen, discussed, or even acknowledged in public. The genital part of the body was considered very private, and the person raised in this kind of culture and according to these customs regards it as so. When this person becomes a patient, his attitude about the privacy of his body does not change much.

As a nursing worker, how can you deal with this problem? First, you need to understand that *you* may have some embarrassment initially if you have been raised in a similar culture with similar customs. Your own embarrassment will be reduced if you remember that your purpose is to *assist the patient*. By regarding the patient as a whole person, you can develop a calm and matter-of-fact attitude, and a nonjudgmental manner while accepting his right to have and express his feelings. Explaining the need for perineal care and the reasons for it can reassure the patient so that he will willingly cooperate in the procedure without undue embarrassment. When performing the procedure, you should be matter-of-fact and objective, and avoid any suggestive conversation or actions.

ITEM 2. PROCEDURE FOR PERINEAL CARE FOR THE FEMALE PATIENT

Important Steps	Key Points
1. Wash your hands. Refer to the unit on handwashing for instructions.	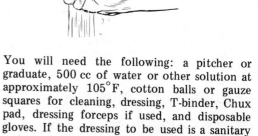
2. Obtain the necessary supplies and equipment. Use the perineal tray if one is provided and take it to the patient's bedside table.	You will need the following: a pitcher or graduate, 500 cc of water or other solution at approximately 105°F, cotton balls or gauze squares for cleaning, dressing, T-binder, Chux pad, dressing forceps if used, and disposable gloves. If the dressing to be used is a sanitary pad, most women will prefer to use an elastic sanitary belt to secure it rather than a T-binder.
3. Approach and identify the patient, explain what is to be done, and enlist her cooperation.	

4. Prepare and position the patient. 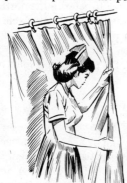	Provide for privacy by closing the door of the room, pulling the cubicle curtain, or using a screen.
	    Position the bed by lowering the siderail if one is used, and elevating the head of the bed slightly. Position the patient by having her lie on her back with her knees flexed and elevated.
	    Drape the patient to avoid undue exposure. Put the bath blanket over her and have her hold the upper edge while you fan-fold the upper covers to the foot of the bed. Raise the lower edge of the bath blanket to her pubic area and place the lower sides of the blanket over each knee as shown in the sketch.
	    Remove the soiled pad or dressing. Observe the amount and type of drainage, then wrap it in paper for discarding. After slipping the Chux under her hips, place the patient on a bedpan.

Important Steps   **Key Points**

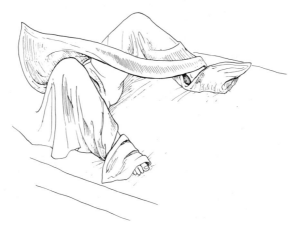

5. Give the perineal care.

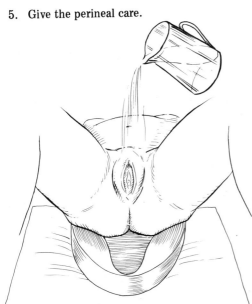

Put on the disposable gloves. Pour warm (105°F) tap water or prescribed solution over the perineal area to rinse off urine, feces or vaginal drainage. Moisten several cotton balls or gauze squares with the remaining solution. Use forceps or your fingers to hold the cotton ball, and wipe from the pubic area down toward the rectum. Make only one downward stroke with each cleansing cotton ball then discard. Cotton balls and gauze clog the plumbing, so they should be discarded by wrapping them in paper and putting them in the trash container, not in the bedpan.

Wipe the perineum dry with fresh cotton balls, gauze squares, or toilet tissues. Remove the bedpan. Dry the lower perineum and the buttocks. Wrap soiled cotton balls or gauze before disposing of them in the trash.

Apply the clean dressing or the pad. Fasten ends of pad to a sanitary belt. Use a T-binder to secure the dressings in place. (The crossbar of the T-binder is fastened around the waist; the tail of the T passes through the legs from the back and is fastened to the waist of the binder in the front.)

U
N
I
T
33

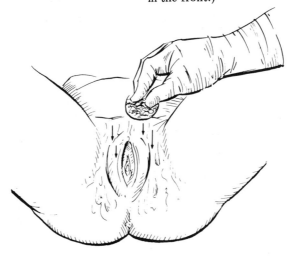

Important Steps	Key Points
6. Replace the top covers and remove the bath blanket.	Fold it and return it ot the bedside stand or the storage place. Remove the Chux.
7. Remove the equipment from the patient's unit.	Wash, rinse, and dry the equipment. Store in the proper place. (In some agencies, the perineal tray is disposable or exchanged daily for clean equipment from Central Supply.)
8. Provide for the patient's comfort.	Leave the signal cord within reach, raise the siderail if used, adjust the position of the bed as desired, and leave the bedside stand and personal articles within easy reach. Tell the patient when you expect to return.
9. Report and record.	Record the procedure on the patient's chart and report to your team leader or the nurse in charge that it has been done. Charting example: 1030. Perineal care given. Moderate amount of lochia, a few small clots. B. Olsen, NA

ITEM 3. PATIENT SELF–CARE OF THE PERINEUM

When the patient is allowed up and is able to care for herself, she should be taught to perform the procedure herself. She can assemble the necessary materials, take them to the bathroom, pour the solution, cleanse and dry herself, and apply a clean pad or dressing.

The following points should be stressed when you given instructions to the patient:

1. Be sure to have a paper or brown bag in which to wrap the soiled pad or dressing, and the cotton balls or gauze used to clean and dry the perineum. All soiled material should be wrapped securely before disposing of it.

2. When cleansing or drying with a cotton ball or gauze, wipe once *from front toward the rectum* with each ball. Discard, and use a clean ball for the next stroke until the entire perineum has been cleaned and dried.

ITEM 4. PERINEAL CARE FOR THE MALE PATIENT

Perineal care may be ordered for the male patient following various types of perineal surgery. Usually the procedure is carried out by a male health worker or orderly since the male patient may be more embarrassed if it is done by a female health worker. However, not all agencies have as many male health workers as they would like, and so it may be necessary

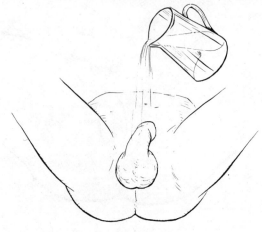

for the female health worker to carry out the procedure for a male patient, until he is able to do it for himself.

The steps of the procedure are the same as those listed in Item 2 for the female patient.

A sanitary pad would not be used for the male patient; his dressings would be held in place by a double-tailed T-binder, which allows for proper support of the scrotum as shown below.

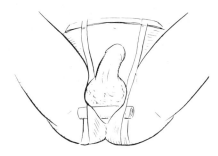

ITEM 5. CONCLUSION OF THE LESSON

After you have practiced the perineal care procedure until you are thoroughly familiar with it and can do it skillfully, arrange with your instructor to take the performance test. You should be able to demonstrate the procedure accurately.

U
N
I
T
33

PERFORMANCE TEST

In the classroom or skill laboratory, your instructor will ask you to demonstrate your skill in carrying out the following procedures without reference to your study guide, notes, or other source material. You are to use Mrs. Chase to simulate the patient.

1. Given a woman patient who has delivered a baby a few hours ago, you are to provide perineal care in order to cleanse the perineum of discharges, and apply a clean sanitary pad without causing her embarrassment or discomfort.

2. Given a male patient who has had perineal surgery, you are to provide perineal care, apply clean dressings, and secure the dressings with a double-tailed T-binder in the proper way. State how you would attempt to reduce his embarrassment about this procedure.

PERFORMANCE CHECKLIST

PERINEAL CARE

GIVING PERINEAL CARE TO A FEMALE PATIENT

Demonstrate the proper way to give perineal care to a female patient.

1. Wash your hands.

2. Obtain all needed supplies.

3. Identify the patient and approach her in a matter-of-fact, reassuring manner.

4. Provide for the patient's privacy by closing the door, pulling the curtain, or using screens.

5. Position the patient on her back with knees bent and elevated.

6. Drape the patient with a bath blanket to prevent undue exposure.

7. Remove the soiled dressing or pad.

8. Place the patient on a bedpan with a Chux under her hips and the pan.

9. Put on disposable gloves.

10. Pour water or a solution of 105°F over the perineal area.

11. Use moistened cotton balls, one at a time, and stroke gently from the pubic area toward rectum once with each to cleanse the perineum. Use gentle strokes to avoid causing discomfort.

12. Use dry cotton balls, gauze, or tissue to dry the perineum, stroking from the front to the rectum once with each ball.

13. Remove the bedpan and apply a clean pad.

14. Discard all soiled dressings, pads, cotton balls, and so forth by wrapping them in paper before disposing of them.

15. Provide for the patient's comfort by removing the bath blanket, adjusting the top covers, placing the signal cord, and elevating the siderail.

16. Remove equipment from the bedside and clean it before returning it to storage.

PERINEAL CARE FOR THE MALE PATIENT

Demonstrate the correct method of perineal care for a male patient.

1. Wash your hands.

2. Obtain all supplies.

3. Identify the patient and approach him in a matter-of-fact, reassuring manner.

4. State ways in which you would attempt to reduce embarrassment, such as an explanation of the procedure and reasons for it, avoiding suggestive conversation or actions.

5. Provide for the patient's privacy by closing the door, pulling the curtain, or using screens.

6. Position the patient on his back with knees bent and elevated.

7. Drape the patient with a bath blanket to prevent undue exposure.

8. Remove the soiled dressing.

9. Place a Chux under his hips and place him on a bedpan.

10. Put on disposable gloves.

11. Pour water or a solution of 105°F over the perineal area.

12. Clean the perineum by using moistened cotton balls and stroking gently from the pubic area toward the rectum once with each one.

13. Dry the perineum by using dry cotton balls, gauze, or tissue, wiping from the front to the rectum once with each one.

14. Remove the bedpan.

15. Apply a clean dressing and secure it with a double-tailed T-binder. Apply a T-binder and dressing correctly to support the scrotum.

16. Discard all soiled dressings, pads, and cotton balls by wrapping them in paper before disposing of them.

17. Provide for the patient's comfort by removing the bath blanket, adjusting the top covers, placing the signal cord, and elevating the siderail.

18. Remove equipment from the bedside and clean it before returning it to storage.

UNIT
33

POST-TEST

Directions: Mark the answer that makes the statement complete.

1. Perineal care is usually referred to as:

    a. sitz care

    c. peri care

    b. Pedi care

    d. trach care

2. The most prevalent feeling that patients receiving perineal care will need to overcome is:

    a. anger

    c. indifference

    b. embarrassment

    d. resentment

3. The position of the patient when receiving perineal care is:

    a. prone with legs extended

    b. on the right side with knees flexed

    c. on the left side with knees extended

    d. lying on his back with knees flexed, elevated, and draped

4. The temperature of the solution used for perineal care is:

    a. $105°F$

    c. $212°F$

    b. $90°F$

    d. $150°F$

5. The most important aspect of perineal care to be carried out by the nurse and the patient is using the following stroke:

    a. start the cleaning stroke from the rectum to the pubic area

    b. use one cotton ball for each cleaning stroke

    c. use one cotton ball for each cleaning stroke, starting from the pubic area toward the rectum

    d. use one cotton ball for all the cleaning strokes

POST-TEST ANNOTATED ANSWER SHEET

1. c.   (p. 683)

2. b.   (p. 683)

3. d.   (p. 684)

4. a.   (p. 685)

5. c.   (p. 685)

ASSISTING WITH SPIRITUAL CARE

I. DIRECTIONS TO THE STUDENT

Please read the unit carefully. You will learn to understand some of the religious needs of your patients while they are in the hospital, the extended-care facility, or the home. You will learn ways in which you can help to meet those needs.

II. GENERAL PERFORMANCE OBJECTIVES

Upon completing this lesson, you will be able to assist the patient to obtain the services of the clergyman for his spiritual needs, provide for the observance of certain religious practices, and help the clergyman as may be needed. You will be expected to show respect for the patient's religious beliefs even though these may differ from your own.

III. SPECIFIC PERFORMANCE OBJECTIVES

When you have finished this unit, you will be able to:

1. Call the religious representative requested or designated by the patient.

2. Assist the patient to observe certain religious paractices during his stay in the hospital if he so wishes.

3. Show your concern for the religious articles belonging to the patient by handling them respectfully and providing for their safekeeping.

4. Demonstrate respect for the patient's religious beliefs in all aspects of your conduct.

IV. VOCABULARY

anointing of the sick—a Roman Catholic sacrament performed by the priest with prayers for recovery and salvation for a critically ill person or one in danger of dying; formerly called the last rites or extreme unction.

agnostic—one who believes that the existence of God or any supreme being is unknown and probably unknowable.

atheist—one who denies the existence of God and rejects all religious faith and practice.

baptism—a sacrament signifying spiritual rebirth and admission into the Christian community through the ritual use of water; many Christian faiths require one to be baptized before death in order to attain grace or to be saved.

chaplain—a clergyman serving the spiritual needs of members of an organization or institution such as a hospital, college, or military unit, regardless of denomination.

clergy—ordained Christian ministers, those ordained to perform ministrations in the church.

communion—
(a) Catholic (Roman and Greek): the sacrament of the eucharist; partaking of a small wafer or piece of unleavened bread that symbolizes the body of Christ.

(b) Protestant: the sacrament of receiving both the unleavened wafer of bread and a drink of wine that symbolize the body and the blood of Christ.

pastor, priest, rabbi—a clergyman; a religious leader of a congregation who guides the spiritual lives of its member.

sacrament—a formal religious ceremony that is sacred; it is performed as a symbol of a spiritual reality, especially those instituted by Christ as a means of grace.

(a) Protestant: two sacraments are generally recognized — baptism and communion.

(b) Catholic: seven sacraments — baptism, confirmation, communion, penance, marriage, anointing the sick, and holy orders.

V. INTRODUCTION

The meaning of religion and God varies among the people of the world. We know that among many religions, and even among followers of the same religion, observance and interpretation of the religious doctrine differ widely. One person may be an active member of an organized religious institution, such as a church or synagogue; another may simply hold a general belief in God or a Supreme Being. Some people may claim to be agnostic or atheistic. The point to remember is that the individual's religious belief or lack of it is his own personal choice.

When the person becomes a patient, he brings with him his religious beliefs and needs as well as his health needs. Because an illness, an operation, or an injury often represents a possible threat to the patient's life, he may turn to religion for comfort and reassurance. The patient's mental and emotional reactions are related to, and have a profound effect on his physical health. Therefore, we must be concerned with helping him to obtain support and peace of mind from his religious beliefs.

As a nurse, you should respect the patient's beliefs even though these may differ from your own. Avoid arguing points of religion, or trying to convert the patient to your own views. It is very important for many patients to talk about their faith and fears when they are facing the stress of illness or surgery. Their fears may have many aspects; fear of pain, of disfigurement, of never being the same again, or of death. The chaplain or clergyman is a valuable member of the health team because of his skills in providing spiritual support for patients who want it. The nurse can also help by listening and helping patients express their feelings. Most health workers find it difficult in the beginning to listen and discuss topics like death because this subject is generally avoided in our society. It becomes easier to handle when you are able to accept the patient's right to feel as he does; then you can proceed from there to talk about possible causes for his feelings. Usually, talking about such fears with someone who does not reject or judge them makes the fears less threatening. As you talk with patients about their feelings, it might be appropriate to ask if they would like to have a chaplain or clergyman visit them. The decision should rest with the patient.

ITEM 1. CARE OF RELIGIOUS ARTICLES

Many patients bring some religious articles with them when they come to the hospital. Although these articles may not seem important to you, they hold great significance for the person who own them. Be sure to treat these possessions with respect and be careful not to drop or misplace them.

Patients who are members of the Catholic faith usually bring crucifixes, religious medals, and rosaries with them. Often, the Catholic patient wishes to wear a medal, but if it is pinned to his hospital gown, it may be lost when the gown is changed. It would be better to tape or tie the medal to the patient.s wrist in order to keep it from being lost.

Protestant patients may bring a Bible, prayer books, or other religious reading materials to the hospital with them. Orthodox and Conservative Jewish men may wear a skull cap (yarmulke) during their daily prayers while they are in the hospital.

ITEM 2. DIETARY REGULATIONS

Certain religious denominations follow special dietary customs. Some of the most common customs you will encounter are described below:

Catholic: Although the Catholic Church has relaxed its dietary regulations, many Roman Catholics still do not eat meat on Fridays and on other specified days.

Protestant: Dietary restrictions vary among denominations, and many have no restrictions that would affect the hospitalized patient. Some, such as the Seventh Day Adventists, are vegetarians (eat no meat) and do not drink stimulants such as coffee, tea, or liquor. Other denominations prohibit smoking, or drinking of alcoholic beverages.

Jewish: Jewish doctrine (law) forbids eating pork and shellfish. The *Orthodox Jew* (strict in observance of law and tradition) eats only kosher foods that are prepared in a manner prescribed by Judaic law. Foods containing milk are not eaten at the same meal with meat. The *Conservative Jew* observes slightly modified dietary regulations and is somewhat less strict in his observances. The *Reform Jew* has no dietary restrictions; his practice of Judaism can be described as a simplified and liberal approach and belief.

ITEM 3. REQUESTS FOR A VISIT BY A CLERGYMAN

The chaplain on the staff of a health agency provides spiritual service for patients on a nondenominational basis. If your agency does not have a resident chaplain, the patient may ask you to have a Protestant minister, a priest, a rabbi, or another religious representative come to see him, or you may ask the patient if he has a preference. After the patient makes his request, call a local church or temple as indicated by the request, and ask that one of its clergymen visit the patient. Many patients will request a visit from a specific priest, minister, or rabbi. In that case, you would obtain the necessary information about his name, the church or temple he represents, and its location.

When making a call to ask a clergyman to visit a patient, you should have the following information:

a. The clergyman — specified by denomination, church or temple, or name.

b. The patient — his name and room number, the name of the hospital or agency, and a general statement about his condition, for example, that he is critically ill or will be undergoing surgery.

c. The service to be performed — a general visit, or an administration of the sacraments of communion, baptism, or anointing of the sick (extreme unction).

After you have called the clergyman, tell the patient that you have contacted him, and give his name and the approximate time of the visit if this is known. By reporting back to the patient, you are letting him know that he can depend on you and that you are concerned about his needs.

ITEM 4. HOW TO ADDRESS A MEMBER OF THE CLERGY

Most clergymen introduce themselves when they arrive at a hospital or agency to see a patient, and they give their title as well as their name so you will know how they are addressed. However, if you are in doubt as to what to call a Protestant minister, the title of Pastor or Mister is customarily used with his surname. If he has a doctor of philosophy he would be called "Doctor." The title "Reverend" is often used incorrectly to address Protestant clergymen.

The Catholic priest is addressed as "Father," and some Episcopal ministers may also use this title. Jewish clergymen are called "Rabbi" which means master or teacher. Rabbis who have a doctoral degree would be addressed with the title of doctor. Any clergyman appointed to serve members of an organization such as a hospital or military unit may be called "Chaplain."

ITEM 5.   THE SACRAMENT OF COMMUNION

As stated earlier, communion is an important sacrament of the Christian faith. It is a spiritual reconfirmation or rededication of faith that provides great consolation for the patient.

In most Catholic hospitals, communion is given daily to those Catholic patients who desire it. Each hospital has a procedure for notifying the priest about patients requesting communion, such as a list that gives the name of the patient and his room number. Catholic patients usually take communion before surgery, and during any serious illness. In other hospitals communion is given on a PRN (as needed) basis, or as requested by the patient. The priest or minister will generally bring whatever he needs for the celebration of communion.

The following procedure is generally used in Catholic hospitals and other agencies to prepare the patient for communion, especially when the priest will be administering the sacrament to a number of patients.

Important Steps	Key Points
1. Wash your hands.	
2. Approach and identify the patient.	Explain that the priest or minister will come in soon to offer communion.
3. Offer the patient the bedpan/urinal, or have him go to the bathroom.	Have him wash his face and hands. He may do this in the bathroom if he is ambulatory. Otherwise, you will assist him to do this.
4. Prepare a work space for the clergyman to conduct communion.	Provide a clear area on the bedside stand or overbed table for the articles used in the sacrament. Cover the table with a clean towel. Place a teaspoon and another folded towel neatly on the towel. (The teaspoon and extra towel may be optional; check your agency procedure.) The towel is used either by the clergyman or the patient if needed. The clergyman will place his special kit on the work area. A glass of water may be needed to assist the patient in swallowing the wafer or unleavened bread.
5. Place the patient in a comfortable supine or semi-Fowler's position.	Pull the curtain around the bed, or close the door of the room.
6. Provide for privacy.	Unless you are requested by the clergyman to assist the patient, leave the immediate area to allow the patient and priest (or minister) privacy, since confession may precede the sacrament of communion.
7. After the sacrament is over and the priest has gone, tidy the room and provide for the patient's comfort.	Following communion, the priest or minister will probably offer a short prayer. Often the patient will meditate or nap following communion.

Important Steps	Key Points
8. Record on the patient's chart.	Charting example: 0730. Communion given by Father John. J. Jones, SN

ITEM 6.   THE SACRAMENT OF BAPTISM

Baptism is a sacrament practiced by the members of the Catholic faith, as well as many Protestant faiths, in which the participant pledges himself to observe the precepts of his faith, and in so doing, becomes a full member of this religion. According to most Christian beliefs, it is essential for an individual to be baptized before dying in order to attain salvation.

In the hospital, the sacrament of baptism is important when a patient, usually a newborn baby, is in danger of dying. When it is a baby born to Catholic parents, the nurse should be prepared to baptize the baby in the absence of a clergyman. Some Protestant parents may also request that the baby be baptized when his life is in danger. The following procedure is used for baptism.

Important Steps	Key Points
Follow steps 1 through 4 in Item 5, communion procedure.	
5. Obtain the baptism tray and place it on a table cleared for that purpose.	Some hospitals use a baptism tray, which contains a vessel or shallow basin, and a bottle of holy water (water that has been blessed by a priest).
6. Pour a small amount of holy water into the vessel.	If the clergyman is baptizing the patient, he will do this; otherwise you would do so.
7. Sprinkle a few drops of water on the patient's head and baptize him.	The clergyman, or you, would then say the words, "I baptize thee in the name of the Father, and of the Son, and of the Holy Ghost. Amen." If the infant is Catholic, it is preferable to have a Catholic nurse baptize him; however, anyone can do it. The important fact is that the child is baptized.
8. Tidy the room and attend to the needs and comfort of the patient.	
9. Record on the patient's chart.	Charting example: 1950. Baptized by A. Jones, SN

U
N
I
T
34

ITEM 7.   ANOINTING OF THE SICK

This is a Catholic sacrament of utmost importance to the Catholic patient because it is intended to prepare his soul for life after death. This sacrament is administered only once during a critical illness or a period of illness when there is danger to the patient's life (e.g., the very aged person), but it can be given several times during one's life. If a Catholic patient dies without receiving this sacrament, the priest should be notified promptly so that he can determine whether the sacrament can still be given.

The following procedure is used in preparing the patient for the sacrament of anointing of the sick.

Important Steps	Key Points

Follow steps 1 through 4 in Item 5, the communion procedure.

5. Remain with the patient and the priest. / You may be needed for assistance. Fold back the bed covers to expose the patient's feet. Stand respectfully at the foot of the bed.

6. The priest anoints the patient. / He will use oil to anoint the patient's forehead, eyes, nose, mouth, hands, and feet.

7. Tidy the room, return supplies to storage, and attend to the needs and comfort of the patient. / Replace the bed covers. If the patient's condition is critical, you may be expected to stay with him and observe him closely.

8. Record on the patient's chart. / Charting example:

0100. Anointed by Father John; or Sacrament of anointing the sick by Father John.
                                                    J. Jones, SN

ITEM 8.   THE JEWISH RITE OF CIRCUMCISION

The Jewish rite of circumcising the male baby is performed much less frequently in hospitals than it was previously when mothers and babies stayed for a week or longer after the baby's birth. You should understand why some Jewish mothers do not have their baby sons circumcised before taking them home. However, it may still occur from time to time.

Circumcision is a surgical procedure of cutting away a portion of the prepuce, or foreskin, of the penis for the purpose of cleanliness. In the Jewish faith, it is a method of purification and is usually done on the 8th day after the baby's birth. Frequently a Mohel (one who has specifically trained for this procedure) performs the circumcision before a prescribed number of witnesses. Following the ceremony, there is usually a celebration at which wine and cakes are served to family and friends. Nowadays, however, the obstetrician frequently performs the circumcision.

ITEM 9.   THE MOSLEM RITE OF CIRCUMCISION

The Moslems also circumcise (Sunnat) their infants, although it may be done anytime during a lifetime.

ITEM 10.   OTHER RELIGIOUS BELIEFS AFFECTING HEALTH CARE

As a part of your job, you may come into contact with patients who have beliefs (religious or personal) different from those previously mentioned. Many individuals and religions stress the "natural order" of life. The "natural order" is a philosophy that believes that our existence depends on the balance found in nature or the environment. Many of these beliefs are beneficial to the health of individuals, but a few may pose problems in the realm of health care.

One belief that you may encounter is that of the Jehovah's Witnesses, which forbids the use of blood transfusions. A patient who holds this belief will refuse to have surgery that may require blood transfusions, or transfusion for medical reasons even though it is a matter of life and death.

Christian Scientists also stress the natural order and the positive power of faith. When someone of this faith becomes sick or disabled, he puts off seeking medical help until the illness or disability becomes quite far advanced.

These are two examples of religious beliefs that may pose difficulties in matters of health care. However, *people have a right to their beliefs and a right to refuse treatment that is contrary to their beliefs.*

ITEM 11. CONCLUSION OF THE UNIT

You have now completed the unit on Assisting with Spiritual Care. Arrange with your instructor to take the performance post-test so that you can demonstrate your skills in assisting the patient with his religious needs.

PERFORMANCE TEST

In the classroom or skill laboratory your instructor will ask you to demonstrate your skill in carrying out the following procedures without reference to your lesson guide, notes, or other source material.

1. Given a Protestant patient who has requested to see a Methodist minister before going to surgery in two days, you are to make a phone call and provide the minister with the necessary information (simulated).

2. Given a critically ill Catholic patient whose family has requested that the priest be called to give the sacraments, you are to prepare the patient and assist as may be necessary in the sacrament of anointing of the sick (simulated).

3. Describe for your instructor what you might say and do in the following situations:

   a. An Orthodox Jewish patient eats only kosher foods and your hospital has no way of providing kosher foods although it does have a selective menu for patients.

   b. A Catholic patient has been prepared for surgery (had all jewelry, false teeth, and so forth removed) but wants to wear a certain religious medal to surgery for his spiritual protection.

PERFORMANCE CHECKLIST

ASSISTING WITH SPIRITUAL CARE

CALLING A CLERGYMAN AT THE PATIENT'S REQUEST

1. Look up the name of a church of the proper denomination in the phone book or a list provided by the agency.

2. Make the phone call and identify yourself.

3. State the purpose of the call. (The following information may be in any order.)

   a. Give the name of the patient, and his room number.

   b. State the name of the hospital.

   c. State that the patient will be going to surgery in two days.

   d. State that the patient wishes to see the clergyman before surgery.

   e. Make a statement about the general condition of the patient.

4. Obtain the name of the clergyman who will visit and the approximate time of his arrival.

5. Report back to the patient that the call has been made, the name of the person who will visit, and the time he will arrive.

6. Record the activity on the nurses' notes.

PREPARING THE PATIENT FOR THE SACRAMENT OF ANOINTING THE SICK

1. Approach the patient and explain that the priest will give the sacrament.

2. Have the patient void, and wash his hands and face; assist him as needed.

3. Clear a space for the sacramental articles and place a towel as a cover. Provide a teaspoon and a second towel if this is part of the agency's procedure.

4. Place the patient in a comfortable position — supine or semi-Fowler's.

5. Pull the curtain to provide privacy.

6. Fold back the bed covers to expose the patient's feet.

7. Stand by respectfully as the priest gives the sacrament.

8. Replace the top bed covers over the patient's feet after the sacrament.

9. Dispose of soiled linen, clean and return the teaspoon to the proper area, and tidy the room.

10. Attend to the needs and comfort of the patient. (Ask if there is anything the patient needs.)

11. Record the sacrament of anointing the sick on the patient's chart with the time, and the name of priest.

DISCUSSION OF SITUATIONS

1. The Jewish patient who eats kosher foods.

    a. Show respect for the other's religious beliefs by discussing alternative ways of meeting his dietary needs.

    b. Might allow the patient's family to bring in some kosher-prepared food (check with agency procedure).

    c. Help the patient to select foods from the menu that he can eat such as fruits and vegetables with milk dishes at one meal, and with meat dishes at the next meal.

    d. Other alternatives include having food sent in from a kosher restaurant, "meals on wheels," or a commercial source.

2. The Catholic patient wearing a medal to surgery.

    a. May be able to tape the medal to the patient's wrist unless it would be in the area where surgery is to be done.

    b. Show respect for the other's religious beliefs by discussing alternative ways of meeting the patient's needs.

    c. Can discuss with the patient other ways in which he can obtain spiritual protection, such as a visit with a priest, and the taking of sacraments before surgery.

    d. Other possible ways suggested by the student.

UNIT 34

Unit 35

THE DYING PATIENT AND POSTMORTEM CARE

I. DIRECTIONS TO THE STUDENT

Proceed through this lesson. When you have finished, practice the preparation of the body on a mannequin, and then ask your instructor to observe you when you go through the procedure again. Complete the post-test.

II. GENERAL PERFORMANCE OBJECTIVES

Following this lesson, you will be able to prepare a body after death. This procedure will involve caring for the skin, body orifices, and tubings, and accounting for valuables left by the patient.

III. SPECIFIC PERFORMANCE OBJECTIVES

When you have completed this lesson, you will be able to:

1. Name and describe the five stages of dying.

2. Demonstrate the correct care of drainage tubes.

3. Demonstrate concern and respect for the patient's body by moving it gently and carefully and without injuring it.

4. Protect the patient's valuables no matter how small and seemingly insignificant.

IV. VOCABULARY

autopsy—the postmortem examination of the organs of a dead body to determine the cause of death or pathological conditions.

coroner—pathologist employed by the city, county, or state (may or may not be a physician) who examines a dead body to determine the cause of death in unusual circumstances as in the case of drownings, shootings, suicides, murders, auto accidents, and so forth.

coroner's case*—the coroner has legal authority to perform an autopsy without family consent in certain cases; examples of coroner's cases include:

1. The death of a person within 24 hours after admission to the hospital.

2. The possibility of death resulting from injury or accident.

3. A person who dies without having seen a physician within 72 hours before death.

deceased—dead or expired.

morgue—a place where dead bodies are kept before they are released to the mortuary.

next of kin—a person related to the deceased who has legal authority to sign documents; see your agency consent manual for more details.

---

*Coroner's cases vary from state to state; check with your particular agency for a list of coroner's cases in your area.

pathologist—a specialist in diagnosing the morbid (death-related) changes in tissues removed during operations and postmortem examinations.

pathology—the study of the nature and cause of disease that involves changes in structure and function.

postmortem—after death.

rigor mortis—temporary rigidity of muscles occurring after death.

shroud—a large sheet, usually muslin or plastic, used to wrap dead bodies.

V. INTRODUCTION

In our society, death and dying are not regarded as part of the life span by most people. Other people may die, but we don't really believe it will happen to us. We avoid thinking or talking about death since it is a depressing subject and makes us feel uncomfortable. From early childhood we have been sheltered from death and any contact with dying people. Death has been cloaked in a conspiracy of silence and of denial. Only in recent years has there been a move to tear away this curtain of silence and denial in order to examine the universal event — the ending of mortal life.

Much of the information and ideas we have about death can be traced to sources such as books, newspapers, and television. Death as shown on most TV news or dramatic programs is a sudden, violent, and mutilative type. This view has contributed to the feelings of shock and fear that we associate with death. However, the truth is that the great majority of deaths are not violent deaths; most people die in their beds.

The major causes of death in the United States are (1) heart diseases, and especially the "heart attack"; (2) all forms of cancer; (3) strokes, which are also called cerebrovascular accidents; (4) accidents of all kinds; and (5) influenza and pneumonia. As you can see, diseases cause most of the deaths, and most occur in sick people who are being treated in hospitals and related health facilities.

Since more than 80 per cent of all deaths in this country occur in hospitals, health workers who care for patients see more of death and dying than do other people. You will be giving care to patients who are in the process of dying. You may also be expected to prepare the body of a patient who has died for the morgue. You will have feelings about the dying patient and death that need to be examined and better understood so that you can cope effectively and help the patient during this trying time.

ITEM 1. COPING WITH APPROACHING DEATH

When a patient suspects or learns that he is dying, he is faced with trying to cope with the ultimate loss — that of his life. Death doesn't come immediately in most cases, but days, weeks, or months later. In the meantime, the dying patient must live each day as it comes. Not only the patient, but his family and those who provide for his care are involved in coping with the loss.

People go through certain stages as they cope with their feelings about death and dying. Five different stages are described as being characteristic of the grieving process for the last crisis of life. These stages are:

Stage 1 — DENIAL	"No, not me." The person cannot believe the fact of death, rejects the information, discounts the seriousness of the illness.
Stage 2 — ANGER	"Why Me"? He looks for cause or fixes blame; he wants to change or reverse the disease, but is powerless to control it.
Stage 3 — BARGAINING	"Yes, me, but — " He has unfinished business or is unable to let go. He pleads to "Make it better" and makes promises in return for longer life.

Stage 4 — DEPRESSION   "It's hopeless." He has feelings that nothing can be done and mourns impending death. He is no longer in control of his own life, he feels.

Stage 5 — ACCEPTANCE   "I am ready." "Yes, me." He has the feeling that this task is finished and that it is right to die.

The stages described here overlap one another. Some patients move back and forth and may skip some stages, while others never move beyond the denial stage. In each case, your understanding of the patient's struggle to cope, and your concern can help the patient and his family.

When a patient dies, nursing personnel often have a variety of different emotions. Some may feel a sense of betrayal because the patient died instead of recovered, especially if they worked very hard to help him. Feelings of relief and guilt may result from the death of a patient who was difficult to care for, had complex procedures to carry out, or had unpleasant odors or drainage. Still others may have feelings of dread and fear caused by the death. If you should have these feelings, talk about them with your instructor, the team leader, or another professional, such as a clergyman.

ITEM 2. CARING FOR THE DYING PATIENT

Nurses who care for terminally ill patients must remember that they are living each day of their lives, just as we are. The main difference is that these patients know their future is very limited. Their plans and goals are concerned with the "here and now", or the immediate future. Even though the patient may not live to celebrate another birthday, or join in a family vacation trip, he can plan on visiting with his loved ones, look forward to a sunny day tomorrow, or appreciate the fragrance of flowers.

One of the prime concerns of the dying patient is the assurance from his family and the nurses that he will not be deserted or left alone. The patient needs to know that others "will stick it out" with him. As a nurse, you will continue to provide care, attention, and support during this time of impending loss. Even though the patient may be very weak, just staying at the bedside a few minutes longer and touching or holding his hand can provide much comfort and reassurance.

Another concern of the dying person is to be spared unnecessary pain and suffering. You should notify the team leader promptly when the patient becomes restless or complains of pain. In addition, there are other nursing measures you can carry out to help make the patient more comfortable. Giving a backrub, changing his position, providing a refreshing drink of water or juice may relieve some discomfort.

ITEM 3. RELIGIOUS BELIEFS AND PRACTICES

As people approach the end of their lives, many receive great comfort from their religious beliefs. Because ideas about death and what is beyond death vary greatly, it is important that you be familiar with some of these beliefs. Members of some religious faiths, such as Catholics and Lutherans, believe that baptism is essential for the soul to go to heaven. They will want dying babies and young children to receive this sacrament. Catholics who are dying may wish to receive the sacraments and the anointing of the sick as described in the unit Assisting with Spiritual Care. When a patient of the Orthodox Jewish faith expires, do not prepare the body until the rabbi has performed the final rites.

You should not press your religious beliefs on the dying patient or his family, but stand by to assist in whatever way you can. This might include such things as getting them coffee, calling the clergyman, or assisting with telephone calls.

ITEM 4. SIGNS OF DEATH

During the terminal stage of life, the patient's body functions slow down. Death occurs when these stop completely. Generally, the patient is considered to have died when he stops breathing or his heart stops beating. When this happens to the hospitalized patient, the cardiopulmonary resuscitation (CPR) team is called to revive the patient, except in cases where there is a doctor's order for no CPR. In spite of the efforts of the CPR team, some patients die.

Signs of approaching death are as follows:

1. The eyes stare, become fixed, and do not respond to light.

2. Circulation slows, and the hands and feet become cold and mottled in color. The pulse becomes weak and thready; the blood pressure falls.

3. The reflexes gradually disappear, and the sphincter muscles relax causing incontinence of the bowel and bladder.

4. Respirations are of the Cheyne-Stokes type with slow, shallow breaths, gradually increasing in depth and rapidity, followed by a short period of apnea (no respiration), then a repetition of the cycle with the periods of apnea becoming longer, until all breathing stops.

5. Hearing is thought to be the last sense to fail. Even though the patient is unconscious, he may still be able to hear, so avoid saying anything in the room of a comatose patient that could adversely affect him.

6. When breathing or the pulse stop, notify the nurse in charge and call the CPR team in accordance with your agency's policy.

ITEM 5. AFTER DEATH OCCURS

Bodies are usually embalmed (chemically preserved) in this country and made to look as natural as possible. Embalming is not carried out in all countries of the world, however. Distortion, discoloration, and scarring of the body are distressing to the family and friends, and therefore should be avoided by moving the body gently and carefully. The body itself should be clean and wrapped in a clean covering when sent to the hospital morgue or to the undertaking establishment, and should be plainly marked to avoid mistakes in identity.

The death certificate, which is sent to the local or state health department, is made out by the physician and the undertaker, and the pathologist if an autopsy is performed. State laws regulate the disposition of unidentified as well as identified bodies. In obtaining permission for autopsies when an unidentified person dies in a hospital, a local agency (police, health or coroner) is notified, and this agency assumes responsibility for trying to determine the identity of the body and for burial arrangements.

When a person has a family or is in the custody of friends, most state laws require that permission of the next of kin or the custodial friend be obtained before an autopsy is performed. If circumstances of death necessitate a coroner's inquest, the state is permitted to conduct an autopsy without the consent of relatives of the deceased.

The family may need a quiet room in which to discuss matters including the choice of the mortuary to handle the funeral services. Because this is a highly emotional ordeal, it is important to provide a quiet, secluded room (often near the chapel) where they can have privacy to release their feelings. Offer them coffee or tea. Stay nearby to help if the need arises.

When a patient dies in the hospital, the RN in charge is responsible for obtaining a form called Release of the Body to the Mortuary and having it properly filled out and signed. There is another form, an autopsy release, which she must also have prepared and signed when circumstances require it.

UNIT
35

ITEM 6. CARE OF THE BODY FOLLOWING DEATH

Upon the pronouncement of death, you will be expected to carry out the following procedure:

Important Steps	Key Points
1. Gather the necessary equipment and take it into the room.	Obtain the "death care kit" consisting of two large shipping tags a clean gown, rubber bands, envelopes or containers for valuables, a shroud, gauze 4 × 4's, cotton balls, paper bags, and a valuables list.
2. Draw the curtains around the bed.	When death occurs in a multi-bed unit, provide others with privacy; close the door to the corridor. Wash your hands.

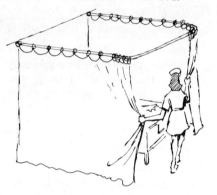

Draw curtains.

Important Steps	Key Points
3. Elevate the bed to working height and set it in a flat position.	Use the proper body alignment, balance, and movement while you work. (Review the lesson if necessary.)
4. Place the body in a supine position as if sleeping.	Close the eyes; you may use cotton gently applied over the eyelids and held in place by tape if the eyes will not stay closed. Straighten the body, with the arms laid to each side, palms down. Some agencies may prefer to have the arms gently crossed over the body at the waist or across the abdomen. Replace the dentures if required and close the mouth. If the mouth will not remain closed, place a towel rolled as a cylinder under the chin to keep the mouth closed. Place a pillow under the head. Move the body gently to avoid bruises and breaks. In general, the body should be put in a sleeping position as soon as possible, so that when stiffness (rigor mortis) occurs, the body will be positioned for an open casket, which many families request during funerals. After rigor mortis sets in, it is difficult to change the position of the body.

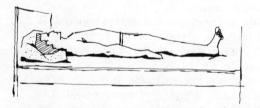

Place body in supine position.

Important Steps	Key Points
5. Remove any jewelry and list all personal articles.	In general, all rings, earrings, bracelets, beads, hairpins, and so forth, should be removed and placed in a container provided for valuables. Include eyeglasses, cards, letters, keys, religious articles.

Important Steps	Key Points
6. Provide security for the deceased patient's valuables.	Follow your agency's policy for the disposition of valuables. *Never* leave valuables unattended. Place them in the nursing station until they can be stored in a more secure place or given to the family. *Nothing* is too small to be listed on the valuables list, for these articles are valuable to the family. Review your agency policy regarding the disposition of these articles. If wedding or other rings worn are too tight to remove, it is advisable to place cotton over the stones, then tape the ring to the finger. Note this on the valuables list as well as on your nursing notes, or wherever your agency requires this to be noted. If the family is present, all personal articles, including the above, should be given to the next of kin. In the nurses' notes, list the items and the name of the person who takes the belongings.
7. Clean the body.	Using plain water, wash the areas of the body that may be soiled with blood, feces, or vomitus. Especially make sure that all body orifices (openings) are cleansed and dried. If leakage occurs around the rectum, urethra or vagina, place a gauze 4 × 4 over each opening and secure it with tape to prevent further soiling. Following death, sphincter muscles relax, often causing incontinence of feces and urine.
8. Arrange the hair.	Brush and comb the hair neatly, so that if the family wishes to see the body before it is moved, grooming will be in order. (Review the lesson on hair care if necessary.) If the family wishes to view the body, place it in a sleeping position, supine, eyes closed, arms gently crossed on the lower abdomen. Straighten the bedding (sheet and spread) as though you had completed a bath and prepared the patient for a nap. Remain with the family during the visit.
9. Care for the tubes.	If there *is* to be an *autopsy*, the tubes are generally left in the body; remove the drainage bottles or bags from the tube and fold the tube over twice; secure the end with a rubber band to avoid leakage. If there is no autopsy, tubes usually may be removed. Make sure you deflate the balloon tips so that you do not injure the body tissues upon removal. (Review your agency policy about tubes after death.)
10. Change the dressings.	Soiled dressings should be replaced with fresh ones. Old adhesive tape marks may be removed with benzene or a similar solution used by your agency.
11. Dress the body. (Follow your agency policy; some do not dress the body in a clean gown.)	If it is your agency's policy, dress the body in a clean gown. Gowning the body is usually done for the family's viewing of the body.

UNIT 35

Important Steps	Key Points
12. Identify the body.	Label the tag(s) with the patient's name, his age, his sex, the date, the hospital number, the room number and the physician's name. Tie the tag to the wrist or ankle according to hospital policy. Tie the tag tight enough so it will not slip off, yet loose enough that it will not cause bruises. Some agencies tape the label to the patient's anterior chest.

13. Place the body on a shroud if this is your agency's policy.

Place the body on the shroud (large square piece of muslin or plastic). As shown in the sketch, wrap side 1 down around the head, followed by side 2 up over the feet. Wrap sides 3 and 4. You may need to tie a bandage lightly under the jaw and up around the head to keep the jaw closed. Also, some agencies lightly bandage the wrists together criss-crossed over the abdomen to prevent the arms from falling off the stretcher when the body is being moved to the morgue. A large safety-pin or masking tape may be used to keep the shroud in place. (If your agency provides instructions for wrapping a body in a shroud, follow those directions.)

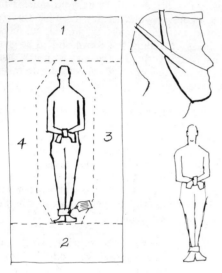

Place body on shroud.

14. Apply the outside label.

Tag the outside of the shroud with the patient's name, age, sex, hospital number, room number, physician's name, and the date. Safety-pin this tag to the outside of the shroud.

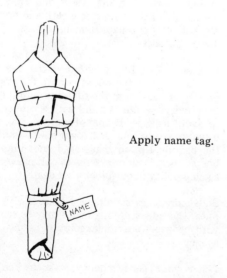

Apply name tag.

15. Transport the body to the morgue. (Some agencies leave the body in the room until a mortician or coroner's officer removes it. Check your agency's policy.)

Using proper body alignment and movement, slide the body gently onto a cart or stretcher. Cover the body with a sheet. In some agencies, the face remains uncovered; others cover the

Important Steps	Key Points

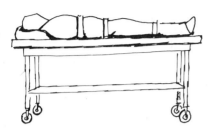

Transport on guerney.

face, particularly when the shroud is used. Follow your agency policy. Secure the body with stretcher straps at the chest and knees. Apply the straps tight enough to prevent the body from slipping off, but loose enough so as not to cause bruising.

When transporting the body, try to use nonpublic elevators and corridors to avoid disturbing visitors. If an elevator is used, secure an elevator key and ask visitors to step off to avoid distress and to make the transfer as fast as possible.

When the assigned personnel have left the body in the morgue, take the stretcher back to the unit, remove the linen and place it in the hamper, wash it (or take it to the central processing area for cleaning), and then put clean linen on the stretcher.

16. Strip the patient's room.

Return to the patient's room. Remove the soiled linen, bottles, pitchers, and other articles, and put them in the place provided for their processing. Call the department for room cleaning, or proceed to clean it yourself, whichever is your agency's policy.

17. Record the entire procedure.

In your nursing notes, record the time and date the body was taken to the morgue or by the undertaker. If valuables were placed in safekeeping, indicate this in writing. If valuables were given to the family or friends, record the name of the person(s) to whom they were given, their relationship to the deceased, the time and the date. Have a co-worker who witnessed this action cosign with you in the notes. Charting example:

0210. Transferred to morgue. Valuables (watch, wedding ring, and 2 nightgowns) sent home with son, John.

J. Jones, SN M. Maye, SN

VII. ADDITIONAL INFORMATION FOR ENRICHMENT

For those who are interested, the instructor will be able to give some additional reading assignments that will be helpful to you as you learn about the dying process. In some agencies, a staff psychiatrist confers with the personnel to help them work through their personal feelings about death. If you have the opportunity to participate in such discussion groups, you might find it interesting and beneficial.

UNIT 35

PERFORMANCE TEST

1. Discuss the five stages of dying with your instructor.

2. In the skill laboratory, prepare the mannequin (Mrs. Chase) as though she were a dead body. You will cleanse her, pack her body orifices, label the body, wrap her in a shroud, label the outside of the shroud, and prepare to transport her to the morgue.

3. Practice charting the activity on the nurses' notes. Your instructor will give you a set of comments that you will record appropriately on the nurses' notes.

PERFORMANCE CHECKLIST

POSTMORTEM CARE

1. Assemble the necessary equipment in the room.

2. Screen the patient (draw the curtains and close the door).

3. Adjust the bed to working height; flatten the bed.

4. Place the body in the supine position with the eyes closed, dentures in place, arms at the sides or across the chest, and pillow under the head.

5. Remove any jewelry and list personal articles.

6. Clean the body and pack all orifices.

7. Arrange the hair.

8. Remove any tubes (if there will be no autopsy). The tubes remain in if an autopsy is to be performed.

9. Change any dressings.

10. Change the patient's clothing according to your agency procedure.

11. Identify the body with a labeled tag on the toe, wrist, or chest (follow your agency procedure).

12. Wrap the body in a shroud and attach a label.

13. Move the body to a stretcher, using correct body movement and alignment.

14. Secure safety belts at the knees and chest.

15. Transport the body to the morgue.

16. Return to the room to strip the bed and a final cleaning.

17. Dispose of all valuables according to your agency procedure.

18. Record your activities on the nurses' notes.

POST-TEST

1. List 2 kinds of cases that are considered to be coroner's cases:

   a. _____

   b. _____ .

2. If an autopsy is to be done, all body tubes are usually _____ in the body.

3. In caring for the body after death, place the body in a _____ position, with eyes _____ and dentures _____ .

4. An autopsy is performed for the purpose of _____ , or _____ , or both.

Circle "T" or "F" if the following statements are true or false:

5. T F Dentures are removed from the body at death.

6. T F Jewelry may be left on the body at death.

7. T F Soiled dressings are changed before the body goes to the morgue.

8. T F Stretcher straps are not necessary when transporting the deceased.

9. T F Identification tags are placed on the body and the shroud.

10. T F Letters and greeting cards of the deceased may be thrown away.

POST-TEST ANNOTATED ANSWER SHEET

1. unidentified bodies; questionable circumstances surrounding the death (p. 700)

2. left (p. 705)

3. supine; closed; in place (p. 704)

4. determining cause of death; determining pathological conditions (p. 700)

5. F (p. 704)

6. T (p. 704)

7. T (p. 705)

8. F (p. 707)

9. T (p. 706)

10. F (p. 704)

UNIT 35

Unit 36

ISOLATION TECHNIQUE
AND TERMINAL DISINFECTION

I. DIRECTIONS TO THE STUDENT

Study the entire unit, write the post-test, and be ready to demonstrate your proficiency in handling direct isolation technique, reverse isolation technique, and terminal disinfection for your instructor.

II. GENERAL PERFORMANCE OBJECTIVE

Upon completion of this lesson, you will correctly employ isolation technique to protect yourself and others when caring for a patient in an isolation unit. You will be able to use reverse isolation technique to protect the patient who is suffering from a denuded skin area, such as after a burn, or a weakened condition such as leukemia or post-organ transplant, from infecting himself. You will know the principles and practices of terminally disinfecting a unit occupied by a patient who has a communicable disease.

III. SPECIFIC PERFORMANCE OBJECTIVES

When you have finished this unit, you will be able correctly to do the following:

1. Prepare a unit for isolation of a patient who has a communicable disease or who needs protection from infection.

2. Use the proper technique to put on and remove a gown worn in an isolation unit.

3. Put on a mask and tell your instructor how to change it in order to retain safe isolation technique practice.

4. Put on and remove rubber gloves using proper technique.

5. Care for contaminated dishes and linen, and dispose of waste.

6. Collect specimens and transfer them to designated places using proper protection.

IV. VOCABULARY

aerobic—requiring the presence of oxygen to live.
anaerobic—life can continue without free oxygen.
autoclave—a mechanical equipment used to render sterile by steam under pressure.
bacteriostatic—arresting (stop or inhibit) bacterial growth.
bactericidal—a solution that destroys bacteria.
carrier—one who carries disease germs (usually not currently ill from the disease), such as Typhoid Mary, a carrier of the typhoid germ who infected others who came in contact with food she handled.
communicable—an illness that may be transferred directly or indirectly from one person to another.

710

denude—removal of a protective layer, as in a 3rd degree burn.

direct contact—communication of a healthy person with a contagious person (one who has a communicable disease) through *touching* an infected part.

germicide—a solution that kills germs, but not resistant spores.

immunity—the state of being resistant to disease; immunity may be brought about by medical practice, such as vaccinations or immunizations.

indirect contact—spread of a contagious disease through some medium other than directly touching the person, such as sputum, dressings, clothing.

isolation—the act of separating, setting apart from others; a method utilized for controlling the spread of communicable or infectious disease.

reverse isolation—a type of isolation technique used for patients suffering from burns or conditions in which the protective mechanisms of the body are defective or inadequate; the patient is protected through use of sterile sheets and other isolation techniques from the worker and other patients.

venereal disease—a disease usually acquired as a result of sexual intercourse with an individual who is infected with gonorrhea, syphilis, chancroid, Vincent's infection of the genitals, or venereal lymphogranuloma.

viruses—minute (very small) microorganisms, some of which can be filtered and studied; others are nonfilterable; many different kinds and strains exist.

V. INTRODUCTION

The prevention of the spread of infections and communicable diseases in hospitals and other health agencies presents one of the most common problems health workers must face. The National Communicable Disease Center in Atlanta, Georgia, states that *"handwashing before and after contact with each patient is the single most important means of preventing the spread of infection."*

However, there are certain additional precautions that must be taken in the case of certain communicable diseases. Federal, state, and local public health agencies set forth specific regulations defining which diseases must be reported and isolated, and to what extent, where, and how long. All health agencies are legally required to carry out these regulations.

The prevention of the spread of infections can be accomplished by controlling one or more of these elements: the source of the infecting organism, the route of transmission of the organism, and a susceptible host. Susceptibility to the disease is also based on the strength and size of the infecting dose, the organism's ability to survive in the environment in which it finds itself (light versus darkness; with oxygen versus without oxygen) and its ability to resist various disinfection methods.

Microorganisms are transmitted by four general routes:

1. Contact:

   a. *Direct*—actual touching of a person with a communicable disease, or an infected animal by a susceptible person. Kissing and sexual intercourse are two means of direct transmission.

   b. *Indirect*—touching of contaminated objects used by an infected person (such as soiled clothing, bed linen, surgical instruments, dressings, handkerchiefs, or toys) and then touching your mouth, nose, or food, and transferring those microorganisms to yourself.

   c. *Droplet spread*—a spray of mist ejected from the nose or mouth when coughing, sneezing, or talking. These droplets do not usually travel more than 3 feet. Most hospital regulations require a distance of at least 6 feet between the beds, as well as the use of proper screening methods.

2. **Vehicle:** Transmission of disease through contaminated food, water, drugs, or blood.

3. **Airborne:** Evaporated droplets of an infectious agent, a disease agent that lodges in dust can remain infectious in the air and may be inhaled or digested by a susceptible host.

4. **Vector borne:** Disease organisms carried by an animal, usually an insect or tick (such as malaria, which is transmitted by the mosquito).

Reservoirs (containers) of infection include man, animals, plants, soil, and objects used in daily living. Man is the most common harborer of infection or disease.

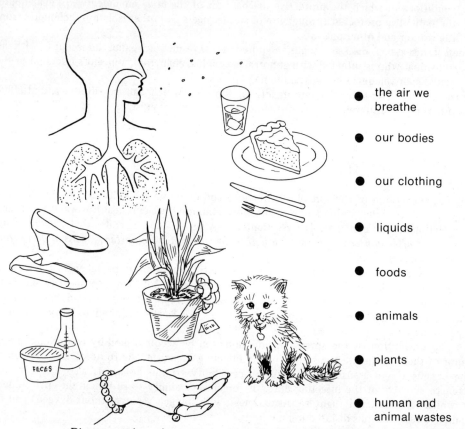

- the air we breathe
- our bodies
- our clothing
- liquids
- foods
- animals
- plants
- human and animal wastes

Disease-causing microorganisms may be found in these places.

Communicable diseases can be controlled by one or more of the following methods:

1. **Disinfection:** An attempt is made to kill pathogenic microorganisms either through chemical or physical means applied directly. Agents used to destroy microorganisms include:

   a. Steam under pressure (best method), as by autoclave.

   b. Boiling (212°F for 20 minutes), which kills most bacteria.

   c. Dry heat, as in an oven (320°F for one hour).

   d. Open flame or fire.

   e. Direct sunlight for 6 to 8 hours.

   f. Drying, which prevents growth and kills some bacteria (because moisture is needed to sustain life).

g. Cold temperature, which retards growth but is not a reliable method of destroying bacteria.

h. Chemicals used to inhibit or destroy bacteria (antiseptics, bacteriostatics, germicides, antibiotics, and ethylene oxide gas sterilization).

Concurrent disinfection—the continuous process of disinfection throughout the hospitalization period.

Terminal disinfection—the destruction of infectious material when the disease is over (after recovery, discharge, or death).

2. **Isolation.** The patient who has the communicable disease is separated from others, either in a private room or a cubicle in a ward area. Everything inside the isolation unit, except the designated clean areas, is considered contaminated.

TYPES OF ISOLATION

There are two main classifications of isolation techniques according to physical set-up. In the *unit type*, a single patient is confined to a location, which may be a room, a cubicle, or a screened area with 6 feet between beds. The *disease type* includes more than one patient in the unit, all with a similar disease; the entire unit is set apart. A tuberculosis unit is an example of the disease type.

Medical and surgical asepsis are involved in the isolation technique. *Medical asepsis* practices reduce the direct or indirect transfer of germs. This is done by using disposable equipment, cleansing the hands, wearing an isolation gown when attending the patient, and sterilizing the dishes. *An effort is made to keep the microorganisms within the unit.*

Surgical asepsis refers to practices that render and keep objects and areas free from microorganisms. This may be done by using sterile equipment, cleansing the hands, and wearing gloves, a gown, a mask and a cap.

Medical Asepsis.

Surgical Asepsis (Protective Technique).

Classifications of Isolation

Protective Isolation

Requirements

1. Private room—door must be closed.

2. Gowns—must be worn by all who enter the room.

3. Masks—must by worn by all who enter the room.

4. Hands—washed on entering and leaving the room.

5. Gloves—worn by all having direct patient contact.

6. Articles of use—suitable to the condition of isolation.

Conditions

1. Agranulocytosis.

2. Severe, noninfected vesicular or eczematous dermatitis.

3. Immunosuppressive therapy.

4. Lymphomas and leukemia.

Wound and Skin Precautions

Requirements

1. Private room

2. Gowns—must be worn by all who have direct contact with patient.

3. Masks—not needed except during dressing change.

4. Hands—washed on entering and leaving the room.

5. Gloves—worn by all having direct patient contact.

6. Articles of use—special precautions for instruments, dressings, and linen. Special dressing techniques must be used in changing dressings.

Conditions

1. Burns—not infected with *Staphylococcus aureus*.

2. Gas gangrene.

3. Impetigo.

4. Staphylococcal skin and wound infections.

5. Streptococcal skin infection.

6. Wound infections that are extensive.

Respiratory Isolation

Requirements

1. Private room—door must be closed.

2. Gowns—worn by all who have direct patient contact.

3. Masks—must be worn by all persons entering the room.

4. Hands—must be washed on entering and leaving the room.

5. Gloves—not necessary.

6. Articles of use—must be disinfected.

Conditions

1. Chickenpox.

2. Herpes zoster (fever blister).

3. Measles (rubeola).

4. Meningococcal meningitis.

5. Mumps.

6. Whooping cough (pertussis).

7. German measles (rubella).

8. Tuberculosis.

9. Venezuelan equine encephalomyelitis.

Enteric Precautions

Requirements

1. Private room—needed for children.

2. Gown—worn by all persons having direct contact with the patient.

3. Masks—not needed.

4. Hands—must be washed on entering and leaving the room.

5. Gloves—worn by all having direct patient contact.

6. Articles—special precautions necessary for articles contaminated with urine and feces.

Conditions

1. Cholera.

2. Enteropathogenic *Escherichia coli* (gastritis from E. coli).

3. Hepatitis (infectious or serum).

4. Salmonellosis (typhoid fever).

5. Shigellosis.

Strict Isolation

Requirements

1. Private room—with door closed.

2. Gowns—worn by all persons entering the room.

3. Masks—must be worn by all persons entering the room.

4. Hands—must be washed on entering and leaving the room.

5. Gloves—must be worn by all persons entering the room.

6. Articles—must be discarded, or wrapped before being sent to Central Supply for disinfection or sterilization.

Conditions

1. Anthrax inhalation.

2. Burns infected with *Staphylococcus aureus* or Group A *Streptococcus.*

3. Diphtheria.

4. Eczema vaccinatum.

5. Draining lesions or draining sinuses.

6. Herpes simplex (neonatal vesicular).

7. Plague.

8. Rabies.

9. German measles.

10. Smallpox.

11. Staphylococcal enterocolitis or pneumonia.

12. Streptococcal pneumonia.

13. Vaccinia that is generalized.

ITEM 1. SETTING UP A UNIT

Use a cubicle or private room with running water. A sign marked "ISOLATION," or a similar designation used in your agency, should be placed on the outside door, or at the entrance to the cubicle. If a cubicle or private room is not available, a selected area of the room can be established as an isolation zone. Screen this area; identify it by hanging an "ISOLATION" sign on the outside of the screens. Acquaint other workers with the limits of the isolation area. Collect these items, and place them properly in the patient's unit:

For Patient Use

1. Thermometer and holder.

2. Paper bags and wipes.

3. Toilet tissue.

4. Paper towels.

5. Bath basin and soap in a holder.

6. Emesis basis, water glass, toothbrush, and dentifrice.

7. Razor, shaving cream, and mirror (if patient is a man).

8. Bedpan and urinal.

9. Wastebasket lined with a plastic bag.

10. Food tray with silverware unless plastic disposable tableware is used. Salt may be included if allowed on the patient's diet.

11. Plastic covering for the pillow and mattress.

12. Linens.

13. Other special equipment designated by the charge nurse as needed.

For Health Worker Use

1. Extra bedside stand to hold rubber gloves, masks, and gowns unless a special cabinet is provided for that purpose.

2. IV standard on which to hang the gown (check with your agency; the "discard gown method" may be used and you may have to put on a new gown every time you enter a different room).

3. If running water and a sink are not available, provide a means to pour 70 per cent alcohol over hands, or use alcohol pledgets to clean them.

4. Hamper for soiled linen.

5. *Floors are contaminated.* Nothing must be used after it is dropped on the floor.

6. Laundry bag and holder

7. Containers for soiled syringes, gloves, needles and instruments.

After you have assembled the supplies and equipment, proceed with the following series of steps.

ITEM 2. PUTTING ON A FACE MASK

Important Steps

1. Take a mask from its container.

2. Put on the mask.

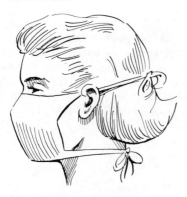

Face mask in place.

Key Points

Masks may be made of cloth or one of a variety of disposable materials. Handle the mask as little as possible because it will be coming in contact with your face, and you will be breathing through it.

Note: The National Communicable Disease Center recommends the use of high-efficiency disposable masks.

Unfold it and put it over your *nose* and *mouth.* Tie the mask with the top strings at the back of your head; be sure the strings pass over your ears. (If you wear glasses, the mask should fit snugly over your nose and under the bottom edge of your glasses. This will prevent your glasses from becoming steamed.) Tie the lower strings of the mask at the back of your head at the neckline. Be sure to fasten the ties securely; if not tied securely over the chin, they may work themselves loose while you are working.

Important Steps	Key Points
3. Wash your hands and remove the mask.	Take it off by untying the lower strings first, then the upper strings. Be careful not to let the strings or mask drop on your gown. Discard the mask in the appropriate container. Proceed to untie the waistband of your gown and follow the gown procedure. *Note:* A mask should never be reused. Therefore, *do not* slide the mask off your nose and mouth down around your neck. Always discard your mask when finished with the procedure. Start with a clean mask each time.
4. Change your mask.	Your mask will become moist as you breathe through it over a period of time. Change your mask whenever it becomes moist. Germs can grow in a wet environment. (A mask becomes moist in about 20 minutes.)
5. Rewash your hands before putting on another mask.	

ITEM 3. PUTTING ON AN ISOLATION GOWN

Important Steps	Key Points
1. Remove any rings, except a plain wedding band, and your wristwatch.	Jewelry may harbor microorganisms that could be carried to others outside the isolation unit. If your watch is needed for the TPR, remove it and place it in a small plastic bag or on a clean paper towel at the patient's bedside. (Take the paper towel from the dispenser in the patient's room.)
2. Wash your hands.	Refer to the unit on handwashing. Use a liquid antimicrobial soap.

Wash hands.

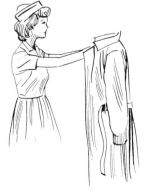

Put on clean gown.

3. Select a clean gown.	Hold the gown at the neck opening and let it unfold downward (gowns are usually folded in thirds for neat storage). The open part at the back should face you. The gown will be full length so it will cover your entire uniform to prevent contamination of your uniform while you work in the isolation unit. *Note:* The National Communicable Disease Center in Atlanta, Georgia, recommends the use of the "individual gown technique." That is, use the gown only once and then discard it.

U
N
I
T
36

Important Steps	Key Points
4. Put your arms through the gown sleeves.	Touch only the *inside* of the gown. Holding the inside of the gown, slip one arm at a time into the appropriate sleeve. Pull the gown on as far as possible.
5. Work inside the sleeves of the gown.	Work carefully to avoid contaminating your hands. Grab the opposite sleeve with your gown-covered hand (see the adjacent diagram); gently pull the sleeve up on your arm and shoulder. When this procedure is completed, go on with the other sleeve in the same manner, always working from the inside of the gown.

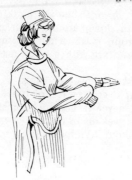

Work hands through ribbed cuffs.

Important Steps	Key Points
6. Adjust the gown on your shoulders.	Place your fingers *inside* the neckband (at the back), and adjust the gown so that it fits comfortably on your shoulders. Remember to work with the *inside* of the gown: keep your hands clean. If you touch the outside of the gown, or your hair, you must repeat the *handwashing procedure.*
7. Tie the neck tapes (ties).	Handle the ties carefully. Keep your hands clean. Do not touch your hair.
8. Draw the edges of the gown together.	The open part of your gown is at your back. Bring the right side of the gown over the left side of the gown. Adjust the gown so that it fits snugly (if you are left-handed, you would proceed from the left; put the right side over the left, then adjust snugly).

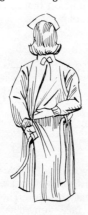

Draw edges together.

Important Steps	Key Points
9. Tie the waist belt.	Grasp the waist belt at the far (distal) ends, draw them together at your back, and tie them snugly.

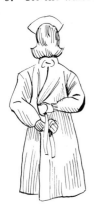

Tie waist belt.

You are now ready to give nursing care unless you need a mask or rubber gloves. If they are required, proceed in the manner prescribed later in the lesson. When you have completed your work in the isolation room, follow the procedure described below.

ITEM 4.   REMOVING AN ISOLATION GOWN

Important Steps	Key Points
1. Untie the waist belt.	Pull the sleeves up above your wrists.
2. Wash your hands.	
3. Untie the neck ties.	Take care not to contaminate your hands by touching your hair or the *outside* of the gown. Remember, it is contaminated. If you do, you must *rewash* your hands.
4. Remove the first sleeve of the gown.	Place your forefinger *under the cuff* of the sleeve and pull the sleeve down over your hand without touching the outside of the gown.
5. Remove the other sleeve.	With your hand inside the first sleeve, working with your gown-covered hand, draw the second sleeve down over your hand.
6. Slip out of the gown.	Discard it carefully in the soiled linen hamper in the patient's room. Remember, the National Communicable Disease Center recommends one-time gown usage.
7. Wash your hands.	Wash them according to procedure; dry them thoroughly. Turn off the faucets with a towel and discard the towel in the designated place. *Avoid touching* anything in the room as you leave. (If you used your wristwatch during the procedure, retrieve it at this time and put it on. Open the door with a paper towel, then discard the towel. Handle it from the top side only. Remember—the underside is contaminated.)

UNIT
36

Important Steps	Key Points
8. Record the nursing tasks that were accomplished.	Note the appropriate information on the patient's chart. Report any unusual signs or symptoms to your team leader. Charting example: Placed in Isolation per order. Explained procedure. Appears to take news very well, is cooperative. B. Bee, SN

For some infectious cases, you may have to wear a mask (see the sample chart, pages 713 to 714). If so, follow the next procedure. *You will put the mask on before washing your hands and putting on a gown, if it is used.* Masks are usually worn in caring for patients who have an airborne disease, draining skin lesions, or who are on Reverse Isolation Technique.

ITEM 5.   PUTTING ON STERILE OR NONSTERILE SINGLE–USE GLOVES

When you work with certain types of infectious cases, you may be required to wear rubber gloves for your protection. (Check the sample chart on pages 713 to 714). Gloves may be used where you will be handling soiled dressings. Your agency will specify the kinds of cases in which you will need rubber gloves.

Important Steps	Key Points
1. Obtain and unfold the glove wrapper.	Lay the glove wrapper on a flat, clean surface and unfold it. (Of course, your hands will have been washed before you put the gloves on. Gloves may be put on inside or outside the room. Check your agency procedure.)
2. Remove the powder packet from the wrapper (if there is one). 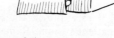 Unfold glove wrapper.	Some gloves are prepowdered. Remove the powder packet, tear it open, and carefully powder your hands. This will make it easier to slip your hand into the glove. Discard the powder packet into the wastebasket. Take care not to spread powder around the room.
3. Remove the glove from its wrapper.	Grasp the folded edge of the left cuff-top with your right hand so that you are touching the inside of the glove with your clean hand. Keep your fingers straight while pulling the glove on your hand.

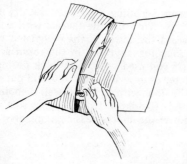

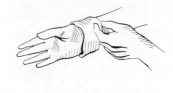

Pick up glove by its folded edge.

Important Steps	Key Points
4. Put on the second glove.	Grasp the folded edge of the cuff-top of the right glove with your left hand so that you are touching the *inside* of the glove with your clean hand. Be sure to keep the fingers of your left hand off the outside of the glove and your skin. Pull the glove on your hand. With your gloved right hand, slip your fingers *under* the folded cuff of the left glove (sterile surface to sterile surface). Pull it up over your hand and cuff to your gown. (Reverse these last two steps if you are left-handed.) Adjust the gloves over the gown cuff. Be careful to avoid touching your skin with the gloved hand—you will contaminate it and need to start at the beginning of the procedure with a new pair of gloves.

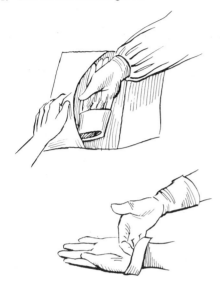

Slip *gloved hand* under cuff of glove.

Important Steps	Key Points
5. Adjust the fingers of the gloves.	When both gloves are in place, you can adjust the fingers of the gloves just as you would regular gloves worn for dress or cold weather.

ITEM 6. REMOVING STERILE OR NONSTERILE SINGLE-USE GLOVES

Gloves must be removed before your gown is removed, if you are wearing one.

Important Steps	Key Points
1. Remove the right-hand glove.	With your left hand, pull the right glove off with its cuff, taking care not to touch your skin with the contaminated glove. Dispose of the gloves in the designated container.
2. Remove the left-hand glove.	Place the fingers of your right hand *inside* the cuff of the left glove. Pull the glove down over and off your hand. Discard it into a designated container. (Reverse the last two steps if you are left-handed.)
3. Wash your hands.	Wash them before removing your mask. Untie the waist belt if you are wearing a gown, and then wash your hands. Follow the gown removal procedure.

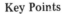

Wash hands.

U
N
I
T
36

ITEM 7.   SERVING A DIET TRAY TO A PATIENT IN ISOLATION

Important Steps	Key Points
1. Take the tray to the isolation door. (*Note:* Check your agency procedure for conditions that require tray isolation.)	Transfer the dishes sent on the cafeteria tray to the tray kept inside the patient's room. Take care not to touch the patient's tray with your hands—it is contaminated. You may do this unassisted or you may have help. Hold the cafeteria tray in your arm as you transfer dishes to the patient's tray.
2. Return the cafeteria tray.	Take it back to the cafeteria or to the unit diet kitchen.
3. Serve the patient's tray.	Unless your agency regulations state otherwise, you do not need to put on a gown if you are careful to touch nothing in the patient's room with your uniform. If you will be assisting the patient to eat, you will need to gown. Identify the patient; compare the identification band with the name card on the diet tray. Place the tray on the patient's overbed table. Assist in cutting foods and pouring milk or coffee. Adjust the bed to semi-Flowler's position if permitted. Move the overbed tray close to the patient.
4. Wash your hands.	Follow the correct procedure before leaving the room.

ITEM 8.   REMOVING THE DIET TRAY

(For patients who are on tray precautions—check your agency Isolation Procedure Manual.) When the patient has finished his meal, return to his room. *Wash your hands.*

Important Steps	Key Points
1. Remove the dishes from the patient's tray.	Usually take one at a time. If disposable dishes are used, empty liquid contents in the patient's toilet and also any soft foods. Fush the toilet. Solid foods such as gristle or bones should be disposed of in waterproof bags provided for that purpose. *Do not* throw them into the toilet. This would stop up the sewer lines. *Disposable dishes* are then placed in the designated containers or wastebasket in the patient's room. If the dishes and utensils are *reusable*, the liquids and solids are disposed of in the above manner. The dishes are then placed in designated bags.
2. Remove the soiled dishes from the isolation room using the double-bagging technique.	You will need a "clean person" on the outside of the room to assist you with this step. Place your carefully wrapped dishes *inside* a clean wrapper that is being held by the "clean person" outside the door (Double-bagged = wrapped in one bag of paper, plastic, or linen inside the room, then inserted into a second clean bag while outside the room.) The other worker will close and secure the edges of the bag with

Important Steps	Key Points
	masking tape. Label the package with the patient's name and identify the package with an isolation label.
3. Return the articles to the processing department (or diet kitchen).	Return the labeled double-bagged package to the processing room or diet kitchen for sterilization. Sterilization may be done either in the dietary department or the central supply; check for your agency's procedure.

ITEM 9.   GENERAL INFORMATION ABOUT USE OF BEDPANS AND URINALS IN ISOLATION

In addition to the usual procedure, you *must follow* these instructions:

Important Steps	Key Points
1. Provide assistance when needed.	
2. Remember to *wear a gown and mask if designated by your procedure manual.*	
3. Contents of the bedpan and urinal are flushed down the toilet unless they must be obtained for a specimen.	Public Health Department Regulations prescribe that the sewage system used in most hospitals and extended-care facilities (ECF) be constructed to take isolation liquids and excretion.
4. Rinse the bedpan or urinal after *each* use.	Dry and return it to storage. If excretions must be emptied in the utility room, transport the bedpan or urinal covered through the hallways. Avoid touching anything with your contaminated hands and equipment. Use the foot pedal to flush the "hopper" (multipurpose sink) usually available in the central utility room.
5. Wash your hands.	

ITEM 10.   COLLECTION OF SPECIMENS IN ISOLATION

Important Steps	Key Points
1. Secure the appropriate container (urine, sputum, etc.).	Obtain it from the storage room. Follow the procedures described in the units on bowel and urine elimination and sputum collection.
2. Label the container.	(See your agency specifications regarding the name and other information needed on the label.)
3. Collect the specimen.	Obtain it in the usual manner. See the previous units on specimen collection.
4. Place the specimen in the container.	Transfer the specimen from the utensil (bedpan, urinal, etc.) to the specimen container.

UNIT 36

Important Steps	Key Points
5. Place the specimen container in a clean, waterproof bag.	Bag should be held by someone "clean" on the outside of the room. Take care not to touch the exterior of the bag. If you touch the bag, you will contaminate it and will need to discard the bag and start over. The "clean person" on the outside of the room will carefully close and secure the opening with masking tape and attach the requisition to the bag.
6. Take it to the designated department.	*Transport* it promptly to the designated department.
7. Record the procedure on the nurses' notes.	Enter the time the specimen was collected, the kind of specimen, the time it was sent to the lab, X-ray, etc.

ITEM 11. SIGNING A DOCUMENT

Important Steps	Key Points
1. Place a clean paper towel on the overbed table.	
2. Place the document on the paper towel.	
3. Place another paper towel with its edge close to the line provided for the patient's signature.	The patient's hand will be resting on the paper towel.
4. When the signature is completed, remove the document from the room.	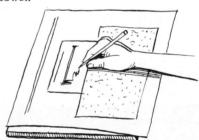
5. Wash the pen with soap and water, or a specified germicidal solution (if it is to be removed from the room; otherwise, place it in the patient's bedside stand).	
	Place paper towel for hand to rest on.
6. Wash your hands.	Wash them before leaving the patient's room.
7. Record the action on the nurses' notes.	Designate the time and type of document that was signed.

ITEM 12. DISPOSAL OF WASTE MATERIALS: DOUBLE–BAG TECHNIQUE

Important Steps	Key Points
1. Empty the wastebasket.	Collect all used dressings, dishes, utensils, and so forth in the designated disposable bags (waxed brown paper or plastic).
2. Seal the bags securely.	Fasten with string, tape, or whatever method is used in your agency.

Important Steps	Key Points
3. Place the soiled bag or bags of materials in a *clean* plastic bag held by someone at the entrance of the room.	*Note:* This same method of transfer at the entrance of the isolation unit may be used for linens, specimens, and waste products to be burned (paper, dressings, etc.). The "clean person" on the outside of the room places his hands under the cuff of the bag to protect himself from being touched by the *contaminated* articles.

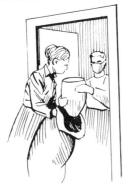

"Clean" nurse holds bag at door of
contaminated unit.

4. The articles are carefully placed inside the plastic or linen bag.	Secure the bag. The "clean person" then carefully secures the bag with tape, safety pin, or tie, labels it "Isolation," and takes it to the disposal area: laundry chute, trash chute, or other area. Isolation linens are frequently color-coded with a yellow marker.

ITEM 13.   REMOVAL OF LINENS

Important Steps	Key Points
1. Place the linen in a hamper.	A laundry hamper with a heavy cloth bag is usually provided in the *clean area* of the patient's room for collection of soiled linens.
2. Remove the linens from the isolation room.	The filled laundry bag in the patient's room is placed in a prelabeled clean bag handled by the clean person *outside* the room. Send soiled linens to the laundry room. Follow the remaining procedure for removal of waste materials from the isolation room (Item 12).

ITEM 14.   TAKING TPR AND BP

Important Steps	Key Points
1. Leave the thermometer and sphygmomanometer in the isolation room until the patient is discharged or removed from isolation.	
2. Wear a gown and mask if indicated.	
3. Follow the regular procedure for taking TPR and BP.	

U
N
I
T
36

Important Steps	Key Points
4. Wash your hands after taking TPR and BP.	
5. Record the procedure.	Note your observations promptly on clean paper in the clean area of the unit. Transfer the notes to the patient's chart at the earliest opportunity.

ITEM 15. TRANSPORTING A PATIENT OUT OF UNIT

Important Steps	Key Points
1. Notify the unit to which the patient is being transferred.	
2. Place a clean sheet over the wheelchair or stretcher.	If the patient goes in a wheelchair, place a clean sheet over the chair and wrap it around the patient after he is seated, for warmth and to protect his modesty. If he goes on a stretcher, place a clean sheet or cotton blanket on the stretcher, then place the patient on it.
3. Put a blanket on or around the patient.	This provides warmth and privacy.
4. Put a mask on the patient.	*Masks* are *always* worn by patients with respiratory diseases or those who are on strict isolation precautions when being transported in the hallways. (Check your agency procedure.)
5. Transport the patient to the designated area.	Remember to use proper body alignment, balance and movement for both you and your patient.
6. Return the patient to his room.	Strip the linen from the stretcher or wheelchair. Dispose of it in the patient's linen hamper.
7. Return the used wheelchair or stretcher for cleansing.	

ITEM 16. TRANSFERRING ISOLATION PATIENT TO ANOTHER HOSPITAL OR UNIT

Important Steps	Key Points
1. Collect the patient's belongings and take them along with the patient.	Remember to take all personal belongings: dentures, glasses, clothing, toilet articles, etc.
2. Place a mask on the patient if indicated.	
3. Prepare a wheelchair or stretcher as needed.	See Item 15.
4. Accompany the patient to his new unit, then settle and orient him in his new room.	Introduce him to the new personnel. Remember your admission procedure. If you have forgotten, review the unit on admissions.
5. Provide for *terminal disinfection* of the room from which the patient came, as well as for the transporting equipment.	Transportation equipment is either washed with a designated germicidal solution by unit personnel as soon as the patient has been returned

Important Steps	Key Points
	to his room, or is sent to the central processing area in your agency for terminal cleaning. After cleaning, the stretcher should be made up with a fresh sheet and ready for use by the next patient. Wash your hands.

6. Record the transfer on the nurses' notes.

ITEM 17. TERMINAL DISINFECTION

This procedure is done to clean the room as well as the supplies and utensils when a patient is discharged, expires, or is removed from isolation. Because this room has been exposed to more germs than are usual in a hospital room, *special precautions* must be taken during the final cleaning process before admitting a new patient.

You will need assistance with this procedure. Your co-worker should remain "clean" outside the room, ready to receive your supplies and equipment in the appropriate receptacles.

Important Steps	Key Points
1. Put on a gown (mask and gloves if required by agency procedure).	Usually at least a gown is required to protect your clothing while you are working in the contaminated room. You will be assisted by a "clean person" who remains outside the isolation room to receive the specially prepared contaminated equipment.
2. Prepare the utensils and supplies for removal from the isolation room.	Articles that can be sterilized in the autoclave must be placed in a special bag and handed to your clean assistant outside of the room. Place your carefully wrapped contaminated articles inside a clean bag held by your outside assistant. Take care to touch only the inside of the bag he is holding. Your clean assistant will label the bag "Isolation" with the patient's name, the room number, and the contents. All linens, clean dressings, metal or glass articles except thermometers can be handled in this way. (Follow your agency disposal procedure.)
3. Prepare a basin with the agency's germicidal solution.	*Delicate instruments* such as sphygmomanometers, otoscopes, scissors, thermometers, and *plastic articles* must be wiped off with a cold germicidal solution. (They would be melted or destroyed by the high temperature used for autoclave sterilization.) If your agency uses disposable thermometers, dispose of them in the trash. Follow the special glass-handling precautions established by your agency. *Aerosol cans* cannot be autoclaved or burned—they would explode. Therefore, they, too, must be wiped off with a cold germicidal solution and sent home with the patient. If an aerosol can is empty, it can be discarded in the trash according to agency procedure. The types of aerosol cans you will handle in this connection are containers for deodorant, hair spray, shave cream, spray cologne.

U
N
I
T
36

Important Steps	Key Points
4. Wash the gown standard (if portable) with germicidal solution.	When it has been wiped clean, roll the standard from the room. The clean assistant will take it to the storage area.
5. Wipe the instruments with germicidal solution.	Give them to your clean assistant to return to the central processing area for further decontamination. Follow the double-bagging and labeling procedure.
6. Remove all burnable supplies.	Burnable items such as paper, dressings, and cotton can easily be burned. You have already been placing them in waterproof bags in the waste containers in the patient's room while working with the patient. Be sure the package is sealed and labeled "Isolation" before sending it to be incinerated.
7. Remove the bags.	Seal the tops carefully by folding them down several times. Place them in a clean bag held by your clean assistant outside the room. Be sure to drop your bags into the center of the clean bag, taking care not to touch the outside of the clean bag—you would contaminate it. Your clean assistant will close the clean bag by rolling the top edge downward. He will fasten it securely with tape, to be taken later to the trash collection area for transfer to the incinerator. From there it will be sent to the incinerator for burning.
8. Remove all other used supplies.	Items such as needles and syringes must be specially disposed of. Follow your agency procedure.
9. Remove all unused supplies or equipment.	Place items that can be autoclaved in a bag for sterilizing. Hand it to your assistant to double-bag, secure the top, and label it for identification: isolation, patient's name, room number, and list of articles in package. Articles that cannot be autoclaved should be scrubbed thoroughly with your agency's disinfectant solution, taken out of the room, and sent back to the central processing room for further decontamination and storage.
10. Remove the bedding and all other soiled linen.	Place soiled linens in a laundry bag in the hamper. *Wash your hands.* Remove your gown and place it in the linen hamper. Carefully close the top of the bag securely by pinning or taping. Without touching your uniform, place it in a clean bag held by the clean assistant who will close and label the bag securely for transportation to the laundry room.
11. Notify the housekeeping department that terminal cleaning is required.	Be sure to notify them that it had been an isolation room. They also must take special precautions.
12. Make a closed bed and set up the unit ready for a new admission.	As soon as the housekeeping personnel have finished cleaning the unit, you can prepare the room for the next procedure.

Important Steps

Key Points

Note: This step may also be done by the housekeeping personnel. Check your agency procedure.

ITEM 18.   REVERSE ISOLATION TECHNIQUE

Reverse isolation technique, sometimes called protective isolation, follows the regular isolation technique in many respects. The difference is the purpose. In *regular isolation* technique, the patient has a communicable disease, and an attempt is made to *protect the health worker* and others from the disease process. In *reverse isolation* technique, the *patient is being protected* from the health worker and others of the health facility.

Persons with extensive burns in which the skin is denuded, patients with open lesions, and those who have very low resistance to infection because of a low white blood count or poor kidney function, benefit from reverse isolation technique. This technique is similar to that of surgical asepsis where all things are kept sterile. In other words, for patients who have low resistance to infection, we must take extra precautions. We set up as near sterile (free from pathogenic organisms) an environment for him as possible.

Set up the unit the same as you would for regular isolation technique. Follow the items listed under general reminders on the next page.

Follow the procedure described in Items 1 through 10 for disposal of waste and soiled linen; however, food trays need not be included since the patient has no contagious disease, but is being protected from others.

In reverse isolation technique, the health worker always wears a gown, gloves in some cases, and *always* a mask. The health facility will advise about each specific case as to the need for gloves.

Terminal disinfection is not needed upon discharge of this patient because the room does not require fumigation as it does when a contagious disease has been involved. The regular hospital facility terminal cleaning of a unit may be followed.

Summary:

1.   The patient in a reverse isolation unit is being protected from *you* and others.

2.   The patient is in a debilitated state and must be protected from any possible respiratory infection or other microorganism that may be brought *to* him.

3.   Reverse isolation care is similar to that of surgical asepsis:

    a.   Hands must be washed carefully and frequently.

    b.   Gown, mask, and sometimes gloves must be worn during care.

    c.   Use sterile equipment for care of the patient.

    d.   Restrict visitors and require that each wear a gown and mask (follow your agency procedure).

    e.   Limit trips in and out of the room. Plan in advance what equipment must be taken into the room.

ITEM 19.   GENERAL ISOLATION REMINDERS

1.   Floors are contaminated. Anything dropped on the floor is contaminated and must be discarded or cleaned carefully before reuse.

2.   Patients with communicable diseases should be grouped according to the epidemiology of transmission:

    a. Contact through respiratory spread.

    b. Gastrointestinal tract.

    c. Direct contact with wound or skin infection.

3. Keep dust down. Sweeping compounds or wet-mops with disinfectants must be used for this purpose.

4. Protect the patient from drafts.

5. Establish contaminated and clean zones. The clean areas should include those used by the health worker. Items like telephones should not be used by the patient outside the unit. There should be a "clean" area in the isolation unit where no contaminated articles are permitted. In other words, items not in the clean area are considered contaminated.

6. Anything that is brought into the isolation area must not be removed except in proper containers, then placed in an outside clean container and labeled "isolation."

7. Never rub your eyes or nose, or put your hands near your mouth when you are taking care of a patient in an isolation unit.

8. Never shake linen when you are removing it or placing it on the bed.

9. Wash your hands often. Refer to the unit on Handwashing Technique for Medical Asepsis.

10. Use clean squares of paper or tissue to touch contaminated articles.

11. Paper towels or clean squares of paper provide a clean area on which to place articles within a unit.

12. Keep a water pitcher and a glass in the room. Ice and fresh water are brought to the door and transferred. (Use the same technique for food.)

13. Faucets should be turned off and on using a paper towel to protect your hands.

14. The same nursing procedures are carried out for these patients as for any patient. However, you have also learned some additional safety precautions (masking, gloving, gowning, and disposal techniques).

15. Inform the charge nurse of skin lesions, sore throat, or other evidence you may have of your own lowered resistance to infection or disease. (She may reassign you to protect you and the patient.)

VI.   ADDITIONAL INFORMATION FOR ENRICHMENT

The health worker may further protect himself from communicable diseases by:

1. Taking a shower daily and shampooing hair as needed (at least once a week).

2. Establishing regular sleeping patterns and sleeping at least 8 hours each night. (Sleep cannot be stored like money in the bank; sleep is required daily for good body resistance to infection and for high performance.)

3. Eating a sensible, well-balanced diet. Avoid crash diets. Use fresh fruits and vegetables for necessary minerals and vitamins. Eat protein foods.

4. Drinking plenty of fluids. Two-thirds of the body consists of water, and because fluid is lost daily by perspiration and elimination, it must be replaced. Drink six to 8 glasses of water daily.

5. Developing good habits of elimination. (Do not deny the body urge to eliminate; this upsets the natural function of the body.)

6. Practicing regular habits of oral hygiene. Never neglect your teeth. See your dentist at least yearly.

7. Balancing hours of activity with recreation. Spend some time out of doors in fresh air. Give your body proper exercise.

8. Taking care of your hands. Apply lotion to keep them soft. Cut off hangnails that may tear and produce a gateway for infection. Protect breaks in the skin that may allow microorganisms to enter.

9. Protecting your eyes when you are in an isolation unit. Do not touch the eyes with your fingers while caring for a patient. (Remember—the most common causes of eye infections are the fingers.) If irrigation fluid happens to get into the eye, rinse the eye immediately with normal saline.

10. Keeping your hands away from your mouth when caring for a patient who is in an isolation unit. Always wash your hands before handling food that enters your mouth.

11. Protecting your hair from contamination. Wear a cap when you are in a highly contagious situation.

12. Removing jewelry when you are caring for a patient in an isolation unit. Rings can harbor microorganisms that may not be removed with regular handwashing. Your watch may also harbor microorganisms and interfere with proper handwashing.

Body Defenses. Human beings are fortunate in natural body defenses. The unbroken skin serves to protect the body from microorganisms. However, microorganisms do enter the body through the respiratory tract, and digestive and genitourinary openings. The defenses that serve to protect these entry sites are body secretions and cilia that act as barriers to bacteria. These barriers include the acid reaction of the urine, digestive juices that kill bacteria, and threadlike projections and mucus that remove dust and bacteria from the respiratory tract.

The skin is called the first line of body defense, and secretions form the second line of defense. If microorganisms break through these two barriers and reach the blood stream, antibodies are formed that fight harmful bacteria.

Fever is another defense. (Fever is the heat that heals.) Moderate fever, from $102°$ to $104°$ F, is a desirable response since few bacteria can survive this temperature. However, fever higher than this may be destructive to the body tissues.

Leukocytes (phagocytes or white blood corpuscles) are wandering cells in the blood that ingest and destroy bacteria. When the body is injured, they increase in number and surround and engulf invading bacteria. Other phagocytes are fixed in the body, in the liver, spleen, bone marrow, and lymph nodes, which are strategic spots of body function. Destruction of bacteria is also carried out here.

The ability to resist contracting a disease is called immunity. There are two different general classifications of immunity—natural and acquired. Natural immunity is the resistance with which one is born. It is inherited and considered permanent. Human beings are subject to many diseases that animals have, but are immune to certain other diseases of animals. Immunity is characteristic of certain races, e.g., yellow fever attacks Caucasians, but native Indians and Negroes are immune to it. Eskimos and Negroes are more susceptible to tuberculosis than the white man.

Acquired immunity is developed during life. This is classified further as active acquired immunity and passive acquired immunity. To develop active acquired immunity, the person must have:

1. contracted the disease and recovered from it. Example: One who has had measles does not ordinarily have them a second time.

2. had a mild (sometimes unnoticed) infection of the disease.

3. been given a suitable vaccine or antigen (a substance that stimulates antibodies within the person's body). Example: One who is vaccinated with smallpox vaccine will not have the disease.

The process of increasing an individual's resistance to a particular infection by artificial means is called *immunization*.

Passive acquired immunity is made possible by injecting into one person the antibodies from the blood of other persons or animals. This type of immunity is immediate in effect, but is of short duration because the human body is not stimulated to produce its own antibodies.

Most microorganisms that invade the body have a substance called antigen. An *antigen* is a substance that causes the body to manufacture antibodies to fight against allergens. An *allergen* is a substance to which the body reacts. Let us say that a microorganism invades a human being; the body reacts to the antigen by producing a protein substance called *antibodies*. These antibodies are formed in the liver, spleen, bone marrow, and other organs. They are carried by the blood and lymph throughout the body and they destroy toxins of the microorganisms, or render them incapable of harming the body.

Gamma globulin injections are another method of providing a defense. This substance consists of a fraction of human blood plasma that contains antibodies against certain diseases. Gamma globulin is often used to modify the effects of hepatitis or measles, although we now have a specific vaccine against measles.

There are ways of *testing immunity*. This is done through skin tests. *Skin tests* determine the presence of certain antibodies in an individual. When immunity is present, a minute (small) amount of the antibody injected under the skin will produce in a given time a localized skin reaction. Skin tests are done for diphtheria (Schick test), scarlet fever (Dick test), tuberculosis (Pirquet's reaction), and histoplasmosis (with histoplasmin). Skin tests are also available to investigate an individual's sensitivity to foods, pollens, and various other substances.

The extent of damage from an infection is the result of two factors: the individual's resistance to injury and the microorganism's power to injure.

The person's resistance is influenced by his age, his state of nutrition, the presence of disease (especially of metabolic origin), the hormones such as glucocorticoids, the adequacy of his blood supply, the location of the infection, and the natural or acquired antibodies.

The microorganism's power to inflict damage to the individual is dependent on its ability to produce certain enzymes. The enzymes may destroy tissues, damage blood vessels and cause hemorrhage, block lymphatic drainage in the body by clot formation, or dissolve blood clots, allowing the infection to spread. In addition, some bacteria are ingested by phagocytes in the body as mentioned earlier. Other bacteria not readily destroyed by the phagocyte's enzymes may be transported to new locations and produce new or additional areas of infection. Rinsing your hands with an antiseptic solution removes harmful bacteria. Common germicidal solutions in use today are phenol, iodine, and hydrogen peroxide. It must be kept in mind, however, that such germicidal solutions can be very injurious to the skin if used in highly concentrated solutions.

To sum up the body's defenses against infection, we are protected by:

1. Healthy unbroken skin and mucous membranes. It is up to you to keep the first line of defense strong.

2. Removal of bacteria by secretions of mucous membranes and by cilia (hair-like projections) in the nose and bronchial tree. The bacteria are removed by coughing and sneezing.

3. Destruction of bacteria by the gastric juices and the acid reactions of urine and vaginal discharges.

4. Filtering action of lymph nodes to remove bacteria from the body system.

5. Increased number of white blood cells upon invasion of bacteria.

6. Antibody formation, which keeps numbers of microorganisms from multiplying.

7. Inflammatory reaction of the body to an invasion of microorganisms. Inflammation represents warfare between the offending organism and the white cells, as well as the body reaction to the invasion.

Psychological Effects of Isolation. It is equally important to think about the patient's attitude and how he may react to being placed in an isolation unit. He may feel not only that he is contaminated, but that he is unacceptable to other members of society. When one considers the high value placed on the capacity to be useful in society and to accomplish what one wishes when and where one chooses, it becomes clear how the image one has of oneself and one's body at this time may influence one's behavior. Can you imagine a more devastating situation than being required to lie totally immobile, completely dependent on someone else to feed you and provide for body elimination—as though you were an infant?

Loss of control of one's activities and functions may cause depression and shame. There is nothing shameful about needing such care, but some patients may view it that way. Society expects the adult to be in control of himself, and being placed in a situation of isolation intensifies his awareness of his inability to be in command of himself. You must therefore understand the patient's right to feel depressed. Make every effort to help him work through this temporary state. Frustration and anger turned inward are sometimes reflected in negative behavior by the patient, and in his use of abusive words and actions. Accept this as a part of his illness. Visit him often so he does not continue to feel so isolated. Some patients may accept isolation willingly. In any event, make every effort to understand your patient's needs.

U
N
I
T
36

PERFORMANCE TEST

1. Discuss with your instructor the differences between isolation technique and reverse isolation technique, as well as the procedure for terminal cleaning following an isolation case.

2. In the skill laboratory with a student partner, correctly demonstrate the isolation technique used in caring for a patient having a staphylococcal wound infection. Demonstrate the procedure for gowning, masking, gloving, removing soiled items from the patient's room, serving, and removing a meal tray.

PERFORMANCE CHECKLIST

ISOLATION TECHNIQUE

GOWNING

1. Remove your rings and wristwatch.

2. Wash your hands.

3. Select a gown (from the cabinet or clothes hook).

4. Put your arms into the sleeves, work the arms on, and adjust the shoulders without contaminating your hands.

5. Tie the neck tapes, close the gown at the back, and tie the waist belt without contaminating your hands.

REMOVING GOWN

1. Untie the waist belt, push up the sleeves, and wash your hands.

2. Untie the neck ties without contaminating your hands.

3. Remove the sleeves of the gown.

    a. Place your forefinger under one cuff of the sleeve.

    b. Pull the sleeve over your hand without touching the outside of the gown.

    c. For the other sleeve, work it off using the gown-covered second hand.

4. Slip out of the gown and dispose of it in a laundry hamper, taking care not to touch your uniform or shake the gown.

5. Wash your hands as you leave the unit, and turn off the faucet with a paper towel.

MASKING

1. Obtain a mask from the container.

2. Unfold the mask, and place it over your nose and mouth.

3. Tie the top strings at the back of your head. (Strings must be *over* the ears and the top edge of the mask under your glasses if worn.)

4. Remove the mask by untying the lower strings, then the top strings, and discard it into the designated receptacle.

5. Change your mask when it becomes moist (or be able to explain when and why you change your mask).

6. Rewash your hands, and put on a clean mask.

GLOVING

1. Obtain and unfold a glove wrapper, and powder your hands if a powder pack is available.

2. Remove the first glove from its wrapper at the folded edge of its cuff, and pull it up on your hand.

3. With your first gloved hand, grasp the second glove under the loose edge of its cuff (sterile surface to sterile surface), and pull the glove up on your hand.

4. Adjust the glove cuffs over the gown cuffs, without contaminating the gloves or gown, and adjust the fingers of the gloves.

5. Remove the gloves before your gown is removed.

    a. Pull the glove off your first hand without contaminating your skin.

    b. Dispose of the glove in a receptacle.

6. Pull the second glove off by placing your fingers inside the cuff of the remaining glove, pull it down over your hand, and discard it into the receptacle.

7. Wash your hands before removing your mask.

REMOVAL OF WASTE MATERIALS

1. Empty waste materials into a designated bag (brown paper or plastic) in the patient's room.

2. Seal the bag securely with string, tape, etc.

3. Place the sealed bag carefully inside a clean bag being held by the clean person outside the room.

    a. Take care to touch only the inside of the bag. (The clean person then closes, secures, and labels the double-bagged package for disposal.)

REMOVAL OF MEAL TRAY

1. Remove all dishes from the tray (one at a time).

2. Dispose of any liquids down the toilet, and flush the toilet.

3. Dispose of solid foods in a brown paper bag(s).

4. Place disposable dishes in the designated receptacle.

5. Place reusable dishes (after foods have been removed) in a brown bag, and seal the bag.

6. Hand the sealed bag to the clean person for double-bagging.

7. Close and secure the bag, label it, and transport it for sterilization.

POST-TEST

True or False: Circle the "T" if the statement is true. Circle "F" if the statement is false.

T F   1. A communicable disease may be transferred from one person to another.

T F   2. All articles of use in an isolation unit are considered contaminated.

T F   3. It is necessary to wear a gown when giving a bedpan.

T F   4. Unused articles and linen in an isolation unit may not be removed and placed with other articles and linen for use by other patients.

T F   5. Microorganisms inflict damage to the patient by their ability to produce certain enzymes.

T F   6. After discharge of an "isolation patient," it is sufficient terminal disinfection practice to air the room for one hour.

T F   7. Linen removed from an isolation unit must be placed in an additional bag as well as the original bag in which it is placed.

T F   8. If your mask slips down from your nose on your neck, it is safe to replace it and wear it.

T F   9. Patients in an isolation unit should not be given a backrub with the bare hands.

T F 10. The faucet in the isolation bathroom is considered clean and suitable to turn on and off without protection.

T F 11. In an isolation ward, a safe distance between beds is 3 feet.

T F 12. In an isolation ward, all patients have communicable diseases and respiratory tract infections; Gi tract infections and skin infections may be placed every other bed for care convenience.

T F 13. Isolation technique dictates that a mask must always be worn.

T F 14. Food trays may be served to the patient in isolation in regular fashion since all dishes are sterilized in the dishwasher.

T F 15. It is all right to give a bedpan in an isolation unit without a gown as long as you do not touch your uniform against anything.

T F 16. TPR may be taken without a gown as long as the uniform does not touch anything.

T F 17. Discarded tissues from an isolation unit may be placed in the regular trash can since all trash is burned anyway.

T F 18. One must wear a mask when doing terminal disinfection.

T F 19. Diseases that can be communicated from one person to another are called isolated.

T F 20. One disease that cannot be contracted through respiration is syphilis.

POST-TEST ANNOTATED ANSWER SHEET

1. T (p. 711)

2. T (pp. 712 and 730)

3. F (p. 723)

4. T (p. 728)

5. T (p. 732)

6. F (p. 712)

7. T (p. 725)

8. F (p. 717)

9. F (p. 730)

10. F (p. 730)

11. F (p. 712)

12. F (p. 712)

13. F (pp. 713–714)

14. F (pp. 722–723)

15. T (p. 723) (Note: This does not include patients on reverse isolation.)

16. T (p. 725)

17. F (pp. 724–725)

18. F (p. 727)

19. F (p. 711)

20. T (p. 711)

Unit 37

CARDIOPULMONARY RESUSCITATION

I. DIRECTIONS TO THE STUDENT

This is one of the most important units in this book because it will introduce you to basic life-saving procedures. The cardiopulmonary resuscitation methods described here are the emergency life support techniques that the American Heart Association recommends for training the general public, beginning with school children in the eighth grade.*

Read the unit carefully, and in the skill laboratory practice the procedures on a mannequin of the Resusci-Annie type until you gain effective skills and speed.

These items are recommended for your study and practice:

1. Filmstrip on CPR, or "The Breath of Life," which may be available to your agency from the American Heart Association local unit.

2. Resusci-Annie type of mannequin.

Please read the following paragraphs carefully. They describe the condition of cardiac arrest and outline step-by-step the actions you should take in basic cardiopulmonary resuscitation. Advanced CPR techniques employing equipment like defibrillators and various drugs are used only by highly trained teams of doctors, nurses, and technicians. When you feel that you have sufficient knowledge and skills to perform the performance test and complete the written test, make arrangements with your instructor to take these tests.

II. GENERAL PERFORMANCE OBJECTIVE

On completion of this lesson, you will be able to recognize the signs of cardiac arrest, and to carry out the emergency cardiopulmonary resuscitation procedures.

III. SPECIFIC PERFORMANCE OBJECTIVES

When you have completed this unit, you will be able to

1. Recognize and describe the signs of cardiac arrest.

2. Palpate the carotid artery for signs of a pulse.

3. Provide a patent airway for the victim.

4. Ventilate the victim through mouth-to-mouth resuscitation.

5. Maintain artificial circulation through closed-chest massage.

---

*American Heart Association, Cardio-Pulmonary Resuscitation and Emergency Cardiac Care Committee, and National Academy of Sciences – National Research Council, Medical Sciences Division, Emergency Medical Services Committee: Standards for Cardiopulmonary Resuscitation (CPR) and Emergency Cardiac Care (ECC). *Journal of American Medical Association*, 277:850, February 18, 1974.

IV. VOCABULARY

Some of the words used in this lesson may be new or unfamiliar to you. These have been listed below with their meanings. Go over this list several times and when you see the word used in the lesson, refer to this section unless you are sure of its meaning.

cardiac arrest—sudden and unexpected loss of cardiac and pulmonary function.
cardiac board—a flat board, usually kept on the cardiac arrest cart, that is placed under the
     patient's back to provide a firm surface for giving external heart massage if he is in bed.
CPR—an abbreviation for cardiopulmonary resuscitation.
myocardial infarction—the heart attack, or blockage of the blood supply to the heart.
pupil—the opening in the center of the iris (the colored portion of the eye).
contracted pupils—pupils become smaller when exposed to light.
dilated pupils—pupils enlarge in darkness (both pupils should be equal in size).
resuscitation—the act of bringing back to life.
sternum—the breastbone; a flat, narrow bone in the midline of the thorax between the ribs.
trachea—the windpipe.
xiphoid process—the lowest portion of the sternum (breastbone).

V. INTRODUCTION TO CARDIOPULMONARY RESUSCITATION

Cardiac arrest is a sudden and dramatic event, regardless of where it occurs. People may become victims of cardiac arrest at any time and at any place. They have been struck down while playing tennis, taking a nap, driving a car, cooking a meal, or being treated in a hospital. The victims appear to be doing fine and have no particular problems until they suddenly collapse and lose consciousness. They die unless the cardiac arrest is recognized and treated in time by someone trained in cardiopulmonary resuscitation (CPR) techniques.

ITEM 1. WHAT IS CARDIAC ARREST?

The term "cardiac arrest" means that the heart has stopped beating and the blood no longer circulates through the body. The victim stops breathing and loses consciousness because the brain lacks the oxygen it needs in order to function. Within 20 to 40 seconds after cardiac arrest, the person is clinically dead. After 4 to 6 minutes, the lack of oxygen has caused permanent and extensive damage to the brain and the heart. "Cardiac arrest" is the term used to refer only to those situations where the loss of heart action and breathing occurs without warning; it is immediate — not gradual — and it is unexpected. You would not refer to deaths resulting from other causes, or from a lingering, fatal disease, as cardiac arrest, even though the heart action does stop.

Causes of Cardiac Arrest

There are a number of conditions that can cause cardiac arrest by interfering with the normal function of the heart or lungs. The underlying reason for cardiac arrest is believed to be a lack of sufficient oxygen to the heart muscle. The heart attack, or myocardial infarction, is a common cause of cardiac arrest. In the heart attack, a segment of the heart muscle is deprived of its blood and oxygen supply. Without oxygen, the heart muscle cells begin to die. As more cells are affected, the heart beats erratically and loses its ability to keep blood circulating adequately in the body. Each year more than one million persons in the United States suffer heart attacks, and more than half of them die. Most of the deaths occur within two hours after the initial attack. Many of these victims of cardiac arrest are adults in the most productive periods of their lives.

Other conditions that may lead to sudden death are associated with hypoventilation. An obstruction of the air passages, infections such as pneumonia, or injury to the chest and lungs all involve some degree of hypoventilation. The reduction in the amount of oxygen available for the body's use exposes the person to a greater risk of cardiac arrest. Extensive burns and hemorrhage that reduce the blood volume, drug intoxication, and metabolic or electrolyte imbalances also increase the risk of cardiac arrest. Electric shock, head injury, and damage to the central nervous system are other causes.

Signs of Cardiac Arrest

When cardiac arrest occurs, the signs of death appear almost immediately, just as if someone had pushed an "off" button. Circulation stops. The heartbeat and pulse are absent. Blood pressure falls to zero. The pupils of the eyes gradually dilate. Respirations cease, and the skin looks pale and greyish in color and feels cool. If respiratory arrest occurs first and the heart continues to beat, the skin color will be bluish or cyanotic. Respiratory arrest rapidly leads to cardiac arrest as a result of the lack of oxygen.

When you observe or are called to help an unconscious person who has probably had a cardiac arrest, first open the airway and feel for a pulse. Palpating the carotid artery for a pulse is recommended rather than trying to find a radial pulse at the wrist or a temporal pulse. The carotid arteries carry blood to the brain and the head, and a pulse can usually be felt here when other pulses have disappeared. The arteries are located on each side of the neck. The pulse can be most easily felt next to the larynx, or voice box. You should practice locating and palpating the carotid pulse on yourself and others.

Important Steps	Key Points
1. Locate the larynx.	It is also called the "Adam's apple" or voice box. It is located in the front center of the neck.
2. Use the tips of your index and middle fingers.	
3. Slide finger alongside the larynx in the grooves formed by the muscles at the side of the neck.	
4. Palpate the pulse.	Avoid compressing the artery and blocking out a weak pulse.

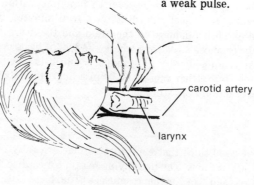

Palpating for carotid pulse.

ITEM 2. THE PURPOSE OF CARDIOPULMONARY RESUSCITATION

The purpose of CPR is to provide basic life support. This means that it is aimed at maintaining the viability, or life, of the victim's central nervous system until the body recovers sufficiently to resume these functions. In other words, you must restore the circulation and breathing. This is done by ventilating the victim's lungs and keeping the circulation going via closed-chest compression until the person revives.

The success or failure of the CPR effort depends on the speed with which the victim's breathing and circulation are restored. The need for CPR is immediate when the person suffers a cardiac arrest. There is no time to waste looking for equipment or drugs, or trying to transport the victim to a doctor or a hospital. What is needed at that moment is someone who is trained and skilled in basic cardiopulmonary resuscitation.

ITEM 3. BASIC CARDIOPULMONARY RESUSCITATION

You are shopping in a department store, waiting for an elevator. The door of the elevator opens and you see passengers gathered around a man who had just collapsed to the floor. They say he is dead. What might you do? Could you carry out cardiopulmonary resuscitation? With prompt CPR, the man may revive and live for years longer.

Basic cardiopulmonary resuscitation relies on the skills of the person who knows how to proceed and who does so promptly. A delay of more than 4 minutes from the onset of cardiac arrest may result in permanent brain damage, if indeed the CPR is successful in reviving the patient at all. However, there are wide variations among people with respect to tolerating lack of oxygen, so it is essential to attempt basic CPR even when more than 4 minutes have elapsed.

Unwitnessed Arrest

When the CPR rescuer has not actually seen the victim collapse and lose consciousness, as with the man in the elevator, the situation is referred to as an unwitnessed arrest, even though other people did see it happen. The rescuer would follow these steps:

1. Place the victim on his back and search for signs of breathing.

2. Open the victim's airway.

3. If he is not breathing, give four quick ventilations by using mouth-to-mouth resuscitation.

4. Palpate the carotid artery for a pulse.

5. If the pulse is absent, begin artificial circulation by using external chest compression.

6. Continue your efforts without pause until the victim revives, or you are relieved by others.

Witnessed Arrest

"Witnessed arrest" is the term used when the victim collapses in the presence and sight of the person who performs the rescue by using CPR. In a witnessed arrest, the rescuer would carry out the following steps:

1. Open the airway and palpate for the carotid pulse.

2. If the pulse is absent, give one precordial thump.

3. If breathing is absent, give four quick ventilations.

4. If breathing and pulse do not begin spontaneously after steps 2 and 3, proceed with CPR, using mouth-to-mouth resuscitation and external chest compression.

UNIT 37

ITEM 4. BEGINNING CPR — OPEN THE VICTIM'S AIRWAY

In the skill laboratory, practice the skills required to begin the cardiopulmonary resuscitation procedure. Some portions of the procedure covered in later items will require the use of the Resusci-Annie mannequin.

Given a person who has collapsed and lost consciousness, and who has no breathing activity or pulse, carry out basic cardiopulmonary resuscitation.

Important Steps	Key Points
1. Remain with the victim and tell others to summon more help.	It is essential to begin CPR without delay. Skilled medical treatment will be needed when the patient revives.
2. Turn the patient on his back.	
3. For a witnessed arrest, palpate for the carotid pulse. If no pulse can be felt, give one precordial thump. For an unwitnessed arrest, omit this step and proceed with step 4.	The majority of arrests are not actually witnessed by the CPR rescuer. (The precordial thump will be described later.)

4. Open the airway.
 	
  a. Tilt the patient's head back as far as possible.
 	
  b. Place one hand under his neck and lift it.
 	
  c. Press his forehead backward with your other hand.
	Often, positioning to open the airway causes the person to resume breathing on his own.
	For infants and small children:
	Avoid tilting the head back in extreme hyperextension because this may collapse and obstruct the breathing passages.
	For accident victims:
	Tilting the neck back in hyperextension should be avoided when dealing with victims of diving or auto accidents where a fracture of the neck is suspected. Avoid any movement of the neck. Immobilize the head in a neutral position with your hands at each side of the head, and raise the lower jaw, or mandible, with your fingers to prevent the tongue from obstructing the back of the throat.

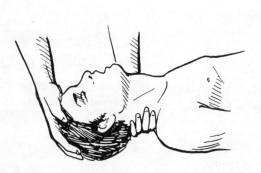

Opening airway in adult victim of cardiac arrest.

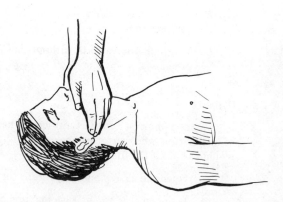

Immobilizing head and bringing chin forward when fracture of neck is suspected.

Precordial Thump

The precordial thump is only used when the rescuer has witnessed the cardiac arrest, and then only during the first minute following the arrest. It is not recommended for use in unwitnessed arrests or in children. If the thump is effective, the heart resumes beating, and a carotid pulse can be felt.

To deliver a precordial thump in a victim with no carotid pulse, follow these steps:

Important Steps	Key Points

1. Locate the middle of the sternum.

2. Raise your fist 8 to 12 inches over the chest.

3. Deliver one sharp, quick blow to the midportion of the sternum, using the bottom and fleshy part of the fist.

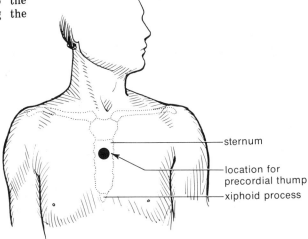

sternum

location for precordial thump

xiphoid process

4. Palpate for the carotid pulse.

If the pulse is absent, begin cardiopulmonary resuscitation at once.

ITEM 5. MOUTH-TO-MOUTH VENTILATION

If the victim does not begin to breathe after the airway is open, artificial ventilation should be done at once. Practice doing mouth-to-mouth resuscitation using the Resusci-Annie or a similar type of mannequin.

Important Steps	Key Points

The first steps were covered in Item 4.

5. If the victim is not breathing, give mouth-to-mouth resuscitation.

Use the hand that had been pressing the forehead back. This helps prevent the escape of air during ventilation.

   a. Pinch the nostrils shut.

   b. Open your mouth wide and take a deep breath.

   c. Place your mouth tightly over the patient's mouth.

Make an airtight seal.

   d. Blow your breath into the patient's mouth.

You should see the patient's chest rise as air fills his lungs; feel and hear the air as it is exhaled.

   e. Remove your mouth and allow the patient to exhale.

   f. Initially, repeat four times.

Do not wait for the lungs to deflate fully. This provides a supply of oxygen while you carry out the next steps of CPR.

UNIT 37

g. Maintain a rate of 16 to 20 respirations per minute if external chest massage is not used.

The respiratory rate will be less when CPR is carried out by one person.

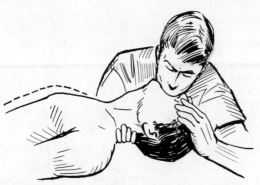

Mouth-to-mouth ventilation requires good airseal of nose and patient's mouth in order to inflate lungs.

Other Methods of Ventilation

Artificial ventilation can also be accomplished by methods other than mouth-to-mouth. Mouth-to-nose ventilation is used when the mouth has been injured, when it is not possible to open the mouth, and when a tight seal around the mouth is difficult to achieve. With infants and small children, the rescuer can cover both the mouth and nose of the victim with his own mouth. Smaller amounts of air are blown into the child's lungs — enough to raise the chest. Mouth-to-stoma ventilation is used for victims who have a permanent tracheostomy. In this case, it is not necessary to tilt the head and hyperextend the neck.

Obstructions

An obstruction of the air passages will prevent the air from reaching the victim's lungs. When there is an obstruction, the chest neither rises with a ventilation breath nor falls when air escapes. The rescuer feels increased resistance while forcing air into the patient's mouth. There is no sound or feeling of air escaping during the exhaling phase.

To check for foreign bodies in the mouth or throat, turn victim on his side and open the patient's mouth. Run your index finger around the inside of the cheek, the base of the tongue, and deep into the throat to remove obstructive foreign objects. If the object is stuck deep in the throat, form a fist and sharply thrust it against the diaphragm in the patient's upper midabdomen, under the sternum and rib cage. Even though the patient is not breathing, often there is enough air in the lungs to dislodge objects such as pieces of food. Striking a blow on the back between the shoulder blades with the palm of the hand will frequently clear an obstruction, especially in small children. After an attempt is made to remove the obstruction, ventilate the patient to see if the air passages are clear.

ITEM 6. ARTIFICIAL CIRCULATION

External chest compression is used to maintain the circulation of a cardiac arrest victim. By this method, a rhythmic pressure is applied over the lower portion of the sternum by using regular, smooth, and uninterrupted motions. This form of artificial circulation produces pulses in the body that can be felt and peaks in the systolic blood pressure over 100 mm Hg, even though diastolic pressure is zero and the carotid arteries carry about one-fourth the normal blood flow to the brain.

In the skill laboratory, practice the steps of external chest compression on the mannequin as you would perform it for a victim with no palpable carotid pulse. Do not practice precordial thump or chest compressions on healthy persons or non-victims as it would interfere with the regular heart rate.

Important Steps   Key Points

For the first steps of the CPR procedure, refer
to Item 4.

6. If there is no carotid pulse, begin artificial
    circulation, using external chest com-
    pression.

    a. Place the patient on his back on a hard   If he is in a bed, insert a board under his back,
        surface.   full-length if possible.

    b. Position yourself at the left side of the   You may need to get on the bed in order to
        patient's chest.   compress the chest.

    c. Locate the lower half of patient's   Avoid putting pressure on the tip of the
        sternum.   sternum (xiphoid process).

    d. Place the heel of your hand over the   Proper positioning of the hands prevents in-
        lower half of his sternum, keeping   juries (e.g., broken ribs from excessive force).
        your fingers off the chest wall.

    e. Put the heel of your second hand on   Keep your arms straight and elbows locked.
        top of the first, and move so that your
        shoulders are lengthwise over the pa-
        tient's sternum.

    f. Exert a firm, heavy force downward   *Adults* — 80 to 120 pounds of pressure are
        on the chest.   required to depress the sternum 1½ to 2 inches.
                                                     By using your entire weight, you should be able
                                                     to compress the chest; this compresses the heart
                                                     and forces blood into the arteries.
                                                     Children — apply pressure at the middle of the
                                                     sternum and depress the chest 3/4 to 1½ inch.
                                                     Infants — use the tips of your index and middle
                                                     fingers to depress the sternum ½ to 3/4 inch.
                                                     Compress 80 to 100 times per minute.

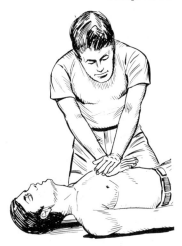

CPR by one rescuer.

    g. Release the pressure, but do not re-   Develop a rhythm by rolling your body for-
        move your hands.   ward to press, and then back to release.

    h. Continue compression at the rate of   Continue until the patient revives, or until you
        80 per minute.   are relieved. Make the change without inter-
                                                     rupting the rhythm. You will need to give two
                                                     lung inflations after each 15 compressions.

UNIT
37

ITEM 7. BASIC RESUSCITATION BY ONE PERSON

Basic cardiopulmonary resuscitation, carried out by one person until additional help arrives on the scene, is life-supporting and essential for the possible survival of the victim of cardiac arrest. The entire basic CPR procedure is outlined below:

1. Remain with the victim and have others summon more help.

2. Turn the patient on his back.

3. For a witnessed arrest only, palpate for the carotid pulse and give a precordial thump if the pulse is absent.

4. Open the airway.

5. If the victim is not breathing, give four quick ventilations by using mouth-to-mouth resuscitation.

6. Palpate the carotid pulse. If it is absent, begin artificial circulation, using external chest compression.

7. After every series of 15 compressions, give two quick lung inflations.

The ratio of compressions to ventilations is 15 to 2.

ITEM 8. BASIC RESUSCITATION BY TWO PERSONS

Basic resuscitation is easier to carry out with two rescuers. When help arrives, one rescuer continues with chest compression and the other one gives artificial ventilation. Two people can continue CPR for several hours if necessary; they can change positions when the one who is doing the chest compressions becomes fatigued. The unusual position required for the hands causes strain when artificial circulation must be maintained over a period of time.

Two rescuers carry out the basic CPR procedure. The first rescuer delivers one ventilation between the fifth compression and the one following it. The compression rate is 60 per minute and the ratio of compressions to ventilations is 5 to 1.

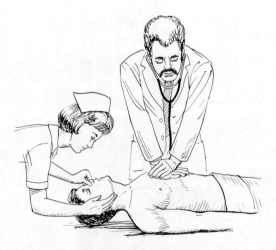

CPR by two rescuers.

ITEM 9. CPR IN THE HOSPITAL SETTING

Cardiac arrest can occur in patients who are already in the hospital for the treatment of some other illness or injury. Patients with conditions known to have a greater risk of cardiac arrest are generally treated in special areas such as the coronary care unit and the intensive care unit. Here the patients are under close observation by skilled nurses and doctors. Monitors are used to keep continuous track of the patient's vital signs — heart action, rate, and blood pressures such as the central venous pressure or the pulmonary arterial pressures. The detection of early changes in heart and lung functions, and prompt treatment of the causes can prevent the disaster of cardiac arrest.

When arrest does occur in the hospital, basic CPR is started immediately by a trained person while the CPR team is summoned. Many hospitals use the loudspeaker or paging system, and the call "Code Blue — CCU" or "Doctor Blue — CCU" to alert members of the CPR team that a cardiac arrest has occurred and to tell them where.

The CPR team consists of doctors and nurses who have had special training in basic and advanced methods of cardiopulmonary resuscitation. They make use of specialized equipment and various drugs to resuscitate and begin treatment of the underlying cause. An emergency cart containing all the supplies and equipment required in advanced resuscitation is rushed to the scene of the cardiac arrest. The CPR team takes over and relieves the person who has been carrying out the basic CPR.

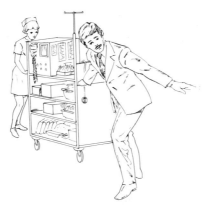

Hospital CPR team springing into action.

As a beginning worker, find out the policy of your hospital or agency regarding what is expected of you in situations where a cardiac arrest has occurred. If there is no policy, these three principles can serve as your guidelines:

1. Act to save a life.

2. Perform what you have been taught or know how to do.

3. Call for help and let the more highly trained and skilled person take over.

IV. ADDITIONAL INFORMATION FOR ENRICHMENT

Those of you who have an interest in problems leading to cardiac arrest and in cardiopulmonary resuscitation may wish to read further. Some subjects of interest in this connection include heart diseases, especially the "heart attack," or myocardial infarction. What are the risk factors for people who might have heart attacks? What is being done in your community to reduce the number of deaths from cardiac arrest? Does your community have mobile emergency units? If so, do they provide basic CPR and advanced life support measures? What people in your community have had training in basic CPR?

Perhaps you might be more interested in learning about the advanced CPR techniques, such as the use of defibrillators, types of drugs, cardiac pacemakers, various kinds of airways, and respirators that assist in ventilation of the patient.

Good sources of information include your local chapter of the American Heart Association, and the library. Many hospitals also have extensive libraries and carry many of the professional journals, such as *Heart and Lung* and *Circulation*, as well as other medical and nursing journals.

UNIT 37

PERFORMANCE TEST

In the classroom or your skill laboratory, your instructor will ask that cardiopulmonary resuscitation be performed in pairs. You and your partner will demonstrate the procedure, using the mannequin, and then change positions. Each of you will demonstrate skill in performing artificial ventilation and artificial circulation.

1. Given a person who has suffered a cardiac arrest, is unconscious, has no pulse, and is not breathing, you and another rescuer are to give basic cardiopulmonary resuscitation. This is an unwitnessed arrest.

PERFORMANCE CHECKLIST

BASIC CARDIOPULMONARY RESUSCITATION

1. Remain with the victim and have others summon more help.

2. Turn the patient on his back.

3. Open the airway.

    a. Tilt his head back.

    b. Place your hand under his neck and lift it.

    c. Press his forehead backward with your other hand.

4. If breathing is absent, give mouth-to-mouth resuscitation.

    a. Pinch his nostrils shut.

    b. Open your mouth and take a deep breath.

    c. Make an airtight seal over the patient's mouth with your own.

    d. Forcefully exhale into the patient's mouth.

    e. Remove your mouth and allow the patient to exhale.

    f. Repeat four times initially, and then between every fifth compression and the one following it.

5. If carotid pulse is absent, maintain artificial circulation, using external chest compression.

    a. Position yourself on the left side of the patient's chest.

    b. Locate the lower half of his sternum.

    c. Place the heel of your hand over the lower half of his sternum.

    d. Keep your fingers elevated from his chest wall.

    e. Put the heel of your other hand on top of the first hand and lean forward so that your shoulders are parallel to and above the patient's sternum.

    f. Exert firm force downward to depress the sternum 1½ to 2 inches.

    g. Release the pressure, but keep your hands in place.

    h. Repeat steps f and g for a compression rate of 80 times per minute with one rescuer, or 60 compressions with two rescuers.

POST-TEST

Multiple choice: For each of the test questions, there is one correct or best answer. Indicate the answer you have selected.

_____ 1. All but one of the following events happen when a person suffers a cardiac arrest. Which one does not apply?

    a. the person's circulation stops

    b. the pulses in the body are absent

    c. systolic pressure is 100 and diastolic is zero

    d. all respirations cease

_____ 2. "Cardiac arrest" is a term that means all but which one of the following?

    a. any death when the heart stops

    b. death due to a heart attack

    c. an immediate and unexpected death

    d. sudden death

_____ 3. Brain tissue is less able to tolerate a lack of oxygen than some other body tissues. Permanent damage results when the brain is deprived of oxygen for more than:

    a. 20 to 40 seconds

    b. 1 to 2 minutes

    c. 2 to 4 minutes

    d. 4 to 6 minutes

_____ 4. If you are called to assist a person who has collapsed and lost consciousness, the first thing you should do is:

    a. look for injuries from the fall

    b. establish an open airway

    c. give a precordial thump

    d. provide warmth and treat for shock

_____ 5. Cardiac arrests are classified either as witnessed arrests or unwitnessed arrests. An unwitnessed cardiac arrest means that:

    a. a doctor was not present to begin CPR

    b. other people were around to see the arrest

    c. the patient was alone and no one was around

    d. the person starting CPR did not see the arrest

_____ 6. The only time a person should use the precordial thump when giving basic CPR is:

    a. within 4 minutes of the time of the arrest

    b. when a pulse is felt faintly in the carotid artery

    c. after actually seeing the person collapse

    d. during the pause in compression when another takes over

_____ 7. In giving mouth-to-mouth resuscitation to an adult, the recommended position for the patient is:

   a. the head tilted backward and the lower jaw raised

   b. lying prone on a hard surface

   c. lying supine on a soft surface

   d. in Sims' position with the head turned to the side

_____ 8. The basic underlying cause of cardiac arrest is believed to be:

   a. infection of the lungs

   b. lack of oxygen

   c. blood clot in the brain

   d. heart attack, or myocardial infarction

_____ 9. Following a cardiac arrest, the clinical signs of death are seen within:

   a. 20 to 40 seconds

   b. 1 to 2 minutes

   c. 2 to 4 minutes

   d. 4 to 6 minutes

_____ 10. The purpose of cardioplumonary resuscitation is to:

   a. give artificial ventilation

   b. give artificial circulation

   c. provide basic life support

   d. stimulate the central nervous system

_____ 11. When giving artificial ventilation, signs that the air passages are open include all of the following except:

   a. air can be felt rushing out of the victim

   b. you can hear the air escape when the lungs deflate

   c. the sternum is depressed 1½ to 2 inches

   d. the chest rises with each ventilation

_____ 12. The number of ventilations used to inflate the lungs at the beginning of CPR is:

   a. one breath

   b. two breaths

   c. three breaths

   d. four breaths

_____ 13. The indication for starting artificial circulation is:

   a. contracted pupils

   b. blood pressure of 100/0

   c. absence of respirations

   d. absence of carotid pulse

_____ 14. As a result of external chest compression, the blood flow to the brain is:

    a. fully restored

    b. one-half of normal

    c. one-fourth of normal

    d. diverted to the heart

_____ 15. While performing artificial circulation, the CPR rescuer applies pressure to what portion of the chest?

    a. the xiphoid process of the sternum

    b. the lower half of the sternum

    c. the left side of the chest

    d. the right side of the chest

_____ 16. When giving CPR to an infant, the rescuer would compress the chest using:

    a. the index and middle fingers

    b. the heel of one hand

    c. the fleshy, bottom part of the fist

    d. both hands as with an adult

_____ 17. A force of 80 to 120 pounds is required during artificial circulation in order to compress the adult's chest:

    a. ½ to ¾ inches

    b. ¾ to 1½ inches

    c. 1½ to 2 inches

    d. 2 to 4 inches

_____ 18. When CPR is performed by one rescuer, after the initial ventilation the ratio of breaths to compressions is:

    a. 1 breath, 5 compressions

    b. 2 breaths, 5 compressions

    c. 1 breath, 15 compressions

    d. 2 breaths, 15 compressions

_____ 19. The ratio of compressions to ventilations when CPR is given by two people is:

    a. 1 breath, 5 compressions

    b. 1 breath, 15 compressions

    c. 2 breaths, 5 compressions

    d. 4 breaths, 15 compressions

_____ 20. The hospital CPR team is highly skilled and trained in the use of:

    a. basic CPR methods

    b. advanced CPR methods

    c. cardiac drugs and equipment

    d. all of the above

    e. all but a

UNIT 37

POST-TEST ANNOTATED ANSWER SHEET

1. c. (p. 740)
2. a. (p. 739)
3. d. (p. 739)
4. b. (p. 741)
5. d. (p. 741)
6. c. (p. 742)
7. a. (p. 742)
8. b. (p. 739)
9. a. (p. 739)
10. c. (p. 740)

11. c. (p. 744)
12. d. (p. 741)
13. d. (p. 741)
14. c. (p. 744)
15. b. (p. 745)
16. a. (p. 745)
17. c. (p. 745)
18. d. (p. 746)
19. a. (p. 746)
20. d. (p. 747)

INDEX

Note: Page numbers in *italics* indicate illustrations.

i